World Health Organization Classification of Tumours

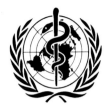

WHO   OMS

International Agency for Research on Cancer (IARC)

4th Edition

WHO Classification of Tumours of Female Reproductive Organs

Edited by

Robert J. Kurman

Maria Luisa Carcangiu

C. Simon Herrington

Robert H. Young

International Agency for Research on Cancer

Lyon, 2014

World Health Organization Classification of Tumours

Series Editors   Fred T. Bosman, MD PhD
Elaine S. Jaffe, MD
Sunil R. Lakhani, MD FRCPath
Hiroko Ohgaki, DVM PhD

WHO Classification of Tumours of Female Reproductive Organs

Editors   Robert J. Kurman, MD
Maria Luisa Carcangiu, MD
C. Simon Herrington, MD FRCPath
Robert H. Young, MD

Technical Editor   Rachel Purcell, PhD

Database   Alberto Machado
Delphine Nicolas

Layout   Stefanie Brottrager

Printed by   Maestro
38330 Saint-Ismier, France

Publisher   International Agency for
Research on Cancer (IARC)
69372 Lyon Cedex 08, France

This volume was produced with support from the

Charles Rodolphe Brupbacher Foundation

MEDIC Foundation

The WHO Classification of Tumours of Female Reproductive Organs presented in this book reflects the views of a Working Group that convened for a Consensus and Editorial Meeting at the International Agency for Research on Cancer, Lyon 13–15 June 2013.

Members of the Working Group are indicated in the List of Contributors on pages 254–259

Published by the International Agency for Research on Cancer (IARC),
150 cours Albert Thomas, 69372 Lyon Cedex 08, France

Distributed by
WHO Press, World Health Organization, 20 Avenue Appia, 1211 Geneva 27, Switzerland
Tel: +41 22 791 3264; Fax: +41 22 791 4857; e-mail: bookorders@who.int

First print run (10 000 copies)

Format for bibliographic citations:
Robert J. Kurman, Maria Luisa Carcangiu, C. Simon Herrington, Robert H. Young, (Eds.): WHO Classification of Tumours of
Female Reproductive Organs.
IARC: Lyon 2014

IARC Library Cataloguing in Publication Data

WHO classification of tumours of female reproductive organs / edited by Robert J. Kurman … [et al.] - 4th edition

(World Health Organization classification of tumours)

1. Genital Neoplasms, Female – classification 2. Genital Neoplasms, Female – genetics 3. Genital Neoplasms, Female – pathology

I. Kurman, Robert J. II. Series

ISBN 978-92-832-2435-8   (NLM Classification W1)

Contents

Preface

R.J. Kurman   C.S. Herrington
M.L. Carcangiu   R.H. Young

"Every generation has the obligation to free men's minds for a look at new worlds… to look out from a higher plateau than the last generation."
Ellison S. Onizuka

Objectives

A histopathological classification should be descriptive, reflect biology and behaviour and fulfil three objectives: 1) serve as a guide for clinical management, 2) provide a framework for organizing diseases that assists in furthering scientific investigation and 3) serve as an educational tool. There is an inherent tension between the first two objectives. For clinical management, a classification with a limited number of categories is more practical as clinicians have only a few therapeutic options. On the other hand, for researchers, a more complex classification is preferred because a concise classification of combined categories may obscure important differences, which may ultimately be shown to have clinical relevance. In this edition of the WHO Classification we have attempted to reconcile these disparate needs. The most salient changes from the last edition are briefly discussed below.

Historical perspective and controversial issues

Epithelial ovarian neoplasia

As is almost invariably the case in medicine, current workers owe a great debt to those who preceded them and that is certainly true in this fourth edition, as it is one of a line dating back to the initial WHO classification of 1973 {1735}, which in major part was prepared under the guidance of the late Dr Robert E. Scully. With the assistance of a group of other distinguished pathologists from several countries, the first, truly well-organized classification of ovarian tumours was presented and it stands the test of time exceptionally well. We would like to acknowledge those who first "blazed the trail" in the difficult area of ovarian tumour classification and to acknowledge the countless other individuals whose

contributions have increased our understanding of this and other gynaecological tumours.

In 1961 the Cancer Committee of the International Federation of Gynaecology and Obstetrics (FIGO) proposed a histopathological classification of the common epithelial ovarian tumours {55}. As part of that classification, a new category was introduced that was designated *"serous cystadenomas with proliferating activity of the epithelial cells and nuclear abnormalities but with no infiltrative destructive growth (low potential malignancy)"*. The entire classification was referred to the Reference Centre of the WHO, composed of the aforementioned pathologists, for their recommendations {1735}. The FIGO classification was accepted by WHO and published in 1973 but the above term was changed to *"tumours of borderline malignancy (carcinomas of low malignant potential)"* {1735}. This term eventually evolved into 'borderline tumour', which has been widely used, the implication being that this group of tumours had morphological features and behaviour between a benign cystadenoma and carcinoma. Since many patients with widespread extra-ovarian disease did well, even when untreated or inadequately treated, extra-ovarian lesions were designated "implants" rather than metastasis. In the late 1970s and early 80s, investigators in Australia {1653} and the US {125} proposed that implants be divided into non-invasive and invasive as the latter were more predictive of an adverse outcome. Subsequent studies called attention to a particular growth pattern of serous borderline tumours (SBTs), characterized by a micropapillary architecture which, unlike the usual type of SBT, was associated with a significantly worse outcome {217,1726,1798}. It was proposed that the usual type of SBT be designated "atypical proliferative serous tumour (APST)" and the micropapillary tumour "non-invasive micropapillary (low-grade) serous carcinoma." This proved to be highly controversial as several investigators acknowledged that, although the micropapillary tumour was more often

associated with advanced stage disease and a greater frequency of invasive implants compared to APST, it was not significantly associated with an adverse outcome {485,633,1521}

In view of the disparate opinions concerning the terminology of this lesion, it is designated "SBT, micropapillary variant/noninvasive low-grade serous carcinoma"; the terms are synonymous. The most important feature that predicts adverse outcome for all the noninvasive serous tumours is the presence of invasive implants, which are now classified as low-grade serous carcinomas (LGSCs) {120,128,1727,1729}. Fatalities from SBTs result from progression to LGSC, which occurs in approximately 5% of cases. Thus, SBTs are tumours with a good prognosis, which very infrequently progress to LGSC {1117}. Accordingly, some pathologists favour the term "SBT" to draw attention to the inherent hazards of sampling, as a large "borderline" tumour might harbour an occult carcinoma. Other pathologists, though cognizant of this concern, prefer "APST" to emphasize the benign nature of most of these neoplasms. Accordingly, it was agreed that both terms are synonymous and either one could be used.

The entire category of borderline tumours for the non-serous types has been revisited. As there are no well documented cases of extra-ovarian disease or deaths from adequately sampled mucinous, endometrioid, clear cell and Brenner borderline tumours, there is little justification in calling them borderline. The designation "atypical proliferative tumour" and "borderline tumour" are considered equivalent and can be applied to all these other cell types.

Recent clinicopathological and molecular genetic studies have shown that LGSC and high-grade serous carcinoma (HGSC) do not represent a morphological spectrum in which well differentiated tumours progress to moderately and then poorly differentiated carcinomas. Rather it has been shown that the low- and high-grade tumours develop along distinctly different pathways and therefore the three tier-grading system of well-, moderately and poorly differentiated has been replaced by two separate categories designated "LGSC" and "HGSC" {1153,1766}. It should be noted, however, that on rare occasion SBTs and LGSCs can progress to an HGSC {182,433}.

Cervical epithelial neoplasia
Mirroring the concepts first developed for the Bethesda System and most recently by the 2012 US-based Lower Anogenital Squamous Terminology (LAST) project, broad agreement was reached to replace the three-tier CIN 1, CIN 2, and CIN 3 terminology with a two-tier system of low- and high-grade intraepithelial lesions (LSIL and HSIL respectively). The rationale for this change is that the two-tier system is more biologically and clinically relevant and histologically more reproducible {412}. As cytology and histology are both morphological representations of a common biological process that impacts the cervix, it is logical that the terms describing these processes be the same, especially given the more biological orientation of the new classification {1840}.
LSIL in tissue is the morphological manifestation of the differentiation-dependent expression of an HPV virion production program on the host squamous cells and therefore encompasses lesions showing koilocytotic atypia with or without features judged to indicate mild dysplasia, CIN 1, VaIN 1 and VIN 1. The inherent difficulty in distinguishing pure HPV infection ("flat condyloma") from CIN 1/VaIN 1 and VIN 1 was vigorously debated but because of issues of interpretive reproducibility and lack of any biologically meaningful criteria or markers for separating them, the spectrum of such lesions are all designated as LSIL. Similarly, exophytic productive HPV infections (condyloma acuminatum) are also a variant of LSIL based on these unifying biologic concepts {465}.
A similar approach defines HSIL as representing lesions that are classified as precancerous, meaning they carry a significant risk of invasive cancer development if untreated. Moderate and severe dysplasia, squamous carcinoma in situ, CIN 2 and CIN 3 are all encompassed by HSIL. Historically, severe dysplasia was recognized as a more mature variant of carcinoma in situ, and both were combined as CIN 3 because of a lack of reproducible histological distinctions. Similarly, no biomarker defines a

distinct intermediate state of CIN 2 and the emerging consensus is that CIN 2 is a mix of biological CIN 1 and CIN 3, the true nature of which is confounded by issues of colposcopic biopsy sampling and pathological interpretive variability {596,1844,1845}.
In general, there are no meaningful management distinctions between CIN 2 and CIN 3. However, in young women, clinicians may request that pathologists try to distinguish HSIL (CIN 2) from HSIL (CIN 3) to allow for the possibility of regression of HSIL (CIN 2), thereby potentially sparing these women complications from cervical excision which might compromise child-bearing.
Similar biological concepts impacted the classification of glandular precancers. Although adenocarcinoma in situ (AIS) is the preferred term, high-grade cervical glandular intraepithelial neoplasia is a synonym. Lesions previously termed endocervical glandular dysplasia or low-grade cervical glandular intraepithelial neoplasia were deemed poorly defined and non-reproducible.
To facilitate clarity and simplicity of communication, the formal reporting diagnosis of LSIL, HSIL or AIS should be used for the cervix, and LSIL and HSIL for the vagina and vulva. The "intraepithelial" synonyms may be reported optionally in parentheses or in a note, but are not necessarily to be included as routine.

Epithelial endometrial neoplasia
Precursors of endometrioid carcinoma have been divided into four groups of hyperplasia by WHO since 1994, according to the degree of architectural crowding (simple/complex), and nuclear alterations (atypical/non-atypical) {1708,1783}. In this edition a two-group system of "hyperplasia without atypia" and "atypical hyperplasia" {901} will replace the four-tier system. An alternate system to hyperplasia without atypia and atypical hyperplasia in which excessively proliferating glandular lesions are divided into two groups, hyperplasia and endometrial intraepithelial neoplasia (EIN) has been proposed, based on studies of clonality, morphometry and cancer risk {1321}. The criteria for the diagnosis of EIN are essentially the same as for atypical hyperplasia and the reproducibility and risk of progression to endometrioid carcinoma are also similar {1020}. The main problem with both systems is the subjectivity in the determination of "atypia" that impairs re-

producibility. This reflects the limitations of histopathology and is an important challenge for investigators to develop a reliable and more objective molecular marker in the future. Patient management is also currently predicated on a two-tier system {1932} and consequently, there was general agreement that a two-tier system would be preferable, either using the terms "hyperplasia without atypia" and "atypical hyperplasia/endometrioid intraepithelial neoplasia." It should be noted that the original term "endometrial intraepithelial neoplasia" has been changed to "endometrioid intraepithelial neoplasia" to clearly indicate that the latter is a precursor of endometrioid carcinoma and not serous carcinoma.

Explanatory notes

General points
As similar lesions can occur in different anatomic sites in the female reproductive organs, for brevity and to avoid redundancy, the more detailed discussion of the entity is presented in the site where it occurs most frequently and is then cross-referenced for the other sites. Also, since almost any type of neoplasm can occur in the female reproductive organs, extremely rare ones are not included in the classification. Finally, as the primary focus of this text is the histological classification, gross photos are only sparingly included.

Terminology
In certain instances, different investigators preferred different terms for the same lesion. When there was scientific evidence to support the use of both terms, they are both listed and are meant to be synonymous. The order in which they appear is based on length of usage and is not intended to indicate a preference.

Immunohistochemistry
Immunohistochemistry has been a valuable adjunct in histopathological diagnosis and in elucidating pathogenesis but as the focus of the text is on histological classification, immunohistochemical images are used sparingly and included only where they illustrate a point that cannot be conveyed in the text.

Molecular genetics
Molecular genetic analyses of tumours have radically changed our understanding of pathogenesis. For example, molecular genetic studies in conjunction with

morphological studies of epithelial ovarian carcinomas have led to a dualistic model (type I and type II) which provides a framework for the study of ovarian neoplasia by taking into account distinctive morphological, clinical and molecular genetic features of the individual tumour types and relating them to their respective precursor lesions {1766}.

Molecular genetic studies will undoubtedly play an important role in the future but at present have not achieved applicability in routine practice and therefore,

in this edition, they are discussed in the context of pathogenesis and where a specific inherited disorder results in a high risk of tumour development.

In conclusion, the fourth edition of the *WHO Classification of Tumours of the Female Reproductive Organs*, like previous editions, is a work-in-progress that attempts to capture the diversity and nuances of gynaecological neoplasia. It represents our understanding of the disease processes at a single point in time,

along a path of evolving knowledge, and therefore there are areas of uncertainty and incomplete understanding that result in questions that cannot be satisfactorily answered. We recognize that this classification is not perfect but we hope it will be useful to pathologists, clinicians, epidemiologists and investigators who seek to obtain a deeper understanding of the nature of gynaecological disease. In so doing, this classification sets the stage for the next one.

CHAPTER 1

Tumours of the ovary

WHO Classification of tumours of the ovary[a,b]

Epithelial tumours
Serous Tumours
Benign
Serous cystadenoma	8441/0
Serous adenofibroma	9014/0
Serous surface papilloma	8461/0

Borderline
Serous borderline tumour / Atypical proliferative serous tumour	8442/1
Serous borderline tumour - micropapillary variant / Non-invasive low-grade serous carcinoma	8460/2*

Malignant
Low-grade serous carcinoma	8460/3
High-grade serous carcinoma	8461/3

Mucinous tumours
Benign
Mucinous cystadenoma	8470/0
Mucinous adenofibroma	9015/0

Borderline
Mucinous borderline tumour / Atypical proliferative mucinous tumour	8472/1

Malignant
Mucinous carcinoma	8480/3

Endometrioid tumours
Benign
Endometriotic cyst	
Endometrioid cystadenoma	8380/0
Endometrioid adenofibroma	8381/0

Borderline
Endometrioid borderline tumour / Atypical proliferative endometrioid tumour	8380/1

Malignant
Endometrioid carcinoma	8380/3

Clear cell tumours
Benign
Clear cell cystadenoma	8443/0
Clear cell adenofibroma	8313/0

Borderline
Clear cell borderline tumour / Atypical proliferative clear cell tumour	8313/1

Malignant
Clear cell carcinoma	8310/3

Brenner tumours
Benign
Brenner tumour	9000/0

Borderline
Borderline Brenner tumour / Atypical proliferative Brenner tumour	9000/1

Malignant
Malignant Brenner tumour	9000/3

Seromucinous tumours
Benign
Seromucinous cystadenoma	8474/0*
Seromucinous adenofibroma	9014/0*

Borderline
Seromucinous borderline tumour / Atypical proliferative seromucinous tumour	8474/1*

Malignant
Seromucinous carcinoma	8474/3*

Undifferentiated carcinoma
	8020/3

Mesenchymal tumours
Low-grade endometrioid stromal sarcoma	8931/3
High-grade endometrioid stromal sarcoma	8930/3

Mixed epithelial and mesenchymal tumours
Adenosarcoma	8933/3
Carcinosarcoma	8980/3

Sex cord-stromal tumours
Pure stromal tumours
Fibroma	8810/0
Cellular fibroma	8810/1
Thecoma	8600/0
Luteinized thecoma associated with sclerosing peritonitis	8601/0
Fibrosarcoma	8810/3
Sclerosing stromal tumour	8602/0
Signet-ring stromal tumour	8590/0
Microcystic stromal tumour	8590/0
Leydig cell tumour	8650/0
Steroid cell tumour	8760/0
Steroid cell tumour, malignant	8760/3

Pure sex cord tumours
Adult granulosa cell tumour	8620/3
Juvenile granulosa cell tumour	8622/1
Sertoli cell tumour	8640/1
Sex cord tumour with annular tubules	8623/1

Mixed sex cord-stromal tumours
Sertoli-Leydig cell tumours
Well differentiated	8631/0
Moderately differentiated	8631/1
With heterologous elements	8634/1
Poorly differentiated	8631/3
With heterologous elements	8634/3
Retiform	8633/1
With heterologous elements	8634/1
Sex cord-stromal tumours, NOS	8590/1

Germ cell tumours

Dysgerminoma	9060/3
Yolk sac tumour	9071/3
Embryonal carcinoma	9070/3
Non-gestational choriocarcinoma	9100/3
Mature teratoma	9080/0
Immature teratoma	9080/3
Mixed germ cell tumour	9085/3

Monodermal teratoma and somatic-type tumours arising from a dermoid cyst

Struma ovarii, benign	9090/0
Struma ovarii, malignant	9090/3
Carcinoid	8240/3
Strumal carcinoid	9091/1
Mucinous carcinoid	8243/3
Neuroectodermal-type tumours	
Sebaceous tumours	
Sebaceous adenoma	8410/0
Sebaceous carcinoma	8410/3
Other rare monodermal teratomas	
Carcinomas	
Squamous cell carcinoma	8070/3
Others	

Germ cell - sex cord-stromal tumours

Gonadoblastoma, including gonadoblastoma with malignant germ cell tumour	9073/1
Mixed germ cell-sex cord-stromal tumour, unclassified	8594/1*

Miscellaneous tumours

Tumours of rete ovarii	
Adenoma of rete ovarii	9110/0
Adenocarcinoma of rete ovarii	9110/3

Wolffian tumour	9110/1
Small cell carcinoma, hypercalcaemic type	8044/3*
Small cell carcinoma, pulmonary type	8041/3
Wilms tumour	8960/3
Paraganglioma	8693/1
Solid pseudopapillary neoplasm	8452/1

Mesothelial tumours

Adenomatoid tumour	9054/0
Mesothelioma	9050/3

Soft tissue tumours

Myxoma	8840/0
Others	

Tumour-like lesions

Follicle cyst	
Corpus luteum cyst	
Large solitary luteinized follicle cyst	
Hyperreactio luteinalis	
Pregnancy luteoma	
Stromal hyperplasia	
Stromal hyperthecosis	
Fibromatosis	
Massive oedema	
Leydig cell hyperplasia	
Others	

Lymphoid and myeloid tumours

Lymphomas	
Plasmacytoma	9734/3
Myeloid neoplasms	

Secondary tumours

---

a The morphology codes are from the International Classification of Diseases for Oncology (ICD-O) {575A}. Behaviour is coded /0 for benign tumours, /1 for unspecified, borderline or uncertain behaviour, /2 for carcinoma in situ and grade III intraepithelial neoplasia and /3 for malignant tumours; b The classification is modified from the previous WHO classification of tumours {1906A}, taking into account changes in our understanding of these lesions; *These new codes were approved by the IARC/WHO Committee for ICD-O in 2013.

TNM and FIGO classification of tumours of the ovary, fallopian tube and primary peritoneal carcinoma

T - Primary Tumour

TNM	FIGO	
TX		Primary tumour cannot be assessed
T0		No evidence of primary tumour
T1	I	Tumour limited to the ovaries
T1a	IA	Tumour limited to one ovary (capsule intact) or fallopian tube surface; no malignant cells in ascites or peritoneal washings
T1b	IB	Tumour limited to one or both ovaries (capsules intact) or fallopian tubes; no tumour on ovarian or fallopian tube surface; no malignant cells in ascites or peritoneal washings
T1c	IC	Tumour limited to one or both ovaries or fallopian tubes with any of the following:
T1c1	IC1	Surgical spill
T1c2	IC2	Capsule ruptured before surgery or tumour on ovarian or fallopian tube surface
T1c3	IC3	Malignant cells in ascites or peritoneal washings
T2	II	Tumour involves one or both ovaries or fallopian tubes with pelvic extension below pelvic brim or primary peritoneal cancer
T2a	IIA	Extension and/or implants on uterus and/or fallopian tubes and/or ovaries
T2b	IIB	Extension to other pelvic intraperitoneal
T3 and/or N1	III	Tumour involves one or both ovaries or fallopian tubes, or primary peritoneal carcinoma, with cytologically or histologically confirmed spread to the peritoneum outside the pelvis and/or metastasis to the retroperitoneal lymph nodes
N1	IIIA1	Retroperitoneal lymph node metastasis only
N1a	IIIA1i	Lymph node metastasis up to 10 mm in greatest dimension
N1b	IIIA1ii	Lymph node metastasis more than 10 mm in greatest dimension
T3a	IIIA2	Microscopic extrapelvic (above the pelvic brim) peritoneal involvement with or without retroperitoneal lymph node
T3b	IIIB	Macroscopic peritoneal metastasis beyond the pelvis up to 2 cm in greatest dimension with or without retroperitoneal lymph node metastasis
T3c	IIIC	Macroscopic peritoneal metastasis beyond the pelvis more than 2 cm in greatest dimension, with or without retroperitoneal lymph node metastasis (excludes extension of tumour to capsule of liver and spleen without parenchymal involvement of either organ)
M1	IV	Distant metastasis excluding peritoneal metastasis
M1a	IVA	Pleural effusion with positive cytology
M1b	IVB	Parenchymal metastasis and metastasis to extra-abdominal organs (including inguinal lymph nodes and lymph nodes outside the abdominal cavity)

N — Regional Lymph Nodes

NX	Regional lymph nodes cannot be assessed
N0	No regional lymph node metastasis
N1	Regional lymph node metastasis
N1a	Lymph node metastasis up to 10 mm in greatest dimension
N1b	Lymph node metastasis more than 10 mm in greatest dimension

M — Distant Metastasis

M0	No distant metastasis
M1	Distant metastasis
M1a	Pleural effusion with positive cytology
M1b	Parenchymal metastasis and metastasis to extra abdominal organs (including inguinal lymph nodes and lymph nodes outside the abdominal cavity)

pTNM Pathological Classification

The pT and pN categories correspond to the T and N categories.

pM1	Distant metastasis microscopically confirmed

Note: pM0 and pMX are not valid categories.

pN0	Histological examination of a pelvic lymphadenectomy specimen will ordinarily include 10 or more lymph nodes. If the lymph nodes are negative, but the number ordinarily examined is not met, classify as pN0.

Stage Grouping

Stage IA	T1a	N0	M0
Stage IB	T1b	N0	M0
Stage IC1	T1c1	N0	M0
Stage IC2	T1c2	N0	M0
Stage IC3	T1c3	N0	M0
Stage IIA	T2a	N0	M0
Stage IIB	T2b	N0	M0
Stage IIC	T2c	N0	M0
Stage IIIA1	T1/T2	N1	M0
Stage IIIA2	T3a	N0/N1	M0
Stage IIIB	T3b	N0/N1	M0
Stage IIIC	T3c	N0/N1	M0
Stage IV	Any T	Any N	M1

References

American Joint Committee on Cancer (AJCC) Cancer Staging Manual, 7th ed. (2011). Edge SB, Byrd DR, Compton CC, Fritz AG, Greene FL, Trotti III eds. Springer: New York

International Union against Cancer (UICC): TNM Classification of Malignant Tumours, 7th ed. (2009) Sobin LH, Gospodarowicz MK, Wittekind Ch eds. Wiley-Blackwell: Oxford

A help-desk for specific questions about the TNM classification is available at http://www.uicc.org.

Prat J, FIGO Committee on Gynecologic Oncology (2014). Staging classification for cancer of the ovary, fallopian tube, and peritoneum. Int J Gynaecol Obstet 124:1-5.

Serous tumours

Introduction to serous tumours - Pelvic serous neoplasia

T.A. Longacre
M. Wells

Historically, almost all serous cancer involving the ovary was considered to arise primarily in the ovary, with early spread to other abdominal sites. Recent developments in our understanding of serous neoplasia have challenged this approach with the result that malignant serous ovarian neoplasia is now considered to represent two separate diseases: low-grade and high-grade serous carcinoma. This is based on a dualistic model of epithelial ovarian cancer, which divides epithelial ovarian carcinomas into two broad categories, designated type I and type II {1766}. The prototypic type I tumour is low-grade serous carcinoma, which has a high frequency of KRAS and BRAF mutations but no TP53 mutations and the prototypic type II tumour is high-grade serous carcinoma, which is characterized by a high level of genetic instability and harbours TP53 mutations in nearly all cases {1008}. The tumours in the two categories develop via separate pathways. The precursor of low-grade serous carcinoma is a borderline serous tumour/atypical proliferative tumour. Non-invasive serous tumours exhibiting an ample micropapillary pattern are more likely to be associated with synchronous or metachronous invasive disease {1117}. Low-grade serous cancers and borderline serous tumours/atypical proliferative tumours demonstrate mutations in KRAS or BRAF and few chromosomal abnormalities. In contrast, high-grade serous carcinomas harbour mutations in TP53 and are, chromosomally, highly unstable. High-grade serous cancers are usually rapidly growing, highly aggressive neoplasms that are often diagnosed at an advanced stage. Although low-grade serous carcinoma may rarely progress to high-grade serous carcinoma, the majority of low-grade serous carcinomas develop along a pathway that is distinct from that implicated in the development of their high-grade counterparts {182,433}.

Based on the traditional model of ovarian carcinogenesis, the ovarian surface mesothelium is the favoured cell of origin for serous neoplasia, presumably as a result of Müllerian metaplastic change to a tubal epithelial type, with subsequent neoplastic transformation related to mutational events occurring as a consequence of ovulatory trauma {75,536}. Conventionally, it has been assumed that the majority of serous epithelial tumours arise primarily from such metaplastic change of the surface mesothelium, despite the apparent rarity of putative precursor lesions. In recent years, an alternative tubal origin has emerged as an important source of high-grade serous carcinomas and initially, was based on the evaluation of risk-reducing salpingo-oophorectomy specimens in women with BRCA mutations {1079}. Although, according to the conventional model of ovarian carcinogenesis, primary fallopian tube carcinoma is extremely rare (estimated incidence of 0.41/100 000 versus 15/100 000 for primary ovarian cancer) {1837}, an increasing number of serous carcinomas are found to involve the fallopian tube at an early stage in these risk-reducing specimens {222,232,233,555,761,1066,1504, 1517,1518}. Based on complete sectioning of the ovaries and fallopian tubes in women at high risk of developing ovarian cancer (including the SEE-FIM protocol), prophylactic salpingo-oophorectomy specimens have revealed small non-invasive and invasive carcinomas much more commonly in the fallopian tube than the ovary {364,1245,1504}.

The non-invasive intraepithelial lesions have been designated serous tubal intraepithelial carcinoma (STIC) or high-grade serous tubal intraepithelial neoplasia. They have cytological features identical to high-grade serous ovarian cancer and also show TP53 mutation and aberrant p53 protein expression, high-proliferation indices and marked genomic instability {1245,1669}. It has also been shown that STIC is present in the fallopian tube in up to 60% of women with high-grade serous cancers that would have been considered to be ovarian or primary peritoneal tumours based on conventional criteria {931,1532,1669}. The fallopian tube is completely obliterated by tumour in an additional 20% of cases and may also be the primary site in such cases. In advanced stage high-grade serous cancer, STIC harbours TP53 mutations identical to the disseminated tumour, establishing that they are clonal {931,988} and a comparison of telomere length in matched STIC and the associated ovarian tumours suggests that the STIC is indeed the earlier lesion, antedating the ovarian tumour {989}.

The possibility of a field change within native or metaplastic tubal-type epithelium, resulting in multifocal lesions must also be considered as a plausible alternative pathogenetic hypothesis {1900}. In approximately 15–30% of cases of high-grade serous cancer, the fallopian tubes are normal, with no demonstrable serous tubal intraepithelial or invasive carcinoma present, despite meticulous histopathological assessment {1532,1669}. In these cases, the ovarian surface epithelium or cortical inclusion cysts are also presumptive sites of potential precursor lesions. Historically, cortical inclusion cysts (CICs) have been considered to be the consequence of entrapment of ovarian surface mesothelium following ovarian surface trauma at ovulation. Although some cortical inclusion cysts are lined by flat cells resembling the ovarian surface mesothelium, the majority of CICs are morphologically and immunohistochemically identical to fallopian tube epithelium leading some to propose that these CICs are derived from implanted tubal epithelium occurring at the time of ovulation {74,536,1008}. A report of aneuploidy in inclusion cysts supports this interpretation {1516}.

Although high-grade, extra-uterine serous carcinomas may arise from the fallopian tube, ovary or rarely, from the peritoneum, the site of origin is often obscured by bulky disease at the time of diagnosis. Nonetheless, these tumours are characterized by common epidemiological features and clinical behaviour {854}. Accordingly, tumours diagnosed as ovarian high-grade serous carcinoma might be viewed as an amalgamation of primary (extra-uterine) *"pelvic high-grade serous carcinomas"* {1753}. FIGO has recently proposed a new staging system to encompass tumours arising in these three sites, with the recommendation that those cases, for which it is not possible to clearly delineate a primary site, be listed as "undesignated." The decision as to primary site should be pragmatic, based on experience and professional judgement. It is considered inappropriate, for example, to base primary site of origin of a tumour on arbitrary *ex cathedra* recommendations based on tumour volume.

While a higher proportion of high-grade serous carcinomas probably arise from the fallopian tube than has been appreciated hitherto, it must be emphasized that definitive proof of a tubal origin for most high-grade serous cancers is lacking. The best evidence is in *BRCA1* mutation carriers who constitute no more than 10–12% of patients. Whether *BRCA2*-associated and sporadic high-grade serous cancers also arise from the tubes awaits further investigation and confirmation. In any event, the molecular genetic features of high-grade serous cancer are sufficiently distinct from those detected in low-grade serous cancer {851,994} that a separate classification scheme for these two tumours is warranted.

Summary of the current WHO classification and definitions

With improvements in our understanding of the molecular alterations involved in serous carcinogenesis, pathologists now recognize two distinct types of serous carcinoma. Therefore, in this fourth edition of the WHO classification, the term low-grade serous carcinoma is used to denote those serous neoplasms that are associated with serous borderline tumours/atypical proliferative tumours and include tumours historically classified as grade 1 serous carcinoma. The term high-grade serous carcinoma is used to encompass the majority of malignant non-uterine serous carcinomas of the female genital tract historically classified as grade 2 or grade 3 serous cancers and do not otherwise require additional grading. Recommendations for assignation of primary site in the pathology report, albeit imperfect, are based on the current conceptual framework including the probable tubal origin of at least a subset of cases.

The consensus meeting in Lyon that preceded the publication of this fourth edition of the WHO classification did not lead to agreement on a single, unifying concept for borderline tumours of the ovary for several reasons. First, borderline serous tumours comprise a unique group of tumours that is biologically distinct from borderline tumours of other histological types. Borderline serous tumours can present at high stage, occasionally with nodal involvement, and are associated with a distinct, albeit low, risk of transformation over time to low-grade serous carcinoma {1117,1778}. In contrast, borderline ovarian tumours of non-serous histology are typically confined to the ovary and generally pose no risk for transformation, provided they are adequately sectioned. Second, there exists a significant difference in opinion among gynaecological pathologists with respect to borderline serous tumours in particular. Some view the borderline serous tumours as essentially benign and favour the term atypical proliferative tumour, while others believe the borderline tumour terminology uniquely captures the unusual nature of these tumours. The application of the borderline tumour terminology to the non-serous types, is problematic, in as much as there are no well documented cases of malignant behaviour in well sampled tumours, leading many pathologists to favour the term atypical proliferative. However, because of its long usage the term borderline has been retained. Accordingly, both terms are accepted terminology in the current (fourth) edition of the WHO classification. In subsequent sections of this edition, the classification of serous epithelial tumours of the ovary and the specific histological, epidemiological and molecular features of these neoplasms are described in more detail.

Serous cystadenoma, adenofibroma and surface papilloma

J.D. Seidman
D.A. Bell
C.P. Crum
C.B. Gilks
R.J. Kurman
D.A. Levine
T.A. Longacre

B. Pasini
C. Riva
M.E. Sherman
I.M. Shih
G. Singer
R. Soslow
R. Vang

Definition
Tumours characterized by epithelial cell types resembling those of the fallopian tube, including ciliated cells. The epithelial component may be associated with a prominent component of stromal cells (cystadenofibroma, adenofibroma), may lack a stromal component (cystadenoma) or be entirely a surface papillary lesion (surface papilloma). Combinations of these growth patterns occur.

ICD-O codes
Serous cystadenoma	8441/0
Serous adenofibroma	9014/0
Serous surface papilloma	8461/0

Clinical features
Patients range in age from 40 to 60 years. Women are frequently asymptomatic, the tumours being detected incidentally. Symptomatic women, usually those with large tumours, present with chronic pelvic pain or acute pain resulting from torsion.

Macroscopy
A cut-off size of 1 cm is used to distinguish between cortical inclusion cysts (< 1 cm) and serous cystadenomas (> 1 cm). Cystic tumours range from 1 to > 30 cm in greatest dimension, have smooth outer surfaces and contain one or more thin-walled cysts filled with clear, watery fluid. Cystadenofibromas are composed of cysts surrounded by a variable amount of fibrotic tissue. Adenofibromas are typically solid whereas surface papillomas are exophytic.

Histopathology
Serous cystadenomas are composed of cysts and papillae lined by non-stratified or stratified cuboidal to columnar cells resembling fallopian tube epithelium. Cilia are almost invariably present though sometimes only focally. When there is a prominent fibrous stroma the tumour is designated an adenofibroma. Some pathologists classify cysts with an otherwise nondescript flattened epithelial lining as serous cystadenoma. Foci that qualify as serous borderline tumour/atypical proliferative serous tumour (SBT/APST) may be present and, if < 10% of the epithelial volume, are designated serous cystadenoma/fibroma with focal epithelial proliferation {1117,1729}. Small papillary growths with bland, serous-type epithelium on the surface of the ovary are designated serous surface papillomas.

Genetic profile
Unlike SBT/APST and low-grade serous carcinoma (LGSC), serous cystadenomas do not contain mutations in either *KRAS*

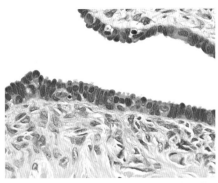

Fig. 1.03 Serous cystadenoma. The cysts and papillae are lined by benign-appearing cuboidal to columnar, focally ciliated cells. The lining may also be flattened or cuboidal without cilia.

or *BRAF*. Most serous cystadenomas are polyclonal but monoclonal cystadenomas occur. Accordingly, it appears that serous cystadenomas develop as a hyperplastic expansion from epithelial inclusions with a clonal/neoplastic transformation occurring in a subset {288}. Only rare serous cystadenomas/adenofibromas show DNA copy number changes in the epithelial cells {794}. Such changes are more common in the fibromatous stromal cells of these tumours.

Genetic susceptibility
No specific genetic predispositions to benign serous tumours have been recognized.

Prognosis and predictive factors
Lesions are benign, although they may occasionally recur after cystectomy. Serous cystadenomas with focal epithelial proliferation are also benign, though published data are very limited.

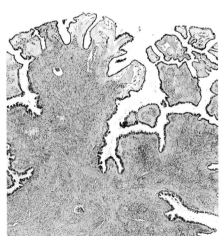

Fig. 1.01 Serous cystadenofibroma. Branching papillae lined by serous epithelium with bland nuclei overlying fibromatous stroma.

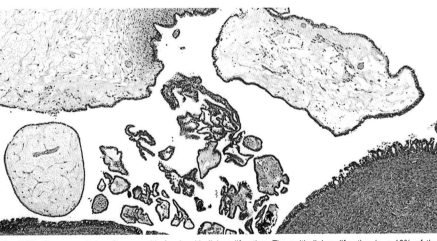

Fig. 1.02 Serous cystadenofibroma with focal epithelial proliferation. The epithelial proliferation is < 10% of the neoplasm.

A surface atypical component is logically more potentially significant than an intracystic one and should be noted in a comment.

Serous borderline tumour / Atypical proliferative serous tumour

Definition
Serous borderline tumours/atypical proliferative serous tumours (SBT/APSTs) are non-invasive tumours that display greater epithelial proliferation and cytological atypia than benign serous tumours but less than low-grade serous carcinoma (LGSC).

ICD-O code   8442/1

Synonym
Serous tumour of low malignant potential (not recommended)

Epidemiology
The mean age of patients is 42 years. The incidence of these tumours is considerably lower than that of high-grade serous carcinoma (HGSC) {1277}. In addition, they occur at a younger age and are not related to mutations in BRCA1/2 {659}. Most studies identify at least some similarities in risk-factor associations to HGSC, notably a protective effect of parity {802,1282,1299,1591}. A history of infertility is more common when compared to women with HGSC.

Clinical features
Patients present with masses that appear to be confined to the ovary in the vast majority of cases {1117}. Imaging studies show greater complexity than benign tumours. Presenting symptoms are similar to benign tumours, but some patients with advanced stage disease may present with ascites.

Macroscopy
The tumours are typically cystic and generally > 5 cm. They often have an additional surface component; rarely is there only a surface component. Velvety, papillary tumour typically involves at least part of the cyst lining or represents the surface component. Tumours are bilateral in about one-third of patients.

Histopathology
A hierarchical branching pattern characterized by irregular papillae that branch from large to progressively smaller papillae terminating in detached tufts of epithelial cells, is typical. The papillae are lined by non-stratified or stratified cuboidal to columnar cells that are typically ciliated. Many tumours have a variable number of polygonal and hobnail cells with eosinophilic cytoplasm containing moderately enlarged, hyperchromatic nuclei and sometimes nucleoli {217,485,1296,1727} but the latter are rarely diffusely prominent. Cells with clear cytoplasm may also be present {1410}.

Some typical SBT/APSTs display foci composed of micropapillae arranged in a non-hierarchical branching architecture simulating non-invasive LGSC. In contrast to the latter, these SBT/APSTs lack the nuclear atypia of non-invasive LGSC and measure < 5 mm in confluent growth and therefore qualify as SBT/APST.

The term "microinvasion" has been applied to clusters of cells in the stroma with abundant eosinophilic cytoplasm, similar to the eosinophilic cells on the surface of papillae, that measure < 5 mm in greatest dimension {123,1296}. These cells are less likely to express oestrogen and progesterone receptors and have a significantly lower Ki-67 labelling index, suggesting they may be terminally differentiated or senescent {1160}. This may explain why most lesions classified as "microinvasion" have no adverse effect on survival {1240,1729,1777}. On rare occasions, small foci of low-grade serous carcinoma, which differ from the clusters of eosinophilic cells that are typically classified as "microinvasion," are detected in the stroma of an SBT/APST. To distinguish these small carcinomas from microinvasion, some pathologists refer to them as "microinvasive carcinoma". There are insufficient data to comment on their clinical significance. The findings should prompt extensive sampling.

Implants
Peritoneal lesions associated with SBT/APST were originally classified as "non-invasive" or "invasive" implants based on whether the lesions were confined to the surface of organs (non-invasive) or infiltrated the underlying tissue (invasive) {125,1200}. Implants that display hierarchically branching papillae or detached clusters of cells associated with non-fibrotic stroma that do not invade have been termed "epithelial-type non-invasive implants," whereas, those composed of clusters of cells embedded in reactive-appearing or dense fibrous tissue that overshadow the epithelial component and appear "tacked on" to the peritoneal surface, have been termed "desmoplastic-type non-invasive implants." Single cells with eosinophilic cytoplasm may be present in the stroma in the latter type but are not indicative of invasion {125,128,1200}. Although the presence of unequivocal invasion is an important prognostic feature, this may be difficult to establish in some cases. Some studies have shown that implants that do not infiltrate underlying tissue but display the cytological features of invasive implants, specifically small, solid nests of cells surrounded by a space, micropapillae and/or cribriform growth, behave in a similar manner to clear-cut invasive implants as described above {128}. Because the latter and invasive implants behave like *low-grade serous carcinoma (LGSC)* they should be designated as

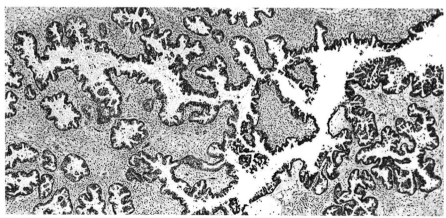

Fig. 1.04 Serous borderline tumour/atypical proliferative serous tumour (SBT/APST). Hierarchical, branching architecture lined by cuboidal to columnar epithelium with minimal cytological atypia.

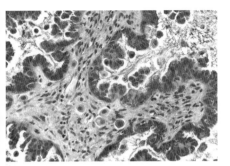

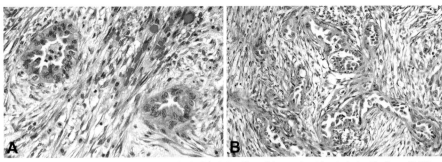

Fig. 1.05 Serous borderline tumour/atypical proliferative serous tumour with microinvasion. Rounded eosinophilic cells are present in the stroma and resemble similar eosinophilic cells on the surface of the papillae. Eosinophilic cells are also present as detached clusters floating above the papillae.

Fig. 1.07 Implant (non-invasive, desmoplastic). **A** Glands lined by mild to moderately atypical epithelium with little or no mitotic activity. Most of the cells contain abundant eosinophilic cytoplasm. **B** The gland-like epithelial structures are surrounded by a granulation tissue-type stroma with reactive spindle cells. The majority of the epithelial cells contain abundant eosinophilic cytoplasm closely resembling the eosinophilic cells lining the papillae of serous borderline tumour/atypical proliferative serous tumour and in foci of microinvasion. The epithelial and spindle cell components appear to blend with one another.

such. All other implants that are non-invasive can be designated *"implants"*.

Pelvic lymph nodes associated with SBT/APST

These can contain a variety of lesions, including endosalpingiosis, clusters of eosinophilic cells, implants and, rarely, LGSC. *Eosinophilic cells*, identical to those described above, in lymph node sinuses have been interpreted as senescent cells and have no adverse effect on survival {1160}. The pathology report can comment on their presence but they should not be classified as metastases and their benign behaviour should be indicated. *Endosalpingiosis* is also frequently found in pelvic lymph nodes as well as implants (non-invasive). The latter resemble the primary ovarian SBT/APST. Neither of these lesions appears to affect survival. Less frequently, lymph node parenchyma can be replaced by LGSC, which is typically associated with an ovarian LGSC but occasionally with an SBT/APST. These lesions should be classified as LGSC.

Immunohistochemistry

Various epithelial markers are expressed including cytokeratin (CAM 5.2, AE1/AE3), EMA, BER-EP4, WT1 and PAX8 {109,1041}. High levels of both ER and PR are frequently observed {506}. These tumours show a p53 wild type pattern (see Introduction p.15). Diffuse p16 staining is absent {38}.

Genetic profile

The most consistent molecular genetic alterations are somatic mutations in *KRAS* and *BRAF* which occur in about 50% of cases {851,1788}. Mutations of *KRAS* and *BRAF* occur in the epithelium of cystadenomas adjacent to SBT/APSTs (but not in cystadenoma without SBT/APST), suggesting that these mutations precede the development of SBT/APST {763}. SBT/APST has a very low level of DNA copy number changes, suggesting that the genome is relatively stable {994}.

Prognosis and predictive factors

The survival of women with SBT/APSTs confined to the ovaries (Stage I) does not

differ from the general population {704}. The presence of "microinvasion" as defined above does not alter this outcome. Patients with implants (non-invasive) may develop adhesions and recurrences that may require surgical intervention. The survival for such patients is greater than 95% {1727}. Extra-ovarian peritoneal implants (Stage II and higher) occur in approximately 13% of patients {704} and most qualify simply as non-invasive implants (implants). Identification of extra-ovarian disease is critical since the most important predictor of adverse outcome is the presence of LGSC (invasive implants) {1727}. Among patients with extra-ovarian disease only 8% qualify as LGSC (invasive implants) {704}. Recent studies have more clearly delineated the long-term behaviour of SBT/APSTs. Most behave in a benign fashion but a minority pursues an indolent course, some as long as 20 years; tumours may recur as SBT/APSTs or as LGSC. Progression to LGSC mirrors the behaviour of tumours that present initially as invasive LGSC

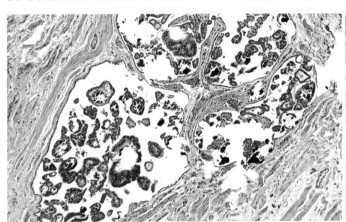

Fig. 1.06 Implant (non-invasive). Branching papillae within smoothly contoured spaces. Numerous psammoma bodies are present.

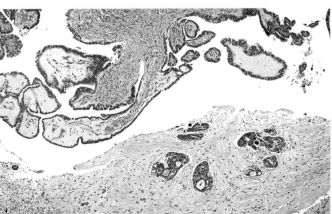

Fig. 1.08 SBT/APST with a small focus of invasive carcinoma. There are multiple small groups of cells measuring < 5 mm in greatest dimension in the stroma. This is not microinvasion.

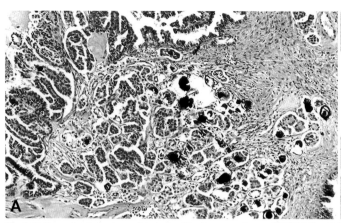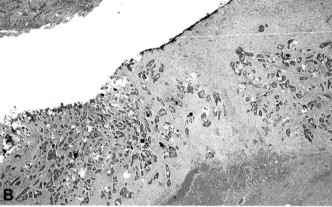

Fig. 1.09 Serous borderline tumour/atypical proliferative serous tumour (SBT/APST) with focus of low-grade serous carcinoma. **A** The focus of tumour cells in the stroma occupying most of the field measures < 5 mm and represents low-grade serous carcinoma. **B** Low-grade serous carcinoma in parametrium (invasive implant). The lesion is identical to primary ovarian low-grade serous carcinoma. Although occasionally associated with a serous borderline tumour/atypical proliferative serous tumour, this lesion is significantly more frequently associated with serous borderline tumour, micropapillary variant/non-invasive low-grade serous carcinoma.

{1770}. Lymph node involvement as described above has no adverse effect on outcome. In summary, deaths from SBT/APSTs are due to progression to LGSC which occurs in about 5% {1117} of cases and non-cancer causes (i.e. bowel obstruction or complications from treatment).

Serous borderline tumour - micropapillary variant / Non-invasive low-grade serous carcinoma

Definition
A non-invasive tumour displaying a non-hierarchical branching architecture featuring micropapillary and/or cribriform patterns composed of rounded cells with scant cytoplasm and moderate nuclear atypia.

ICD-O code   8460/2

Epidemiology
Similar to serous borderline tumour/atypical proliferative serous tumour (p. 18).

Clinical features
Similar to serous borderline tumour/atypical proliferative serous tumour (p. 18). The mean age of patients is 45 years.

Macroscopy
Similar to serous borderline tumour/atypical proliferative serous tumour (p. 18)

Histopathology
These tumours are characterized by a non-hierarchical branching architecture in which a myriad of fine, micropapillae, usually five times taller than they are wide, emanate directly from large, often fibrotic papillae. The micropapillae have scant or no stromal cores and in contrast to serous borderline tumour/atypical proliferative serous tumour (SBT/APST), which contain columnar cells that are frequently ciliated, the cells in these tumours are cuboidal to polygonal with a high nuclear to cytoplasmic ratio and small, uniform, more atypical nuclei. Small but prominent (often cherry-red) nucleoli are seen and cilia are conspicuously absent.

The mitotic index is low but typically higher than in SBT/APST. Some tumours display a cribriform pattern on the surfaces of the papillae and occasional tumours are purely cribiform and/or show a slit-like glandular pattern without micropapillae. The micropapillary/cribriform features may coexist with usual SBT/APST. A diagnosis of non-invasive LGSC requires at least one confluent area of micropapillarity measuring 5 mm in one dimension and nuclear atypia greater than that allowed in a SBT/APST. Tumours with lesser micropapillarity and atypia can be classified as SBT/APST with focal micropapillary features {217,485,1117,1726}.

Immunohistochemistry
Various epithelial markers are expressed including cytokeratin (CAM 5.2, AE1/AE3), EMA, BER-EP4, WT1 and PAX8 {109,1041}. High levels of both ER and PR are frequently observed {506}. These tumours show a p53 wild type pattern (see Introduction p.15). Diffuse p16 staining is absent {38}.

Genetic profile
Like SBT/APSTs, the most consistent molecular genetic alterations are somatic mutations in *KRAS* and *BRAF* which occur in about 50% of cases {851,1788}. Gene expression profile studies have shown differential gene expression between SBT/APST and the non-invasive LGSC but no differential expression between the latter and invasive LGSC. This supports the view that despite morphological similarities, SBT/APST differs at a molecular level from non-invasive LGSC and invasive LGSC and represents an intermediate step in progression to LGSC. In addition, a recent molecular profiling study showed that a subgroup of SBT/APSTs can be classified into tumours with a benign- or malignant-like methylation profile that may help in identifying tumours more likely to progress to LGSC {1190A,2151A}. The genome of the tumour is relatively stable and chromosomal 1p36 loss is the most significant DNA copy number change. The deletion of tumour suppressors in that locus may contribute to tumour progression from SBT/APST and non-invasive LGSC to invasive LGSC {994}.

Prognosis and predictive factors
The survival of women with a tumour confined to the ovaries (Stage I) does not differ from the general population {704}. However, compared to SBT/APST, which presents with advanced stage disease in 13% of cases, non-invasive LGSC presents with advanced stage disease in 27% (*P* < 0.003). In addition, among patients with extra-ovarian disease, non-invasive LGSC is associated with LGSC

(invasive implants) in 50% of cases compared to 8% of women with SBT/APSTs ($P < 0.0001$) {704}. In a study of 56 women with advanced stage non-invasive LGSC involving greater than 10% of what was otherwise a SBT/APST, patients developed recurrence in 92% of cases and were alive with disease or died of disease in 80% of cases, which was the same as women who had invasive LGSC {1614}. In summary, non-invasive LGSC is a more aggressive tumour than SBT/APST.

Low-grade serous carcinoma

Definition
An invasive carcinoma, usually with distinctive patterns showing low-grade malignant cytological atypia.

ICD-O code   8460/3

Epidemiology
Low-grade serous carcinomas (LGSCs) account for about 5% of all serous carcinomas {951}. Analyses of risk factors for low-grade tumours are limited by case numbers and its recent recognition as a distinct tumour type {1183}.

Clinical features
Patients with LGSC present approximately one decade earlier than patients with high-grade serous carcinoma (HGSC) {1974}. Ovarian masses may be symptomatic or detected incidentally. Most patients present with advanced stage disease. Ascites and other features similar to HGSC may be present but the volume of disease is generally less in LGSC. Ovarian masses are usually cystic on imaging,

but may contain thick septae or nodular components with increased vascularity.

Macroscopy
LGSC is often bilateral and exhibits fine papillary growth. Compared with HGSC, necrosis is rarely, if ever, observed. Calcification is frequently present and may be extensive. Extra-ovarian lesions may be gritty on palpation due to calcification.

Histopathology
LGSC is characterized by a variety of architectural patterns including single cells and irregularly shaped small nests of cells haphazardly infiltrating stroma, micropapillae or less commonly, macropapillae surrounded by an unlined clear space; different patterns of invasion often coexist {2084}.
A significant proportion of LGSCs have an associated component of serous borderline tumour/atypical proliferative serous tumour (SBT/APST) {1152}. The cells of LGSC show mild to moderate nuclear atypia, and may contain a single prominent nucleolus {1152,1153,1974}. In contrast to HGSC, LGSC is composed of a more uniform population of small cells with limited nuclear pleomorphism. Necrosis is almost never detected, psammoma bodies are much more frequent and mitotic activity is significantly lower (usually < 2–3 mitotic figures per 10 HPF) than in HGSC {1152}.

Immunohistochemistry
The immunohistochemical profile is identical to serous borderline tumour/APST except for lower PR expression which is observed in about 50% of cases {506}. Ki-67 proliferation index is typically low-

er compared to HGSC. In cases where distinction between LGSC and HGSC is problematic, aberrant p53 expression can be useful, as this pattern is consistent with mutant *TP53* and supports a diagnosis of HGSC (see Introduction to serous tumours, p. 15) {38}.

Genetic profile
Exome sequencing analysis {851} demonstrates a significantly lower number of somatic mutations in LGSC than other types of human cancer and confirms the frequent *KRAS* and *BRAF* mutations (in approximately 50–60% of cases) {1772,1788}. Advanced stage LGSCs harbour *BRAF* mutations less frequently {2046}. As compared with HGSC, the LGSC genome is relatively stable and chromosomal 1p36 loss appears as the most significant DNA copy number change. Methylation profiling shows that LGSC is more closely related to SBT/APST than HGSC {1765}.

Prognosis and predictive factors
Prognosis of tumours confined to the ovary is excellent with surgical therapy alone. Five- and ten-year survival rates in advanced stage are approximately 85% and 50%, respectively {627,733}. Over 2 cm of residual disease after surgery portends a poor outcome {385}. LGSCs do not respond well, but are not refractory, to conventional platinum-based chemotherapy in the neoadjuvant, adjuvant or recurrent settings {195,628,1696}.

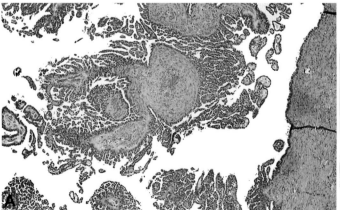
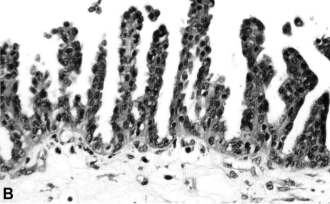

Fig. 1.10 Serous borderline tumour, micropapillary variant. Non-invasive low-grade serous carcinoma. **A** The tumour is characterized by a non-hierarchical architecture in which a myriad of micropapillae emanate directly from large papillary cores. **B** The micropapillae are at least five times as long as they are wide. The cells lining the micropapillae are rounded with a high nuclear:cytoplasmic ratio and unlike serous borderline tumour/atypical proliferative serous tumour have greater nuclear atypia and lack cilia.

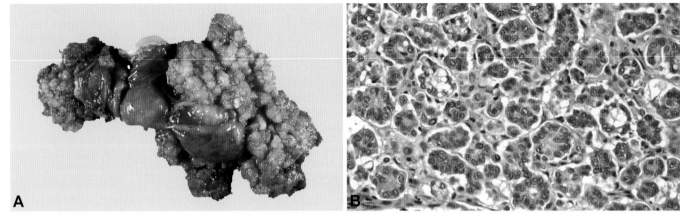

Fig. 1.11 A Low-grade serous carcinoma. Bilateral tumours with extensive exophytic papillary growth. **B** Stromal invasion is characterized by micropapillae infiltrating stroma in a haphazard pattern. Nuclei are relatively small, rounded and uniform in size and often contain a single, small but prominent nucleolus. Note the absence of mitotic figures in this field.

High-grade serous carcinoma

Definition
A carcinoma composed of epithelial cells displaying papillary, glandular (often slit-like) and solid patterns with high-grade nuclear atypia.

ICD-O code   8461/3

Epidemiology
Annually, there are about 225 000 newly diagnosed ovarian carcinomas and 140'000 related deaths worldwide, the majority of which are high-grade serous carcinoma (HGSC) {546}. HGSCs disproportionately affect women in western nations {546} with cumulative lifetime risks in the US of 1.38%, which is higher among white women as compared to black women. In the US, rates have been declining for many years, and this trend accelerated after 2002.

Etiology
Studies have variably identified relationships between several intertwined menstrual and reproductive factors and lower ovarian cancer risk, including parity, later age at menarche, earlier age at menopause and oral contraceptive use {792,1485,1489,1855}. In aggregate, these factors are associated with shorter lifetime number of menstrual cycles; however, other mechanisms may mediate the protective effects of these individual factors. The protective effect of parity increases with greater numbers of births, whereas infertility may increase risk independently. Tubal ligation also provides long-term protection for serous carcinoma (although its effects may be stronger for endometrioid carcinomas) and likely reduces risk among *BRCA1/2* mutation carriers {319}. Oestrogen-only hormonal therapy and combined oestrogen and progestin regimens are associated with

increased risk, although the association is attenuated with the latter preparation {1480}. It is unclear whether this overall risk applies equally to serous carcinoma as compared with other histological types. Oral contraceptives afford strong protection against HGSC, which is related directly to duration of use and wanes slowly, persisting for decades following discontinuation {135}. It is estimated that use of these medications has prevented over 200'000 cancers worldwide over the past several decades {135}. Infertility treatments do not seem to affect risk independently of other factors {1987}; however, data are limited by small numbers and the comparatively young age of exposed cohorts.

Clinical features
The mean age of patients is 63 years. Presenting symptoms are relatively nonspecific but are often gastrointestinal,

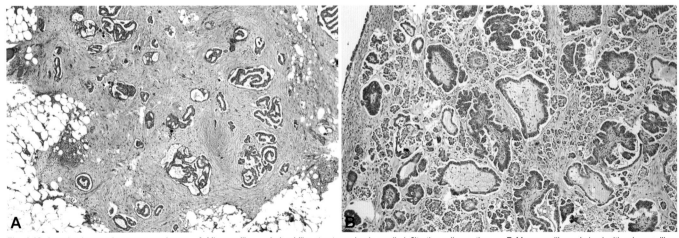

Fig. 1.12 Invasive low-grade serous carcinoma. **A** Micropapillae and gland-like structures haphazardly infiltrating adipose tissue. **B** Macropapillae admixed with micropapillae, displaying a haphazard pattern of infiltration {2084}.

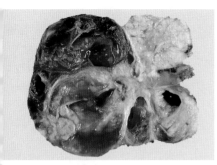

Fig. 1.13 High-grade serous carcinoma. Note the solid growth and large fluid filled cysts.

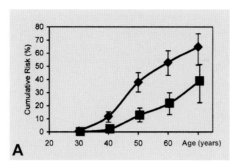

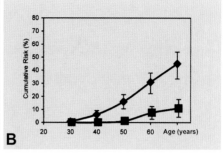

Fig. 1.15 A Cumulative risk of breast (♦) and ovarian (■) cancer in *BRCA1*-mutation carriers. **B** Cumulative risk of breast (♦) and ovarian (■) cancer in *BRCA2*-mutation carriers. Reprinted from {55B}.

including nausea, anorexia, early satiety, abdominal distension, bloating, pain, tenesmus and constipation as well as back pain and urinary frequency {648}. When associated with malignant pleural effusion, cough and dyspnea are common. Diagnosis is often delayed because symptoms are non-specific. Imaging studies reveal large, complex, hypervascular pelvic masses, ascites and omental/peritoneal nodules. Serum CA-125 is usually elevated with median values in the range of 500–1000 U/ml for advanced stage disease {2175}.

Macroscopy

HGSCs are variable in size. Although often large, in over one-third of cases the ovaries are either grossly normal or display surface nodules of tumour < 1 cm. Tumours are often bilateral, exophytic and demonstrate solid and papillary growth and fluid-filled cysts. The solid regions are tan-white and typically contain extensive necrosis and haemorrhage. The fallopian tube may be macroscopically involved and not readily identifiable

or a small, firm, sometimes polypoid lesion may be seen at its fimbriated end. The fimbriae may be splayed over the tumour surface.

Histopathology

HGSCs are typically composed of solid masses of cells with slit-like spaces. In addition, papillary, glandular and cribriform areas are common. Necrosis is frequent. Nuclei are large, hyperchromatic and pleomorphic, often with large bizarre or multinucleated forms. Nucleoli are usually prominent and may be very large and eosinophilic. Mitoses are numerous and often atypical. Psammoma bodies are variably conspicuous. A papillary pattern or one of thick undulating bands of epithelial cells closely resembling urothelial carcinoma (transitional cell carcinoma) may be present and occasionally predominates. Immunohistochemical studies have shown that these are variants of HGSC and less commonly of high-grade endometrioid carcinoma and not a distinct entity {1885}. Well sampled "transitional cell carcinoma" usually shows areas of typical

serous carcinoma. A very small proportion of HGSCs are intracystic and lack apparent invasion and in the past have erroneously been classified as "borderline" tumours. These tumours display marked nuclear atypia and high mitotic activity, similar to their invasive counterparts.

Immunohistochemistry
Nuclear expression of WT1 is considered a useful marker for HGSC (absent in most endometrial serous carcinomas). p53 expression can demonstrate two different patterns which correlate with a *TP53* mutation. The usual pattern, and the one most commonly observed, is strong diffuse nuclear staining in approximately 60% of cells or greater. This pattern correlates with a missense mutation. The other pattern is complete absence of staining (it is important to confirm that the stain is working properly), which correlates with a nonsense mutation resulting in a truncated protein that is not detected by the p53 antibody. Accordingly, both patterns correlate with a *TP53* mutation and since mutated *TP53* occurs in

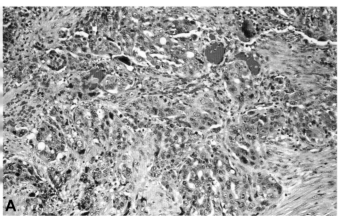

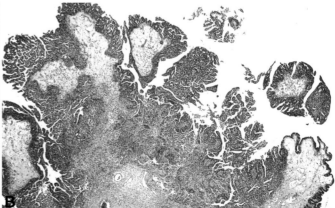

Fig. 1.14 A High-grade serous carcinoma, invasive. Solid masses of cells with slit-like spaces, high-grade nuclear atypia. **B** High-grade serous carcinoma. This low-magnification view displays a complex papillary serous proliferation which architecturally does not appear to be infiltrating the underlying stroma. The cytological features at higher magnification (not shown) are identical to typical high-grade serous carcinoma and warrant such a diagnosis.

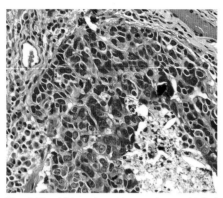

Fig. 1.16 High-grade serous carcinoma. Marked cytological atypia, mitotic figures and necrosis are seen.

Table 1.1 Immunohistochemical staining of ovarian carcinoma types {38,506,951A,953,1169A,1772A,2085}

Carcinoma Type	PAX8, positive	WT1, positive	TP53 aberrant*	CDKN2A, diffuse#	ER pos.	PR pos.
LGSC	100%	100%	0	0	96%	50%
HGSC	98%	92%	93%	60%	80%	30%
MC	50-60%	0%	50%	14%	6%	0
EC	84%	4%	11%	6%	86%	72%
CCC	99%	0%	12%	9%	13%	6%

* Aberrant expression (associated with *TP53* mutation) refers to either overexpression (strong nuclear expression > 60% of tumour cell nuclei) or complete absence (< 5% of tumour cell nuclei), which is different from the TP53 wild type pattern (not associated with *TP53* mutation); # diffuse bloc staining in > 90% staining; LGSC, low-grade serous carcinoma; HGSC, high-grade serous carcinoma; MC, mucinous carcinoma; EC, endometrioid carcinoma; CCC, clear cell carcinoma

virtually all HGSC this stain is considered helpful in confirming the diagnosis of an HGSC (see Table 1.1)

Genetic profile

The most prominent molecular changes include alterations in *TP53*, nearly always mutations, in virtually all HGSCs and inactivation (germline or somatic mutation or promoter methylation) of *BRCA1* and *BRCA2* in nearly one-half of HGSCs {226}. Another distinctive feature of HGSC is the high level of chromosomal alterations as manifested by prominent DNA copy number changes {990,994}. The amplified DNA regions in HGSC always harbour well known oncogenes such as *CCNE1* (encoding Cyclin E1), *NOTCH3*, *PIK3CA* and *AKT*.

Genetic susceptibility

Hereditary predisposition to ovarian cancer can explain up to 15–20% of newly diagnosed HGSC, mostly due to germline mutations in *BRCA1* (17q21.31) and *BRCA2* (13q13.1) genes. *BRCA1* mutations cause a 50% life-time risk of ovarian cancer (20%–65%) with average age at diagnosis of 49–53 years. The risk as-

sociated with *BRCA2* mutations is lower (11–37%) and the age at diagnosis later (55–58 years). Virtually all *BRCA*-associated ovarian cancers exhibit high-grade serous morphology {1190}. An increased risk for ovarian cancer occurs with mutations in other DNA-repair genes involved in homologous recombination/Fanconi anaemia pathway (*BARD1, BRIP1, PALB2, RAD51C, RAD51D, RAD50, MRE11A, NBN*) accounting for up to 6% of additional germline mutations {1998} in ovarian cancer.

Prognosis and predictive factors

Almost all patients with HGSC receive cytotoxic chemotherapy. There is no subset of patients with a sufficiently favourable prognosis for whom chemotherapy can routinely be withheld {952}.

The most important prognostic factor for patients with HGSC is stage; by the time patients become symptomatic, they have advanced stage disease in approximately 75–80% of cases, and < 25% of patients with stage III/IV HGSCs will be cured by current therapies {167}. In advanced stage patients, the amount of residual tumour after staging and debulking

is the most important prognostic factor. Patients in whom all macroscopic disease can be completely resected (completely debulked) have a significantly better prognosis {491}. There is some prognostic stratification based on size of residual disease (i.e. < 1 cm, 1–2 cm, > 2 cm) in patients with macroscopic residual disease, but it is relatively minor {776}. It is not clear at this time whether resectability reflects an intrinsically more favourable disease type, or whether increased surgical effort leads to better outcomes independent of intrinsic tumour characteristics.

Molecular markers of prognosis in HGSC are relatively few and none have entered into routine clinical practice. The presence of tumour infiltrating lymphocytes, specifically CD3+ or CD8+ T-cells, are a marker of favourable prognosis in patients with HGSC {322,1067,2159}. *BRCA1* and *BRCA2* germline mutations are associated with a more favourable prognosis, although this effect is less pronounced for mutations near the 5" end of the *BRCA1* gene, compared to the 3" end {165}.

Mucinous tumours

T.A. Longacre
D.A. Bell
A. Malpica

J. Prat
B.M. Ronnett
J.D. Seidman
R. Vang

Mucinous cystadenoma / adenofibroma

Definition
A benign, cystic tumour lined by mucinous gastrointestinal-type epithelium or rarely, having prominent fibrous stroma (adenofibroma).

ICD-O codes
Mucinous cystadenoma   8470/0
Mucinous adenofibroma   9015/0

Epidemiology
Mucinous cystadenomas account for approximately 80% of all primary ovarian mucinous tumours. Mucinous adenofibromas are uncommon {119,711}.

Clinical features
These tumours are seen in patients with a wide age range. Mean age is 50 years. The most common symptoms are abdominal/pelvic pain and the presence of an abdominal or pelvic mass. Some cases present with oestrogenic or androgenic effect due to luteinization of the stromal cells.

Macroscopy
Typically, these are unilateral (95%) with a smooth surface and are multilocular or,

less often, unilocular, cystic neoplasms. They range in size from a few centimetres to > 30 cm; with a mean of 10 cm. Adenofibromas are solid and usually smaller.

Histopathology
The typical tumour is composed of multiple cysts and glands lined by simple, non-stratified mucinous epithelium resembling gastric foveolar-type or intestinal epithelium containing goblet cells and sometimes neuroendocrine cells or Paneth cells. Focal papillae may be seen. The ovarian stroma immediately adjacent to the epithelium may be cellular with areas of stromal luteinization. At times, small areas of extravasated mucin or mucinous granulomas are present in the stroma, secondary to rupture of the cysts. Mucinous cystadenomas may be associated with a dermoid cyst or Brenner tumour in around 10% of cases. Rarely, a benign mucinous tumour has a dense fibromatous stroma (mucinous adenofibroma).

Histogenesis
The association of some mucinous cystadenomas with dermoid cysts indicates that some are of germ cell origin and an association with Brenner tumours indicates a surface epithelial origin for another subset {1725}.

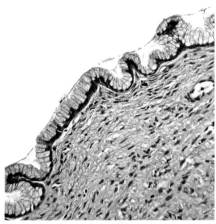

Fig. 1.18 Mucinous cystadenoma. Uniform gastro-intestinal-type mucinous cells with minimal or no cytological atypia. Mild pseudostratification may be present but mitotic figures are rare or absent.

Genetic profile
KRAS mutations have been found in up to 58% of cases {391}.

Prognosis and predictive factors
These tumours are benign; however, recurrences may be seen in cases treated with cystectomy {101}.

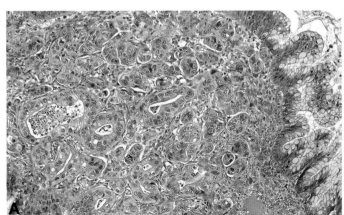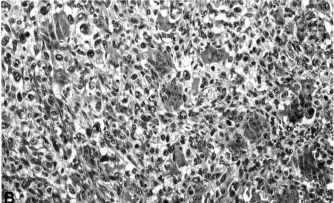

Fig. 1.17 A Mucinous borderline tumour / Atypical proliferative mucinous tumour (MBT/APMT) with microinvasive carcinoma. Mucinous glands and solid epithelial nests, with the architectural and cytological features of carcinoma, are present in the stroma. **B** Mural nodule (sarcoma-like). The nodule is composed of a heterogeneous cell population with numerous multinucleated cells of the epulis type.

Mucinous borderline tumour / Atypical proliferative mucinous tumour

Definition

Tumours composed of mild to moderately atypical gastrointestinal-type, mucin-containing epithelial cells that show proliferation greater than that seen in benign mucinous tumours. Stromal invasion is absent.

ICD-O code   8472/1

Synonyms

Mucinous tumour of low malignant potential (not recommended)

Epidemiology

These are the second most common type of borderline/atypical proliferative tumour in North America and Europe, comprising 30–50% of such tumours, but are the most common form in Asia making up about 70% of borderline/atypical proliferative tumour {915}.

Clinical features

The tumours occur across a wide age range from 13–88 years, with a mean age of 40–49 years {915, 923, 1060, 1595, 1791}. Patients most often present with an abdominal mass that is nearly always unilateral and confined to the ovary; although a few bilateral cases have been reported {915,923,1060,1595,1613,1791}. Bilaterality should prompt consideration of a metastatic carcinoma. There are no well-documented cases of a mucinous borderline/atypical proliferative mucinous tumour (MBT/APMT) associated with peritoneal implants and consequently all are stage I. Acellular mucin can sometimes be detected on peritoneal surfaces {923,1060}.

Macroscopy

The tumour size ranges from several centimetres to 50 cm in greatest dimension (mean, 21.5 cm) {2086}. The tumours are nearly always unilateral and have smooth external surfaces. They are composed of small to large cysts containing mucinous material but solid areas may be seen. The cysts usually have smooth walls but some may be ulcerated or have areas of solid growth {915,923,1060,1595,1613,1791}. Adequate sampling of these tumours is crucial since they are typically hetero-

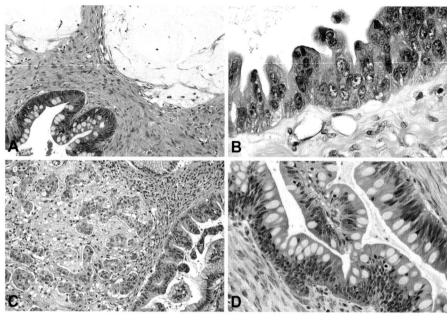

Fig. 1.19 Mucinous borderline tumour / Atypical proliferative mucinous tumour (MBT/APMT). **A** Pools of mucin are present in the stroma. **B** Intraepithelial carcinoma. The cells are markedly atypical, with loss of polarity. **C** Stromal microinvasion. Small nests of low-grade mucinous epithelium, resembling the adjacent borderline mucinous tumour are suspended in mucin within the ovarian stroma. **D** Stratified columnar mucin-containing cells are present with many goblet cells. Mild to moderate nuclear atypia is present.

geneous and can harbour occult foci of carcinoma. Sampling should consist of 1 section per cm of greatest tumour dimension in tumours that measure less than 10 cm, focusing on solid or grossly unusual areas. Once the tumour reaches 10 cm or shows microinvasion or intraepithelial carcinoma, the sampling should be increased to 2 sections per cm of greatest tumour dimension {1129}.

Histopathology

The cysts are lined by gastrointestinal-type epithelium in the form of gastric pyloric-type epithelium, goblet cells, neuroendocrine cells and, occasionally, Paneth cells. The epithelium exhibits varying degrees of stratification, tufting and villous or slender filiform papillae. The cells show mild to moderate nuclear enlargement, hyperchromasia and sometimes pseudostratification, but high-grade nuclear features are not seen. Proliferative areas must comprise greater than 10% of the epithelial volume of the tumour to qualify as MBT/APMT. The mitotic index varies from slight to brisk {1060,1613}. Pseudomyxoma ovarii (acellular pools of mucin in the stroma) is present in about 20% of tumours {1060} and a granulomatous stromal response to gland rupture and mucin is common (mucin granuloma) {1060,1613}.

MBT/APMT with intraepithelial carcinoma displays features of MBT/APMT and in addition has foci with marked nuclear atypia confined to the epithelium. There is usually appreciable architectural proliferation but a cribriform pattern on its own or epithelial stratification of greater than three cell layers in absence of severe atypia does not qualify {711,915, 975,1618}.

MBT/APMT with microinvasion is defined as small foci of stromal invasion measuring less than 5 mm in greatest linear extent, with no requirement regarding the number of such foci allowed in a given tumour {676, 768, 914, 915, 1060, 1337, 1595,1613}. It is characterized by single cells, glands, clusters/nests, small foci of confluent glandular or cribriform growth displaying mild to moderate atypical mucinous epithelial cells within the stroma. Similar growth patterns with cells displaying more marked cytological atypia should be classified as *"microinvasive carcinoma"* {1618}.

Grossly evident so-called *mural nodules* can be associated with MBT/APMT or carcinomas. Three varieties of mural nodules have been described, including *reactive sarcoma-like mural nodules, foci of anaplastic carcinoma* and *sarcomatous nodules* {92,1523,1531,1940}. The size of the nodules ranges from microscopic to about 10 cm and they may be single or multiple and sharply demarcated from the adjacent mucinous epithelium. Reactive nodules are typically haemorrhagic and neoplastic nodules solid and white, but there is overlap.

Sarcoma-like mural nodules show a heterogeneous cell population with numerous multinucleated cells of the epulis type, atypical spindle cells and inflammatory cells. In some nodules, the predominant elements are spindle-shaped cells of moderate size with hyperchromatic nuclei and pleomorphic mononucleated or binucleated giant cells. The mitotic index in the most cellular areas is often brisk. Sarcoma-like mural nodules usually show weak/focal cytokeratin staining {92}. Their circumscription and extensive inflammatory cell component suggest that they represent a reaction to haemorrhage or to the mucinous content of the cysts. All tumours with *sarcoma-like mural nodules* have had a benign clinical course {92}. *Nodules of anaplastic carcinoma* and *sarcoma* are discussed elsewhere (see section on mucinous carcinoma).

Immunohistochemistry
CK7 is typically diffusely positive whereas CK20 displays variable positivity (usually less extensive than CK7 expression). CDX2 is variable and ER and PR are almost always negative, while PAX8 is expressed in up to 50–60% of tumours {1963,1965,1967}.

Histogenesis
These tumours appear to arise from mucinous cystadenomas and have similar associations with dermoids and Brenner tumours.

Genetic profile
KRAS mutations are present in 30–75% of the tumours {391,616,803,1285}. In tumours with benign, atypical proliferative and malignant components in the same neoplasm, identical *KRAS* mutations have been identified in each, suggesting that *KRAS* mutations are an early event with progression from benign tumours to MBT/APMT to carcinoma {391,616,1156}.

Prognosis and predictive factors
The prognosis is excellent; only a few cases of progression to carcinoma have been reported and these tumours were not adequately sampled. Therefore, the possibility that occult areas of carcinoma were missed cannot be excluded. Since some of the patients who had recurrences of MBT/APMT were treated by incomplete excision or cystectomy, surgical removal of the entire ovary is the treatment of choice. Unilateral salpingo-oophorectomy is an option because of the low frequency of bilaterality {299,915}.

Overall survival for women with *MBT/ APMT with intraepithelial carcinoma* is 95% with most recent studies showing 100% survival. Rare tumour deaths have been reported in stage I {1060} and advanced stage tumours. The extent to which these latter cases were evaluated to exclude an extra-ovarian primary is unclear.

Based on limited data, the recurrence rate for MBT/APMT with microinvasion is 5% and the tumour-related death rate is < 5% with adverse behaviour restricted to FIGO stage IC tumours {923}. There are insufficient data to describe the behaviour of "microinvasive carcinoma".

Mucinous carcinoma

Definition
A malignant epithelial tumour composed of gastrointestinal-type cells containing intra-cytoplasmic mucin.

ICD-O code   8480/3

Epidemiology
Mucinous carcinoma accounts for 3–4% of all primary ovarian carcinomas {951}.

Clinical features
The mean age at presentation is 45 years. Patients typically present with abdominal swelling or pain. Most tumours are confined to the ovary at presentation. Advanced stage primary mucinous ovarian carcinoma is very rare {2137}.

Macroscopy
Mucinous carcinomas form large, typically unilateral, complex, solid and cystic masses. Surface ovarian involvement is not identifiable in most cases, although large tumours may exhibit areas of rupture and/or adhesions.

Histopathology
There is often a continuum of architectural and cytological atypia that includes benign, borderline and frankly carcinomatous areas. Invasive carcinoma is characterized by two different patterns of invasion, which may co-exist in a single tumour. The confluent glandular or expansile invasive pattern is recognized by marked glandular crowding with little intervening stroma, creating a labyrinthine appearance. A cribriform pattern may be present. The destructive stromal invasive

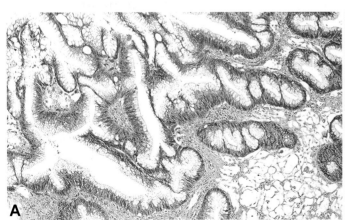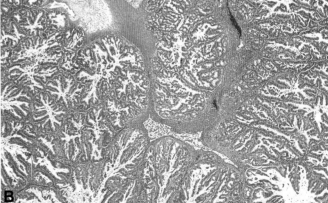

Fig. 1.20 A Mucinous tumour associated with teratoma. Low-grade adenomatous mucinous tumour with pseudomyxoma ovarii is indistinguishable from an appendiceal low-grade mucinous neoplasm secondarily involving the ovary in the setting of pseudomyxoma peritonei. Tumour is CK7-/CK20+ (not shown). **B** Mucinous carcinoma, confluent (expansile) invasion. Complex glands with cytological atypia form a confluent or expansile pattern.

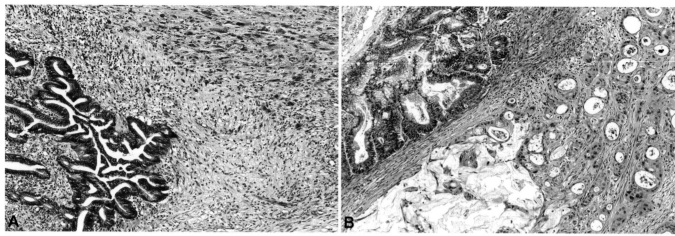

Fig. 1.21 A Mucinous borderline tumour/atypical proliferative mucinous tumour with malignant mural nodule (anaplastic carcinoma). Markedly atypical, malignant spindle cells adjacent to mucinous borderline/atypical proliferative tumour. **B** Mucinous carcinoma, destructive (infiltrative) pattern. Malignant glands invade ovarian stroma in small nests, cords and single cells, right bottom.

pattern, which is less common, is recognized by irregular glands, nests and single cells with malignant cytological features infiltrating stroma, which is often desmoplastic. An infiltrative pattern, particularly in the setting of bilateral ovarian involvement, should raise suspicion for metastatic mucinous carcinoma and prompt evaluation for an extra-ovarian source. Mitotic activity is often quite high and abnormal mitotic figures are frequently present. Tumour heterogeneity is common in mucinous neoplasms, so that areas of benign and borderline histology may coexist in the tumour, often in the same section. Areas of anaplastic carcinoma may be present, usually focally, often forming so-called *mural nodules*. They may show: 1) large rhabdoid cells with abundant eosinophilic cytoplasm; 2) sarcomatoid spindle cells often exhibiting a herringbone pattern; or 3) pleomorphic cells {1531}. Frequently, there is invasion of the surrounding tissue and, occasionally, vascular space invasion {1531}. In contrast to *sarcoma-like mural nodules*, the tumour cells react strongly for cytokeratin. Mural nodules of different types may be present in the same neoplasm and individual nodules may exhibit mixed morphological features. Negativity

for cytokeratins does not exclude anaplastic carcinoma, as the anaplastic cells may have lost cytokeratin expression.

Histogenesis

Mucinous carcinomas develop from mucinous borderline tumour/atypical proliferative mucinous tumours, although some may arise from a teratoma and some from a Brenner tumour. Tumours derived from teratomas include low-grade mucinous tumours similar to those secondarily derived from primary appendiceal low-grade mucinous neoplasms associated with pseudomyxoma peritonei (see metastatic ovarian tumours, p. 83); they exhibit a similar CK7-/CK20+ immunoprofile. This subset is often associated with the presence of pseudomyxoma ovarii and occasionally, pseudomyxoma peritonei. Distinction from secondary involvement of the ovary by a primary appendiceal neoplasm is made when teratomatous elements are identified {1241,1968}.

Genetic profile

The most consistent molecular genetic alterations are somatic mutations in *KRAS* {391,616,803,1285}. In tumours with benign, borderline and malignant

components in the same neoplasm, identical *KRAS* mutations have been identified in each, suggesting that *KRAS* mutations are an early event {391,616,1156}. *HER2* amplification is seen in 15–20% of tumours; most such tumours do not harbour mutations in *KRAS* {53}.

Prognosis and predictive factors

The majority of invasive mucinous carcinomas are confined to one ovary (stage I) at presentation and the prognosis is very favourable. Invasive carcinoma with a confluent glandular pattern is associated with a better prognosis than those displaying destructive stromal invasion. Recurrences tend to occur early (within 3 years of diagnosis, and often less) and do not appear to respond well to chemotherapy or radiotherapy {1692}. Most patients with extra-ovarian disease at presentation die of disease {2137}. Tumours containing anaplastic carcinoma (anaplastic mural nodules) have a reasonably good prognosis. Recent data indicate that nodules of anaplastic carcinoma, when found within unruptured stage I mucinous cystic tumours, may be associated with a favourable prognosis {1531}.

Endometrioid tumours

L.H. Ellenson
S.G. Carinelli
K.R. Cho

K.-R. Kim
J. Kupryjanczyk
J. Prat
G. Singer

Endometriotic cyst

Definition
Endometriotic cysts (endometriomas) are cystic forms of endometriosis. They may or may not be associated with endometriosis elsewhere in the pelvis.

Epidemiology
They are among the more common causes of ovarian enlargement in the fourth and fifth decades {483}.

Clinical features
Endometriotic cysts can present, like other large adnexal masses, with pain. It is not unusual for them to be associated with conspicuous endometriosis elsewhere, in which case they often lead to infertility.

Macroscopy
The cysts range in size up to 15 cm. The cyst lining is usually irregular with areas of haemorrhage. The cyst contents are typically dark brown due to old haemorrhage (chocolate cyst).

Histopathology
The classic endometriotic cyst is lined by endometrial epithelium overlying endometrial stroma and is associated with haemorrhage. The endometrial stroma typically contains many small blood vessels. Haemosiderin-laden macrophages and fibrosis are other hallmarks. In older lesions pseudoxanthoma cells may be a prominent feature. When endometrial stroma is not clearly evident the tumour may be classified as an *endometrioid cystadenoma* (see following section).

The epithelium lining of the cyst may show significant nuclear atypia characterized by enlargement, hyperchromasia and some pleomorphism. Mitotic figures may be present. Mucinous metaplasia and prominent ciliated metaplasia are frequently present.

Histogenesis
Morphological and molecular genetic studies have implicated endometriotic cysts and endometriosis in the development of endometrioid, clear cell and seromucinous tumours {18,1655,1656,1980,2028,2053}.

Molecular genetics
Identical mutations of *ARID1A* and *PIK3CA* and as well as loss of heterozygosity of *PTEN* are detected in the normal-appearing epithelium of endometriotic cysts adjacent to clear cell and endometrioid carcinomas and in the carcinomas themselves, suggesting that molecular alterations of those genes play an important role in tumour development. Similarly, loss of expression of *ARID1A* has been detected in seromucinous borderline/atypical proliferative tumours and in the epithelium of endometriotic cysts adjacent to these tumours {79,1688,2070}.

Prognosis and predictive factors
These are benign tumours which can occasionally undergo malignant transformation.

Endometrioid cystadenoma / adenofibroma

Definition
Endometrioid cystadenoma is a cystic lesion lined by benign endometrioid epithelium lacking the stroma, typical vasculature and other stigmata of endometriosis. When associated with a dense fibromatous component the tumour is an endometrioid adenofibroma.

ICD-O codes
Endometrioid cystadenoma   8380/0
Endometrioid adenofibroma   8381/0

Epidemiology
In comparison to serous cystadenomas endometrioid adenofibromas are uncommon. Endometrioid cystadenomas are very rare and some probably represent endometriomas in which the endometrial stroma is indistinct.

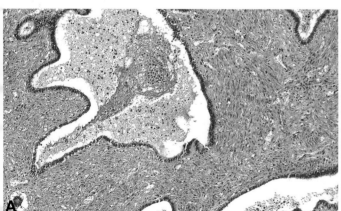 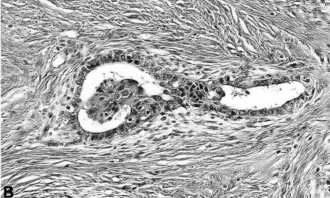

Fig. 1.22 Endometrioid adenofibroma. **A** Cystically dilated glandular structures surrounded by dense fibrous stroma. **B** Focal squamous metaplasia in an endometrioid gland lined by benign appearing epithelium.

Clinical features

The average age of patients is 55 years {1780}. The tumours are often unilateral and clinical symptoms are usually non-specific. Acute pain may be due to torsion of a relatively large cyst or bleeding into an underlying or adjacent endometriotic cyst, as these tumours are often associated with endometriosis.

Macroscopy

Adenofibromas are solid but may be associated with an endometriotic cyst. Cystadenomas resemble other cystadenomas except that associated endometriosis is more common.

Histopathology

Endometrioid adenofibromas are characterized by a predominance of fibrous stroma. The glandular component is composed of tubular and cystic glands lined by benign, proliferative-type epithelium. Cystadenomas are lined by endometrioid epithelium which is cuffed by cellular non-specific stroma that merges with non-specific fibroma-like stroma. Dystrophic stromal calcifications may be present. Squamous differentiation in the form of squamous morules can occur. These tumours may develop within an endometriotic cyst as observed with other endometrioid tumours of the ovary {121}.

Prognosis and predictive factors

The tumours are benign.

Endometrioid borderline tumour/ Atypical proliferative endometrioid tumour

Definition

A solid or cystic tumour composed of crowded glands lined by atypical endometrioid-type cells and lacking destructive stromal invasion and/or confluent glandular growth.

ICD-O code   8380/1

Synonym

Endometrioid tumours of low malignant potential (not recommended)

Epidemiology

Endometrioid borderline tumours/atypical proliferative endometrioid tumours (EBT/APET) of the ovary are uncommon and constitute only 0.2% of all epithelial ovarian tumours. Many patients have associated endometriosis (63%). In addition, coexisting endometrial hyperplasia and/or carcinoma is common (39%) {1634}.

Clinical features

The average age of patients is 51 years. Most patients present with a pelvic mass. The majority of tumours are unilateral; bilateral disease is rare (4%).

Macroscopy

There is a wide range in size; the average size is 9 cm. Tumours are typically solid but may be cystic. Cystic tumours typically have friable tumour focally involving the cyst lining. The cyst fluid is usually brown with the appearance of altered blood due to haemorrhage. Solid tumours are associated with a dense fibromatous stroma.

Histopathology

EBT/APETs exhibit two major growth patterns: adenofibromatous and intracystic. In approximately one-half of cases an adenofibroma is present in the background. The glandular proliferation may consist of crowded, back-to-back endometrioid glands with mild or moderate cytological atypia, often with epithelial stratification, analogous to atypical hyperplasia/endometrioid intraepithelial neoplasia. The epithelial proliferation may result in bridging and approximately 30% of the tumours will show a cribriform growth pattern. If the cytological atypia is severe the diagnosis of "intraepithelial carcinoma" is justified {1634}. Squamous (morular) metaplasia is common and may lend an appearance of solid growth that should not be mistaken for invasion. In the cases without an adenofibromatous background, the epithelial proliferation may show back-to-back proliferation or a papillary growth pattern protruding into a cystic structure. Confluent glandular growth (expansile) measuring > 5 mm or unequivocal invasion warrants a diagnosis of carcinoma. Microinvasion has been defined in two ways; either confluent glandular growth < 5 mm or haphazardly infiltrating single cells, glands or nests of cells with cytological atypia. A small study suggested that microinvasion of either type does not adversely affect patient outcome {127}.

Histogenesis

The common association of EBT/APETs with endometriosis and endometrioid adenofibromas suggests that they arise

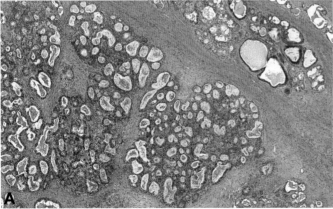 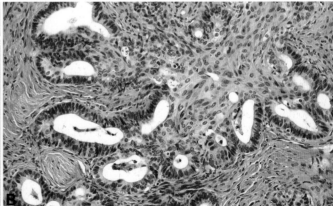

Fig. 1.23 Borderline endometrioid tumour/atypical proliferative endometrioid tumour. **A** Crowded glands lined by endometrioid epithelium with mild to moderate cytological atypia embedded in dense fibrous stroma. **B** Mild cytological atypia is present in both the endometrioid glands and the squamous morules {1724A}.

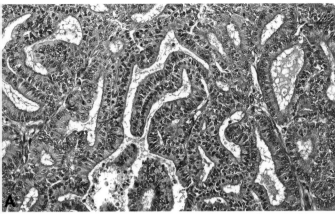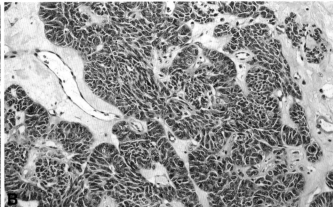

Fig. 1.24 A Well-differentiated endometrioid adenocarcinoma. Confluent glandular growth with loss of intervening stroma. The tumour resembles well-differentiated endometrioid carcinoma of the uterine corpus. **B** Endometrioid carcinoma resembling sex cord-stromal tumour (sertoliform endometrioid carcinoma).

from these lesions. Progression directly from endometriotic cysts may explain why some tumours lack an adenofibromatous background.

Genetic profile
There are limited studies on the molecular alterations of EBT/APETs.

Prognosis and predictive factors
The prognosis is excellent. Malignant behaviour has not been reported in well documented cases.

Endometrioid carcinoma

Definition
A malignant, epithelial tumour resembling endometrioid carcinoma of the uterine corpus.

ICD-O code   8380/3

Epidemiology
Endometrioid carcinoma accounts for 10–15% of ovarian carcinomas, representing the second most common form of ovarian epithelial malignancy. It is most common in the fifth and sixth decades of life. Up to 42% of the tumours are associated with endometriosis in the same ovary or elsewhere in the pelvis {447,1307} and 15–20% co-exist with endometrial carcinoma {817,946,2142}. The frequent association of ovarian endometrioid carcinomas with endometriosis, endometrial carcinoma or both suggests that some ovarian endometrioid carcinomas may share risk factors with endometrial carcinomas {408}. Patients whose tumours occur in association with endometriosis are 5–10 years younger on average than

patients without associated ovarian endometriosis {1849}.

Clinical features
The mean patient age is 58 years, slightly lower than that for serous carcinoma {1849}. Many endometrioid carcinomas are asymptomatic. Some present as a pelvic mass, with or without pain. The stage distribution of endometrioid carcinomas differs from that of serous carcinomas. Most tumours are confined to the ovary at presentation (Stage Ia) but are bilateral in 17% of the cases (Stage Ib). Serum CA125 is elevated in over 80% of the cases {945,1052}.

Macroscopy
Endometrioid carcinomas have a mean size of 15 cm and have a smooth outer surface. The cut surfaces show friable soft masses or papillae partly filling cystic spaces that may contain blood-stained fluid. They may be completely solid, exhibiting haemorrhage or necrosis. If the carcinoma has arisen in an endometriotic cyst, it tends to be a polypoid nodule projecting into the lumen of a thick-walled, blood-filled cyst.

Histopathology
Most tumours show a back-to-back arrangement of the glands with confluent or cribriform proliferations of round, oval or tubular glands; villoglandular patterns also occur. Although generally the glands are lined by stratified non-mucin-containing epithelium with well-defined luminal margins, foci lined by mucinous epithelium are not unusual. Less frequently, the tumours exhibit destructive growth characterized by obvious stromal invasion in the form of glands, cell clusters or individual cells, disorderly infiltrating the

stroma and frequently associated with a desmoplastic or inflammatory stromal reaction {284}.

Squamous differentiation occurs in 30–50% of cases, most often in the form of morules (cytologically benign-appearing squamous cells) {190}. Occasionally, aggregates of spindle-shaped epithelial cells undergo a transition to clearly recognizable squamous cells suggesting that the former represent abortive squamous differentiation {1930}.

Secretory changes in the form of vacuolated cells resembling those of early secretory endometrium are seen in about one-third of cases and luteinized stromal cells in 12% of cases. Rare examples of mucin-rich, ciliated cell, oxyphilic and spindle cell types have been described {488,739,1509}. Foci of mucinous epithelium are present in some endometrioid carcinomas and should not lead to the diagnosis of mucinous carcinoma. The *oxyphilic variant* has a prominent component of large polygonal tumour cells with abundant eosinophilic cytoplasm and round central nuclei with prominent nucleoli {1509}.

Sex cord-stromal type patterns also occur. One such pattern is characterized by solid areas punctuated by tubular or round glands or small rosette-like glands (microglandular pattern) simulating an adult granulosa cell tumour. Another variant displays focal to extensive areas resembling Sertoli and Sertoli-Leydig cell tumours {1431,1638,2117}. They contain small, hollow or solid tubules or, rarely, thin cords resembling sex cords. Furthermore, the stroma may appear cellular and fibrous, resembling the spindle cell component of stromal tumours. These tumours are designated as *"sertoliform endometrioidcarcinoma"* or *"endometrioid carcinoma resembling sex cord-stromal tumour"*. About 10% of endometrioid carcinomas contain argyrophilic cells of neuroendocrine type. Endometrioid carcinomas may show transitional cell-like differentiation {878}. On occasion, foci indistinguishable from moderate to poorly differentiated squamous carcinoma can be seen.

Grading
The grading of endometrioid carcinoma of the ovary is the same as for endometrial adenocarcinoma of the uterus. Most ovarian endometrioid carcinomas are well differentiated, and show low-grade nuclei. Thus, nuclear grade is the best discriminator. Poorly differentiated endometrioid carcinomas are predominantly solid with focal microglandular areas. Haemorrhage and/or necrosis are prominent. Distinguishing high-grade endometrioid carcinoma from high-grade serous carcinoma may be difficult and immunohistochemical staining more characteristic of serous carcinoma may aid in this distinction. Non-specific gland differentiation should not lead to the designation "endometrioid" {950}.

Immunohistochemistry
See Table 1.1 (p. 24)

Histogenesis
The presence of shared molecular genetic changes in endometriosis, endometrioid borderline/atypical proliferative tumours and low-grade endometrioid carcinoma supports endometriosis as a precursor lesion. The histogenesis of high-grade endometrioid carcinoma is not as clear, since many tumours that have been classified as such in the past, probably are high-grade serous carcinomas showing glandular differentiation. Clear-cut high-grade endometrioid carcinomas exist and some share molecular alterations with low-grade endometrioid carcinomas as well as *TP53* mutations,

suggesting that they have evolved from low-grade neoplasms.

Genetic profile
β-catenin-mediated canonical Wnt pathway signalling is dysregulated in 16–38% of endometrioid carcinomas {1300,1665, 2050,2054,2055}. Several studies have noted the association of *CTNNB1* mutation with squamous differentiation, low tumour grade and favourable outcome {599,1663,2033,2054}. Inactivating mutations of the tumour suppressor gene *PTEN* have been reported in 14–21% of ovarian endometrioid carcinomas {252,1403}. An alternative mechanism by which PI3K signalling is activated in endometrioid carcinomas is through activating mutations of *PIK3CA*, which have been identified in up to 20% of ovarian endometrioid carcinomas {225}. Concomitant *PIK3CA* and *PTEN* mutations are sometimes observed in the same tumour {2033,2054}.
Inactivating mutations of *ARID1A*, which encodes a subunit of the SWI/SNF chromatin remodelling complex, have been observed in 30% of endometrioid carcinomas {2028}. The mutations are typically frameshift or nonsense mutations that result in loss of protein expression.
TP53 mutations have been reported in upwards of 60% of endometrioid carcinomas arising in the ovary, most often in high-grade tumours. However, more recent studies indicate that many ovarian tumours previously diagnosed as high-grade endometrioid carcinomas lack mutations characteristic of low-grade endometrioid carcinoma and have gene expression profiles indistinguishable from high-grade serous carcinoma {1704,2054}. These findings, along with the high prevalence of *TP53* mutations in high-grade serous carcinoma, suggest that many tumours diagnosed previously as high-grade endometrioid carcinomas might be more appropriately classified as high-grade serous carcinomas {304,305,1205}. Microsatellite instability

has been observed in 13–20% of ovarian endometrioid carcinomas, and is usually associated with loss of hMLH1 or hMSH2 expression {252,1108}. Activating mutations in *KRAS* and *BRAF* have also been reported in ovarian endometrioid carcinomas, but the frequency of mutations in these genes is less than 7% {46,219,503,1192,2054}.

Prognosis and predictive factors
The 5-year survival of patients with stage I carcinoma is 78%; stage II, 63%; stage III, 24%; and stage IV, 6%. Patients with grade 1 and 2 tumours have a higher survival than those with grade 3 tumours. Peritoneal foreign body granulomas containing keratin have been found in cases of endometrioid carcinomas with squamous differentiation do not affect the prognosis adversely in the absence of viable-appearing tumour cells and do not warrant upstaging {925}.
Endometrioid carcinoma of the ovary associated with carcinoma of the endometrium occurs in 15–20% of cases {523,946,1755,2142}. Usually, both tumours are well differentiated and resemble each other. The criteria for distinguishing metastatic from independent primary carcinomas rely mainly on the clinicopathological findings. Accordingly, in cases of low-grade endometrial carcinoma associated with hyperplasia and minimal or no myometrial invasion, the ovarian tumour can be regarded as an independent primary, particularly if endometriosis, adenofibroma or an EBT/APET is also present. In these patients, however, the 5-year survival is 70–92%, and the median survival is 10 years or longer {1807,1849}; thus, follow-up favours two independent adenocarcinomas since most patients survive without recurrence {523,1481,1522}. In contrast, bilaterality and multinodular growth, as well as vascular space and tubal invasion, are characteristic of ovarian metastases.

Clear cell tumours

C.B. Gilks   R. Soslow
D.A. Bell   H. Tsuda
D. Huntsman   G.F. Zannoni
T.A. Longacre   C. Zhao
E. Oliva   X. Zhou

Clear cell cystadenoma / adenofibroma

Definition
A tumour composed of glands or cysts lined by bland cuboidal to flattened cells with clear or eosinophilic cytoplasm embedded in a fibromatous stroma.

ICD-O codes
Clear cell cystadenoma   8443/0
Clear cell adenofibroma   8313/0

Epidemiology
These are very rare tumours, with only a few cases reported in the literature {122,1636}.

Clinical features
They may present as an incidental finding or with non-specific symptoms. There may be a palpable pelvic mass.

Macroscopy
Adenofibromas form a solid mass ranging from 3–16 cm, with a smooth, lobulated external surface and on sectioning, small cysts can be seen within a solid background.

Histopathology
In adenofibromas, widely spaced simple glands, often cystically dilated, are embedded in a fibromatous stroma. The glands are lined by cells that can be cuboidal to flattened, with clear or eosinophilic cytoplasm. The nuclei in both the epithelial and stromal components are cytologically bland. Mitotic figures are rare to absent {122}. There is often associated endometriosis. The diagnosis should only be made after thorough, preferably complete, sampling to exclude a clear cell borderline tumour/atypical proliferative clear cell tumour (CCBT/APCCT) or carcinoma. The rare cystadenomas have bland lining cells that at least focally have clear cytoplasm but are often compressed with scant cytoplasm.

Prognosis and predictive factors
These tumours are benign.

Clear cell borderline tumour / Atypical proliferative clear cell tumour

Definition
These are clear cell adenofibromatous tumours with atypia of the glandular epithelium but without stromal invasion.

ICD-O code   8313/1

Epidemiology
Clear cell borderline tumours/atypical proliferative clear cell tumours (CCBT/APCCT) comprise less than 1% of borderline/atypical proliferative tumours. Almost all the women are post-menopausal (mean age, 59–68 years) {122,874, 1636,1867,1952}.

Clinical features
Most patients present with a mass or abdominal enlargement {122,1636}. All tumours have been confined to the ovaries and almost all are unilateral {122,874,1952,2164}.

Macroscopy
Their size is variable with a mean of about 6 cm. On sectioning, they are solid but may contain tiny cysts; rarely, large cysts are seen {122,1636,1867,2164}. Thorough sampling is indicated to exclude a clear cell carcinoma component.

Histopathology
The glands are typically round to oval and relatively evenly spaced in a fibromatous stroma. Some degree of compaction of glands may be evident but stromal invasion, and hence small foci of invasive clear cell carcinoma, should only be diagnosed when a clearly abnormal architecture indicative of invasion, sometimes associated with a stromal reaction, is present. The cysts and glands are lined by cuboidal, hobnail, or flattened cells with clear or eosinophilic cytoplasm. Cellular stratification may be seen and gland lumens may be filled with neoplastic cells. The lining cells show moderate nuclear atypia. Mitotic figures are infrequent {122,1636,2164}. Foci of endometriosis are often found in association with these tumours. These tumours have a similar immunoprofile to that of clear cell carcinomas {2164}.

Genetic profile
When CCBT/APCCTs co-exist with clear cell carcinoma, they share genetic abnormalities (LOH, loss of *ARID1A* expression) indicating that the tumours are clonally related {2069,2071,2073}.

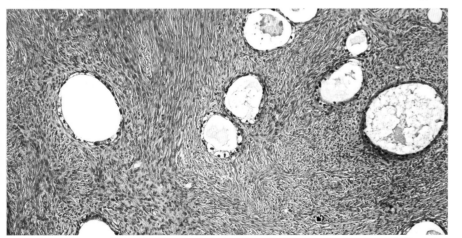

Fig. 1.25 Clear cell adenofibroma. Widely spaced glands, without significant crowding, are present in fibromatous stroma.

Prognosis and predictive factors

All well documented cases have been benign {122,1867,1952}.

Clear cell carcinoma

Definition

A malignant tumour composed of clear, eosinophilic and hobnail cells, displaying a combination of tubulocystic, papillary and solid patterns.

ICD-O code   8310/3

Epidemiology

Mean patient age is 55 years {264}. This tumour arises from endometriosis in 50–70% of cases {584,1408}. Clear cell carcinoma accounts for a higher percentage of ovarian carcinomas in Japan relative to western countries {264,821,1856}. It has been associated with Lynch syndrome {221,610,835,908,1126}.

Clinical features

Clear cell carcinoma is the ovarian tumour most frequently associated with ovarian or pelvic endometriosis {393,584, 1316,1408}. It is also the most common epithelial carcinoma associated with paraneoplastic hypercalcaemia {1689} and venous thromboembolism {478,649, 1186}.

Macroscopy

These tumours are typically unilateral with a mean size of 15 cm. They range from solid, to solid and cystic, to mainly cystic with fleshy, pale yellow nodules lining an endometriotic cyst {1407}. The solid foci may be purely carcinoma or in part may represent a background of adenofibroma.

Histopathology

This tumour displays tubulocystic, papillary and solid patterns admixed in varying degrees {438,1407}. Occasionally, markedly dilated cysts lined by flattened cells are seen, imparting a deceptively benign appearance. The papillae are generally relatively regular and small but may be large with prominent fibrovascular cores that are frequently hyalinized {886}. Solid areas are composed of sheets of polyhedral cells, separated by delicate septa. The tumour cells vary from polygonal to cuboidal to flattened and the cytoplasm ranges from clear

to less commonly eosinophilic. Most tumours also contain cells with apical hyperchromatic nuclei (hobnail cells). Nuclei are hyperchromatic, often eccentric, with conspicuous nucleoli. Mitotic figures are relatively uncommon. The tubules and cysts most often contain eosinophilic secretions that sometimes appear dense and rounded ("targetoid") and may be intracytoplasmic. Intraluminal basophilic material (positive for mucin) may also be seen, as may intracytoplasmic mucin, rarely resulting in a signet-ring cell appearance.

The clear cells have glycogen-rich cytoplasm that is PAS positive and diastase sensitive, although diastase resistant material may be present along the apical cell membranes. Psammoma bodies and eosinophilic hyaline bodies can be seen. There is no well validated grading system for clear cell carcinomas. At present they are all considered high-grade.

Immunohistochemistry
See Table 1.1 (p. 24)

Histogenesis

Most ovarian clear cell carcinomas occur in association with endometriosis {2028}. A minority appear to arise from borderline clear cell/atypical proliferative clear cell tumours and adjacent atypical endometriosis, supporting endometriosis as the precursor {79,2028}.

Genetic profile

The most common mutations identified in ovarian clear cell carcinoma include *ARID1A* mutation (46–57%) {852,2028}, *PIK3CA* activating mutation (40%) {225,995,2070} and *PTEN* mutation (8.3%) {1688}. *ARID1A* somatic inactivating mutations correlate with loss of BAF250a expression (the protein encoded by *ARID1A*) {852,2028}. *ARID1A* mutations and BAF250a loss are also seen in contiguous endometriotic lesions but not in endometriosis at distant sites lending further support to endometriosis as a precursor lesion {2028}. Most *PIK3CA* activating mutations (71%) occur in *ARID1A*-deficient carcinomas {2071}. These results suggest that the loss of *ARID1A*-associated protein occurs as a very early event, similar to *PIK3CA* mutation, and loss of *ARID1A* can cooperate with *PIK3CA* mutations during oncogenesis.

Genetic susceptibility

Clear cell carcinoma is associated with Lynch syndrome, most commonly in association with germline mutations in *MSH2* {221,610,835,835,908,1126}, but not with hereditary ovarian-breast cancer syndrome (e.g. *BRCA1* or *BRCA2* mutation).

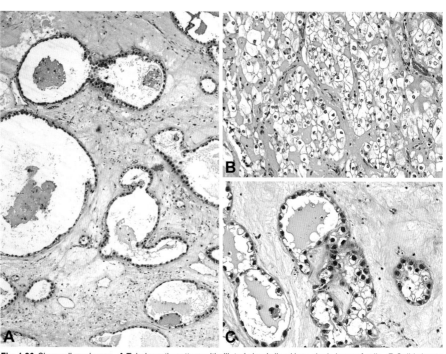

Fig. 1.26 Clear cell carcinoma. **A** Tubulocystic pattern with dilated glands lined by a single layer of cells. **B** Solid sheets composed of cells with clear cytoplasm. Note the stromal hyalinization. **C** Tubules lined by a single layer of cuboidal cells with clear cytoplasm.

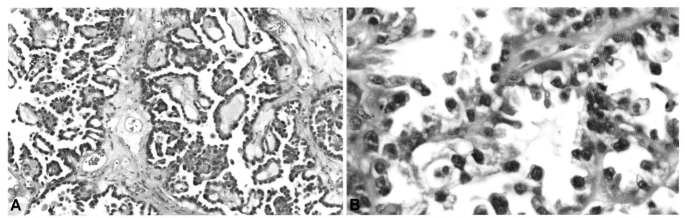

Fig. 1.27 Clear cell carcinoma. **A** Papillary architecture, with mostly small, relatively regularly shaped papillae. **B** Hobnail cells with apical hyperchromatic nuclei projecting into cyst lumens.

Prognosis and predictive factors

Stage is the single most important prognostic factor. Stage Ia tumours have a very good prognosis. Stage Ic tumours have a poorer prognosis. Poor responsiveness to platinum-based chemotherapy has been shown in high-stage disease, resulting in poor overall- and disease-specific survival {52,264,1856}.

Brenner tumours

C.B. Gilks
S.G. Carinelli
A. Liu
J. Prat
J.D. Seidman
R. Soslow

Brenner tumour

Definition

A tumour composed of nests of bland, transitional-type cells (resembling urothelial cells) within a fibromatous stroma.

ICD-O code   9000/0

Epidemiology

Brenner tumours account for approximately 5% of benign ovarian epithelial tumours {484,968}.

Clinical features

The majority of these tumours arise in adults in the fifth to seventh decades, although they may occur in patients younger than thirty or older than eighty years {571, 2093}. Most patients are asymptomatic and the tumours are typically found incidentally in ovaries removed for other reasons {168}. A few patients with larger tumours may present with abdominal enlargement or pain {2007}. Occasionally, Brenner tumours with functioning stroma are associated with endocrine symptoms {424,698}.

Macroscopy

Most of benign Brenner tumours are < 2 cm, and only rarely are > 10 cm in dimension {1649}. Fever than 10% are bilateral {571,1030}. They are solid with firm rubbery consistency and circumscribed. The sectioned surface is grey-white or yellowish. Calcification can be seen in some cases. Small cysts are common, and rarely, the tumour is predominantly cystic {99}. One-quarter of Brenner tumours are associated with other tumour types (mucinous is most common) {212,2095}.

Histopathology

Benign Brenner tumours are characterized by oval or irregular nests of transitional-type cells within a fibromatous stroma. The nests may be solid or exhibit central cavities containing mucin or eosinophilic material. The lumina may be lined by transitional-type, mucinous, ciliated or cuboidal or flat cells. The transitional-type cells are polyhedral to elongate, with pale to clear cytoplasm. The nuclei are ovoid, with fine chromatin. Nucleoli may be prominent and, in some cases, nuclei contain longitudinal grooves. The mucinous cells overlying the transitional-type cells are considered metaplastic {1637}. Epithelial atypia is inconspicuous and mitoses are rare. Focal or extensive calcification is often present and in these cases there is sometimes prominent hyalinization of the stroma.

Immunohistochemistry

Brenner tumours express CK7, p63, S100P, GATA3, uroplakin and thrombomodulin, but do not express, or only focally express, CK20 {507,1587,1679}.

Histogenesis

The histogenesis of these tumours is not well characterized {102,1725,1756,2007}. Some may be derived from Walthard rests which are nests of metaplastic transitional epithelium that have invaginated into underlying paratubal tissue, as that is where most are located. An extra-ovarian Brenner tumour has been reported {701,1533}. The rare cases associated with a teratoma may originate from germ cells {189,1630}.

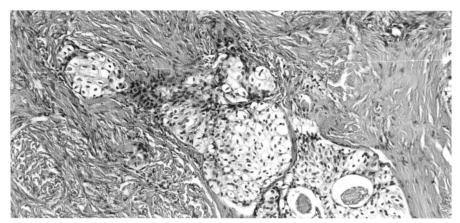

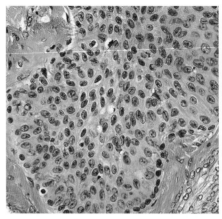

Fig. 1.28 Benign Brenner tumour. Nests of bland transitional-type epithelial cells within an abundant fibromatous stroma.

Fig. 1.29 Benign Brenner tumour. The tumour nuclei are uniform, with some showing prominent nuclear grooves.

Genetic profile

KRAS mutations at codon 12 have been identified in three of five benign Brenner tumours in one study {390} and amplification of 12q14–21 is reported in another study {1483}.

Borderline Brenner tumour / Atypical proliferative Brenner tumour

Definition

A neoplasm of transitional cell type (resembling non-invasive, low-grade urothelial neoplasms) displaying epithelial proliferation beyond that seen in benign Brenner tumours and lacking stromal invasion.

ICD-O code   9000/1

Clinical features

The mean patient age is 59 years. Patients often present with a pelvic mass. Tumours are unilateral and confined to the ovary.

Macroscopy

These are typically large, cystic tumours measuring, on average, 18 cm (range 10–28 cm). Papillary masses project into the cyst lumens. Solid areas often reflect a benign Brenner component. Rarely, the tumour is completely solid.

Histopathology

The papillary component closely resembles low-grade non-invasive papillary transitional cell (urothelial) tumours. High-grade cytological features rarely occur and, in the absence of invasion, can be diagnosed as borderline Brenner tumour/atypical proliferative Brenner tumour with intraepithelial carcinoma.

Mucinous metaplasia is often present. A solid area of benign Brenner tumour is nearly always present, helping to confirm the cell type. An uncommon pattern is one with marked crowding of the transitional nests, which may be large and tortuous. In addition, there is increased mitotic activity and/or cytological atypia but unequivocal stromal invasion is not detected.

Immunohistochemical stains for p63 and GATA3 are usually positive. WT1 is consistently negative {389,507,1094,1113}.

Histogenesis

These tumours are presumed to arise from benign Brenner tumours.

Genetic profile

A small number of cases analysed for *PIK3CA*, *KRAS*, *BRAF*, *CTNNB1* and *TP53* showed no mutations {389}.

Prognosis and predictive factors

The behaviour is benign, although local recurrence may rarely occur.

Malignant Brenner tumour

Definition

An ovarian carcinoma usually of transitional cell type, resembling an invasive urothelial carcinoma. Rarely, the tumour is of squamous type. In either case the tumours are associated with a benign or borderline/atypical proliferative Brenner tumour.

ICD-O code   9000/3

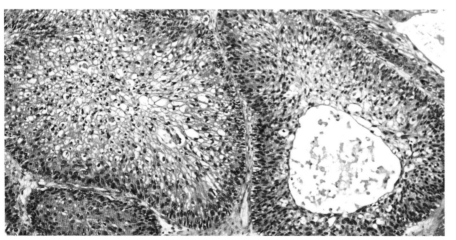

Fig. 1.30 Borderline Brenner tumour/atypical proliferative Brenner tumour. Large, crowded nests and masses of cells beyond what would be expected in a benign Brenner tumour.

Epidemiology

Malignant Brenner tumours account for less than 5% of Brenner tumours {694,1271,1779}.

Clinical features

These tumours occur in women over 50 years of age. Patients present with an abdominal mass or pain. Some may have abnormal vaginal bleeding {76,1631}.

Macroscopy

The tumours are usually large with a median size of 16–20 cm. They may be solid or cystic with mural nodules. Typically, they exhibit a benign Brenner tumour component which may be fibromatous and calcified. About 80% of cases are confined to the ovary (stage I) at the time of diagnosis, of which 12% are bilateral {76}.

Histopathology

The tumour is composed of irregularly shaped masses of malignant transitional-type cells and rarely of squamous cells. Cystic areas within the tumour are lined by multilayered epithelium exhibiting hyperchromatic and pleomorphic nuclei and prominent mitotic activity. Invasion

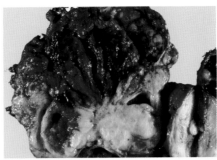

Fig. 1.31 Malignant Brenner tumour. A large solid and cystic tumour with polypoid masses of fleshy and haemorrhagic tissue. A fibroma-like component of benign Brenner tumour is seen at the bottom.

may be difficult to detect because of the densely fibromatous background of the tumour but a desmoplastic stromal reaction is helpful in identifying unequivocal stromal invasion. Rarely, the invasive component appears to arise directly from a benign Brenner tumour, without an atypical proliferative (borderline) component {1819}. Mucinous glandular elements and, more rarely, mucinous adenocarcinoma may coexist with the Brenner component. Lack of a benign or atypical proliferative (borderline) Brenner component should raise the possibility of high-grade serous or endometrioid carci-

nomas with transitional cell-like differentiation {33,878}.

Immunohistochemistry

The immunoprofile resembles that of benign Brenner tumours (see above) with a variable pattern of expression in the invasive component {33,389}.

Genetic profile

PIK3CA mutations (exon 9) have been demonstrated in a case of malignant Brenner tumour {389}. It has been suggested that malignant Brenner tumours are low-grade carcinomas with activation of the PI3K/AKT pathway through *EGFR*; however, *EGFR* amplification was not encountered in the reported case {389}. The genetic profile differs from that of transitional-like carcinoma of high-grade serous type, in which *TP53* mutations result in chromosomal instability {389}.

Prognosis and predictive factors

Patients with stage Ia tumours have an 88% 5-year survival. Tumours with extra-ovarian spread behave similarly to other ovarian cancers, based on the limited data {76}.

Seromucinous tumours

M. Köbel
D.A. Bell
M.L. Carcangiu
E. Oliva

J. Prat
I.M. Shih
R. Soslow
R. Vang

Seromucinous cystadenoma / adenofibroma

Definition
A benign cystic neoplasm with two or more Müllerian cell types, all accounting for at least 10% of the epithelium. Rare tumours have more prominent fibrous stroma (adenofibroma).

ICD-O codes
Seromucinous cystadenoma   8474/0
Seromucinous adenofibroma   9014/0

Synonym
Müllerian cystadenoma of mixed cell types

Epidemiology
These tumours account for approximately 1% of benign epithelial neoplasms; they are typically seen in adults with a peak in the late reproductive age group.

Clinical features
The signs and symptoms are non-specific; these tumours are usually diagnosed incidentally.

Macroscopy
These tumours typically present as a unilocular cyst with a smooth surface and inner lining. They may contain serous or mucinous fluid, and rarely may have a solid component with a white homogenous cut surface.

Histopathology
The cysts are lined by a variable admixtures of serous and mucinous cells (endocervical-type) but endometrioid and less often transitional or squamous cells may be seen. If present, the stroma is bland and fibromatous.

Histogenesis
They are likely derived from endometriosis.

Prognosis and predictive factors
These are benign tumours.

Seromucinous borderline tumour / Atypical proliferative seromucinous tumour

Definition
A non-invasive, proliferative, epithelial tumour composed of more than one epithelial cell type, most often serous and endocervical-type mucinous; however, endometrioid, and less often, clear cell, transitional or squamous may be seen.

ICD-O code   8474/1

Synonyms
Endocervical-type mucinous borderline tumour, Müllerian mucinous borderline tumour, atypical proliferative (borderline) Müllerian tumour

Epidemiology
In the past they have been considered a subset of mucinous tumours (endocervical type) and therefore of all mucinous atypical proliferative (borderline) tumours, they account for 15% of cases {1656}.

Clinical features
Most patients have FIGO stage I disease, but a minority have advanced stage disease in the form of implants and/or lymph node involvement. The average age of patients is 34–44 years {474,1612,1655,1656,1743}. They present with non-specific signs and symptoms related to an adnexal mass.
Tumours are associated with endometriosis in about a third of cases {2053}.

Macroscopy
Mean size is 8–10 cm {474,1612,1655, 1656,1743}. These tumours are typically unilocular, smooth-surfaced and contain viscid fluid. Friable papillary excrescences occupy variable proportions of the cyst lining. Granular to haemorrhagic foci may be present, often indicating an association with endometriosis. Solid areas are occasionally seen. Up to 40% are bilateral.

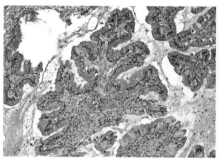

Fig. 1.32 Seromucinous borderline tumour / atypical proliferative seromucinous tumour. The papillae are lined by endocervical-like mucinous epithelium with columnar cells containing abundant cytoplasm and basally situated low-grade nuclei.

Histopathology
These tumours have architectural features similar to serous borderline/atypical proliferative serous tumours {1729}. They show complex papillary architecture which branches in a hierarchical manner into progressively smaller papillae, terminating in small detached epithelial tufts. The larger papillae tend to have oedematous stroma containing neutrophils. The epithelium lining the papillae is typically stratified and is composed mostly of endocervical-type mucinous or serous epithelium, but endometrioid and squamous epithelium is not unusual. Rarely, clear or transitional cells are seen. Goblet cells are not present. Cytoplasmic eosinophilia is often conspicuous and the nuclei are low-grade; mitotic figures are infrequent. Microinvasion, intraepithelial carcinoma and micropapillary features may occur {474,1326,1612,1743}. A portion of the cyst lining may exhibit features of an endometriotic cyst.

Immunohistochemistry
These tumours typically exhibit a CK7(+)/CK20(-)/CDX2(-) coordinate immunoprofile {1101,1964}. They usually express ER and PR; most tumours are negative for WT-1 {1101,1964,2081}.

Histogenesis
Although data on pathogenesis are limited, these tumours are associated with endometriosis in at least one-third of

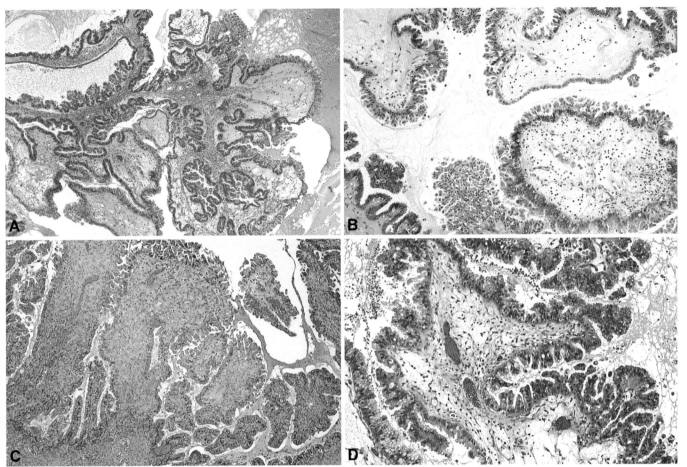

Fig. 1.33 Seromucinous borderline tumour/atypical proliferative seromucinous tumour. **A** Complex branching papillary architecture. **B** Epithelial stratification with cells showing mild nuclear atypia. Hobnail cells with abundant eosinophilic cytoplasm are prominent and a neutrophilic infiltrate is present in the stroma of the papillae. **C** Intracystic complex papillary architecture. **D** Large papillae with oedematous stroma.

cases and frequently appear to arise in an endometriotic cyst. Endometrial-type tissue in general and endometriosis may undergo mucinous metaplasia, which then sequentially evolves into a cystadenoma and a borderline/atypical proliferative tumour {1059}. The pathogenesis of these tumours is unrelated to borderline/atypical proliferative mucinous tumours, gastrointestinal type. The association with endometriosis, ER positivity and lack of WT1 expression suggests a close relationship to endometrioid and clear cell neoplasms {1964,2053}, which is further supported by the finding of *ARID1A* mutations and loss of expression in a proportion of these tumours similar to endometrioid and clear cell carcinomas {2053}.

Genetic profile
Loss of *ARID1A* expression, which closely corresponds to a mutation of the *ARID1A* gene, has been reported in one-third of these tumours, which is similar to

the frequency found in endometrioid and clear cell carcinomas, further supporting their close relationship {2053}.

Prognosis and predictive factors
These tumours are associated with a good outcome even in the presence of peritoneal implants {474,1612,1655,1656,1743}.

Seromucinous carcinoma

Definition
A carcinoma composed predominantly of serous and endocervical-type mucinous epithelium. Foci containing clear cells and areas of endometrioid and squamous differentiation are not uncommon.

ICD-O code   8474/3

Synonyms
Endocervical-type mucinous and mixed epithelial carcinomas of Müllerian type

Epidemiology
These tumours are quite uncommon and therefore data on the epidemiology are not available.

Clinical Features
The mean age in one reported series {1743} was 45 years. Most patients presented with a pelvic mass and 57% of the women had peritoneal endosalpingiosis.

Macroscopy
The mean tumour size in one series was 12 cm and over half the tumours were bilateral {1743}. Tumours were unilocular or multilocular and contained solid areas. Papillary excrescenses were present on the inner lining of the cysts and on the surface.

Histopathology
Tumours are generally papillary and display epithelial stratification closely resembling serous tumours. The most common pattern of invasion is cribriform and

confluent (expansile), although destructive infiltrative growth also occurs. By definition, these tumours contain endocervical-type mucinous and serous-type epithelium, but cells with clear cytoplasm (not displaying patterns of clear cell carcinoma), as well as foci of endometrioid differentiation, including squamous cells may also be present {1743}. The mitotic index is variable but tends to be low (< 5 mitotic figures/10 HPF).

The immunohistochemical profile is similar to the borderline/atypical proliferative group of seromucinous tumours.

Parenthetically, it should be noted that besides seromucinous carcinomas, which can show a variety of cell types, all the epithelial ovarian tumours can also show mixtures of cell types. They are classified by the predominant type but the smaller components can be included in the diagnosis. For example, a high-grade serous carcinoma with an endometrioid component showing clear-cut squamous differentiation could be classified as a "high-grade serous carcinoma with endometrioid differentiation".

Histogenesis
The histogenesis is uncertain because of the small number of reported cases but in view of their frequent co-existence with seromucinous borderline/atypical proliferative tumours and endometriosis, it is likely that endometriosis is the precursor lesion.

Prognosis and predictive factors
In one series with a small number of patients, the outcome was favourable for women with stage I disease, but half of the patients with advanced stage tumours died of disease {1743}.

Undifferentiated carcinoma

M. Köbel
D.A. Bell
M.L. Carcangiu
E. Oliva
J. Prat
I.M. Shih
R. Soslow

Definition
A malignant, epithelial tumour showing no differentiation of any specific Müllerian cell type.

ICD-O code   8020/3

Epidemiology
These are uncommon tumours.

Clinical features
Patients are diagnosed at a mean age of 55 years {951,1875}. Tumours are usually high stage at presentation.

Macroscopy
They usually appear as solid masses with extensive necrosis.

Histopathology
These tumours usually display sheet-like growth, frequently associated with geographic necrosis. Nests, cords, clusters and single cells may be seen. The tumour cells are often monotonous and non-cohesive. They are typically round but they may be spindle-shaped. The mitotic activity is high {1875}.

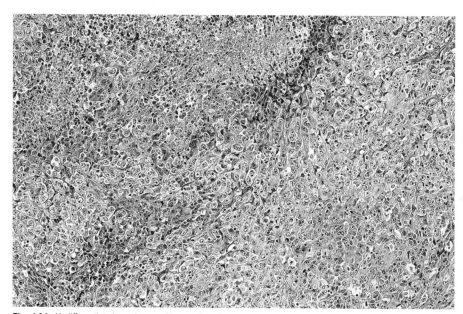

Fig. 1.34 Undifferentiated carcinoma. Sheets of ovoid, monotonous, mitotically active tumour cells with areas of necrosis.

Histogenesis
Association with low-grade endometrioid carcinoma suggests a progression from endometrioid carcinoma in a subset of tumours.

Genetic profile
Deficient mismatch repair proteins have been found in almost half of the tumours {1875}.

Prognosis and predictive factors
These are highly aggressive neoplasms.

Mesenchymal tumours

L.H. Ellenson
S.G. Carinelli
K.R. Cho
K.-R. Kim

J. Kupryjanczyk
J. Prat
G. Singer
R. Soslow

Low-grade endometrioid stromal sarcoma

Definition
A mesenchymal tumour identical to low-grade uterine endometrial stromal sarcoma.

ICD-O code   8931/3

Epidemiology
Less than 100 cases have been reported to date {1169B,1710,2118}. The patient age ranges from 11–76 years; most of these tumours occur during the fifth and sixth decades of life.

Clinical features
Most patients present with abdominal distension and/or pain, back pain, palpable mass {1031} or elevated serum CA125 level {619}. Tumours can be unilateral or bilateral. Tumour extension beyond the ovary at the time of exploratory laparotomy is a frequent finding {2118}.

Macroscopy
These tumours are solid, solid and cystic or, rarely, predominantly cystic. The cysts are usually filled with haemorrhagic fluid {2118}. The sectioned surfaces are tan or yellow-white and have a soft consistency.

Histopathology
Low-grade endometrioid stromal sarcoma (LGESS) is typically composed of sheets of small, closely packed cells resembling the stromal cells of the proliferative endometrium, with scanty cytoplasm, round to oval nuclei and small blood vessels resembling the spiral arterioles of late secretory endometrium. Secondary changes, including storiform fibrosis, a "starburst" pattern of hyaline plaques, foamy cell change, sex cord-like differentiation and myxoid change may occur. Focally, a few benign-appearing endometrioid glands may be present, and such cases should be distinguished from endometriosis {1083}. The differential diagnosis includes adult granulosa cell tumour, fibroma, fibrosarcoma and in rare cases when gland-like structures are present, Müllerian adenosarcoma and malignant mixed Müllerian tumour (MMMT). In contrast to a granulosa cell tumour, LGESS displays a characteristic vascular pattern and lacks expression of α-inhibin and calretinin. Sex cord-like and endometrioid glandular elements do not show the high-grade nuclear atypia characteristic of MMMT {1418A}.

Immunohistochemistry
LGESS exhibits diffuse, strong positivity for CD10 but this is not specific for an endometrioid stromal tumour {1420}.

Histogenesis
LGESS may originate from ovarian endometriosis, as endometriotic foci are identified adjacent to the tumour in almost half of the cases. Approximately 30% of cases are accompanied by a similar tumour in the uterus and most likely the ovarian involvement is metastatic. A number of extrauterine LGESS have the same genetic alterations as their uterine counterpart, including fusions of *JAZF1-JJAZ1 (SUZ12)*, *EPC1-PHF1* and *PHF1* rearrangement {298,1138,1687}, suggesting that ovarian LGESS has a similar histogenesis as the uterine tumour {298}.

Genetic profile
JAZF1-SUZ12 gene fusion and *PHF1* gene rearrangement, typical of uterine LGESS has been detected in some ovarian LGESSs.

Prognosis and predictive factors
Hysterectomy with bilateral salpingo-oophorectomy is the primary treatment of choice. As with the comparable uterine tumours, delayed recurrences may occur. Radiation, chemotherapy and progestin treatment have been used for treatment of recurrent disease {267,1031,1098,2118}. The behaviour of LGESS of the ovary is reminiscent of advanced-stage uterine LGESS {267}. At times, patients with widespread disease respond favourably to progestin treatment {619,1098,1418A}.

High-grade endometrioid stromal sarcoma

Definition
A mesenchymal tumour with some evidence of endometrial stromal differentiation, but showing high-grade cytologic atypia with brisk mitotic activity. In the high-grade regions a resemblance to proliferative endometrial stromal cells seen in low-grade areas is lost.

ICD-O code   8930/3

Histopathology
These rare tumours demonstrate only modest endometrial stromal differentiation without marked nuclear pleomorphism as seen in undifferentiated sarcomas. The tumour cells are larger than the tumour cells of LGESS with increased cytoplasm and nucleomegaly. Mitotic activity is high and tumour cell necrosis is usually present.

Genetic profile
The *YWHAE-FAM22* resulting from translocation t(10;17)(q22,p13) that is seen in the corresponding uterine tumours has not been reported.

Prognosis and predictive factors
The prognosis is poor.

Mixed epithelial and mesenchymal tumours

Adenosarcoma

Definition
A rare biphasic tumour with malignant mesenchymal and benign to atypical epithelial components.

ICD-O code   8933/3

Clinical features
Patients present at a mean age of 54 years and have non-specific symptoms/signs of an ovarian mass. About two-thirds of the tumours are confined to the ovary at the time of diagnosis {489}.

Macroscopy
Most tumours are unilateral, large and predominantly solid but may be solid and cystic; surface excrescences may be present.

Histopathology
There is a biphasic arrangement of glands in a stroma, which is often more cellular around the glands ("cuffs") showing mild to moderate cytological atypia. The glands are uniformly distributed and often lined by endometrioid-type epithelium, which is benign or atypical but not frankly malignant. Papillary to polypoid fronds of stroma often project into cystic glands or project from the surface of the tumour, imparting a phyllodes-like appearance. Heterologous, as well as sex cord-like elements, may be seen. The stromal component is typically CD10, ER and PR positive. Typically, the stroma is low-grade but can be high-grade malignant with high mitotic activity, reminiscent of endometrioid stromal neoplasia. In these cases the stromal cells often lose expression of CD10, ER and PR. Stromal overgrowth can also display rhabdomyomatous differentiation, in which case the cells are positive for desmin and myogenin. These tumours are designated *adenosarcoma with sarcomatous overgrowth*.

Prognosis and predictive factors
Outcome is less favourable than for its uterine counterpart (25% 5-year recur-

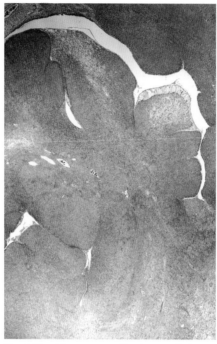

Fig. 1.35 Adenosarcoma. The tumour displays a characteristic leaf-like (phyllodes) pattern. Close application of the stromal to the epithelial component is evident.

rence-free survival). Worse prognosis is associated with age < 53 years, tumour rupture, high-grade stroma and sarcomatous overgrowth {489}.

Carcinosarcoma

Definition
Biphasic neoplasm composed of high-grade, malignant, epithelial and mesenchymal elements.

ICD-O code   8980/3

Synonyms
Malignant mixed mesodermal tumour; malignant mixed Müllerian tumour (MMMT)

Epidemiology
This tumour accounts for approximately 2% of all ovarian malignancies.

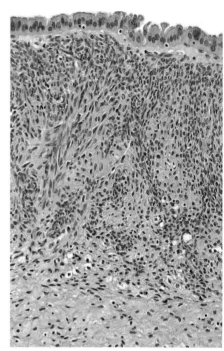

Fig. 1.36 Adenosarcoma. The epithelium is bland and the underlying stromal cells show only minimal atypia. Mitotic activity is variable but often relatively low.

Clinical features
Most patients are older than 60 years and often have high-stage tumours at the time of diagnosis {200,992}.

Macroscopy
These tumours are large (mean size, 14 cm) and predominantly solid with frequent cystic degeneration and extensive haemorrhage and necrosis {992}.

Histopathology
These tumours are composed of high-grade carcinoma and sarcoma. One or the other may predominate. Both components are distinct but are typically intermingled with one another. The carcinomatous component is most often a high-grade serous carcinoma but other histological types may be seen {992}. The sarcomatous elements are classified as homologous when the stromal component has a non-specific appearance or heterologous when rhabdomyosarcoma, chondrosarcoma (these being the most

common), osteosarcoma, rarely liposarcoma or angiosarcoma are present.

Immunohistochemistry
As high-grade serous carcinoma can lose cytokeratin expression but express vimentin, whereas the sarcomatous component may express cytokeratins, the use of these markers is not recommended to establish the diagnosis. The presence of heterologous components can be confirmed by immunohistochemistry including desmin, myogenin and myoD1 for rhabdomyosarcoma or S100 for chondrosarcoma.

Histogenesis
The tumours are of epithelial cell origin and molecular studies endorse a monoclonal origin by showing concordant *TP53* abnormalities within the carcinoma and sarcoma component {7,577,840}. Further

indirect evidence supporting the epithelial origin is that recurrences are usually high-grade serous carcinoma {597} and that the metastatic pattern is similar to that of high-grade serous carcinomas.

Genetic profile
High-grade serous carcinomas and MMMT share several molecular abnormalities including *TP53* mutations and CDKN2A (p16) overexpression {7}. The carcinomatous component of MMMT almost always expresses PAX8 and WT1.

Genetic susceptibility
There has been occasional evidence of germline *BRCA2* mutation {1811}.

Prognosis and predictive factors
The median survival is < 24 months and the 5-year survival 15–30%,

which compares unfavourably with that of high-grade serous carcinoma {200,992,1070,1563}. Most tumours are diagnosed at advanced stage (stage III) and optimal tumour debulking is the most important prognostic factor {200}. The presence of extra-ovarian sarcomatous elements is thought to be an adverse prognostic factor {992}.

Sex cord-stromal tumours - pure stromal tumours

W.G. McCluggage   P.N. Staats
T. Kiyokawa   R.H. Young

Fibroma

Definition
A fibroma is a benign stromal tumour composed of spindled to ovoid fibroblastic cells producing collagen.

ICD-O codes
Fibroma   8810/0
Cellular fibroma   8810/1

Epidemiology
Fibroma is the most common pure ovarian stromal tumour, accounting for 4% of all ovarian neoplasms.

Clinical features
It may occur at any age, but is most frequent in middle age (average 48 years) and is less common before the age of 30. Almost all are unilateral but bilateral cases occasionally occur, especially in patients with nevoid basal cell carcinoma syndrome (NBCCS) (Gorlin syndrome) {656}. In this syndrome, fibromas tend to occur at a younger age, often in children. Fibromas most commonly present with symptoms referable to an ovarian mass but sometimes are incidental findings. Meigs syndrome (ascites and pleural effusion) occurs in 1% of cases. Ascites alone may also occur, especially with fibromas > 10 cm in diameter {656,1670}.

Macroscopy
The ovarian capsule is usually smooth and intact and the sectioned surfaces are typically hard, chalky and white or yellowish white. Areas of oedema and cystic degeneration may be present, especially when the tumour is large. Haemorrhage or necrosis can be present, secondary to torsion.

Histopathology
Fibromas are composed of cells with spindled to ovoid nuclei and scant cytoplasm. The nuclear features are bland. The cells are arranged in intersecting bundles, sometimes with a storiform pattern. Collagen bands or hyalinized plaques are often present. Occasional tumours show greater vascularity than usual. The cytoplasm of the neoplastic cells may contain small amounts of lipid or eosinophilic hyaline globules {1260}. Mitoses are uncommon in most cases. The cellularity varies from case to case and within individual tumours; some are hypocellular with oedema.

Approximately 10% of fibromas are densely cellular with scant collagen. In the presence of only mild nuclear atypia these are referred to as *cellular fibromas* {815,1524}. Cellular fibromas may have mitotic activity of > 4 per 10 HPF (mitotically active cellular fibroma) {815}. Haemorrhage and necrosis may

occur, sometimes secondary to torsion. This is particularly so in cellular fibromas and the infarct-type necrosis should not be mistaken for coagulative tumour cell necrosis. Focal or diffuse calcification is present in some cases. Diffuse calcification is characteristic of fibromas in patients with NBCCS, as is a multinodular pattern {656}. Rarely, collections of luteinized cells are present in fibromas or there is a minor component of sex cord elements, by definition comprising < 10% of the neoplasm. The lutein cells rarely contain crystals of Reinke. Some fibromas have zones that resemble thecoma, but the tumour should be classified based on its predominant appearance. Fibromas may be immunoreactive for inhibin, calretinin and other sex cord markers {373,431,963}.

Genetic profile
Trisomy and/or tetrasomy 12 are often found in tumours in the fibroma-thecoma group, although not specific for these tumour types {600}. Loss of heterozygosity at 9q22.3 (PTCH) and 19p13.3 (STK11) have been reported to be frequent in cellular fibromas {1938}.

Genetic susceptibility
Fibromas are common in NBCCS, occurring in approximately 75% of females with this syndrome {656}.

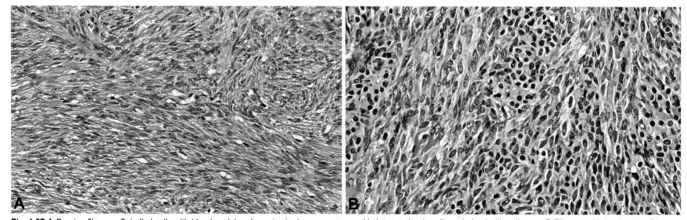
Fig. 1.37 A Ovarian fibroma. Spindled cells with bland nuclei and scant cytoplasm are arranged in intersecting bundles admixed with collagen. **B** Fibroma with lutein cells. Clusters of steroid-type cells with eosinophilic cytoplasm are admixed with spindle cells.

44   Tumours of the ovary

Prognosis and predictive factors

Most of these tumours are benign. A small proportion, especially cellular fibromas, is associated with ovarian surface adhesions, rupture, or extra-ovarian involvement at the time of presentation {815}. Those with adhesions or rupture are at risk of local recurrence, often after a long interval.

Thecoma

Definition
Thecomas are stromal tumours containing a significant number of cells with appreciable cytoplasm resembling to varying degrees theca cells.

ICD-O code   8600/0

Epidemiology
Thecomas are uncommon accounting for no more than 1% of ovarian tumours.

Clinical features
Most thecomas (97%) are unilateral and typically occur in postmenopausal women (mean 59 years); no more than 10% arise in women younger than 30 years {156}. Patients may have symptoms referable to an ovarian mass or present with hormonal manifestations. Thecomas are often estrogenic and rarely androgenic {156}, the latter usually contain variable numbers of lutein cells.

Macroscopy
Thecomas are usually 5–10 cm in diameter. The cut surface is most often solid and yellow but occasionally focally white. Cystic degeneration, haemorrhage, necrosis and calcification are uncommon.

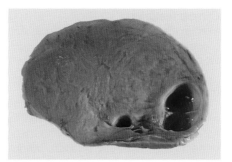

Fig. 1.38 Ovarian thecoma. The cut surface shows a well circumscribed solid yellow-orange tumour with vague lobulation and focal cysts.

Histopathology
Thecomas are composed of sheets of uniform cells with oval to round nuclei and pale greyish-pink cytoplasm with ill-defined borders. The cytoplasm is only rarely conspicuously lipid rich. The tumours usually exhibit little or no nuclear atypia and mitoses are infrequent. Rarely, they may have bizarre degenerative nuclei without mitotic activity, resembling those seen in some leiomyomas {2119}. Hyaline plaques are common and focal calcification may be seen. Extensively calcified thecomas occasionally occur, especially in young women {2108}. Some thecomas contain individual or clusters of steroid-type cells with eosinophilic or clear cytoplasm. In the past such tumours have been referred to as "luteinized thecomas", but all stromal tumours, and many other ovarian neoplasms, can have lutein cells in the stroma and, if extensive, it may merit comment but should not alter the overall pathological designation. Therefore, the term "luteinized thecoma" is no longer recommended, except in the context of a distinctive lesion discussed in the next section. Rarely, a minor component of sex cord elements is present. Many thecomas have zones that resemble fibroma. These tumours can be classified as fibrothecomas. In thecomas, reticulin usually surrounds individual cells. Most tumours are immunoreactive for inhibin, calretinin and other sex cord markers {373,431,963}.

Prognosis and predictive factors
Thecomas are benign with rare exceptions. Rarely, a tumour with nuclear atypia and elevated mitotic activity may metastasize {2008,2158}.

Luteinized thecoma associated with sclerosing peritonitis

Definition
A distinctive stromal tumour typically associated with sclerosing peritonitis {343}.

ICD-O code   8601/0

Epidemiology
This is a rare lesion.

Clinical features
This lesion occurs mostly in premenopausal women (median, 28 years), is almost always bilateral and usually presents with abdominal swelling, ascites and symptoms of bowel obstruction {343,1821}. Hormonal manifestations are usually absent.

Macroscopy
The tumours are usually bilateral and typically soft, sometimes cerebriform and often with a tan to red sectioned surface.

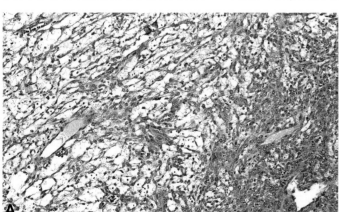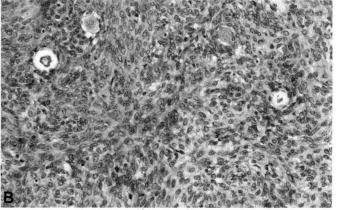

Fig. 1.39 A Luteinized thecoma with sclerosing peritonitis. A cellular spindle cell proliferation is associated with a microcystic pattern secondary to oedema. B The tumour entraps pre-existing primordial follicles and it is composed of spindled and weakly luteinized cells.

Histopathology

The tumours are hypercellular, usually with scattered, sometimes conspicuous zones of oedema occasionally imparting a microcystic appearance. Most of the tumour cells are spindled but a minority are rounded with pale cytoplasm, representing weakly luteinized cells {343,1821}. Brisk mitotic activity is typical. Entrapment of ovarian follicles and diffuse involvement of the cortex with sparing of the medulla may be conspicuous. The spindle cells in luteinized thecomas associated with sclerosing peritonitis are usually negative with sex cord markers while the luteinized cells are positive.

Histogenesis

The sparing of pre-existing follicles and predominant cortical involvement suggests a non-neoplastic process in some cases and the term thecomatosis has been proposed {1821}.

Prognosis and predictive factors

Several patients have died of complications related to intestinal obstruction (due to the sclerosing peritonitis) but there has been no recurrence or metastasis of the ovarian lesion {343,1821}.

Fibrosarcoma

Definition

A malignant, fibroblastic tumour of the ovary.

ICD-O code   8810/3

Epidemiology

These are rare ovarian neoplasms.

Clinical features

Most patients are postmenopausal and present with symptoms referable to a pelvic or abdominal mass {1524}.

Macroscopy

These tumours are usually unilateral and are typically large and predominantly solid, often with areas of haemorrhage or necrosis. There may be extra-ovarian spread.

Histopathology

These neoplasms are usually hypercellular and composed of long fascicles of spindle cells. The nuclei exhibit moderate to marked atypia and mitotic figures, often including abnormal forms, are easily identified. Mitotic activity of 4 per 10 HPF in an ovarian cellular fibromatous neoplasm in the absence of moderate to severe atypia does not signify a fibrosarcoma. In such cases, a diagnosis of mitotically active cellular fibroma is made {815}. Areas of haemorrhage and necrosis are common.

Genetic profile

Trisomy 12 and trisomy 8 have been reported in one case {1939}.

Genetic susceptibility

Ovarian fibrosarcomas are rarely associated with Maffucci syndrome and nevoid basal cell carcinoma syndrome {311,983}.

Prognosis and predictive factors

These are aggressive neoplasms with a poor prognosis {1524}.

Sclerosing stromal tumour

Definition

A benign, stromal tumour composed of admixed rounded and spindled cells, arranged in cellular nodules in a hypocellular, oedematous or collagenous background stroma.

ICD-O code   8602/0

Epidemiology

These tumours are uncommon.

Clinical features

Most occur in young females with a mean age of about 27 years {259,1547,2151}. Patients typically present with symptoms referable to an ovarian mass. Hormonal symptoms are uncommon. Almost all tumours are unilateral.

Macroscopy

Most are < 10 cm, are well circumscribed and usually show a solid, yellow to white cut surface {259,2151}. Oedema is common and cyst formation may be seen.

Histopathology

The tumour has a pseudolobular architecture with cellular lobules in a background of hypocellular collagenous or oedematous to occasionally myxoid stroma. Dilated, sometimes branching, thin-walled vessels are typical. The cellular areas are composed of bland spindle-cells admixed with rounded cells. The latter have small, regular nuclei and eosinophilic or vacuolated cytoplasm; some may have a signet-ring appearance. Mitotic activity is low. Inhibin and other sex cord markers are usually positive {2151}.

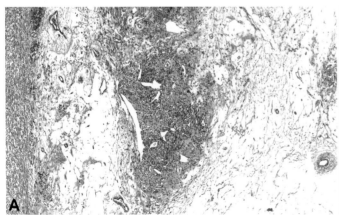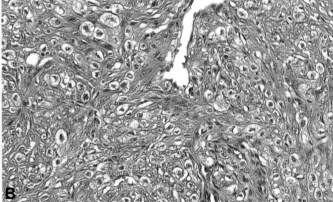

Fig. 1.40 Sclerosing stromal tumour. **A** Cellular pseudolobules are present in an oedematous stroma; dilated, thin-walled vessels are present. **B** The cellular regions are composed of spindle and rounded cells with pale to lightly eosinophilic cytoplasm (luteinized).

Genetic profile

FISH studies on a small number of cases have revealed a subpopulation of tumour cells (13–30% of cells) with trisomy 12 {892,977}.

Prognosis and predictive factors

The sclerosing stromal tumour is benign.

Signet-ring stromal tumour

Definition

A benign, stromal tumour containing cells with signet-ring morphology but without intracytoplasmic mucin, glycogen or lipid, in a background fibromatous stroma.

ICD-O code   8590/0

Epidemiology

These tumours are rare.

Clinical features

They have occurred in adults, ranging from 21–83 years. Presentation is usually referable to an ovarian mass. Hormonal symptoms have not been reported.

Macroscopy

In all but one case the tumours have been unilateral {566}. The tumours are predominantly solid but sometimes have a cystic component.

Histopathology

Variable numbers of signet-ring cells with eccentric nuclei and a single large cytoplasmic vacuole are present, in a background often resembling cellular fibroma {453,1962}. The signet-ring cells have bland nuclei and there is little or no mitotic activity. The cytoplasmic vacuoles are clear and do not contain mucin, glycogen or lipid. Eosinophilic hyaline globules are sometimes present. Immunohistochemically, the signet-ring cells express vimentin and smooth muscle actin and may display focal broad spectrum cytokeratin positivity, but they are negative for EMA and mucin stains. Inhibin has been negative in all cases tested.

Prognosis and predictive factors

Reported cases have had benign follow-up.

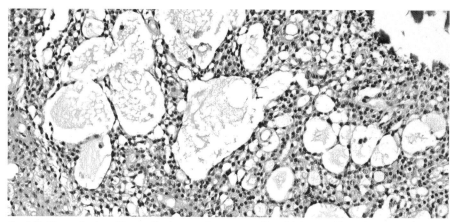

Fig. 1.41 Microcystic stromal tumour. The tumour cells are arranged in solid sheets and form microcysts.

Microcystic stromal tumour

Definition

A rare, benign, ovarian tumour which is probably of stromal origin and characterized by a distinctive microcystic appearance.

ICD-O code   8590/0

Clinical features

The patients have ranged from 26–63 years (mean 45 years) and typically presented with symptoms of a pelvic mass {819}. Hormonal manifestations are rare.

Macroscopy

The tumours are typically unilateral with a mean size of about 9 cm {819}. They are usually solid-cystic and less commonly solid or cystic. The solid component is usually firm and tan or tan-white.

Histopathology

There are three components that vary in amount: microcysts, solid cellular zones and collagenous stroma. Microcysts usually predominate and this pattern is characterized by small rounded to oval cystic spaces, in areas coalescing to larger irregular channels; intracytoplasmic vacuoles are also frequently present. The solid cellular areas are often intersected by collagenous stroma with hyaline plaques. The cells contain a moderate amount of finely granular, lightly eosinophilic cytoplasm, with generally bland, round to oval or spindle-shaped nuclei with small indistinct nucleoli. Bizarre nuclei are often present. Mitotic activity is low. The tumour cells are usually CD10 positive while inhibin and calretinin are typically negative {819}. Broad spectrum cytokeratins are sometimes focally positive while epithelial membrane antigen is negative {819}. WT1 and β-catenin nuclear immunoreactivity has been described {1139}.

Histogenesis

These are presumed to be of ovarian stromal origin, although the histogenesis is not firmly established.

Genetic profile

Mutation analysis in two cases revealed an identical point mutation in exon 3 of β-catenin (CTNNB1) {1139}. This suggests that dysregulation of the Wnt/β-catenin pathway plays a role in the pathogenesis of ovarian microcystic stromal tumour.

Prognosis and predictive factors

Malignant behaviour or extra-ovarian spread has not been reported {819}.

Leydig cell tumour

C.J. Zaloudek　　P.N. Staats
E.E. Mooney　　R.H. Young

Definition
A steroid cell tumour composed of Leydig cells, as proven by the presence of cytoplasmic crystals of Reinke. The diagnosis is occasionally tenable in the absence of crystals when other classic features are present.

ICD-O code
8650/0

Synonym
Hilus cell tumour

Epidemiology
Leydig cell tumours account for 20% of steroid cell tumours {1454,1643,1832}.

Clinical features
They occur at an average age of 58 years and are commonly androgenic and only rarely oestrogenic. They are unilateral in most cases.

Macroscopy
The tumours are usually small (mean, 2.4 cm) with a solid cut surface. They range from red-brown to yellow to occasionally black. Most arise in the ovarian hilus, but rarely they originate within the ovarian stroma ("non-hilar type").

Histopathology
They are well circumscribed and composed of cells with abundant eosinophilic, but occasionally pale, lipid-rich cytoplasm. Lipochrome pigment is commonly seen. Clustering of nuclei, creating intervening eosinophilic nuclear-free zones, is a characteristic feature. Cytoplasmic Reinke crystals (rod-shaped elongated eosinophilic inclusions) prove the diagnosis, but may be rare. Nuclei are typically round with a single prominent nucleolus; nuclear pseudoinclusions may be present, and sometimes bizarre nuclear atypia can be seen. Mitoses are rare or absent. In one-third of cases, fibrinoid necrosis of blood-vessel walls is seen. Hyperplasia of non-neoplastic hilus cells is commonly present in the uninvolved ovarian hilus. Occasional tumours have conspicuous fibrous stroma.

A diagnosis of "steroid cell tumour, probably Leydig cell tumour" is appropriate in tumours that lack identifiable Reinke crystals but have a hilar location and display nuclear clustering, fibrinoid necrosis of vessels and associated hilus cell hyperplasia.

Immunohistochemistry
Leydig cell tumours are positive for sex cord-stromal markers, such as inhibin, calretinin and steroidogenic factor-1. They are usually positive for Melan-A.

Prognosis and predictive factors
Leydig cell tumours are benign.

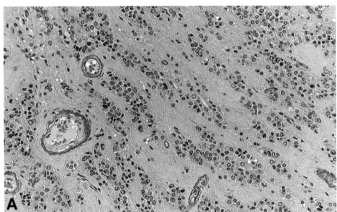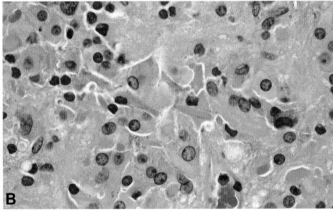

Fig. 1.42 Leydig cell tumour. **A** The tumour cells have uniform round nuclei and abundant eosinophilic cytoplasm. The tumour cell nuclei tend to cluster, leaving zones of eosinophilic nuclear-free cytoplasm. The eosinophilic fibrinoid changes in the walls of the blood vessels are a characteristic finding, but are not present in every case. **B** The tumour cell nuclei are rounded with vesicular chromatin and medium-sized nucleoli. The nuclear size is relatively uniform, although some larger nuclei are present. There are no mitotic figures. The cytoplasm is abundant and eosinophilic. Some cells contain intracytoplasmic eosinophilic rod-like structures called crystals of Reinke (centre of picture). These are not present in every case and can be difficult to find when they are present. Some cells contain round eosinophilic inclusions, which could be precursors of Reinke crystals, or cross sections of crystals.

Steroid cell tumour

Definition
A tumour composed entirely of cells resembling steroid-secreting cells that lack Reinke crystals.

ICD-O codes
Steroid cell tumour   8760/0
Steroid cell tumour, malignant 8760/3

Synonyms
Lipid cell tumour; lipoid cell tumour

Epidemiology
Steroid cell tumours account for 0.1% of ovarian neoplasms. About 80% of steroid cell tumours fall into the "not otherwise specified" (NOS) category.

Clinical features
These occur over a wide age range, but their mean age (43 years) is substantially younger than for Leydig cell tumours {724}. About half of patients present with androgenic symptoms, 10% with oestrogenic symptoms (more commonly in tumours formerly designated as stromal luteomas), and rare cases show progestational changes or Cushing syndrome. Most tumours are unilateral.

Macroscopy
Steroid cell tumours, NOS are circumscribed with a mean diameter of 8.4 cm {724}. They are solid and may be yellow, orange, red, brown or black. Haemorrhage is more common than in cases of Leydig cell tumour. Small tumours, usually < 1.0 cm and confined to the ovarian cortex were formerly designated "stromal luteoma" {725}.

Histopathology
The cells are most commonly arranged in a diffuse pattern, but can grow in nests or cords. Stroma may range from scant to prominent with fibrous bands. The tumour cells are polygonal and have abundant cytoplasm that ranges from eosinophilic (lipid-poor) to pale and vacuolated (lipid-rich); the latter is much more common than in Leydig cell tumour. Variable amounts of intracytoplasmic lipochrome pigment can be present. The nuclei are typically round with a prominent central nucleolus; rarely there is substantial nuclear atypia, usually accompanied by increased mitotic activity. In some small steroid cell tumours, particularly when small, stromal hyperthecosis is seen in the adjacent ovarian stroma.

Immunohistochemistry
These tumours are positive for sex cord-stromal markers, such as inhibin, calretinin and steroidogenic factor-1. They are usually positive for Melan-A {845} and negative for FOXL2.

Histogenesis
These tumours are presumably of stromal cell origin.

Prognosis and predictive factors
Steroid cell tumours, NOS exhibit malignant behaviour in approximately one-third of cases. Features that predict malignant behaviour include size > 7 cm, > 2 mitoses/10 HPF, necrosis, haemorrhage and significant nuclear atypia {724}.

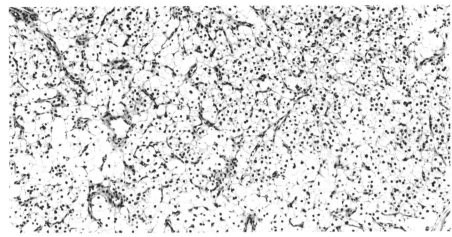

Fig. 1.43 Steroid cell tumour. The tumour consists of diffuse sheets of steroid cells with foamy, lipid-rich cytoplasm.

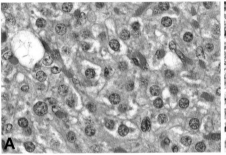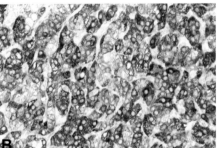

Fig. 1.44 Steroid cell tumour. **A** Tumour cells are polygonal with central round nuclei and abundant eosinophilic cytoplasm. **B** There is diffuse strong cytoplasmic staining for inhibin.

Sex cord-stromal tumours - pure sex cord tumours

C.J. Zaloudek   P.N. Staats
E.E. Mooney   R.H. Young

Adult granulosa cell tumour

Definition
A low-grade malignant, sex cord-stromal tumour composed of granulosa cells often with a variable number of fibroblasts and theca cells.

ICD-O code   8620/3

Epidemiology
Adult granulosa cell tumour accounts for about 1% of all ovarian tumours.

Clinical features
Adult granulosa cell tumours occur over a wide age range with an average age of 53 years {1864}. The typical clinical presentation is postmenopausal bleeding in older women and menorrhagia, metrorrhagia, or amenorrhea in younger patients. Rupture or torsion of the tumour causes acute abdominal symptoms in about 10% of patients. The tumour is typically unilateral and confined to the ovary at diagnosis.

Macroscopy
Granulosa cell tumours vary greatly in size, but the average diameter is about 10 cm. They are most typically solid and cystic, but may be solid or rarely entirely cystic. The solid areas are usually soft and tan to yellow. The cysts typically contain clotted blood and some tumours, particularly those associated with rupture, exhibit conspicuous haemorrhage.

Histopathology
A variety of growth patterns occur and are often admixed. The most common pattern is diffuse, in which the tumour cells grow in sheets. Tumour cells often grow in cords and trabeculae, in undulating ribbons and in nests (insular pattern). A microfollicular pattern (Call-Exner bodies), in which granulosa cells surround small spaces containing eosinophilic secretion, sometimes with nuclear debris or occasionally hyaline material, is seen in a minority of tumours and is uncommonly conspicuous. Occasionally larger follicles are seen (macrofollicular pattern). The cysts of granulosa cell tumours are lined by granulosa cells, often underlain by theca cells. In some tumours, the cells are spindled and can mimic cellular fibroma. A pseudopapillary architecture may be seen. The tumour cells usually have scant pale cytoplasm, but rarely the cytoplasm is abundant and eosinophilic (luteinized). The nuclei are typically uniform, pale and round to oval. Nuclear grooves are a characteristic feature but in many tumours are not conspicuous. Nuclear atypia is usually absent except for occasional (about 2%) cases which show bizarre nuclei, unassociated with increased mitotic activity. Mitotic activity is variable, and sometimes brisk. Rare granulosa cell tumours contain heterologous mucinous epithelium or exhibit hepatoid differentiation. Granulosa cell tumours contain a variable amount of fibromatous or thecomatous stroma. In granulosa cell tumours, reticulin fibres surround nests of tumour cells, except in stromal regions. Some adult granulosa cell tumours have a component of juvenile granulosa cell tumour; the tumour should be classified based on its predominant histology.

Immunohistochemistry
Granulosa cell tumours usually exhibit inhibin, calretinin, FOXL2, steroidogenic factor-1 (SF-1), WT1 and CD56 positivity {25,253,2163}. They may be positive for broad spectrum and low-molecular weight (8 and 18) keratins but are typically negative for CK7 and EMA. They may be positive for smooth muscle actin, desmin, CD99 (membranous) and S-100 protein.

Histogenesis
Granulosa cell tumour is presumed to develop from the granulosa cells of ovarian follicles but its histogenesis is unproven.

Genetic profile
The most common abnormalities reported have been trisomy 12, trisomy 14, monosomy 16 or deletion of 16q and

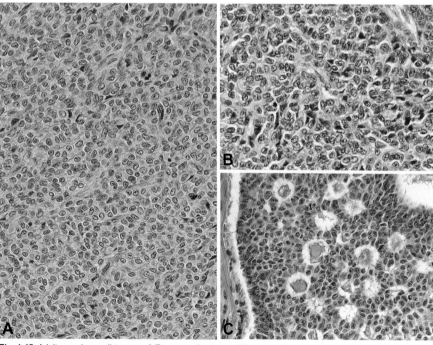

Fig. 1.45 Adult granulosa cell tumour. **A** Tumour cells show a diffuse growth pattern. **B** Sheets of monotonous small cells with scant cytoplasm and nuclei with occasional longitudinal grooves are seen. **C** In the microfollicular pattern (Call-Exner bodies), the tumour cells surround small, rounded spaces filled with eosinophilic material.

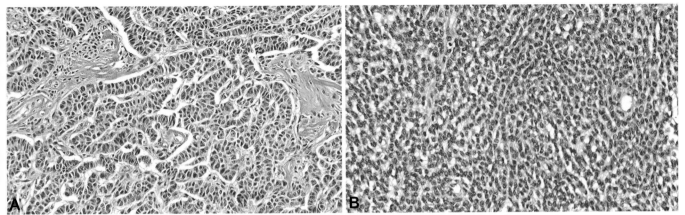

Fig. 1.46 Adult granulosa cell tumour. **A** Inter-anastomosing trabeculae in a collagenous background. **B** Delicate cords of tumour cells are present.

monosomy 22 {620,1102}. There is a missense somatic point mutation in the *FOXL2* gene (402 C to G) in more than 90% of adult granulosa cell tumours {830,927,1741}.

Prognosis and predictive factors
The recurrence rate is 10–15% for stage Ia tumours and 20–30% overall. Metastases/recurrences are often detected > 5 years after initial treatment, sometimes after intervals of > 20 years. Extraovarian spread is to the peritoneum and omentum and rarely to liver or lungs {1920}. Lymph node metastases are uncommon. Unfavourable factors include advanced stage (most important), large size (> 15 cm), bilaterality and tumour rupture. There is no correlation between microscopic appearance, including mitotic activity, and outcome.

Juvenile granulosa cell tumour

Definition
A distinctive type of granulosa cell tumour that occurs mainly in children and young adults.

ICD-O code   8622/1

Epidemiology
It accounts for 5% of granulosa cell tumours.

Clinical features
This variant occurs usually in the first three decades (average age is 15 years), but can be seen in older patients {1699}. Young girls typically have isosexual pseudoprecocity. Older children and premenopausal women present with menorrhagia or amenorrhea or with non-specific symptoms such as abdominal or pelvic pain, distension or a palpable mass. Torsion or rupture of the tumour causes acute abdominal symptoms. Juvenile granulosa cell tumours are typically unilateral, and more than 95% of them are confined to the ovary (stage I).

Macroscopy
The average size is about 12 cm and most are solid and cystic, but some are uniformly solid or cystic. The solid areas are yellow or tan. Haemorrhage may be conspicuous within cysts and solid foci of the neoplasm, particularly in tumours that have ruptured.

Histopathology
The tumour has a nodular or diffuse growth punctuated, in most cases, by follicles of varying sizes and shapes. Sometimes they are round and uniform but they more often have irregular shapes. They contain secretions that may be eosinophilic but are, more often, basophilic and may stain for mucin. Sometimes a basophilic matrix is present in the background stroma. The cells lining the follicles and in the solid areas characteristically have abundant eosinophilic but occasionally pale amphophilic cytoplasm. The nuclei are round and lack grooves with rare exceptions. Mitotic figures are typically frequent and striking nuclear atypia is seen in 10–15% of the tumours. Pseudo-papillae lined by granulosa cells are seen in some tumours {818}. The stroma is generally less conspicuous in these tumours compared to adult granulosa cell tumours but it is occasionally prominent and in rare cases there is striking sclerosis which may obscure the underlying neoplastic cells. Some juvenile granulosa cell tumours have a component of adult granulosa cell tumour; the tumour should be classified based on its predominant histology.

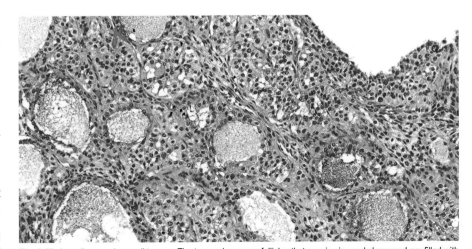

Fig. 1.47 Juvenile granulosa cell tumour. The tumour has many follicles that vary in size and shape and are filled with basophilic secretion.

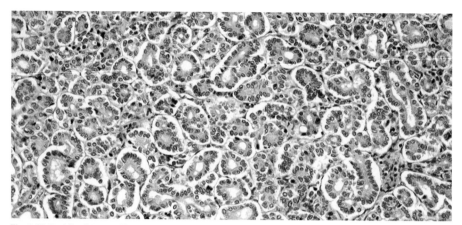

Fig. 1.48 Sertoli cell tumour. The tumour shows hollow tubules lined by cuboidal to columnar cells.

Immunohistochemistry
These tumours are usually positive for inhibin, calretinin, SF-1, CD99 and CD56 {25}. A small minority express FOXL2. Low molecular weight cytokeratin may be positive while EMA is only rarely weakly and focally positive {1204}.

Histogenesis
This tumour is presumed to develop from the granulosa cells of ovarian follicles but its histogenesis is unproven. The frequent absence of FOXL2 in these tumours compared to its presence in nearly all adult granulosa cell tumours suggests that they are distinctive.

Genetic profile
The most common cytogenetic abnormality associated with this tumour is trisomy 12, which is present in most cases {695,1700}. *FOXL2* (C402G) mutation is absent in these neoplasms {401,1741}.

Genetic susceptibility
Juvenile granulosa cell tumour has been associated with the hereditary conditions Ollier disease (enchondromatosis) and Mafucci syndrome (enchondromatosis and multiple subcutaneous haemangiomas) {1590,1898,1979,2110}.

Prognosis and predictive factors
Juvenile granulosa cell tumour is typically limited to the ovary at diagnosis and has a good prognosis. Recurrences usually occur within three years of diagnosis. Patients with ruptured tumour, positive peritoneal cytology or extra-ovarian tumour spread have a higher risk of recurrence {2110,2143}.

Sertoli cell tumour

Definition
A neoplasm composed of Sertoli cells arranged in a variety of patterns, but most commonly as hollow or solid tubules.

ICD-O code   8640/1

Epidemiology
Sertoli cell tumours are rare {1412}.

Clinical features
Tumours can occur at any age (mean 30 years). Patients may present with abdominal pain, swelling or vaginal bleeding and approximately 40% have hormonal manifestations, usually estrogenic {1909}.

Macroscopy
These are unilateral neoplasms with a mean size of 8 cm. They are usually solid, but may be solid and cystic or less commonly cystic. Solid areas are tan to yellow, and areas of haemorrhage and necrosis may be seen.

Histopathology
Sertoli cell tumours may show a broad range of patterns. A tubular pattern, either hollow or solid, is seen in most tumours at least focally. Other patterns include trabecular, diffuse, alveolar, pseudopapillary, retiform and rarely, spindled. Cells usually have cytoplasm that ranges from pale and lipid-rich to eosinophilic. Nuclei are typically oval or round with a small nucleolus and are cytologically bland in most instances. The presence of an occasional Leydig cell within the tumour does not exclude the diagnosis of Sertoli cell tumour.

Most tumours are positive for WT1, SF-1, broad spectrum keratins, inhibin, calretinin and CD99. Smooth muscle actin and S-100 are positive in a minority of neoplasms while EMA is negative {2160,2162}.

Genetic susceptibility
Rare tumours (mostly lipid-rich and oxyphilic variants) are seen in patients with Peutz-Jeghers syndrome.

Prognosis and predictive factors
Sertoli cell tumours are usually benign and confined to the ovary at the time of diagnosis. Rare tumours are malignant and factors that may influence outcome are size (> 5 cm), > 5 mitoses/10 HPF, nuclear atypia and necrosis {1412}.

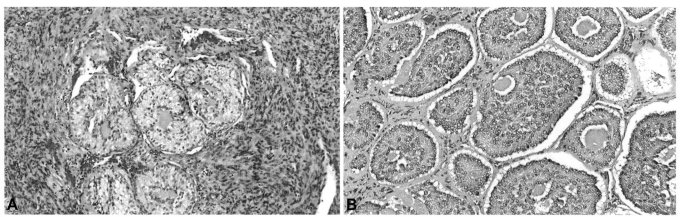

Fig. 1.49 Sex cord tumour with annular tubules. **A** A typical microscopic focus in the ovarian cortex of a woman with Peutz-Jeghers syndrome. **B** This sporadic example shows numerous nests of tumour cells forming annular tubules.

Sex cord tumour with annular tubules

Definition
An uncommon, sex cord-stromal tumour with a distinctive pattern of simple and complex annular tubules.

ICD-O code   8623/1

Epidemiology
These are rare, comprising < 1% of sex cord-stromal tumours.

Clinical features
These occur in two settings; sporadically or in association with Peutz-Jeghers syndrome. They occur over a wide age range. Patients with Peutz-Jeghers syndrome are slightly younger (average age 27 years) than those without the syndrome (average age 36 years). The tumours are generally an incidental finding in women with Peutz-Jeghers syndrome, whereas in the sporadic cases, general symptoms of ovarian neoplasia may be present. The non-syndromic tumours may secrete progesterone.

Macroscopy
Tumours that occur in patients with the Peutz-Jeghers syndrome are small, multifocal, and usually bilateral; many are not visible. Those that can be seen are solid tan to yellow and measure < 3 cm, sometimes with a gritty texture due to calcification. Sporadic tumours are generally unilateral and typically > 3 cm. Most tumours are solid, some are solid and cystic and rare examples are uniformly cystic. They have a tan or yellow cut surface.

Histopathology
The tumour is composed of individually dispersed or nodular aggregates of simple or complex annular tubules {2131}. Tubules typically lack lumens and the lining cells have an antipodal arrangement of the nuclei. The stroma is fibrous and the nests of tumour cells are surrounded by eosinophilic hyaline material that is continuous with the hyaline cores within the nests. Calcification is typically present in the syndrome-associated tumours, in which the nests are typically multifocal and may lie on the background of normal ovarian stroma. Sporadic tumours exhibit more complex growth patterns including elongated tubules, coalescent nests of tumour cells, solid growth, cysts or acellular zones of eosinophilic hyaline material. The tumour cells are columnar and have clear or foamy cytoplasm and round or oval hyperchromatic nuclei with small nucleoli. Atypia and mitotic figures are uncommon. Small foci of granulosa cell or Sertoli cell differentiation, particularly in the non-syndromic examples, are occasionally present.

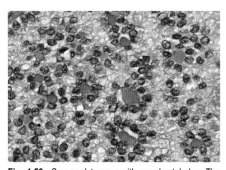

Fig. 1.50 Sex cord tumour with annular tubules. The tumour shows an antipodal arrangement of the nuclei within the tubules. The latter contain hyaline material.

Immunohistochemistry
The tumour cells are usually positive for inhibin, calretinin, FOXL2, SF-1, WT1 and CD56 {431}. There may be positive staining for broad spectrum cytokeratins, but EMA is negative.

Histogenesis
The tumour presumably arises from ovarian sex cord cells.

Genetic profile
Germline mutations of *STK11* result in LOH in the 19p13.3 region in tumours associated with the Peutz-Jeghers syndrome {368}. Somatic mutations of the *STK11* gene are not detected in sporadic tumours.

Genetic susceptibility
About a third of tumours are detected in women with the Peutz-Jeghers syndrome {117,2131}.

Prognosis and predictive factors
Tumours in women with the Peutz-Jeghers syndrome are benign, but approximately 20% of those unassociated with the syndrome have had a low-grade malignant course. Lymph node spread is more common than with other sex cord-stromal tumours.

Mixed sex cord-stromal tumours

C.J. Zaloudek   P.N. Staats
E.E. Mooney   R.H. Young

Sertoli-Leydig cell tumours

Definition
Tumours composed of variable proportions of Sertoli cells, Leydig cells and in the case of moderately and poorly differentiated neoplasms, primitive gonadal stroma and sometimes heterologous elements.

ICD-O codes
Sertoli-Leydig cell tumour,
   well differentiated   8631/0
Sertoli-Leydig cell tumour,
   moderately differentiated   8631/1
Sertoli-Leydig cell tumour,
   moderately differentiated
   with heterologous elements   8634/1
Sertoli-Leydig cell tumour,
   poorly differentiated   8631/3
Sertoli-Leydig cell tumour,
   poorly differentiated with
   heterologous elements   8634/3
Sertoli-Leydig cell tumour,
   retiform   8633/1
Sertoli-Leydig cell tumour, retiform,
   with heterologous elements   8634/1

Synonyms
Androblastoma; arrhenoblastoma

Epidemiology
Sertoli-Leydig cell tumours are rare, accounting for < 0.5% of ovarian neoplasms; moderately and poorly differentiated forms are the most common. Sertoli-Leydig cell tumours have been reported in females from 1–84 years of age with a mean age of 25 years {2124,2144}. Those occurring in patients with a germline *DICER-1* mutation occur at a younger median age of 13 years {1593}. Tumours with a prominent retiform pattern also occur at a younger age, median 15 years.

Clinical features
Between 40% and 60% of patients are virilised, while occasional patients have oestrogenic manifestations {677,2144}. Androgenic manifestations include amenorrhoea, hirsutism, breast atrophy, clitoral hypertrophy and hoarseness, whereas estrogenic effects include isosexual pseudoprecocity and menometrorrhagia. Patients may present with abdominal pain, ascites or tumour rupture. About 2–3% of tumours have spread beyond the ovary at presentation, but lymph node metastases are rare.

Imaging
A solid or solid and cystic mass may be identified on ultrasound, computed tomography or magnetic resonance imaging.

Macroscopy
Over 97% of Sertoli-Leydig cell tumours are unilateral. The size ranges from 2–35 cm (mean 12–14 cm). They may be solid, solid and cystic or rarely, cystic. Solid areas are fleshy and pale yellow, pink or grey. Areas of haemorrhage and necrosis are occasional and torsion and infarction may be seen.

Histopathology
In well differentiated Sertoli-Leydig cell tumours, Sertoli cells are present in open or closed tubules and lack significant nuclear atypia or mitotic activity. There is a delicate fibrous stroma in which Leydig cells are found in small clusters, cords, and singly. Hyalinization and ossification are rare findings {1295}. In tumours of moderate differentiation cellular lobules composed of darkly staining Sertoli cells, typically with scant cytoplasm, and admixed in a jumbled fashion with Leydig cells, are typically separated by an edematous stroma. A nested to alveolar arrangement of Sertoli cells may be present in some cases and the overall picture is punctuated to varying degrees by hollow and solid tubules lined by Sertoli cells. The latter usually exhibiting only modest cytologic atypia although bizarre degenerative type atypia may be rarely seen. This is not of adverse prognostic import. Tubules in neoplasms of well and moderate differentiation may mimic an endometrioid neoplasm {1230}. Mitotic figures average 5/10 HPF in tumours of moderate differentiation. Leydig cells are found in clusters at the periphery of the cellular lobules or admixed with other elements. They may be vacuolated, contain lipofuscin or rarely have Reinke crystals. Mitotic figures are rare among the Leydig cells, which also lack cytological atypia. In poorly differentiated neoplasms, a sarcomatoid stroma resembling primitive gonadal stroma, is the dominant feature and the lobulated arrangement of Sertoli-Leydig cell tumour of moderate differentiation is typically present to only a minor degree such that significant areas of the tumour, in isolation, cannot be diagnosed as Sertoli-Leydig cell tumour. The mitotic rate in poorly differentiated tumours is variable, but in many regions high, often being up to 20/10 HPF. Sertoli-Leydig cell tumours are subdivided into well differentiated, moderate and poorly differentiated forms based on the degree of tubular differentiation of the Sertoli cell component (decreasing with increasing grade) and the quantity of primitive gonadal stroma (increasing with increasing grade). Leydig cells also decrease with increasing grade. Heterologous elements and/or a retiform pattern may be seen in all but the well differentiated variant.

When the tumour contains substantial areas of anastomosing, slit-like spaces resembling the rete testis, the term "retiform Sertoli-Leydig cell tumour" is used. Retiform tubules are not seen in well differentiated Sertoli-Leydig cell tumours. Patients with retiform tumours tend to be younger, and virilization is less common. The retiform pattern varies from slit-like spaces lined by cuboidal or columnar epithelium, to areas with a papillary pattern, to a multicystic pattern with sieve-like spaces lined by flattened cells.

Some Sertoli-Leydig cell tumours contain tissue types not regarded as intrinsic to the sex cord-stromal category. Such elements include epithelial and/or mesenchymal tissues and tumours arising from these elements. The presence of heterologous elements does not alter the presentation, but patients may have a raised serum α-fetoprotein (AFP) due in some cases to hepatocytes as a heterol-

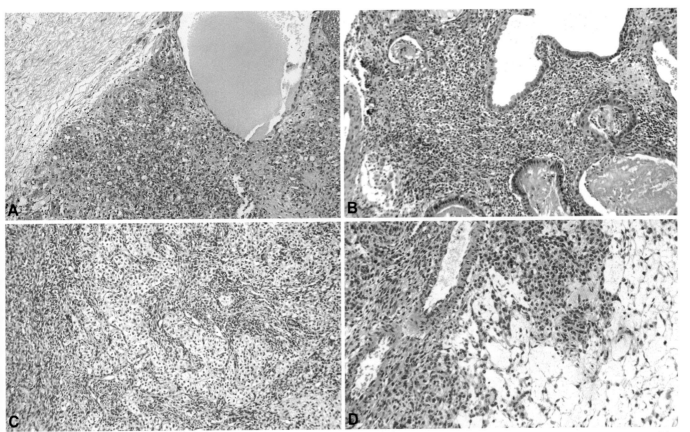

Fig. 1.51 A Sertoli-Leydig cell tumour of moderate differentiation, partly cystic. **B** Sertoli-Leydig cell tumour with heterologous elements. Mucinous glands and cysts, some containing eosinophilic secretion, are embedded in the background of an otherwise typical Sertoli-Leydig cell tumour. **C** Sertoli-Leydig cell tumour, moderate differentiation. The tumour shows mainly Sertoli cells in a nested to solid tubular pattern. **D** Sertoli-Leydig cell tumour, moderate differentiation. Alternating hypo- and hypercellular areas are noted with the latter showing darkly staining Sertoli cells admixed with Leydig cells.

ogous element. Heterologous elements are seen in up to 20% of Sertoli-Leydig cell tumours. They occur only in those of moderate or poor differentiation or in retiform tumours. The most common element is mucinous epithelium of enteric type. This is usually bland, but proliferation, borderline change and carcinoma may be seen. Close apposition of the gonadal stromal element and mucinous epithelium may be the only clue that what appears to be a mucinous cystadenoma is, in fact, a Sertoli-Leydig cell tumour with a prominent heterologous element. Rarely, carcinoid occurs as a heterologous epithelial element. Heterologous mesenchymal elements are less common than epithelial elements and usually consist of cartilage or skeletal muscle, often cellular and of fetal type. They may be admixed with the sex cord areas of the tumour or present as dis-

crete areas. While bile plugs or acini may enable hepatocytes to be distinguished from Leydig cells, immunohistochemistry is usually necessary {1294}.

Serous neoplasms, carcinosarcomas and yolk sac tumours may resemble a retiform Sertoli-Leydig cell tumour, and the differential diagnosis of tumours of well and moderate differentiation includes an endometrioid adenocarcinoma with "sertoliform" glands. The presence of gonadal stroma and/or heterologous elements assists in making the diagnosis.

Immunohistochemistry

Positivity for vimentin, keratin, α-inhibin and calretinin is seen, with differing intensity of expression between sex cord and stromal areas. Sertoli-Leydig cell tumours are positive for CD 56, SF-1 and WT-1; 50% express CD 99, which does not stain the Leydig cell compo-

nent {2163}. Sertoli-Leydig cell tumours express FOXL2 in at least 50% of cases {25}. Leydig cells in Sertoli-Leydig cell tumours show either no or minimal staining for FOXL2, WT-1 and CD 99, but express Melan-A. Dicer1 immunohistochemistry shows strong staining of Sertoli cells and weak staining of Leydig cells {1593}.

Heterologous elements show the immunoprofile of their constituent tissues, with mucinous epithelium positive for CK 7 and CK 20. Leydig cells are negative for keratins and α-fetoprotein, and positive for vimentin and α-inhibin. Hepatocytes are positive for keratins and α-fetoprotein and negative for vimentin and inhibin. Alpha-fetoprotein positivity may be seen in endodermal-like structures.

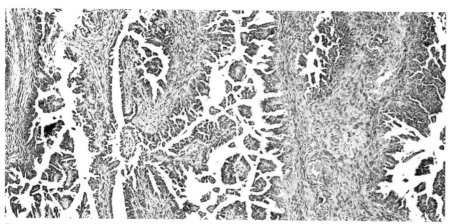

Fig. 1.52 Sertoli-Leydig cell tumour, retiform. Florid retiform pattern mimicking a serous papillary neoplasm.

Genetic profile
Clonality studies on the Sertoli, Leydig and heterologous elements in Sertoli-Leydig cell tumours have yielded varying results. Leydig cells are felt to be reactive stromal cells in some cases and possibly neoplastic in others {497,1292}.

Genetic susceptibility
Mutations in *DICER1*, a gene encoding an RNase III endoribonuclease, are found in 60% of Sertoli-Leydig cell tumours. Germline mutations in this gene are seen in familial multinodular goitre with Sertoli-Leydig cell tumour, and tumour susceptibility includes pleuropulmonary blastoma in childhood {741,1593,1703}. Sertoli-Leydig cell tumour has been reported in association with cervical embryonal rhabdomyosarcoma in four cases {1201}.

Prognosis and predictive factors
The prognosis of Sertoli-Leydig cell tumours is overall favorable but related in significant part to the grade. Well differentiated tumours have close to 100% survival and tumours of moderate differentiation, with or without heterologous elements are clinically malignant in about only 10% of the cases. The presence of a retiform component may have a slightly adverse impact on prognosis of tumours of moderate differentiation although conclusive proof is lacking. Poorly differentiated tumours and, less commonly, those of moderate differentiation may behave in a malignant fashion; recurrence is usually within two years and occurs in the peritoneal cavity {1773}. Tumour rupture and the presence of mesenchymal heterologous elements, along with stage II or higher disease are associated with a poorer outcome.

Sex cord-stromal tumours, NOS

Definition
A sex cord-stromal tumour that lacks definitive characteristics of a specific tumour type.

ICD-O code   8590/1

Epidemiology
These neoplasms represent < 5% of sex cord-stromal tumours {1723}. Tumours removed during pregnancy are more likely to fall into this category {2111}.

Clinical features
They may be oestrogenic, androgenic or non-functioning.

Histopathology
Histological features are variable, but distinctive features of a specific sex cord-stromal tumour are not identifiable or are rare. Changes seen in pregnancy include prominent oedema, luteinization and prominent Leydig cells {2111}. Tumours reported in two patients with Peutz-Jeghers syndrome are included in this category; they resembled, to a limited degree, retiform Sertoli-Leydig cell tumour, but contained prominent cells with abundant eosinophilic cytoplasm {2109}.

Prognosis and predictive factors
Behaviour appears to be similar to granulosa and Sertoli-Leydig cell tumours, with a 92% 5-year survival {1723}.

Germm cell tumours

J. Prat
D. Cao
S.G. Carinelli

F.F. Nogales
R. Vang
C.J. Zaloudek

Dysgerminoma

Definition

Dysgerminoma is a primitive germ cell tumour composed of cells showing no specific pattern of differentiation.

ICD-O code   9060/3

Epidemiology

Dysgerminoma is the most common malignant primitive germ cell tumour of the ovary, but comprises only 1–2% of all malignant ovarian tumours.

Clinical features

It occurs almost exclusively in children and young women. The average patient age is 22 years {798,1984}. The clinical presentation is with abdominal distension, an abdominal mass or abdominal pain. The serum lactic dehydrogenase (LDH) is often elevated and 3–5% of patients have a modest elevation of human chorionic gonadotropin (hCG). Rare patients have paraneoplastic hypercalcaemia. About 10% of the tumours are grossly bilateral and if a grossly normal contralateral ovary is biopsied, an additional 10% will be discovered to be bilateral. A small subset of tumours occurs in patients with an intersexual disorder.

Macroscopy

Dysgerminoma is usually > 10 cm diameter with a solid, fleshy tan or white cut surface. Foci of haemorrhage, necrosis or cystic degeneration may be present.

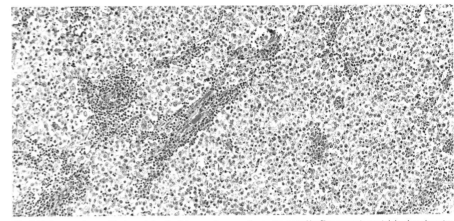

Fig. 1.53 Dysgerminoma. Nests and sheets of dysgerminoma cells are separated by fibrous septa containing lymphocytes

Histopathology

Dysgerminoma typically consists of sheets or nests of polygonal cells with abundant granular eosinophilic or clear cytoplasm and distinct cell membranes. Less commonly, cords, trabeculae, solid tubules, pseudoglands and an unusually prominent collagenous stroma are seen. The tumour cells have uniformly medium-sized nuclei with vesicular chromatin and prominent nucleoli. The nuclear membrane is characteristically angulated ("squared off"). Mitotic figures are numerous. The tumour is typically intersected by fibrous septa that contain lymphocytes (mostly T-cells) {455,1836} and epithelioid histiocytes that can form sarcoid-like granulomas. Lymphocytes and, less often, epithelioid histiocytes are also sprinkled among the tumour cells. About 3% of dysgerminomas contain syncytiotrophoblastic giant cells unassociated with cyto-

trophoblast. Some tumours exhibit extensive necrosis which may show dystrophic calcification. The latter, if unassociated with necrosis, may indicate the presence of an underlying gonadoblastoma which gives rise to dysgerminoma in some cases and rigorous sampling may show definitive features of gonadoblastoma.

Immunohistochemistry

The tumour cells show cytoplasmic and membranous placental alkaline phosphatase (PLAP) and membranous CD117 (c-KIT) and D2–40 (podoplanin) immunoreactivity {268,1737}. Diffuse positive nuclear staining for the stem cell/primitive germ cell nuclear transcription factors OCT-4, NANOG, and SALL4 is seen {229,268,290}. There can be limited cytoplasmic dot or rim-like staining for cytokeratin but EMA is negative. The syncytiotrophoblastic giant cells are positive for hCG.

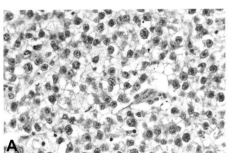
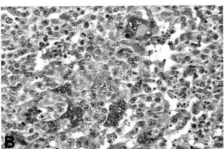
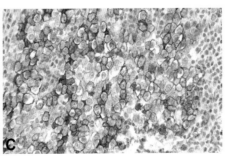

Fig. 1.54 A Dysgerminoma. The tumour cells have round vesicular nuclei with prominent eosinophilic macronucleoli, abundant pale cytoplasm, and well-defined cell membranes. A few lymphocytes with small dark nuclei are scattered among the dysgerminoma cells. **B** Scattered among the dysgerminoma cells are syncytiotrophoblastic giant cells, which have multiple nuclei and abundant purple cytoplasm. **C** Dysgerminoma. CD117 (c-kit) immunoreaction shows crisp membrane staining of the tumour cells.

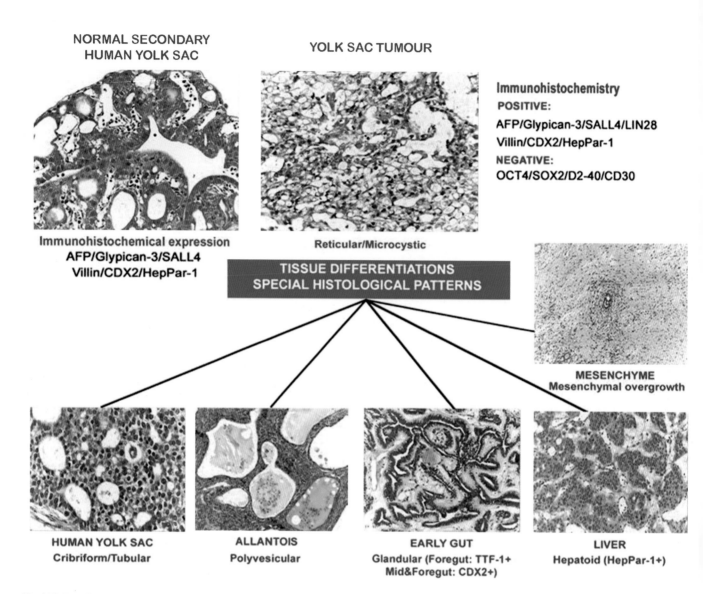

NORMAL SECONDARY HUMAN YOLK SAC

Immunohistochemical expression
AFP/Glypican-3/SALL4
Villin/CDX2/HepPar-1

YOLK SAC TUMOUR

Reticular/Microcystic

Immunohistochemistry
POSITIVE:
AFP/Glypican-3/SALL4/LIN28
Villin/CDX2/HepPar-1
NEGATIVE:
OCT4/SOX2/D2-40/CD30

TISSUE DIFFERENTIATIONS
SPECIAL HISTOLOGICAL PATTERNS

MESENCHYME
Mesenchymal overgrowth

HUMAN YOLK SAC
Cribriform/Tubular

ALLANTOIS
Polyvesicular

EARLY GUT
Glandular (Foregut: TTF-1+
Mid&Foregut: CDX2+)

LIVER
Hepatoid (HepPar-1+)

Fig. 1.55 Normal tissue differentiation and parallel morphology in yolk sac neoplasia. Primitive endodermal areas (top centre) with classical reticular, microcystic and mesoblastic patterns can differentiate into and co-exist with various somatic tissues with corresponding histological patterns such as human yolk sac (cribriform/tubular), allantois (polyvesicular), early gut (glandular), liver (hepatoid) and mesenchyme. The normal human secondary yolk sac (top left) is shown for comparison purposes. The immunophenotypes of the human yolk sac and of the various histological patterns of yolk sac tumours are shown.

Histogenesis
Dysgerminoma develops from germ cells in the ovary.

Genetic profile
The majority of dysgerminomas show isochromosome 12p {372}. *c-KIT* mutations are seen in 25–50% of tumours {289,750,766}, most commonly in exon 17, not in the exon 11 location that confers susceptibility to imatinib therapy.

Genetic susceptibility
Dysgerminoma is the most common malignant gonadal tumour in patients with gonadal dysgenesis and a partial or complete Y chromosome. It typically arises in a gonadoblastoma in this setting.

Prognosis and predictive factors
The overall survival for optimally treated patients with dysgerminoma is greater than 90% {798,1984}. Stage and size (< 10 cm) are the most important prognostic factors. If the tumour recurs, it does so in the first few years after primary treatment.

Yolk sac tumour

Definition

Yolk sac tumour is a primitive germ cell tumour with a variety of distinctive patterns which may also exhibit differentiation into endodermal structures, ranging from the primitive gut and mesenchyme to the derivatives of extra-embryonal (secondary yolk sac and allantois) and embryonal somatic tissues (intestine, liver and mesenchyme) {1373}.

ICD-O code   9071/3

Synonyms

Endodermal sinus tumour (not recommended); primitive endodermal tumour (a recently proposed term that defines more accurately the epithelial and mesenchymal differentiation that occurs in these neoplasms) {1373}

Macroscopy

These tumours are large, soft and usually well encapsulated {1000}. The cut surface is grey-yellow with frequent areas of necrosis, haemorrhage and cystic degeneration {1372}; rarely, they are almost entirely cystic {345}. A subset may co-exist with a grossly recognizable benign cystic teratoma or they may be a component of a primitive mixed germ cell tumour in which a second component is grossly identifiable, usually dysgerminoma {1373,1988}.

Histopathology

Two or more patterns often co-exist, the most common being reticular, in which a labyrinth of channels lined by primitive cells focally expand to form microcysts lined by clear or flattened, atypical epithelial cells. Typically the stroma is hypocellular, loose and myxoid; the latter may focally predominate. Other patterns include long arching cords (festoon pattern) and papillary growth (no more than 20% of cases). In classic form, these are papillary fibrovascular structures in which a central blood vessel is mantled by the tumour cells and projects into a space lined by tumour cells (endodermal sinuses, Schiller-Duval bodies) {1373}. Less common histological patterns include solid {872}, polyvesicular vitelline, cribriform-tubular {1373}, glandular {345,359}, parietal {409} and hepatoid {1328,1520}. In the polyvesicular vitelline variant, cystic spaces {1373} lined by flattened cells and separated by prominent fibrous stroma are seen; the flattened cells may merge with columnar mucinous epithelium {1372,2130}.

The solid pattern shows cells with abundant clear cytoplasm or in some cases, smaller cells with scant cytoplasm (blastema-like). Focal differentiation into somatic endodermal gland-like structures, as well as embryonal liver can occur in one-third of cases {1329,1946} and rarely, they may predominate. The glands and papillae are lined by columnar cells and surrounded by loose stroma {1373}. Characteristically, the epithelial cells exhibit subnuclear and apical vacuoles resembling early secretory endometrium {345}. The stroma may show hyaline basement membrane material (parietal pattern) {1000}. Hyaline globules may be conspicuous both within cells and in the stroma {921}.

These tumours are usually pure but may be part of a mixed germ cell tumour, usually with dysgerminoma. In older patients, there is rarely an association with a surface epithelial tumour, usually endometrioid {1373,1646}.

Immunohistochemistry

These tumours express AFP (often only focally), glypican-3 (stronger than AFP but less specific) {1527,2177}, SALL4 {229} and LIN28 {2061}. Villin is also expressed in membranes and cytoplasms of epithelial cells. Endodermal elements may be immunoreactive for their corresponding tissue markers i.e. hepatic components for hepatocyte paraffin antigen 1 {1367,1508}, intestinal elements for CDX2 {1373} and foregut-derived epithelia for thyroid transcription factor 1 {607}. However, yolk sac tumour is negative for OCT4, SOX2, D2–40 and CD30.

Histogenesis

Most of these tumours are derived from germ cells but may originate from somatic tumours, usually endometrioid epithelial tumours {1373,1646}.

Genetic susceptibility

Rarely, tumours have arisen from a gonadoblastoma in patients with gonadal dysgenesis.

Prognosis and predictive factors

Yolk sac tumours generally have a favourable response to chemotherapy. However, if associated with a somatic neoplasm, they are less responsive to chemotherapy {1365,1646}.

Embryonal carcinoma

Definition

A rare, primitive, germ cell neoplasm that shows rudimentary epithelial differentiation and is morphologically identical to its testicular counterpart.

ICD-O code   9070/3

Epidemiology

Embryonal carcinoma is rare in pure form or as a component of a mixed germ cell tumour.

Clinical features

Embryonal carcinoma occurs almost exclusively in children and young women < 30 years (average 15 years) {999}. The most common clinical presentation is pelvic or abdominal pain, abdominal mass or menstrual abnormalities. Precocious pseudopuberty can occur in children. The serum Beta-HCG level is often increased.

Macroscopy

It is typically a large, solid tumour with an average diameter of 15 cm. The cut surface is soft and fleshy with variably sized cysts. The tumour is tan or grey and there are generally prominent areas of haemorrhage and necrosis.

Histopathology

The tumour grows in sheets or nests with focal gland differentiation and, less commonly, papillae. The polygonal cells have vesicular nuclei with coarse, basophilic chromatin and one or two prominent nucleoli. The cell membranes are well defined and the cytoplasm is abundant and usually amphophilic but occasionally focally clear. Mitotic figures and apoptotic bodies are numerous. Syncytiotrophoblast cells are present in most cases.

Immunohistochemistry

The tumour cells are typically positive for wide spectrum cytokeratin (AE1/AE3), CD30, OCT4, SALL4 and glypican 3. SOX2 is variably positive {229,268,291}. Epithelial membrane antigen is negative. Syncytiotrophoblastic giant cells, if present, are cytokeratin and HCG positive {999}.

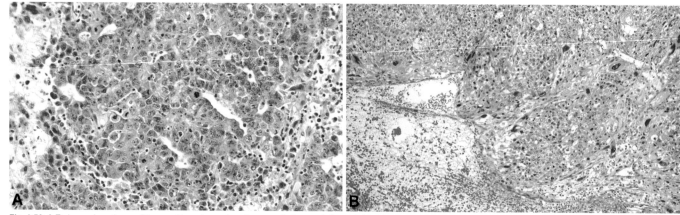

Fig. 1.56 A Embryonal carcinoma. Pleomorphic embryonal carcinoma cells line poorly formed glandular clefts. **B** Non-gestational choriocarcinoma. Mononucleate trophoblastic cells and syncytiotrophoblastic cells are arranged in a plexiform pattern.

Histogenesis
Embryonal carcinoma derives from ovarian germ cells.

Genetic profile
The genetic profile of most embryonal carcinomas contains an isochromosome, i12p {291}.

Genetic susceptibility
A rare embryonal carcinoma has arisen in a gonadoblastoma in a patient with gonadal dysgenesis.

Prognosis and predictive factors
These are aggressive tumours but they respond to chemotherapy.

Non-gestational choriocarcinoma

Definition
A malignant neoplasm of germ cell origin composed of cytotrophoblast and syncytiotrophoblast cells.

ICD-O code   9100/3

Epidemiology
Non-gestational choriocarcinoma is rare and accounts for < 1% of ovarian malignant germ cell tumours {1003}, either pure or as a component in mixed germ cell tumours {658,1133}.

Clinical features
Patients are typically children and young adults, but rarely are postmenopausal {658,1133,1461}. Most patients present with precocious pseudopuberty, vagi-

nal bleeding and/or signs mimicking an ectopic pregnancy. Serum β-hCG levels range from hundreds to > 2'000'000 mIU/ml {1133}.

Macroscopy
The tumour is typically large with a solid or solid and cystic cut surface, often with haemorrhage and necrosis.

Histopathology
Mononucleate trophoblastic cells and syncytiotrophoblastic cells are arranged in a characteristic plexiform pattern, often with haemorrhage; the latter may predominate and obscure a sometimes minor component of neoplastic cells. Some tumours may be predominantly composed of mononucleate cells. Choriocarcinoma rarely may be seen in association with carcinoma {688,1413}. These latter tumours occur in older patients.

Genetic susceptibility
Two of 45 patients with pure non-gestational choriocarcinoma had gonadal dysgenesis (46XY, 45XO/46XY) {310,658}.

Prognosis and predictive factors
The prognosis is less favourable than that of gestational choriocarcinoma.

Mature teratoma

Definition
A tumour composed exclusively of mature tissues derived from two or three germ layers (ectoderm, mesoderm and endoderm). Tumours are usually cystic (mature cystic teratoma), but rarely solid (mature solid teratoma).

ICD-O code   9080/0

Synonyms
Mature cystic teratoma; dermoid cyst

Epidemiology
Mature teratomas account for approximately 20% of all ovarian neoplasms {1497,1644,1710}.

Clinical features
The age distribution is wide, but most occur during the reproductive years. Patients present with abdominal pain, abdominal mass or swelling; many tumours are incidental findings on imaging studies or at the time of operation. Ten percent are bilateral {1497,1644,1710}.

Macroscopy
Most tumours are cystic (mature cystic teratomas) and usually measure from 5–10 cm {1497}. The cut surface of the tumour, which is usually unilocular, reveals a cyst filled with sebaceous material and hair; teeth may be seen. A solid nodule (Rokitansky protuberance) is commonly present. Rarely, the tumours are predominantly solid with interspersed cysts (mature solid teratoma) {1495,2037}. The rare fetiform teratoma resembles a malformed human foetus with the caudal portion being more developed {1}.

Histopathology
Ectodermal derivatives represented by squamous epithelium and other adnexal structures, as well as brain tissue (e.g. glia, ependymal tubules and cerebellum), are the most abundant component. Mesodermal derivatives such as bone, cartilage, smooth muscle and adipose

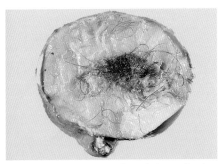

Fig. 1.57 Mature teratoma. Gross features of mature cystic teratoma: the cut surface shows a unicystic mass filled with sebaceous material and hair.

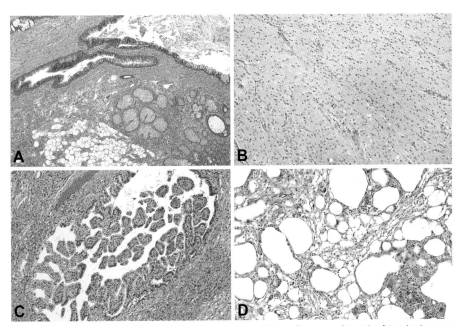

Fig. 1.58 Mature teratoma. **A** The cyst is lined by respiratory epithelium. The cyst wall contains fat and sebaceous glands. **B** Neural tissue within mature cystic teratoma. **C** Choroid plexus within mature cystic teratoma. **D** Lipogranulomatous reaction within mature cystic teratoma.

tissue are usually seen. Endodermal derivatives such as gastrointestinal and respiratory/bronchial epithelium, thyroid and salivary glands are less common. Rarely, prostate {689}, pituitary, adrenal and parathyroid tissue have been reported. Rarely, microscopic foci of immature neural tissue may occur {2074}. Fat necrosis imparts a cystic appearance (sieve-like pattern) in many cases, and may be the only evidence of the tumour.

Histogenesis
The most widely accepted explanation is the parthenogenetic theory, which suggests an origin from the primordial germ cell {1104,1105,1467,1561}.

Prognosis and predictive factors
These tumours are benign except if malignant transformation occurs. The presence of rare, microscopic foci of immature neural tissue is associated with an excellent outcome {2074}. Peritoneal implants composed entirely of mature glial tissue may occasionally be observed in cases of mature solid teratoma, but do not adversely affect prognosis {1601}. Rarely, immature teratoma develops in residual ovary after excision of a dermoid cyst, particularly if the latter was multiple or had ruptured {2074}.

Immature teratoma

Definition
A teratoma containing variable amounts of immature (typically primitive/embryonal neuroectodermal) tissues, including, in its most primitive forms, embryoid bodies.

ICD-O code   9080/3

Epidemiology
It is the second most common malignant ovarian germ cell tumour {1802}, and can be pure or rarely as a component of a mixed germ cell tumour.

Clinical features
It is seen most frequently in the first three decades of life {1368}. The signs and symptoms are the usual ones associated with an adnexal mass. Low serum AFP levels may occur.

Macroscopy
It is typically unilateral, large, predominantly solid, fleshy, grey-tan in colour and may contain cysts, haemorrhage and necrosis {1382}.

Histopathology
Variable amounts of immature embryonal-type tissues, mostly in the form of neuroectodermal tubules and rosettes, but sometimes with a conspicuous component of cellular mitotically active glia, are admixed with ectodermal and endodermal elements, with varying degrees of maturation. The tubules are lined by overlapping, hyperchromatic cells with numerous mitoses and may be pigmented. Immature cartilage, adipose tissue, bone and skeletal muscle are often present. Endodermal structures including hepatic tissue, immature gastrointestinal tract and embryonic renal tissue are less common. The most primitive component of immature teratoma is in the form of embryoid bodies constituted by yolk sac epithelium and a germ disk whose epithelium resembles that of embryonal carcinoma (tumours dominantly composed of embryoid bodies have been termed polyembryoma). A conspicuous reactive vascular proliferation may be seen in immature teratomas

Table 1.2 Grading of ovarian immature teratomas using a three-tiered grading system compiled from {1382}

Grade	Histological criteria
Grade 1	Tumours with rare foci of immature neuroepithelial tissue that occupy < 1 low power field (40x) in any slide (low-grade).
Grade 2	Tumours with similar elements, occupying 1-3 low power fields (40x) in any slide (high-grade).
Grade 3	Tumours with large amount of immature neuroepithelial tissue occupying > 3 low power fields (40x) in any slide (high-grade).

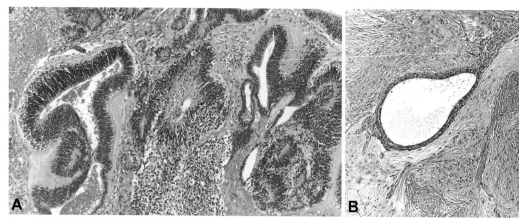

Fig. 1.59 A Immature teratoma. Immature neuroectodermal tubules co-exist with sheets of immature neural cells (lower centre). **B** Gliomatosis peritonei. Mature astrocytes from a peritoneal implant of gliomatosis peritonei occasionally may exist with foci of endometrial glands and stroma.

{98,1363}. Based on the relative amounts of immature neuroectodermal component, immature teratomas have been graded from one to three {1382}, but a two-tiered (low- and high-grade) system is now more commonly used {1401} (see Table 1.2, p. 61).

Immunohistochemistry
The intestinal and immature neural elements are SALL4 positive {1551}. SOX2 and glypican 3 are positive in the neuroepithelium. AFP may stain immature gastrointestinal-type glands.

Genetic profile
Immature teratomas probably originate from premeiotic germ cells {2172} and do not usually exhibit a gain of 12p or i(12p) {984,1596}.

Prognosis and predictive factors
Although chemotherapy has improved prognosis of immature teratomas, stage and grade of the primary tumour and metastases remain important predictive factors. In approximately one-third of cases, innumerable miliary nodules of mature

glia occur in the peritoneum (gliomatosis peritonei) and abdominal lymph nodes, but the prognosis remains favourable.

Mixed germ cell tumour

Definition
A tumour with two or more types of malignant, primitive, germ cell components. The most common admixture is that of dysgerminoma and yolk sac tumour.

ICD-O code   9085/3

Epidemiology
They represent about 8% of malignant germ cell tumours.

Clinical features
The average age of the patients is 16 years and about one-third of premenarchal girls affected have precocious pseudopuberty. LDH, AFP and β-hCG serum levels are usually elevated {21,1288}.

Histopathology
The individual components are similar to

those seen in pure form and may be intimately admixed or form relatively discrete zones within the neoplasm. Embryoid bodies (representing a component of immature teratoma) may be a component, usually being associated with overgrowth of the yolk sac or embryonal carcinoma epithelium. A panel of immunomarkers including OCT4, CD30, glypican 3 and GDF3 is useful for characterizing the tumour components {291,655}. The components present should be specified in the diagnostic report.

Prognosis and predictive factors
The proportion of each tumour type influences prognosis {626,1001,1802,1915}. Tumours composed of more than one-third yolk sac tumour, choriocarcinoma or grade 3 immature teratoma were historically associated with poor prognosis; however, with the advent of modern chemotherapy, differences in outcome have become less overt and stage is the most important prognostic factor {1058,1802,1915}.

Monodermal teratomas and somatic-type tumours arising from a dermoid cyst

J. Prat
D. Cao
S.G. Carinelli

F.F. Nogales
R. Vang
C.J. Zaloudek

Struma ovarii

Definition
A mature teratoma composed either exclusively or predominantly of thyroid tissue.

ICD-O codes
Struma ovarii, benign   9090/0
Struma ovarii, malignant   9090/3

Epidemiology
Struma ovarii is the most common type of monodermal teratoma {1604,2048}.

Clinical features
Most patients are in the reproductive years {1644,1645,2048}. The clinical findings are similar to those observed in patients with mature cystic teratoma. A rare patient has symptoms related to hyperfunction of the thyroid tissue. Up to one-third of patients have ascites.

Macroscopy
Struma ovarii is usually unilateral and solid. It varies in size but typically measures < 10 cm. The cut surface is beefy-red to brown or green and may be lobulated. Some tumours may be predominantly or, rarely, entirely cystic, sometimes containing soft, green-brown tissue {1873}.

Histopathology
Struma ovarii is typically composed of acini filled with colloid and resembling eutopic thyroid. Variations include intensely

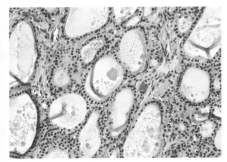

Fig. 1.60 Struma ovarii. The tumour is composed of acini lined by a single layer of eosinophilic, low-cuboidal cells with round nuclei and filled with colloid, as seen in the eutopic thyroid.

cellular regions composed of numerous tiny acini (microfollicular), sertoliform tubules as well as solid areas in which the cells may have abundant eosinophilic or clear cytoplasm {1874}. The acini may be separated by a prominent oedematous to less often fibromatous stroma. In those that have gross cysts, microscopic examination shows them to be lined by cuboidal cells with non-descript features, whose nature may only be proven by immunohistochemistry {1873}. Occasional tumours have a prominent band of lutein cells at the periphery.

Most thyroid-type carcinomas arising in struma are of the papillary type, including its follicular variant, followed by follicular carcinoma {613,1604,1640}. Whether malignant struma ovarii should be diagnosed based on the same criteria used for tumours in the eutopic thyroid is unclear. Struma ovarii associated with recurrence or extra-ovarian metastasis that histologically resemble non-neoplastic thyroid tissue have been designated "highly differentiated follicular carcinomas" {1635}. This entity, however, had previously been considered benign strumosis {879}.

Tumour cells show immunohistochemical expression of thyroglobulin and TTF1.

Genetic profile
BRAF mutations and RET/PTC rearrangements, as seen in papillary thyroid carcinoma of the eutopic thyroid, have been identified in papillary thyroid carcinoma arising in struma ovarii {179,1698}.

Prognosis and predictive factors
Most cases of typical struma ovarii are benign. The outcome of histologically and biologically malignant thyroid-type tumours in struma is favourable {1604,1739}; only a small subset of patients with thyroid-type carcinomas in struma ovarii die of disease {1640}. The size of the strumal component correlates with malignant outcome, and abundant peritoneal fluid, numerous adhesions or ovarian serosal defects are more common in clinically malignant tumours {1604,1647,1739}. In general, however, it is not possible to reliably determine which cases will develop progressive disease {1740}.

Carcinoid

Definition
Well-differentiated neuroendocrine neoplasms that resemble carcinoids of the gastrointestinal tract.

ICD-O codes
Carcinoid   8240/3
     Strumal carcinoid   9091/1
     Mucinous carcinoid   8243/3

Synonym
Well-differentiated neuroendocrine tumour, grade 1

Epidemiology
Ovarian carcinoids are uncommon tumours {1805}.

Clinical features
The patients range in age from 14-79 years (mean, 53 years) {97,1599,1602,1603}. Many tumours are incidental findings. One-third of insular carcinoids have been associated with the carcinoid syndrome despite the absence of metastases {415,1599,1805}.

Macroscopy
The tumours are unilateral and range from uniformly solid to being represented by a nodule/mass within a dermoid cyst, struma ovarii or, rarely, a mucinous cystic tumour. Mucinous carcinoids may have a glistening cut surface.

Histopathology
Insular carcinoid is the most common type of primary ovarian carcinoid tumour (26–53%). It is composed of small acini and solid nests of uniform, polygonal cells with round or oval, centrally located hyperchromatic nuclei. The acini are often at the periphery of the solid nests, but may punctuate them. Trabecular

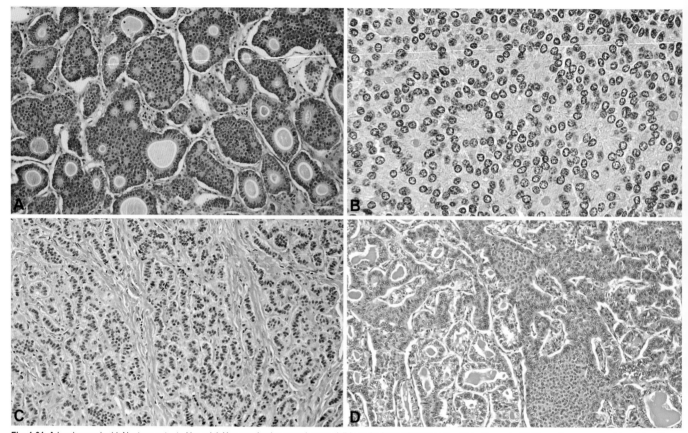

Fig. 1.61 **A** Insular carcinoid. Nests punctuated by acini. Neuroendocrine granules are visible at the base of many cells. **B** Insular carcinoid. The cells are arranged in acini and have abundant lightly eosinophilic cytoplasm. The nuclei are round, uniform, and display a "salt and pepper" chromatin. **C** Trabecular carcinoid. Cords and ribbons of tumour cells are separated by fibrous stroma. **D** Strumal carcinoid. The tumour has insular and trabecular patterns and colloid is seen.

carcinoid is less common (23-29%) and shows long, often wavy ribbons or parallel trabeculae of cells surrounded by fibrous stroma. The designation of strumal carcinoid refers to an insular or trabecular carcinoid associated with struma ovarii (26–44%). The carcinoid and strumal components can be relatively discrete or intimately admixed. Strumal carcinoid differs from non-strumal forms by having a frequent component of intestinal-type mucinous glands (approximately 40% of cases). The tumour cells of carcinoids have lightly eosinophilic cytoplasm, often with identifiable, basally located red to brown argentaffin granules and round and regular nuclei with stippled chromatin. Mucinous (goblet cell) carcinoid is rare and shows numerous small glands or acini lined by uniform columnar or cuboidal epithelium with variable numbers of goblet cells, some cells containing red to brown argentaffin granules and small round or oval to compressed nuclei. Atypical and carcinomatous forms with variable microscopic features have been described {97}. Stroma in carcinoids can

be striking and often fibromatous.

Immunohistochemistry
Carcinoids are positive for one or more neuroendocrine markers (variable extent and intensity) and often for CDX2 {2161}. Insular and trabecular carcinoids are CK7 positive and CK20 negative; in contrast, mucinous carcinoids more frequently show a CK7(-)/CK20 diffuse profile {1968}. In strumal carcinoids, TTF1 and CK7 are usually expressed in the strumal component with no expression in the carcinoid component {1550}.

Histogenesis
These tumours are considered monodermal teratomas.

Prognosis and predictive factors
Insular, trabecular and strumal carcinoids are almost invariably benign {415,1603,1888}, while mucinous carcinoids, particularly if associated with atypical features, may have an aggressive behavior {30,97,1887}.

Neuroectodermal-type tumours

Definition
Tumours consisting exclusively or almost exclusively of neuroectodermal tissue with similar morphology and differentiation as neuroectodermal tumours of the central nervous system. Less often these tumours resemble peripheral-type tumours (Ewing sarcoma/primitive neuroectodermal tumour).

Epidemiology
These tumours are rare {944,1304,1848, 1942}.

Clinical features
Tumours occur in patients with a wide age-range (6–69 years), but most are young. They are typically unilateral {239,1304}. Most patients present with abdominal/pelvic pain or an abdominal mass {944,1304}. Other presenting symptoms include menstrual irregularity, weight loss and signs of excess androgens {944}.

Macroscopy

The tumours are typically large, solid or solid and cystic {944,1304,1942}. The solid component is soft and grey to white. The cysts may contain papillary excrescences. Haemorrhage and necrosis may be prominent {944}.

Histopathology

These tumours are morphologically identical to their counterparts of the central or peripheral nervous system. They are divided into differentiated, primitive and anaplastic groups {944}. The differentiated group includes ependymoma, astrocytoma and oligodendroglioma. The primitive tumours are neuroectodermal tumours (PNETs), neuroblastoma, ependymoblastoma, medulloblastoma and medulloepithelioma. Glioblastoma multiforme represents the anaplastic group. In contrast to the other differentiated tumour types, ependymoma is only rarely associated with a teratoma {944,1848,1942}. Primitive tumours of the central type may be associated with teratomas {944,1304}.

Immunohistochemistry

These tumours show immunoprofiles similar to their CNS or peripheral counterparts except ependymomas. Primary ovarian ependymomas are more likely to express various cytokeratins, ER and PR {804}.

Histogenesis

Given the association of many with teratomas, most tumours are thought to originate from germ cells. The histogenesis of ependymomas as well as peripheral PNET is obscure.

Genetic profile

Peripheral PNET may show t(11;22) (q24;q12) {889}.

Prognosis and predictive factors

Clinical stage is the most important prognostic factor {944,1304}. Primitive and anaplastic tumours are more likely to present with extra-ovarian disease than differentiated tumours and consequently may pursue a more aggressive course {944,1304}.

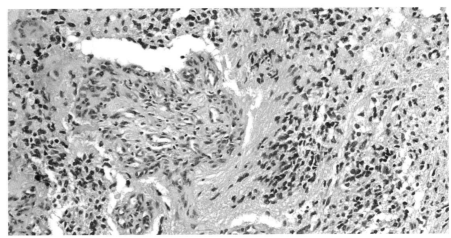

Fig. 1.62 Neuroectodermal-type tumour. Glioblastoma multiforme arising in mature teratoma. Microvascular proliferation is present.

Sebaceous tumours

Definition

Neoplasms resembling various forms of cutaneous sebaceous gland tumours (sebaceous adenoma, basal cell carcinoma with sebaceous differentiation, sebaceous carcinoma) that may arise within a dermoid cyst {317}.

ICD-O codes

Sebaceous adenoma   8410/0
Sebaceous carcinoma   8410/3

Epidemiology

These tumours are exceedingly rare.

Clinical Features

The patients are typically middle-aged to elderly and usually have symptoms referable to a pelvic mass.

Macroscopy

The tumours are predominantly cystic and are typically associated with a dermoid cyst.

Microscopy

The tumours are identical to their cutaneous counterparts with large numbers of mature, foamy or bubbly sebaceous cells that stain with oil red-O being their most distinctive feature.

Histogenesis

These tumours represent overgrowth of the sebaceous elements of a dermoid cyst.

Prognosis

Most tumours are benign, but those with features of carcinoma may be clinically malignant.

Other rare monodermal teratomas

Prolactinoma and corticotroph cell adenoma, responsible respectively for hyperprolactinema with amenorrhea and Cushing syndrome, may arise within a dermoid cyst and have a benign clinical course {77,866,1449}. Tumours resembling retinal anlage tumour have rarely been described, one of them having an association with an immature teratoma; these tumours are aggressive {934}. Rare cysts lined by mature glial tissue, ependymal, respiratory or melanotic epithelium also fall in the monodermal teratoma group.

Carcinomas

Squamous cell carcinoma

Definition
Malignant transformation of squamous epithelium within a dermoid cyst.

ICD-O code   8070/3

Epidemiology
Squamous cell carcinomas account for about 80% of cases of malignant transformation within a dermoid cyst {1496}.

Clinical features
The tumours occur over a wide age range (19–87 years, average 55 years) {282,467,687,1496}. They occur in patients two decades older than those with uncomplicated dermoid cysts.

Large tumours may present with signs and symptoms related to adherence to surrounding organs {467,759,1809}. Diameter > 10 cm and elevated CEA in patients 45 years or older are suspicious of malignancy and imaging may be confirmatory {282,467}. Squamous cell carcinomas arising in dermoid cyst are typically unilateral {1506}.

Macroscopy
Tumours are typically large, solid or solid and cystic and may have a recognizable component of dermoid cyst. They may protrude into the wall of the cyst or be represented by thickening of the cyst wall {282,467}.

Histopathology
Various patterns of squamous cell carcinoma may be seen, ranging from conventional, well differentiated, keratinizing to poorly differentiated, sometimes having a prominent component of cells with abundant eosinophilic cytoplasm, to anaplastic (including sarcomatoid) {1506,1809}. Extension through the wall of the parent dermoid cyst and overt extra-ovarian spread are common {919}.

Histogenesis
They arise from the squamous epithelium of dermoid cysts.

Prognosis and predictive factors
Prognosis is highly dependent on stage and tumours limited to the ovary have a favourable outcome. The overall 5-year survival is 15–52% for all stages {759} and 75.7% for stage I tumours {282,297,467,687}. Prognosis of patients with advanced disease is poorer than that of common ovarian cancer {282,467,687,797}.

Others

Adenocarcinoma is the second most common malignancy arising in dermoid cysts accounting for 7% of cases {183, 354, 1496, 1559, 1583, 1863}, with most tumours arising from gastrointestinal {1082} and respiratory-type epithelium {1810,1863,1944,2064}. Mucinous cystadenomas arising within mature teratomas have a homozygous teratomatous genotype, supporting their germ cell origin, but by convention, are not considered in this group. Endodermal variants of mature teratoma lined exclusively by respiratory epithelium {331} and ovarian epidermoid cysts {525} may fall into the category of monodermal teratoma. Mesodermal derived tumours such as lipoma, composed of mature adipocytes with scattered benign sweat glands, may occur {608}. Glomus tumour may rarely arise within a typical dermoid cyst {1781}. Sarcomas account for 8% of cases of malignancies in dermoid cysts and are more often seen than squamous cell carcinoma in younger patients. Leiomyosarcoma, angiosarcoma {1357}, osteosarcoma {1348}, chondrosarcoma, fibrosarcoma, rhabdomyosarcoma and malignant fibrous histiocytoma have been reported {1710}. Primary ovarian melanomas are much less common than metastatic ovarian melanomas {414,684,1211}. Overall, one-half of the patients with stage I dermoid-associated melanoma are alive at two years {236}. Melanocytic naevi of various types may arise within a typical dermoid cyst {1012}. Pigmented progonoma and malignant tumours derived from retinal anlage within ovarian teratomas, have grossly pigmented areas that correspond to solid nests, tubules and papillae composed of atypical melanin-containing cells {699,934,1790}.

Germer cell - sex cord-stromal tumours

J. Prat
D. Cao
S.G. Carinelli
F.F. Nogales
R. Vang
C.J. Zaloudek

Gonadoblastoma, including gonadoblastoma with malignant germ cell tumour

Definition
A tumour consisting of a mixture of immature sex cord cells and germ cells which can be viewed as an "in situ" form of malignant germ cell tumour {1889}.

ICD-O code   9073/1

Epidemiology
Gonadoblastomas are rare.

Clinical features
It occurs predominantly in phenotypic females with gonadal dysgenesis and an abnormal karyotype, but also exceptionally in apparently normal females with a 46 XX karyotype. Gonadoblastoma is discovered in young patients (average 18 years). Most tumours are found when a patient is evaluated for primary or secondary amenorrhea or for an abnormally formed genital tract. Some are incidental findings or are discovered when adnexal calcifications are seen on imaging studies. More than half of female patients with gonadoblastoma are at least mildly virilised. More than 40% of gonadoblastomas are bilateral.

Macroscopy
Most tumours are small solid tan or white and measure up to 2–3 cm. A gritty cut surface is common. A gonadoblastoma can be a component of a larger mass, the latter representing an invasive, malignant germ cell tumour that has arisen from the gonadoblastoma.

Histopathology
The usual growth of gonadoblastoma is as rounded nests separated by fibrous stroma that contains lutein or Leydig cells in about two-thirds of cases. The nests are composed of sex cord-type cells that form small acini that encircle primitive germ cells {1707}. Hyalinization (basement membrane-type material) and

calcification may occur within the acini and the latter may become confluent (mulberry-like masses). The germ cells are similar to dysgerminoma cells. They are large and round with abundant clear or amphophilic cytoplasm, vesicular nuclei and prominent nucleoli. Mitotic figures may be present {208}. The sex cord cells have small dark nuclei and variable amounts of amphophilic cytoplasm. The acini may become distended by proliferating germ cells and in some cases early invasion of the stroma is identified as part of the progression to germinoma, which often arises in gonadoblastoma; rarely, yolk sac tumour, embryonal carcinoma and choriocarcinoma have also been reported.

The germ cells are positive for placental alkaline phosphatase, CD117 (c-Kit), and D2–40 (podoplanin), OCT-4, NANOG and SALL4 {229,290}. Cytoplasmic and membrane staining for TSPY is present in the germ cells {1089}. The sex cord-type cells usually stain with inhibin, calretinin, WT-1 and FOXL2, but they are negative for SOX9 {208,749}.

Histogenesis
Gonadoblastoma almost always arises in the abnormal gonads of an intersex individual, most of whom have a partial or complete Y chromosome. The tumour presumably arises from abnormal germ cells.

Genetic profile
FISH testing may reveal a Y chromosome {766} and the presence of the *TSPY1* region in all conventional gonadoblastomas arising in intersex individuals {752}. 12p abnormalities such as an

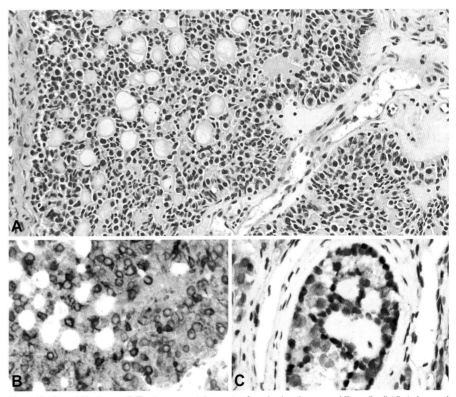

Fig. 1.63 Gonadoblastoma. **A** The tumour contains nests of predominantly sex cord-like cells distributed around hyalinized acini. Large germ cells are also visible in smaller numbers. **B** The germ cells in a gonadoblastoma are positive for germ cell tumour markers, in this case placental alkaline phosphatase (PLAP), while the sex cord-stromal cells are negative. **C** The sex cord-stromal cells show positive nuclear staining for FOXL2 while the germ cells are negative.

isochromosome have not been identified in gonadoblastoma, but few cases have been studied {372}.

Genetic susceptibility

Most patients have some form of gonadal dysgenesis. The most common karyotypes are 46 XY (Swyer syndrome) and 45X/46XY. A Y chromosome or a Y chromosome fragment is almost always present although rare patients with a 46 XX karyotype have been reported. Some patients with Turner syndrome can be shown to harbour Y chromosome material and they, like patients with gonadal dysgenesis, are at risk for gonadoblastoma. In situ hybridization studies performed on gonadoblastomas in patients with mosaic karyotypes show that the gonadoblastoma is derived from cells that have a Y chromosome. The GBY locus, a portion of the centromeric region of the long arm of the Y chromosome, contains the testis-specific protein Y 1 gene *(TSPY1)* which is associated with susceptibility to gonadoblastoma in patients with dysgenetic gonads {1040}. Several syndromes that include mutations in the Wilms tumour gene *(WT1)* can occur in patients with gonadal dysgenesis and be associated with gonadoblastoma, including the Frasier syndrome, the Denys-Drash syndrome and the WAGR syndrome; the association with gonadoblastoma is strongest with the Frasier syndrome {751}.

Prognosis and predictive factors

Pure gonadoblastoma is benign. The prognosis of tumours with malignant transformation is dependent on the tumour type, size and stage of the secondary component {1707}.

Mixed germ cell - sex cord-stromal tumour, unclassified

Definition

A neoplasm composed of germ cells and sex cord elements occurring in genetically and phenotypically normal females

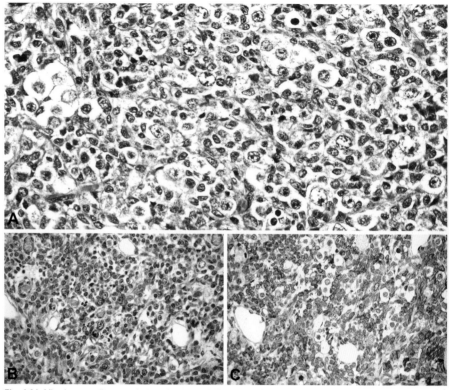

Fig. 1.64 Mixed germ cell-sex cord-stromal tumour. **A** The tumour is composed of an admixture of smaller sex cord cells and larger germ cells with clear cytoplasm in a haphazard fashion. **B** The germ cells react for c-Kit (CD117), while the sex cord-stromal cells are negative. **C** The sex cord-stromal cells show positive cytoplasmic staining for alpha-inhibin while the germ cells are negative.

and without the distinctive appearance of a gonadoblastoma {1889,1890}.

ICD-O code   8594/1

Epidemiology

These tumours are rare.

Clinical features

Most tumours occur in infants or children younger than 10 years. Occasionally, tumours are associated with isosexual pseudoprecocity.

Macroscopy

The tumours are typically large, unilateral, solid masses with a grey-pink or yellow to pale-brown cut surface.

Histopathology

Microscopically, the proportions of sex cord and germ cell components vary. Sex cord cells may form cords or trabeculae, hollow or solid tubules (sometimes resembling sex cord tumours with annular tubules), cysts or grow diffusely. The sex cord elements are typically immunoreactive for inhibin. The germ cells resemble dysgerminoma cells and are immunoreactive for PLAP, OCT4 and c-Kit protein {1261}.

Prognosis and predictive factors

Most of the lesions are clinically benign and development of malignant germ cell tumours and metastasis are rare {1889}. Dysgerminoma or another malignant germ cell tumour develops in about 10% of all patients, more frequently in post-pubertal patients {1889}.

Miscellaneous tumours

W.G. McCluggage   A. Malpica
D. Daya   E. Oliva
P. Ip   R.H. Young

Tumours of rete ovarii

Definition
Tumours arising from the rete ovarii.

ICD-O codes
Adenoma of rete ovarii   9110/0
Adenocarcinoma of rete ovarii   9110/3

Epidemiology
Rete ovarii cysts (cystadenomas) represent less than 1% of ovarian cysts {1654}. Adenomas are uncommon and adenocarcinomas are extremely rare {728,1366,1654}.

Clinical features
Rete cysts are most commonly seen in postmenopausal patients. Symptoms and signs include abdominal or pelvic discomfort/pressure, virilization, hirsutism, and pelvic mass. Adenomas are usually an incidental finding; the only case of rete ovarii adenocarcinoma presented with abdominal swelling and ascites in a 52 year old woman.

Macroscopy
Rete cysts are usually unilateral, unilocular, smooth-lined, and filled with serous fluid. They have ranged in size from 1–24, mean 8.7 cm. Adenomas are usually not grossly evident but rarely, have been seen as a solid or solid and cystic mass. The single reported case of adenocarcinoma of the rete ovarii was bilateral with 5.5 cm and 8.5 cm solid/cystic tumours.

Histopathology
Rete cysts are lined by bland, mitotically inactive, flat, cuboidal or columnar cells with scant eosinophilic cytoplasm. Rarely, cilia, focal transitional cell metaplasia and pseudostratification are seen. Adenomas are circumscribed lesions composed of closely packed tubules which can become cystic and contain simple papillae. Rare cases are exclusively papillary. The tubules are lined by bland, mitotically inactive cuboidal or columnar cells with a rare case exhibiting

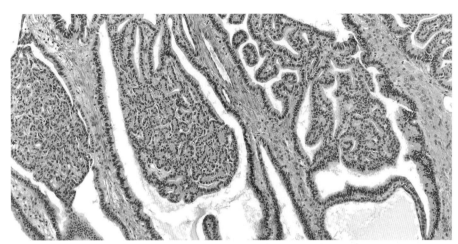

Fig. 1.65 Adenoma of rete ovarii. Closely packed tubules with cyst formation and simple papillae.

focal mild atypia. Adenocarcinoma of the rete ovarii shows a predominant retiform pattern with papillary areas and solid tubules. The tumour cells are atypical and exhibit mitotic activity.

Prognosis and predictive factors
Rete cysts and adenomas are benign. The only reported case of adenocarcinoma presented with advanced stage disease.

Wolffian tumour

Definition
A tumour of Wolffian origin, arising in the ovary or adjacent to it and expanding into it.

ICD-O code   9110/1

Synonym
Female adnexal tumour of probable Wolffian origin

Epidemiology
This is an uncommon ovarian neoplasm {1989,2120}.

Clinical features
Patients have ranged in age from 24–87 years; most are postmenopausal. Symptoms and signs include abdominal enlargement, abdominal pain, abdominal mass, postmenopausal vaginal bleeding and urinary frequency {528,2120}.

Macroscopy
Tumours are unilateral, solid or solid and cystic, grey-white, tan or yellow and have ranged in size from 2–20 cm.

Histopathology
A combination of the following patterns is seen: cysts of variable size (sieve-like pattern); closely packed, sometimes retiform, tubules; and solid foci in which the cells are somewhat spindled. The tumour cells are cuboidal or columnar, although those lining the cysts may be flattened. Hobnails cells can be seen. The cells are usually bland and mitotic rate is usually low.

Immunohistochemistry
The tumour cells are positive for broad spectrum cytokeratins and vimentin and often for calretinin. There is variable expression of cytokeratin 7, estrogen and progesterone receptors, SMA, CD10, androgen receptor, inhibin, c-kit and EMA. The tumour cells are usually negative for monoclonal CEA {528,1989}.

Histogenesis
The tumours are presumed to arise from Wolffian remnants in the adnexal region.

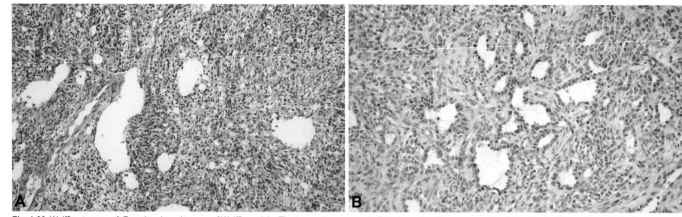

Fig. 1.66 Wolffian tumour. **A** Female adnexal tumour of Wolffian origin. The tumour is composed of tubular and solid arrangements of bland cells with ovoid to spindle shaped nuclei. **B** Typical sieve-like pattern.

Prognosis and predictive factors

This tumour is usually benign and confined to the ovary. However, rare cases have presented with advanced stage disease or behaved in a malignant fashion following resection. Features associated with malignant behaviour include cytological atypia and increased mitotic activity. Occasional tumours with minimal nuclear atypia and a very low mitotic rate have recurred {432,528,1557,2120}.

Small cell carcinoma, hypercalcaemic type

Definition

An undifferentiated neoplasm, predominantly composed of small cells, but occasionally with a large cell component, and which is often associated with paraneoplastic hypercalcaemia. The tumour is unrelated to small cell carcinoma of neuroendocrine (pulmonary) type.

ICD-O code   8044/3

Epidemiology

This is a rare tumour.

Clinical features

This neoplasm typically occurs in young women (mean age, 23 years), most commonly in the second and third decades, and is associated with paraneoplastic hypercalcaemia in two-thirds of cases {452,2116}. Most patients present with symptoms referable to an ovarian mass, although occasionally, presentation is with metastatic disease; symptoms due to hypercalcaemia are rare. There is usually unilateral ovarian involvement with extra-ovarian spread typically in the form of peritoneal disease in about one-half of cases.

Macroscopy

The tumours are usually large and predominantly solid, pale, white to grey. Necrosis, haemorrhage and cystic degeneration are common.

Histopathology

A diffuse growth pattern usually predominates, but in most cases there are focal follicle-like spaces containing luminal eosinophilic or rarely basophilic fluid {452,2116}. Nested, corded or trabecular growth may also be present. Spindle cell morphology is occasionally seen. Usually the nuclei are monotonous and hyperchromatic with coarsely clumped chromatin and small nucleoli. Mitotic activity is conspicuous and there are often areas of necrosis. In most cases, the tumour cells contain scant cytoplasm but occasionally it is focally clear. A component of large cells with abundant eosinophilic cytoplasm is also often present; it can be focal, predominant or exclusive (large cell variant). The large cells often have a rhabdoid appearance with eccentric nuclei, prominent nucleoli and glassy eosinophilic cytoplasm. Small foci of mucinous epithelium, either benign mucinous glands or cysts or, rarely, signet-ring cells are present in up to 15% of cases {2116}. Usually, the stroma is minimal but rarely there is an appreciable amount

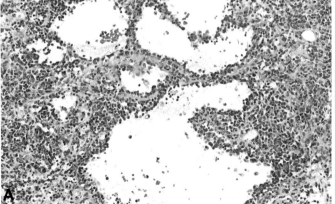
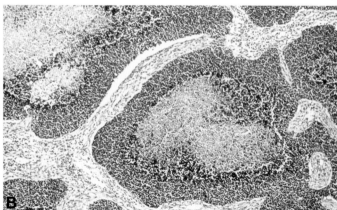

Fig. 1.67 A Small cell carcinoma, hypercalcaemic type. Small cells grow in sheets and are punctuated by follicle-like spaces. **B** Small cell carcinoma, pulmonary type. Aggregates of small cells with scant cytoplasm and conspicuous necrosis.

of myxoid or oedematous stroma. Most cases exhibit diffuse nuclear staining with antibodies against the N-terminal of WT1 {1223}. There is often focal staining with broad spectrum cytokeratins, epithelial membrane antigen, CD10 and calretinin {16,1223,1594}. Parathyroid hormone-related protein may be positive {452}. Flow cytometric studies have demonstrated that the cells are diploid {486}.

Histogenesis
The histogenesis is unknown, but thought to be epithelial.

Genetic susceptibility
Occasional familial cases have been reported. The familial tumours were often bilateral, in contrast to the usual unilateral involvement {452,1029,1118}.

Prognosis and predictive factors
These are highly aggressive neoplasms. Tumour stage is the most important prognostic factor. In the largest reported series, one-third of patients with stage Ia disease were alive and disease free 1–13 years post-surgery {2116}. The remainder either died of disease or had recurrent tumour. Almost all patients with a stage higher than Ia died of disease. Features in stage Ia tumours that were associated with a more favourable outcome included age > 30 years, a normal pre-operative calcium level, tumour size < 10 cm and an absence of large cells.

Small cell carcinoma, pulmonary type

Definition
A small cell carcinoma, resembling pulmonary small cell carcinoma of neuroendocrine type.

ICD-O code   8041/3

Synonym
Small cell carcinoma of neuroendocrine type

Epidemiology
This is a rare tumour.

Clinical features
Most patients are postmenopausal and present with symptoms referable to a pelvic or abdominal mass {490,581,662, 805,1099}.

Macroscopy
These tumours are typically large and predominantly solid, with frequent areas of necrosis. They are often bilateral and extra-ovarian spread is common.

Histopathology
The growth pattern is usually predominantly diffuse but nests, trabeculae, glandular and rosette-like structures are sometimes present. In most cases, a component of usual surface epithelial-stromal tumour, most commonly endometrioid or mucinous, is present {490,581,662,805,1099}. The tumour cells have round, ovoid or slightly spindled hyperchromatic nuclei, often with a "salt and pepper" chromatin and exhibit moulding. The cytoplasm is scant. There is usually abundant mitotic activity and frequent apoptosis. Necrosis is often conspicuous. Rarely these neoplasms arise in an ovarian teratoma {805,1099}. The tumours are variably positive with the neuroendocrine markers chromogranin, CD56, synaptophysin and PGP9.5. Chromogranin positivity may be very focal with punctuate cytoplasmic immunoreactivity. A diagnosis of small cell carcinoma of pulmonary type can be made in the absence of neuroendocrine marker positivity if the morphological appearance is typical. Small cell carcinoma of pulmonary type may be only focally positive (often punctuate cytoplasmic staining) or even negative with broad spectrum cytokeratins. Some cases exhibit nuclear immunoreactivity with TTF1 and this result does not indicate a metastasis from a pulmonary primary {662}. (See cervix, high-grade neuroendocrine carcinoma, p. 197)

Histogenesis
These are probably of surface epithelial-stromal origin in most cases.

Prognosis and predictive factors
These are highly aggressive neoplasms, which usually present at advanced stage and the overall prognosis is poor {490}.

Wilms tumour

Definition
A primary ovarian tumour with features similar to those of the kidney tumour of the same name.

ICD-O code   8960/3

Synonym
Nephroblastoma

Epidemiology
These are rare with less than five cases reported {820,1427,1488,1667}.

Clinical features
This tumour has been reported in children and adults in the third and sixth decades. Symptoms and signs include abdominal pain with or without abdominal distension, pelvic or abdominal mass and ascites.

Macroscopy
The tumour is unilateral and in the reported cases has ranged from 12–19 cm. They are usually solid with cystic and necrotic areas but can present as a multilocular cyst.

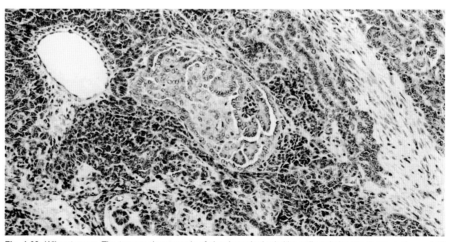

Fig. 1.68 Wilms tumour. The tumour shows a mix of closely packed primitive cells, tubular structures, a glomeruloid structure and spindle cells.

Histopathology

All cases have been found to contain a mix of blastema, epithelium (including tubular and glomeruloid structures) and mesenchymal tissue. No teratomatous elements or anaplasia have been reported.

Histogenesis

The tumours appear to originate from metanephric tissue, which is occasionally seen in the ovary, or primitive mesoderm.

Prognosis and predictive factors

All the reported patients have been alive with no evidence of disease after a follow-up that ranged from 6 months to 9 years {820,1427,1488,1667}.

Paraganglioma

Definition

A neuroendocrine neoplasm usually arising in specialized neural crest cells associated with autonomic ganglia (paraganglia).

ICD-O code   8693/1

Synonym

Phaeochromocytoma

Epidemiology

This is a rare tumour.

Clinical features

Patients with ovarian paraganglioma may present with symptoms referable to an ovarian mass or with hypertension secondary to elaboration of adrenaline or noradrenaline {494,533,1145,1229}. The age in the reported cases has ranged from 15–68 years {494,533,1145,1229}. Two cases, one a typical paraganglioma and the other a gangliocytic paraganglioma, were incidental findings within an ovarian teratomatous neoplasm {494,145}.

Macroscopy

The tumours ranged up to 22 cm and have been solid with a brown, tan or yellow colour. One case was an incidental microscopic finding in a teratoma {494} and another was grossly visible as a mural nodule in a teratoma {1145}.

Histopathology

They are composed of groups of polygonal cells with an epithelioid appearance arranged in nests ("zelballen") separated by stroma containing many thin-walled vascular channels. The polygonal cells usually have central regular nuclei and abundant granular eosinophilic or sometimes clear cytoplasm; multinucleate giant cells may be present. Mitotic activity is usually low.

The cells are positive with the neuroendocrine markers chromogranin, synaptophysin and CD56 and negative with cytokeratins and EMA. In some cases, S100 staining highlights a population of slender spindle shaped sustentacular cells around the periphery of the nests of polygonal cells {494,1229}. Some cases have been inhibin or calretinin positive {1229}.

Histogenesis

Two paragangliomas have arisen in a teratoma suggesting a germ cell origin for at least some tumours {494,1145}. An origin from extra-adrenal paraganglia in the region of the ovary, with subsequent expansion into the ovarian parenchyma is also a possibility.

Prognosis and predictive factors

In the only reported series of three cases, there was extra-ovarian involvement in two {1229}, but long-term follow up is lacking.

Solid pseudopapillary neoplasm

Definition

A tumour morphologically identical to the neoplasm of the same name in the pancreas.

ICD-O code   8452/1

Synonym

Solid and pseudopapillary tumour

Epidemiology

This is a rare tumour.

Clinical features

Patients have ranged in age from 17–57 years and presented with non-specific symptoms related to an ovarian mass {294,448}.

Macroscopy

Tumours are often large (> 10 cm). They have a solid and cystic cut surface, the former being friable and yellow to tan {294,448}.

Histopathology

The neoplastic cells grow in sheets and nests, and less frequently in cords and pseudopapillae. The nests and sheets are surrounded by septa that may be hyalinized and contain a delicate vascular network. The pseudopapillae have myxoid or myxohyaline cores and are lined by one to several cell layers. Microcysts filled with colloid-like material may be present. Cells have moderately abundant pale (sometimes foamy) to bright eosinophilic cytoplasm often containing paranuclear vacuoles and intracellular (as well as extracellular) eosinophilic globules. Nuclei are uniform and round, may contain grooves, and have dispersed chromatin and typically rare to absent mitoses ({294,448}.

Tumour cells show nuclear and cytoplasmic β-catenin positivity and lack E-cadherin. They are diffusely CD56 positive

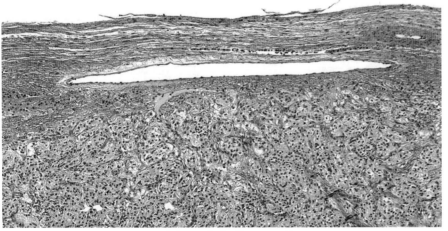

Fig. 1.69 Ovarian paraganglioma composed of nests of cells with an organoid arrangement.

and can be focally CD117 (membranous) and CD10 positive but negative for cytokeratins, chromogranin, inhibin and calretinin {294,448}.

Prognosis and predictive factors
One of three patients with follow-up died of disease and that tumour exhibited necrosis and lymphovascular invasion and had a much higher mitotic rate than the other reported neoplasms {294,448,1870}.

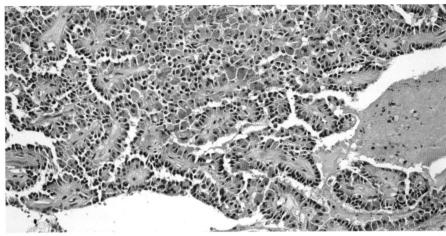

Fig. 1.70 Solid pseudopapillary neoplasm. The tumour exhibits a pseudopapillary architecture and the tumour cells contain abundant eosinophilic globules.

Mesothelial tumours

W.G. McCluggage   A. Malpica
D. Daya   E. Oliva
P. Ip   R.H. Young

Adenomatoid tumour

Definition
A rare, benign, ovarian tumour of mesothelial origin.

ICD-O code   9054/0

Synonym
Benign mesothelioma

Epidemiology
These are not associated with asbestos exposure.

Clinical features
In the ovary, it is often an incidental finding but occasionally presents with symptoms referable to a pelvic mass {2128}.

Macroscopy
Most are small and located in the hilus. They are usually solid but may be multicystic.

Histopathology
They are composed of multiple anastamosing gland-like spaces and tubules with cytoplasmic vacuoles containing basophilic material {2128}. The spaces can be dilated or alternatively tiny and mimic signet-ring cells, or there may be solid growth. The spaces are lined by a single layer of cuboidal or attenuated cells. There is minimal nuclear atypia or mitotic activity. The cytoplasm is usually relatively scanty but occasionally is abundant and eosinophilic {1501}.

Immunohistochemistry
The cells are positive for mesothelial markers such as calretinin, CK5/6, WT1, HBME1 and thrombomodulin {1673,1705}.

Histogenesis
They are of mesothelial origin.

Prognosis and predictive factors
These are benign lesions.

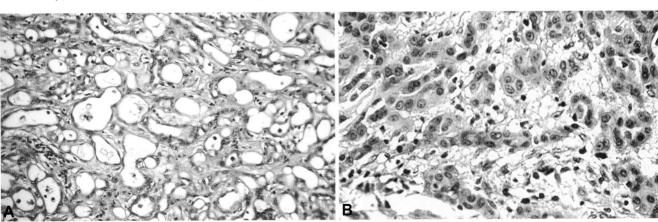

Fig. 1.71 A Ovarian adenomatoid tumour composed of small tubular structures many of which are dilated. **B** Ovarian mesothelioma composed of cords and tubules lined by cells with abundant eosinophilic cytoplasm.

Mesothelioma

Definition
A malignant, mesothelial neoplasm.

ICD-O code
9050/3

Epidemiology
Mesothelioma may be associated with asbestos exposure.

Clinical features
The patient age ranges from 16–63, median 52 years {349}. Symptoms are usually referable to an ovarian mass, such as abdominal or pelvic pain, or abdominal swelling.

Macroscopy
Tumours are typically bilateral, solid and of variable size {349}.

Histopathology
There is usually involvement of both the ovarian surface and parenchyma {95,349,1158}. The neoplasms may be exclusively epithelial-type with papillary, tubular/glandular and solid patterns, or biphasic (epithelial and sarcomatoid-types). The cells in epithelial-type are usually cuboidal with modest amounts of eosinophilic cytoplasm and exhibit only moderate nuclear atypia and a relatively low mitotic rate. The spindle-cell elements range from relatively bland to high-grade.

Immunohistochemistry
Mesotheliomas usually stain for calretinin, CK5/6, WT1, HBME1, thrombomodulin, D2–40 and, sometimes, h-caldesmon, but are typically negative for BerEP4, MOC31, B72.3, LeuM1 and ER {71,367,1041,1434}.

Histogenesis
These lesions are of mesothelial origin.

Prognosis and predictive factors
Outcome is likely similar to its peritoneal counterpart.

Soft tissue tumours

W.G. McCluggage
D. Daya
P. Ip
A. Malpica
G.P. Nielsen
E. Oliva
R.H. Young

Myxoma

Definition
A benign, mesenchymal neoplasm composed of bland spindle-shaped cells embedded in an abundant myxoid matrix.

ICD-O code
8840/0

Epidemiology
This is a very rare tumour.

Clinical features
Most occur in reproductive aged women with symptoms and signs related to an ovarian mass and they are typically unilateral {487}.

Macroscopy
Tumours have ranged from 5–22, mean 11 cm, and have a soft, gelatinous cut surface, sometimes with cystic degeneration.

Histopathology
These neoplasms are paucicellular and composed of bland cells with spindle or stellate-shaped nuclei and scanty cytoplasm, sometimes with tapering cell processes. The cells are embedded in an abundant myxoid matrix which often contains many delicate blood vessels. Focally, the stroma may be collagenous. There is little or no mitotic activity. The stromal matrix stains with alcian blue and is sensitive to pretreatment with hyaluronidase. The tumour cells are positive for smooth muscle actin, but desmin, S100, cytokeratins and epithelial membrane antigen are negative {376,377}.

Histogenesis
It has been speculated that some of these represent massive myxoid change of ovarian stromal tumours {376}.

Prognosis and predictive factors
When strict criteria are applied, these tumours are benign.

Others

A variety of other soft-tissue tumours have been reported arising as primary ovarian neoplasms. All are rare and the morphological features are identical to when these occur at more usual locations. Tumours reported include leiomyoma, haemangioma, neural tumours, lipoma, lymphangioma, epithelioid angiomyolipoma, chondroma, osteoma, ganglioneuroma, fibromatosis, leiomyosarcoma (including myxoid variants), angiosarcoma, low-grade fibromyxoid sarcoma, extra-renal rhabdoid tumour, osteosarcoma, chondrosarcoma, rhabdomyosarcoma and synovial sarcoma {1076,1351,1354,1355, 1357,1364,1391,1799,2036}.

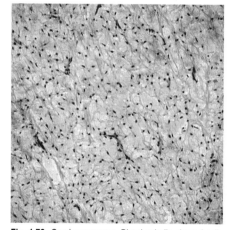

Fig. 1.72 Ovarian myxoma. Bland spindle-shaped cells are present in a myxoid stroma containing thin-walled blood vessels.

Tumour-like lesions

W.G. McCluggage A. Malpica
D. Daya E. Oliva
P. Ip R.H. Young

Follicle cyst

Definition
A physiological cyst lined by granulosa cells, usually underlain by theca cells.

Synonyms
Follicular cyst; functional cyst

Epidemiology
Follicle cysts have three peaks; in the neonatal period, around the time of the menarche and the premenopausal era. Most occur in the reproductive years {411,2103}.

Clinical features
Most follicle cysts are asymptomatic but vague abdominal symptoms may be present. Rarely, they may rupture and result in intra-abdominal haemorrhage. Large neonatal cysts may be complicated by torsion. Isosexual pseudoprecocity may be seen in older children {10}. They may be a component of McCune-Albright syndrome and also may be associated with pseudoprecocity in these cases {411}.

Macroscopy
Follicle cysts are usually solitary, ranging from 3–8 cm in diameter. They have a smooth surface and thin walls and contain clear fluid. Those associated with the McCune-Albright syndrome may be multiple and bilateral.

Histopathology
These cysts are lined by one to several layers of granulosa cells, which typically have moderately conspicuous eosino-philic cytoplasm; theca cells are usually present beneath the granulosa cells. The granulosa cells may be denuded resulting in an apparent lining of only theca cells.

Histogenesis
Follicle cysts usually develop as a result of disordered hypothalamic-pituitary-ovarian function, with abnormal levels of luteinizing or follicle stimulating hormones or due to exogenous hormonal agents.

Prognosis and predictive factors
Most symptomatic follicle cysts resolve spontaneously or with administration of hormonal preparations. Neonatal follicle cysts usually regress spontaneously in the first four months except if associated with McCune-Albright Syndrome in which instance they may recur, as may symptoms of pseudoprecocity.

Corpus luteum cyst

Definition
A cystic corpus luteum > 3 cm in diameter.

Epidemiology
These are common.

Clinical features
Corpus luteum cysts usually affect women of reproductive age. They are rarely found in neonates and may follow sporadic ovulation in a postmenopausal woman. Most patients are asymptomatic. Some may have a palpable adnexal mass or abnormal menstrual bleeding. Occasionally the cyst may rupture and result in pain and intra-abdominal haemorrhage {693,2014}.

Macroscopy
The lumen is usually filled with blood while the wall is convoluted and yellow.

Histopathology
The wall is composed of a thick, convoluted layer of large luteinized granulosa cells and a discontinuous layer of smaller luteinized theca interna cells.

Histogenesis
Excessive haemorrhage in a corpus luteum after ovulation results in a delay in involution with resultant cystic change.

Prognosis and predictive factors
Corpus luteum cysts usually resolve spontaneously.

Large solitary luteinized follicle cyst

Definition
A large, unilateral and solitary cyst occurring during pregnancy or the puerperium and lined by luteinized cells, including some with bizarre nuclei.

Epidemiology
They are typically discovered during late pregnancy or the puerperium.

Clinical features
The cyst usually presents as a palpable

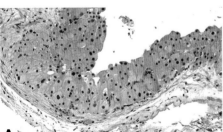
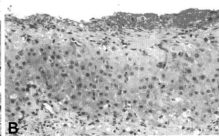
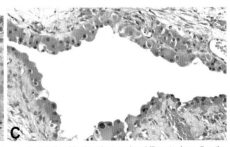

Fig. 1.73 A Follicle cyst. The cells lining the cyst have abundant eosinophilic cytoplasm. **B** Corpus luteum cyst. Luteinized granulosa cells with abundant eosinophilic cytoplasm line the cyst. **C** Large solitary luteinized follicle cyst. Luteinized granulosa cells including a few cells with large atypical nuclei are present lining the cyst.

adnexal mass. There are no endocrine manifestations. Large cysts may undergo torsion or rupture {527}.

Macroscopy
These are large (mean size, 25 cm), unilocular, thin-walled and contain watery fluid.

Histopathology
The cyst is lined by one to many layers of granulosa cells with typically copious eosinophilic to vacuolated cytoplasm. They may invaginate into the wall of the cyst and may be associated with a usually inconspicuous theca cell component. Typically, some cells have large pleomorphic hyperchromatic nuclei which are mitotically inactive {336}.

Histogenesis
It is unknown, but postulated to result from an abnormal response to hCG stimulation.

Prognosis and predictive factors
All patients have had an uneventful outcome following surgical removal.

Hyperreactio luteinalis

Definition
Bilateral enlargement of the ovaries due to numerous luteinized follicle cysts, occurring during pregnancy or ovulation induction (ovarian hyperstimulation syndrome).

Synonym
Multiple follicle cysts

Epidemiology
Overall this is uncommon, but more frequently encountered in patients undergoing infertility treatment.

Clinical features
Pregnant women, with either a normal singleton or multiple pregnancies may be affected. In 10–40% of cases there is associated gestational trophoblastic disease. Hyperreactio luteinalis may also complicate in-vitro fertilization, referred to as ovarian hyperstimulation syndrome, and be seen in rhesus isoimmunization and fetal hydrops {1291}. Patients may be asymptomatic but ovarian enlargement is detected during pregnancy, at Caesarean section or, rarely, in the puerperium. It may be complicated by torsion, rupture and intra-abdominal haemorrhage. Virilization, but not of the female infant, has been reported in 15% of patients and is related to elevated testosterone {1993}. Ovarian hyperstimulation syndrome may occur after ovulation induction by administration of FSH, hCG, or clomiphene. Severe cases are usually seen in those who have successfully conceived, in which the ovaries are huge and there may be massive ascites and/or hydrothorax. Haemoconcentration with secondary oliguria and thromboembolic phenomena is a life-threatening complication in these cases {703}.

Macroscopy
The ovaries are enlarged, up to 15 cm. They contain multiple thin-walled cysts ranging from 1–4 cm that are filled with clear or bloody fluid.

Histopathology
The cysts are found within an oedematous stroma in which clusters of luteinized stromal cells are present. The cysts are lined by markedly luteinized granulosa cells, in turn mantled by prominent theca cells, which are also luteinized.

Histogenesis
It is associated with conditions accompanied by elevated hCG levels, such as

gestational trophoblastic disease, fetal hydrops and multiple gestations. Germline mutations involving the FSH receptor and subsequent undue activation have been described in recurrent ovarian hyperstimulation syndrome {439,1977}.

Genetic profile
FSH receptor missense mutations involve the transmembrane serpentine domain, and result in decreased ligand specificity, leading to activation of the receptor by hCG and thyroid-stimulation hormone {1608}.

Prognosis and predictive factors
Regression typically occurs during the puerperium but may take up to six months postpartum. Other examples regress spontaneously during pregnancy, while others, particularly those secondary to gestational trophoblastic disease, may persist for longer despite normalization of hCG. Treatment is needed only in cases of massive haemorrhage or ovarian infarction.

Pregnancy luteoma

Definition
One or more hyperplastic nodules of large, luteinized cells developing during the latter half of pregnancy and involuting spontaneously during the puerperium.

Synonym
Luteoma of pregnancy

Epidemiology
It is an uncommon, tumour-like lesion of pregnancy.

Clinical features
The patients are typically in their third or fourth decade and 80% are multiparous {1381,1584,1831}. Most are asymptomatic and it is usually an incidental finding during Caesarean section or postpartum tubal ligation. There may be hirsutism or virilisation of the mother in 25% of cases, and 70% of female infants born to masculinized mothers are also virilized due to elevated testosterone {606,740}.

Macroscopy
These are discrete, solid, tan to brown, haemorrhagic nodules ranging up to 20, mean 7 cm. In half of the cases, there are multiple lesions, and one-third of cases are bilateral.

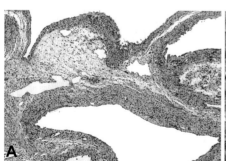
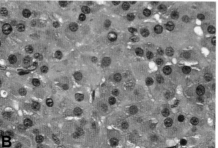

Fig. 1.74 A Hyperreactio luteinalis. Two of many cysts have the characteristics of a follicle cyst. **B** Pregnancy luteoma. The mass is composed of a uniform population of polygonal cells with round nuclei that have finely granular chromatin and medium-sized nuclei. The cytoplasm is abundant and eosinophilic and frequently contains small vacuoles. Although none are shown here, occasional mitotic figures are typically present in luteomas of pregnancy. No crystals of Reinke are seen.

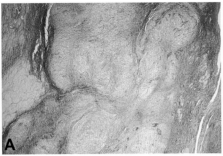
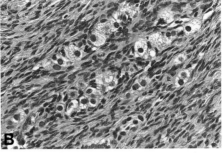

Fig. 1.75 A Stromal hyperplasia. Nodules of stromal cells involve the ovarian parenchyma. **B** Stromal hyperthecosis. Luteinized cells with abundant vacuolated cytoplasm and round nuclei are embedded in the background ovarian stromal cells.

Histopathology

The nodules are typically large, well circumscribed and uniformly solid, but there may be spaces containing colloid-like fluid. The cells are luteinized with ample eosinophilic, lipid-poor cytoplasm, central nuclei, often with prominent nucleoli and can be mitotically active (up to 7 mitoses/10 HPF). Intracellular hyaline globules are occasionally found {963}. Lesions taken out in the postpartum period appear different. Typically, they show regressive changes characterized by a degenerative appearance of the lesional cells; the eosinophilic cytoplasm being replaced by frothy pale cytoplasm. Additionally, collagenous bands tend to be conspicuous {210A}.

Histogenesis

Their occurrence during pregnancy implicates a role for hCG but this is unlikely to be the only factor, as they have not been described in gestational trophoblastic disease or early pregnancy, when the serum hCG is at its highest level.

Prognosis and predictive factors

These are benign and undergo spontaneous postpartum regression.

Stromal hyperplasia

Definition

A non-neoplastic, benign proliferation of ovarian stromal cells without associated luteinized stromal cells.

Epidemiology

This is an uncommon lesion.

Clinical features

Typically an incidental finding in perimenopausal or postmenopausal women, but rarely presents with androgenic or estrogenic manifestations {175}.

Macroscopy

Both ovaries may be normal in size or slightly enlarged. The cortex, medulla or both may be expanded by ill-defined white or yellow nodules or there may be diffuse enlargement with a firm, whitish to pale yellow cut surface.

Histopathology

There is a dense proliferation of uniform, small, oval to spindle-shaped, stromal cells with scanty non-luteinized cytoplasm replacing the ovarian medulla and less frequently the cortex with a vaguely nodular or diffuse growth. Pre-existent ovarian structures may be present, especially in early stages. Luteinized cells are not present in the ovarian parenchyma (otherwise this is referred to as stromal hyperthecosis) but Leydig cell hyperplasia can be seen at the hilus.

Stromal hyperthecosis

Definition

Presence of luteinized cells in the ovarian stroma, typically associated with stromal hyperplasia.

Epidemiology

It has been documented in approximatly one-third of patients > 55 years old in autopsy studies.

Clinical features

This occurs in the reproductive age and in postmenopausal women. Patients may be asymptomatic but frequently present with endocrine manifestations, more often androgenic premenopausal and estrogenic postmenopausal. Patients with androgenic manifestations may have insulin intolerance, hyperinsulinemia, obesity and hypertension {1684}.

Macroscopy

The ovaries may be normal in size or enlarged (up to 8 cm). On sectioning, the parenchyma is firm and tan to yellow and vague nodules may be noted.

Histopathology

The luteinized stromal cells are seen as single cells, clusters and rarely nodules < 1 cm.

Histogenesis

Hormonal factors, including hyperinsulinism, overproduction of androgens and abnormal gonadotropins appear to play a role.

Genetic susceptibility

Rarely, stromal hyperthecosis can be familial {857} or may be associated with HAIR-AN syndrome (hyperandrogenism (HA), insulin resistance (IR) and acanthosis nigricans (AN) {108,476}.

Prognosis and predictive factors

This is a benign process.

Fibromatosis

Definition

A tumour-like enlargement of one or both ovaries due to a fibroblastic proliferation associated with collagen deposition within the ovarian stroma. There is typically preservation of pre-existing ovarian structures {2122}. This process is unrelated to fibromatosis of soft-tissue type, which rarely involves the ovary.

Epidemiology

This is a rare lesion.

Clinical features

Patients are typically premenopausal and present with menstrual abnormalities, abdominal pain or androgenic manifestations {2122}. Rarely, patients may have ascites {1426}.

Macroscopy

One (80%) or both ovaries can be affected. They are enlarged (average 8 cm) with a smooth nodular surface. They have a firm, white to grey cut surface that may contain variably sized cysts {2122}.

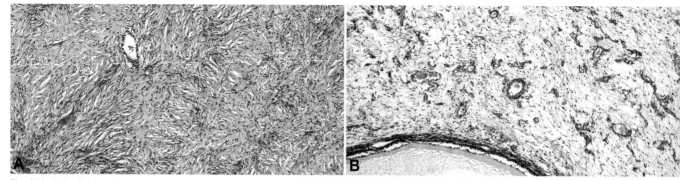

Fig. 1.76 A Ovarian fibromatosis. A hypocellular fibroblastic proliferation of banal spindle cells is associated with collagen production that entraps a pre-existing inclusion cyst. **B** Massive ovarian oedema. Abundant oedema fluid is present within the ovarian stroma. It is also surrounding a pre-existing ovarian follicle.

Histopathology

There is partial (more commonly involving the cortex) or diffuse (more frequent) involvement of the ovary by bland spindle cells forming short intersecting fascicles, sometimes with a storiform pattern, associated with variable amounts of collagen deposition. The fibroblastic proliferation is typically of low cellularity and reminiscent of a paucicellular fibroma. It typically spares pre-existing follicles and other ovarian structures. Oedema, luteinized stromal cells or focal sex cord-like proliferations can be seen {586,2122}.

Histogenesis

It is thought to be of ovarian stromal origin {2122}.

Prognosis and predictive factors

This is a benign lesion.

Massive oedema

Definition

A tumour-like enlargement of one or both ovaries due to accumulation of oedema fluid within the ovarian stroma, usually with preservation of pre-existing follicles {2122}.

Epidemiology

This is a rare lesion.

Etiology

When idiopathic, it is thought to be related to ovarian torsion, as in approximately 50% of cases torsion of the ovarian pedicle is noted {1371,2122}.

Clinical features

It usually affects reproductive-age women (average 22 years) who present with abdominal pain (frequently acute), abdominal swelling and rarely hormonal (including androgenic) manifestations or Meigs-like syndrome {1371,2122}. Ninety percent of cases are unilateral and 10% bilateral. The right ovary is more commonly affected than the left.

Macroscopy

The ovaries are variably enlarged (average 8 cm) and have a smooth surface. On sectioning, an oedematous cut surface exuding watery fluid is seen. Areas of haemorrhage and subcapsular cysts, representing pre-existing follicles, are often present {1371,1633,2122}.

Histopathology

Abundant oedema replaces ovarian stroma with preservation of pre-existing ovarian structures and sometimes sparing the outer cortex {2122}. Luteinized stromal cells and foci of fibromatous stroma can occasionally be seen {1633,2122}. There are often dilated veins and lymphatics {1371,2122}. Massive oedema may be seen with other ovarian pathology, including benign and malignant (primary or metastatic) tumours {116}.

Prognosis and predictive factors

This is a benign lesion.

Leydig cell hyperplasia

Definition

An increased number of Leydig cells in the hilar region of the ovary.

Synonym

Hilar cell hyperplasia

Clinical features

The lesion is most common in pregnant women or in the perimenopausal and postmenopausal age groups. Androgenic or estrogenic manifestations may be present and related to the degree of hyperplasia. This can be a physiological event due to elevated serum hCG or LH levels.

Macroscopy

The lesion is not grossly visible.

Histopathology

There are ill-defined nodules of Leydig cells within the ovarian hilus that may encircle nerve fibres and rete ovarii. The cells are typically polygonal with central round nuclei with prominent nucleoli and abundant eosinophilic cytoplasm that may contain lipofuscin pigment as well as Reinke crystals. Rarely, nuclear atypia, including hyperchromatic and multinucleate forms, may be seen. There may be associated stromal hyperplasia or stromal hyperthecosis.

Others

Other rare, ovarian, tumour-like lesions include granulosa cell proliferations of pregnancy, ectopic decidua, inflammatory and infectious lesions, autoimmune oophoritis, artefactual displacement of granulosa cells {107,347,1429,1990} and mesothelial hyperplasia. The latter occurs around and on the surface of the ovary in association with a variety of gynaecological disorders, particularly endometriosis {342,1429}. The most characteristic morphological appearance is of small, bland tubules, nests and cords of cells, sometimes with a linear arrangement, often embedded in fibrous tissue. In some cases, papillae and/or psammoma bodies are present. Rarely, the mesothelial cells may seem to exhibit lymphovascular invasion (likely an artefact) or are surrounded by spaces or clefts closely simulating lymphovascular invasion.

Lymphoid and myeloid tumours

J.A. Ferry
W.G. McCluggage
D. Daya
P. Ip
A. Malpica
E. Oliva
R.H. Young

Lymphomas

Definition
Malignant neoplasms composed of lymphoid cells.

Epidemiology
Primary ovarian lymphomas are rare. Less than 1% of lymphomas present with ovarian involvement {456,574} and less than 0.5% of neoplasms arising in the ovary are lymphomas. However, in countries where Burkitt lymphoma is endemic, this is a common type of childhood ovarian malignancy. Rare patients are HIV positive {1033} but most patients with ovarian lymphoma have no predisposing factors.

Clinical features
Ovarian lymphomas affect patients over a wide age range, from early childhood to advanced age, with the median age in the fourth or fifth decade {456,1973,2165}. The most common complaints are abdominal pain and increasing abdominal girth {456,1341,1973}. Some patients have weight loss, fatigue, fever or abnormal vaginal bleeding {456,2165}. Ascites is common {2165}. Occasionally, ovarian lymphomas are an incidental finding {1973}. The ovary can also be involved secondarily, in the setting of widespread systemic involvement or as a site of relapse; these scenarios are more common than primary ovarian lymphoma {1970}.

Macroscopy
Primary ovarian lymphoma is unilateral in the majority of cases {2165}. On gross examination, ovarian lymphomas range from microscopic (representing an incidental finding) {1973} to large neoplasms with a mean diameter of 8–15 cm in different series {1970,1973,2165}. They typically have an intact external surface, which may be smooth or nodular. The consistency ranges from soft and fleshy to firm and rubbery, depending on the degree of associated sclerosis. On sectioning, the tumours are usually white, tan or grey-pink. A minority have cystic degeneration, haemorrhage or necrosis. Secondary ovarian lymphomas are bilateral in approximately 50% of cases and are, on average, smaller than primary ovarian lymphomas {1970}.

Histopathology
The most common primary ovarian lymphoma is diffuse large B-cell type, followed by Burkitt lymphoma and follicular lymphoma {456}, with rare cases of B and T lymphoblastic lymphoma {972}. Adolescents and children almost always have diffuse, aggressive lymphomas, in-

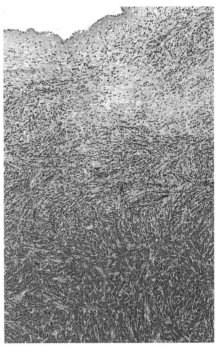

Fig. 1.78 Burkitt lymphoma. Low power shows a dense, diffuse infiltrate of lymphoid cells; the ovarian surface is uninvolved.

cluding Burkitt lymphoma, lymphoblastic lymphoma and diffuse large B-cell lymphoma {972,1970,2165}. Ovarian lymphomas typically obliterate the normal ovarian parenchyma but, on occasion, may spare corpora lutea, corpora albicantia, and developing follicles and a peripheral rim of uninvolved cortical tissue may be seen. Diffuse large B-cell lymphoma is the most common type of secondary lymphoma {1970}. Occasional ovarian lymphomas have been associated with dermoid cysts {601}.

Diffuse large B-cell lymphoma
The histological appearance of this lymphoma in the ovary is similar to that seen in extra-ovarian sites, although in the ovary there may be associated sclerosis and the neoplastic cells may occasionally grow in cords and clusters and mimic carcinoma or may have an elongate shape and grow in a storiform pattern, resembling a spindle cell sarcoma (see Table 1.3, p. 80) {1341,1973}.

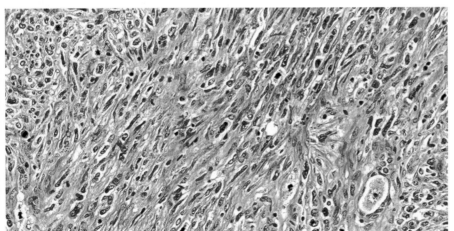

Fig. 1.77 Diffuse large B-cell lymphoma of the ovary. The lymphoma is associated with interstitial sclerosis and is composed of spindle cells, mimicking a spindle cell sarcoma. An entrapped ovum is seen in the lower right corner of the image.

Table 1.3 Haematolymphoid neoplasms of female reproductive organs

Type of lymphoma	Cellular composition	Usual immunophenotype*	Genetic features*	Differential diagnosis
B-cell lymphomas				
Diffuse large B-cell lymphoma	Centroblasts, immunoblasts, spindle cells and/or anaplastic large B-cells; sclerosis is common, especially in cervix and vagina	Monotypic sIg+, CD20+, bcl-6+/−, CD10−/+, bcl2+/−, MUM1/IRF4+/−, CD43+/−	*IGH* clonal, other changes variable	Poorly differentiated carcinoma; florid reactive lymphoid hyperplasia ("lymphoma-like lesion") especially in cervix; spindle cell sarcoma; sex cord tumour in cases with cord-like growth
Intravascular large B-Cell lymphoma	Centroblasts, immunoblasts	CD20+, subset CD5+	*IGH* clonal	Leukaemia, carcinoma
Follicular lymphoma	Mixture of centrocytes and centroblasts, follicular dendritic cells; sclerosis is common	Monotypic sIg+, CD20+, CD10+, bcl6+, CD5−, CD43−, cyclin D1−; Bcl2+/−	*IGH* clonal; t(14;18) (*IGH-BCL2*) found in some cases	Chronic inflammatory process
Extranodal marginal zone lymphoma of mucosa-associated lymphoid tissue (MALT lymphoma)	Marginal zone B-cells, small lymphocytes, plasma cells, reactive follicles, lymphoepithelial lesions	Monotypic sIg+, cIg+/− (IgM > IgG or IgA), CD20+, CD5−, CD10−, bcl6−, bcl2+, CD43−/+, cyclin D1−	*IGH* clonal; t(11;18)(q21;q21) (*API2-MALT1*), t(14;18)(q32;q21) (*IGH/MALT1*), t(1;14)(p22;q32) (*BCL10/IGH*) or t(3;14)(p14.1;q32) (*FOXP1/IGH*) in some cases; Trisomy 18 or trisomy 3 in some cases	
Burkitt lymphoma	Medium-sized atypical lymphoid cells with round nuclei, coarse chromatin, basophilic cytoplasm, numerous mitoses, tingible body macrophages	Monotypic sIgM+, CD20+, CD10+, bcl-6+, bcl-2−, Ki67~100%	*IGH* clonal; t(8;14), t(2;8) or t(8;22) (*MYC*); endemic cases: EBV+; sporadic and immunodeficiency-associated cases: minority EBV+	Other high-grade lymphomas
B lymphoblastic lymphoma	Small to medium-sized blasts with scant cytoplasm	CD19+, CD20−, TdT+, CD10+, CD3−, MPO−	*IGH* clonal; other changes variable	Other high-grade lymphomas

Burkitt lymphoma

Ovarian Burkitt lymphoma is most common among children and adolescents {972}, although occasional cases affect adults. Sporadic, endemic and immunodeficiency-associated Burkitt lymphoma may present with ovarian involvement. In contrast to other primary ovarian lymphomas, Burkitt lymphoma is often bilateral {1023}. The histological, immunophenotypic and genetic features are similar to those seen in other sites (see Table 1.3) {972,1023}.

Follicular lymphoma

Ovarian follicular lymphoma mainly affects older patients. Follicular lymphomas of all three grades occur in the ovary. Some follicular lymphomas have conspicuous diffuse areas {1023}.

Other rare Lymphomas

B and T lymphoblastic lymphomas rarely present with ovarian involvement {824,972,1973}. ALK-positive anaplastic large cell lymphoma presenting with an ovarian mass has been reported, although extra-ovarian involvement by lymphoma was also found on staging {307}. Involvement of the female reproductive organs by Hodgkin lymphoma is vanishingly rare; however, ovarian involvement by classical Hodgkin lymphoma in the setting of advanced stage disease has been documented {155}.

Genetic profile

See Table 1.3

Prognosis and predictive factors

With optimal treatment the prognosis appears similar to that of nodal lymphomas of comparable stage and histological type {443,1163,1973}. Among primary ovarian diffuse large B-cell lymphomas, features associated with an unfavourable outcome include bilateral ovarian involvement, large ovarian masses, widespread disease on staging, and high International Prognostic Index (IPI) score {2165}.

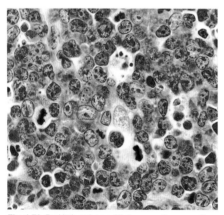

Fig. 1.79 Burkitt lymphoma. High power shows medium-sized, oval to slightly irregular cells with coarsely clumped chromatin and one to several nucleoli per cell. There are numerous mitoses and tingible body macrophages containing apoptotic debris.

Table 1.3 Haematolymphoid neoplasms of female reproductive organs (continued)

Type of lymphoma	Cellular composition	Usual immunophenotype*	Genetic features*	Differential diagnosis
Plasma cell neoplasms				
Plasmacytoma	Small mature plasma cells and/or large immature plasma cells; B lymphocytes and lymphoid follicles absent or very rare	CD138+, Pax5–, CD19–, monotypic cytoplasmic immunoglobulin+, IgG > IgA	Variable; EBV–	Marked chronic inflammation, B-cell lymphomas with plasma-cytic differentiation including plasmablastic lymphoma; poorly differentiated carcinoma
T and NK-cell lymphomas				
Peripheral T-cell lymphomas (PTCL)	Variable; small, medium-sized and/or large cells	Variable expression pan-T-cell antigens, often loss of one or more T-cell antigens, CD4 or CD8 often +	TCR clonal; other changes variable	For low-grade PTCL, chronic inflammatory process; for high-grade PTCL, other poorly differentiated neoplasms
T lymphoblastic lymphoma	Small to medium-sized blasts with round, irregular or convoluted nuclei, finely dispersed to dark chromatin, variably prominent nucleoli, scant cytoplasm and frequent mitoses.	CD3+, CD7+, TdT+, CD1a+, CD10+/–, often CD4/CD8 double+	TCR clonal; IGH clonal in a minority	Other high-grade lymphomas
Extranodal NK/T-cell lymphoma, nasal-type	Small, medium-sized and/or large atypical lymphoid cells, necrosis, vascular damage	cCD3+, CD2+, CD5–, CD56+, granzyme B+, perforin+	NK-lineage cases: TCR germline; EBV+	Other high-grade lymphomas; inflammatory process if necrosis is extensive and viable lymphoma is sparse
Hodgkin lymphoma				
Classical Hodgkin lymphoma	Reed-Sternberg cells and variants in a reactive background	CD15+/–, CD30+, CD20–/+, Pax5+, MUM1/IRF4+, CD3–	EBV+ in approximately half of cases	Other high-grade lymphomas if tumour cell are abundant; inflammatory process if tumour cells are scarce
Myeloid neoplasms				
Acute myeloid leukaemia, Myeloid sarcoma	Variably sized, usually medium-sized blasts with fine chromatin and nucleoli; maturing myeloid elements admixed in some cases	Lysozyme+, CD68+/–, MPO+, CD34+/–, CD117+/–, CD43+, CD20–, CD3–, CAE+	Varied	Large cell lymphoma; carcinoma, especially metastasis from the breast; extramedullary haemato-poiesis

EBV, Epstein-Barr virus; Ig, immunoglobulin; sIg, surface immunoglobulin; cIg, cytoplasmic immunoglobulin; IGH, immunoglobulin heavy chain gene; MPO, myeloperoxidase; TCR, T-cell receptor genes; CAE, chloroacetate esterase
*Most data derived from neoplasms outside the female genital tract

Plasmacytoma

Definition
A clonal proliferation of plasma cells that manifests as a localized growth.

ICD-O code   9734/3

Clinical features
The ovary is rarely involved by plasmacytoma. Ovarian involvement may occur in women with an established diagnosis of plasma cell myeloma or who subsequently develop myeloma. The ovary is rarely involved by apparently isolated extramedullary plasmacytoma {369,498,2168}. Patients usually present with symptoms related to the ovarian mass.

Macroscopy
Isolated extramedullary plasmacytomas are typically unilateral (rarely bilateral), solid tumours usually > 12 cm in diameter {498}. The left ovary appears more commonly involved than the right ovary.

Histopathology
Plasmacytomas are composed of relatively monotonous sheets of plasma cells, which may be small and mature with eccentrically placed nuclei with clock-face chromatin, moderately abundant cytoplasm and a distinct perinuclear hof. In other cases, the plasma cells are large and immature with more open chromatin and with distinct nucleoli, although still typically with an eccentric nucleus and cytoplasm with a recognizable hof.

Genetic profile
See Table 1.3, p. 80.

Prognosis and predictive factors
The prognosis for patients with ovarian plasmacytoma is dependent on whether they develop plasma cell myeloma; outlook is excellent if myeloma does not develop.

Myeloid neoplasms

Definition
Malignant neoplasms of haematopoietic origin, including myeloid leukaemias and myeloid sarcoma, a mass-forming lesion composed of primitive myeloid cells.

Synonyms
Myeloid sarcoma is also known as chloroma, granulocytic sarcoma or extramedullary myeloid tumour.

Clinical features
Myeloid sarcoma of the ovary is rare and patients of any age can be affected. Ovarian myeloid sarcoma may be an isolated finding, but in some cases, staging reveals bone marrow involvement by acute myeloid leukaemia or myeloid sarcoma in other extramedullary sites including breast and lymph nodes {605,1419}. Patients usually present with symptoms related to the ovarian mass.

Macroscopy
Ovarian involvement may be unilateral or bilateral. Lesions have measured from 5–14 cm in diameter {1419}. They are typically circumscribed with a lobulated, firm or fleshy cut surface and are sometimes green {1419}. Disease may be confined to the ovary, but there may be concurrent involvement of other sites within the female genital tract, including the fallopian tube and uterus {605}.

Histopathology
Neoplasms are composed of a diffuse population of primitive, medium-sized cells with oval or irregular nuclei, fine chromatin, distinct to prominent nucleoli and a scant to moderate amount of cytoplasm. Maturing cells with recognizable myeloid differentiation (indented nuclei, more abundant cytoplasm with distinct pink or red colour) may be seen. Primitive cells with folded nuclei and complex nuclear contours suggest monocytic differentiation of the tumour cells. In some cases, occasional eosinophil precursors are identified, which may be a clue to the myeloid lineage of the tumour {605}. Sclerosis is common, and may be fine or coarse. Neoplastic cells may infiltrate normal tissue in a single file pattern, thus potentially mimicking a metastasis from lobular carcinoma of the breast. Rarely there is a pseudoacinar pattern of growth. Mitoses are frequent in most cases. A minority of cases show zonal necrosis {605,1419}.

Genetic profile
See Table 1.3, p. 80.

Prognosis and predictive factors
Outcome is variable. Some patients die of acute myeloid leukaemia after a short period while others treated with therapy directed against acute myeloid leukaemia achieve a remission and have long-term disease-free survival {605,1419}.

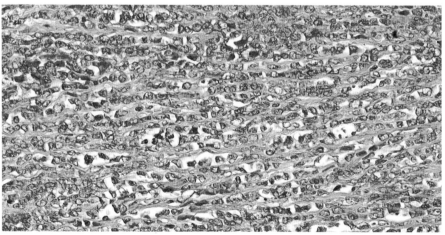

Fig. 1.80 Myeloid sarcoma of the ovary. Neoplastic cells have fine, pale chromatin and scant cytoplasm; they grow in cords and strands associated with delicate sclerosis, mimicking carcinoma.

Secondary tumours

R. Vang
A.N.Y. Cheung
F. Kommoss
X. Matias-Guiu
B.M. Ronnett
R.H. Young

Introduction

These are neoplasms that spread to the ovary from extra-ovarian sites. The proportion of malignant neoplasms of the ovary that are of metastatic origin varies according to the geographic region, ranging from 3–15% in western countries {426,443,1298,1795} to 21–30% in eastern nations {918,2063}. Metastases in the ovaries can present synchronously or metachronously with the primary neoplasm. In some cases, an ovarian mass represents the first manifestation of disease from a clinically occult non-ovarian primary.

As most of the challenging problems regard mucinous tumours, the features described herein pertain mainly to that histological type. Gross features that favour metastases include small size (often < 10–12 cm), bilaterality, a nodular growth pattern and presence of tumour on the surface and/or in the superficial cortex of the ovary {1061,1728,2086}. In contrast, primary ovarian tumours are unilateral and large (> 10–12 cm). Not infrequently, however, metastases can be large, unilateral and cystic, simulating a primary ovarian neoplasm. Histological features that favour metastases include an infiltrative growth pattern with stromal desmoplasia, a nodular growth pattern, involvement of the ovarian surface and superficial cortex and hilar and lympho-vascular space involvement {1061}. In contrast, primary ovarian tumours lack these features and have a confluent, glandular growth pattern. However, some metastatic carcinomas grow in confluent patterns. For endometrioid-like tumours, an adenofibromatous background, squamous differentiation and endometriosis favour primary ovarian origin. The presence of signet-ring cells almost invariably indicates metastatic carcinoma of gastrointestinal tract or breast origin, with rare exceptions {1232,1573,1968}. Certain features that might suggest origin of a neoplasm in the ovary are non-specific and can be seen in metastatic carcinomas, which include the finding of histologically benign-appearing and low-grade proliferative (cystadenomatous and borderline/ atypical proliferative type) mucinous epithelium and stromal luteinization.

For *Immunohistochemical Features* see Table 1.4, p. 85 {315,672,1963,1965}.

Intestinal tract

Definition
Metastatic colorectal adenocarcinoma.

Epidemiology
This is one of the most common secondary ovarian tumours {443,1194,918,1795}.

Clinical features
The age of most patients ranges from the fifth to ninth decades. A small percentage of patients present with adnexal masses (up to 10%).

Macroscopy
Up to 60% of tumours are bilateral with a mean size of 12.5 cm {418A,1036A, 1083A, 2086}. The cut surface is typically friable and/or cystic. Haemorrhage and necrosis are common.

Site of origin
Most originate from the large bowel or rectum but occasionally from the small bowel.

Histopathology
Most tumours are composed of glands of moderate size, but they range from small and tubular to large and cystically dilated {418A,1036A,1083A,857A}. A characteristic pattern, in which the epithelium is draped along the periphery of luminal eosinophilic necrotic material containing karyorrhectic debris ("garland pattern" with "dirty necrosis"), is often seen. There may be simple individual glands or, more often, a complex architecture with cribriform growth. The epithelium is typically stratified and highly atypical and is usually not overtly mucinous. Stromal condensation and luteinization around the glands is common.

For *Immunohistochemical features* see Table 1.4, p. 85.

Prognosis and predictive factors
These neoplasms qualify as stage IV disease and have a poor outcome, but isolated ovarian spread may be associated with prolonged survival {1063A}.

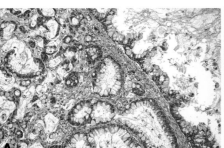
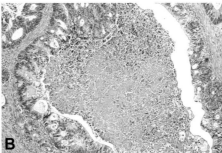
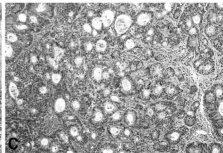

Fig. 1.81 Metastatic colonic carcinoma. **A** The appearance simulates a primary ovarian well-differentiated mucinous carcinoma. **B** Garland pattern with "dirty necrosis". **C** Cribriform pattern with endometrioid-like differentiation mimicking a primary ovarian endometrioid carcinoma.

Gastric

Definition
Metastatic gastric adenocarcinoma.

Synonyms
Krukenberg tumour (this designation refers to metastatic signet-ring cell carcinomas, which may originate from many anatomic sites, stomach most commonly)

Epidemiology
The relative frequency varies according to geographic population (more common in non-western countries) {965,1941,2063}.

Clinical features
The mean age is about 43 years. The majority of patients have symptoms related to an adnexal mass, with most of the remainder having gastrointestinal symptoms.

Macroscopy
The tumours are bilateral in approximately 80% of cases. Most tumours are large and solid with firm, white to yellow cut surfaces. Oedema may be conspicuous, particularly centrally.

Histopathology
Tumours are usually predominantly composed of signet ring cells {769,942}. However, glands, tubules, trabeculae, nests, sheets of cells {210}, and intestinal-type glands may be encountered {1077}. There is often a variably conspicuous stromal component which may range from densely cellular to acellular, resembling a fibroma, to strikingly oedematous. The oedema tends to be seen centrally. Stromal luteinization is relatively common.
For *Immunohistochemical features* see Table 1.4.

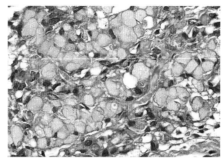

Fig. 1.82 Metastatic gastric carcinoma. The tumour is composed of numerous signet-ring cells (Krukenberg tumour).

Prognosis and predictive factors
These neoplasms qualify as stage IV disease and have a poor outcome.

Pancreatobiliary

Definition
Metastatic adenocarcinoma from the pancreas, gallbladder, or intra- or extrahepatic bile ducts, including Ampulla of Vater.

Epidemiology
This is a relatively uncommon secondary ovarian tumour {443,918,1194,1795, 1835A}.

Etiology
It spreads from a primary in the pancreaticobiliary system.

Clinical features
The reported mean ages range from 56–63 years. Patients frequently present with adnexal masses, but they may have abdominal pain or discomfort, vomiting, fever, chills, jaundice and/or weight loss.

Macroscopy
The tumours are often bilateral and range widely in size. They are usually solid and cystic masses, with or without surface involvement; however, uniformly solid or dominantly cystic masses may be seen, the latter mimicking a primary neoplasm.

Histopathology
They are usually composed of variably sized, well formed glands ranging from small and tubular to large and cystic {913,917,1253,2113,2126}. Well differentiated mucinous glands may be conspicuous. The glands may be infiltrative within a desmoplastic stroma or can form dilated cysts with simple or papillary architecture. Nuclear atypia can vary from minimal to marked. Rare metastases from pancreatic acinar cell carcinoma have been described {1953}. Metastatic neuroendocrine carcinomas from the pancreas also may occur rarely.

For *Immunohistochemical features* see Table 1.4 {838,1199,1901}.

Prognosis and predictive factors
These neoplasms qualify as stage IV disease and have a poor outcome.

Appendix

Definition
Ovarian involvement, secondary to a ruptured appendiceal, low-grade, mucinous neoplasm or adenocarcinoma.

Epidemiology
This is less common than metastatic colorectal or breast carcinoma {443, 918,1194,1795}.

Clinical features
These tumours typically occur in middle-aged women. Low-grade mucinous neoplasms usually present with abundant

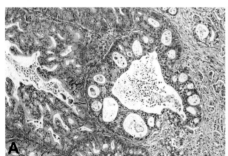
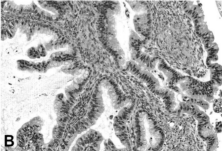
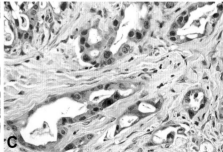

Fig. 1.83 Metastatic pancreatic carcinoma. **A** Mucinous glands and small nests and clusters irregularly infiltrating the stroma. **B** Mucinous differentiation with lack of overtly carcinomatous cytology and unaltered stroma mimics a primary ovarian mucinous tumour of borderline/atypical proliferative type. **C** Infiltrating glands of this type should always raise concern for metastasis.

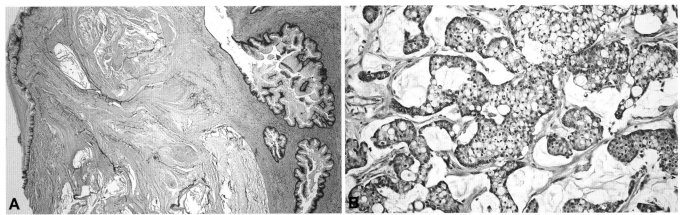

Fig. 1.84 A Secondary involvement by an appendiceal low-grade mucinous neoplasm. Note the dissecting mucin (pseudomyxoma ovarii) with hypermucinous cells. **B** Metastatic appendiceal carcinoma. The tumour is poorly differentiated and shows signet-ring cell differentiation. Note the extracellular mucin.

jelly-like mucinous material in the abdomen (pseudomyxoma peritonei) and variably prominent mucoid nodules of peritoneal tumour. Many women present with adnexal masses. Metastatic carcinoma often presents as a pelvic/adnexal mass or with generalized symptoms of abdominal disease.

Macroscopy

Both types of appendiceal tumours are bilateral in 90% of cases. Low-grade neoplasms involving the ovary have had a mean diameter of 15 cm. They are most often multicystic and mucoid. The mean size is 11 cm for metastatic carcinoma, and the cut surfaces are usually solid and firm; however, a cystic component may be present, particularly in low-grade carcinomas.

Histopathology

Involvement by low-grade mucinous neo-plasm usually shows abundant, dissecting, extracellular mucin (pseudomyxoma ovarii) and hypermucinous epithelium which forms haphazardly and irregularly distributed, incomplete glands that often exhibit retraction from the adjacent basement membrane {1620,1624}. Metastases of appendiceal carcinomas most commonly display a nested (goblet cell carcinoid-like) appearance and signet-ring cell differentiation but can have cords, trabeculae and intestinal-type glands {779,1619}.

For *Immunohistochemical features* see Table 1.4 {1621,1965}.

Prognosis and predictive factors

Low-grade mucinous neoplasms involving the ovary are more indolent and have a significantly better prognosis than metastatic appendiceal adenocarcinomas, which are usually high-grade and have a poor outcome {1620,1622}.

Breast

Definition

Involvement of ovary by a tumour that originates in the breast.

Epidemiology

Overall these are uncommon in surgical specimens, but common at autopsy {918,1298,1941}.

Clinical features

The mean age is 49 years. Patients can present with a pelvic mass, but most often the tumour is an incidental finding.

Macroscopy

Two-thirds of the tumours are bilateral. They are usually < 5 cm and typically solid. Large masses with cysts may be seen.

Table 1.4 Typical immunohistochemical features of primary and secondary ovarian tumours with endometrioid/endometrioid-like and/or mucinous differentiation

Primary site of origin	CK7	CK20	Dpc4	p16	PAX8, ER, PR
Ovarian	Positive (CK7 > CK20)*	Positive/negative (~75% of cases positive)*	Positive	Negative/ focal positive	Endometrioid: positive[†] Mucinous: ~50% positive[†]
Colorectal	Negative (~90% of cases)	Positive (CK20 > CK7)	Positive (~90% of cases)	Negative/ focal positive	Negative
Appendiceal	Negative (70–90% of cases)	Positive (CK20 > CK7)	Positive	Negative/ focal positive	Negative
Pancreatobiliary	Positive (CK7 > CK20)	Positive/negative (~80% of cases positive)	Negative (~50% of cases)[‡]	Negative/ focal positive	Negative
Gastric	Positive/negative	Positive/negative	Positive	Negative/positive	Negative
Endocervical	Positive (CK7 > CK20)	Negative/positive	Positive	Diffuse positive[¶]	PAX8 positive; ER/PR negative

*, A rare subset of primary ovarian mucinous tumours of teratomatous origin is CK7-negative/ CK20-positive; †, primary ovarian mucinous tumours are usually negative for ER and PR while endometrioid ones are often positive; ‡, loss of Dpc4 is relatively specific for pancreatobiliary origin, but retained expression does not exclude that origin; and ¶, HPV-related tumours are positive by in situ hybridization, and HPV-unrelated tumours lack diffuse p16 expression.

Histopathology

Ductal and lobular carcinomas represent 75% and 25% of metastases, respectively. A variety of growth patterns can be encountered, with ductal carcinomas often displaying glandular, papillary, cribriform or diffuse patterns and lobular carcinomas exhibiting characteristic single-file linear cords, trabecular and diffuse patterns, occasionally with signet-ring cell differentiation {594,2104}.

Immunohistochemistry

Breast carcinomas are usually diffusely positive for CK7 and often express ER, PR, GATA-3, mammaglobin and GCDFP-15, but are typically negative for CK20, PAX 8 and WT-1.

Prognosis and predictive factors

These neoplasms qualify as stage IV disease and have a poor outcome.

Others

Definition

Relatively common neoplasms in this category include metastatic adenocarcinomas of the endocervix and endometrium. Uncommon metastases include other carcinomas (lung, urinary bladder, kidney, and cervical squamous cell carcinoma, as well as other rare primary sites), melanoma, carcinoid, various non-gynecologic sarcomas, and uterine mesenchymal tumours (most notably, endometrial stromal sarcoma) and secondary involvement by malignant mesothelioma {2101}. The epidemiologic, clinical, macroscopic, histopathologic, and immunohistochemical features, and prognosis for these tumours vary depending on the primary site.

Epidemiology

These are uncommon to rare {443,918, 1194,1795}.

Clinical features

The clinical presentation may mimic that of

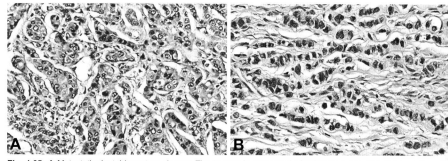

Fig. 1.85 A Metastatic ductal breast carcinoma. The tumour is composed of cohesive nests, trabeculae and cords. The histological features are non-specific and can suggest primary ovarian tumours, such as serous carcinoma. **B** Metastatic lobular breast carcinoma. The uniform tumour cells are arranged in single-file, linear cords.

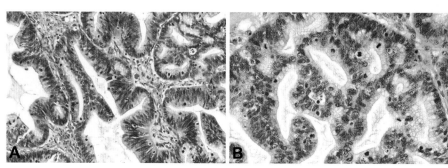

Fig. 1.86 Metastatic endocervical adenocarcinoma of usual type. **A** Confluent growth resembling a primary ovarian mucinous carcinoma (or endometrioid carcinoma with mucinous differentiation). **B** Hybrid endometrioid-like/mucinous differentiation with oval to columnar nuclei with coarse chromatin, basal apoptotic bodies and mitotic figures.

a primary ovarian neoplasm. Rare tumours in this group may occur in childhood.

Macroscopy

Endocervical adenocarcinomas involving the ovary are usually unilateral, and the mean size is 13 cm. Endometrial carcinomas involving the ovary are usually smaller than 5 cm and bilateral. Both types of tumours can be nodular, solid, and/or cystic.

Histopathology

Endocervical adenocarcinomas commonly exhibit variable admixtures of villoglandular, papillary, and confluent glandular growth patterns {493,1623}. The "usual type" endocervical adenocarcinomas are high-risk HPV-related and are characterized by glands exhibiting endometrioid and/or mucinous differentiation with enlarged, elongated, and hyperchromatic atypical nuclei, basal apoptotic bodies, and numerous apical mitotic figures. Rarely, endocervical adenocarcinomas are of the minimal deviation adenocarcinoma (adenoma malignum) subtype, which are unrelated to high-risk HPV.

The two most common histological types of endometrial carcinoma involving the ovaries are endometrioid and serous, resembling their uterine counterparts. For *Immunohistochemical features* see Table 1.4, p. 85 {1966,2019}.

Prognosis and predictive factors

Most ovarian metastases of endocervical adenocarcinoma have a favorable prognosis {1623}. Ovarian metastases of endometrial carcinoma qualify as FIGO stage IIIa endometrial tumours. The prognosis of other tumours depends largely on the primary site of origin.

CHAPTER 2

Tumours of the peritoneum

Mesothelial tumours

Epithelial tumours of Müllerian type

Smooth muscle tumours

Tumours of uncertain origin

Miscellaneous primary tumours

Tumour-like lesions

Secondary tumours

WHO Classification of tumours of the peritoneum[a,b]

Mesothelial tumours

Adenomatoid tumour	9054/0
Well-differentiated papillary mesothelioma	9052/0
Malignant mesothelioma	9050/3

Epithelial tumours of Müllerian type

Serous borderline tumour / Atypical proliferative serous tumour	8442/1
Low-grade serous carcinoma	8460/3
High-grade serous carcinoma	8461/3
Others	

Smooth muscle tumours

Leiomyomatosis peritonealis disseminata	8890/1

Tumours of uncertain origin

Desmoplastic small round cell tumour	8806/3

Miscellaneous primary tumours

Solitary fibrous tumour	8815/1*
Solitary fibrous tumour, malignant	8815/3
Pelvic fibromatosis	8822/1
Inflammatory myofibroblastic tumour	8825/1

Calcifying fibrous tumour	8817/0
Extra-gastrointestinal stromal tumour	8936/3
Endometrioid stromal tumours	
Low-grade endometrioid stromal sarcoma	8931/3
High-grade endometrioid stromal sarcoma	8930/3

Tumour-like lesions

Mesothelial hyperplasia	
Peritoneal inclusion cysts	9055/0
Transitional cell metaplasia	
Endometriosis	
Endosalpingiosis	
Histiocytic nodule	
Ectopic decidua	
Splenosis	
Others	

Secondary tumours

Metastatic carcinoma	
Low-grade mucinous neoplasm associated with pseudomyxoma peritonei	
Metastatic sarcoma	
Gliomatosis	

---

[a] The morphology codes are from the International Classification of Diseases for Oncology (ICD-O) {575A}. Behaviour is coded /0 for benign tumours, /1 for unspecified, borderline or uncertain behaviour, /2 for carcinoma in situ and grade III intraepithelial neoplasia and /3 for malignant tumours; [b] The classification is modified from the previous WHO classification of tumours {1906A}, taking into account changes in our understanding of these lesions; *These new codes were approved by the IARC/WHO Committee for ICD-O in 2013.

TNM and FIGO classification of tumours of the ovary, fallopian tube and primary peritoneal carcinoma

T - Primary Tumour

TNM	FIGO	
TX		Primary tumour cannot be assessed
T0		No evidence of primary tumour
T1	I	Tumour limited to the ovaries
T1a	IA	Tumour limited to one ovary (capsule intact) or fallopian tube surface; no malignant cells in ascites or peritoneal washings
T1b	IB	Tumour limited to one or both ovaries (capsules intact) or fallopian tubes; no tumour on ovarian or fallopian tube surface; no malignant cells in ascites or peritoneal washings
T1c	IC	Tumour limited to one or both ovaries or fallopian tubes with any of the following:
T1c1	IC1	Surgical spill
T1c2	IC2	Capsule ruptured before surgery or tumour on ovarian or fallopian tube surface
T1c3	IC3	Malignant cells in ascites or peritoneal washings
T2	II	Tumour involves one or both ovaries or fallopian tubes with pelvic extension below pelvic brim or primary peritoneal cancer
T2a	IIA	Extension and/or implants on uterus and/or fallopian tubes and/or ovaries
T2b	IIB	Extension to other pelvic intraperitoneal
T3 and/or N1	III	Tumour involves one or both ovaries or fallopian tubes, or primary peritoneal carcinoma, with cytologically or histologically confirmed spread to the peritoneum outside the pelvis and/or metastasis to the retroperitoneal lymph nodes
N1	IIIA1	Retroperitoneal lymph node metastasis only
N1a	IIIA1i	Lymph node metastasis up to 10 mm in greatest dimension
N1b	IIIA1ii	Lymph node metastasis more than 10 mm in greatest dimension
T3a	IIIA2	Microscopic extrapelvic (above the pelvic brim) peritoneal involvement with or without retroperitoneal lymph node
T3b	IIIB	Macroscopic peritoneal metastasis beyond the pelvis up to 2 cm in greatest dimension with or without retroperitoneal lymph node metastasis
T3c	IIIC	Macroscopic peritoneal metastasis beyond the pelvis more than 2 cm in greatest dimension, with or without retroperitoneal lymph node metastasis (excludes extension of tumour to capsule of liver and spleen without parenchymal involvement of either organ)
M1	IV	Distant metastasis excluding peritoneal metastasis
M1a	IVA	Pleural effusion with positive cytology
M1b	IVB	Parenchymal metastasis and metastasis to extra-abdominal organs (including inguinal lymph nodes and lymph nodes outside the abdominal cavity)

N — Regional Lymph Nodes

NX Regional lymph nodes cannot be assessed
N0 No regional lymph node metastasis
N1 Regional lymph node metastasis
N1a Lymph node metastasis up to 10 mm in greatest dimension
N1b Lymph node metastasis more than 10 mm in greatest dimension

M — Distant Metastasis

M0 No distant metastasis
M1 Distant metastasis
M1a Pleural effusion with positive cytology
M1b Parenchymal metastasis and metastasis to extra abdominal organs (including inguinal lymph nodes and lymph nodes outside the abdominal cavity)

pTNM Pathological Classification

The pT and pN categories correspond to the T and N categories.
pM1 Distant metastasis microscopically confirmed
Note: pM0 and pMX are not valid categories.

pN0 Histological examination of a pelvic lymphadenectomy specimen will ordinarily include 10 or more lymph nodes. If the lymph nodes are negative, but the number ordinarily examined is not met, classify as pN0.

Stage Grouping

Stage IA	T1a	N0	M0
Stage IB	T1b	N0	M0
Stage IC1	T1c1	N0	M0
Stage IC2	T1c2	N0	M0
Stage IC3	T1c3	N0	M0
Stage IIA	T2a	N0	M0
Stage IIB	T2b	N0	M0
Stage IIC	T2c	N0	M0
Stage IIIA1	T1/T2	N1	M0
Stage IIIA2	T3a	N0/N1	M0
Stage IIIB	T3b	N0/N1	M0
Stage IIIC	T3c	N0/N1	M0
Stage IV	Any T	Any N	M1

References

American Joint Committee on Cancer (AJCC) Cancer Staging Manual, 7th ed. (2011). Edge SB, Byrd DR, Compton CC, Fritz AG, Greene FL, Trotti III eds. Springer: New York

International Union against Cancer (UICC): TNM Classification of Malignant Tumours, 7th ed. (2009) Sobin LH, Gospodarowicz MK, Wittekind Ch eds. Wiley-Blackwell: Oxford

A help-desk for specific questions about the TNM classification is available at http://www.uicc.org.

Prat J, FIGO Committee on Gynecologic Oncology (2014). Staging classification for cancer of the ovary, fallopian tube, and peritoneum. Int J Gynaecol Obstet 124:1-5.

Mesothelial tumours

D. Daya   K.-R. Kim
A.N.Y. Cheung   J. Prat
S. Khunamornpong   R.H. Young

Adenomatoid tumour

Definition
A benign tumour of mesothelial origin.

ICD-O code   9054/0

Clinical features
These tumours may be seen at any age, but are usually found in adults. They may arise from extragenital peritoneum such as the omentum or mesentery. The more common sites are the fallopian tube, ovary and myometrium. The lesions are often an incidental finding.

Macroscopy
These typically appear as small firm nodules. Rarely, particularly when larger, they may show cystic change.

Histopathology
The tumour has a distinctive pattern, composed of mesothelial cells with cytoplasmic vacuoles and bland, round to oval nuclei with absent, or only rare, mitotic figures. The tumour is typically composed of anastomosing, gland-like spaces which show, at least to a minor degree, cystic dilatation. The second most common pattern is a solid arrangement of neoplastic cells which may have abundant eosinophilic cytoplasm; rarely, papillae may be encountered.
The neoplastic cells are typically positive for cytokeratin, vimentin, WT1 and calretinin, CK5/6, HBME1 and thrombomodulin. Differential diagnosis includes vascular tumours and metastatic carcinoma {2000,2083}.

Well-differentiated papillary mesothelioma

Definition
Well-differentiated papillary mesothelioma (WDPM) is a rare papillary tumour of mesothelial origin which typically exhibits an indolent behaviour.

ICD-O code   9052/0

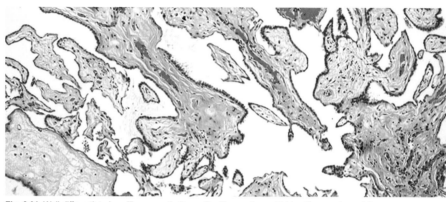

Fig. 2.01 Well-differentiated papillary mesothelioma. Papillary pattern with bland low-grade nuclei.

Clinical features
Eighty per cent occur in females, mostly in their reproductive years, but occasionally may occur in postmenopausal women. Well differentiated papillary mesotheliomas usually present as an incidental finding at laparotomy but rarely tumours are associated with abdominal pain and/or ascites {418,650,1154}.

Macroscopy
The tumours are usually solitary but may be multiple. They are grey to white, firm, papillary or nodular lesions, often < 2 cm.

Histopathology
Common patterns include papillary, tubulopapillary, adenomatoid-like areas and branching cords. The papillae are lined by a single layer of flattened to cuboidal mesothelial cells with bland nuclei. Mitoses are rare. Psammoma bodies are encountered in occasional cases. The main differential diagnoses include malignant mesothelioma, which may focally have a well differentiated papillary pattern, and serous borderline tumour/atypical proliferative serous tumour. The presence of stromal infiltration, areas of solid growth, extensive pseudostratification of nuclei, nuclear enlargement, more than mild atypia or more than a few mitoses is indicative of malignant mesothelioma.

Immunohistochemistry
Tumour cells are positive for EMA, CK7, CK5/6, Calretinin, D2–40 and HBME1.

In contrast to carcinoma, WDPMs are usually negative for CEA, B72.3, Ber EP4, Leu M1, ER, PR and MOC31 {111,286,318,1435}.

Histogenesis
The histogenesis is unknown but, in one series, there were two sisters who had exposure to asbestos {418}.

Prognosis and predictive factors
Tumours that tend to behave in a benign fashion are usually solitary, asymptomatic, occur as an incidental finding, are < 2 cm in diameter, are purely tubulopapillary and have low-grade nuclei {650}. When multiple, the behaviour is less clear but they may pursue an aggressive course in some cases.

Malignant mesothelioma

Definition
Malignant mesothelioma (MM) is a malignant tumour arising from the mesothelial lining of the peritoneal cavity.

ICD-O code   9050/3

Etiology
Over 80% of the patients in one series were men with occupational exposure to asbestos. In contrast, in two recent series of malignant mesotheliomas in women, there was no association with asbestos exposure.

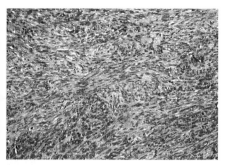

Fig. 2.02 Malignant mesothelioma. Sarcomatous pattern.

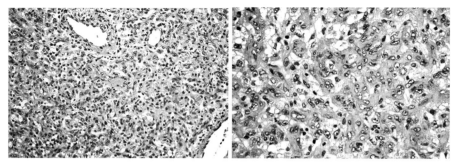

Fig. 2.03 Malignant mesothelioma. Low power showing ill-defined clusters (left). High power showing uniform cytology (right).

Clinical features

One-third of the patients are females, usually middle-aged or elderly. Occasional tumours may occur in young adults. Patients often present with abdominal discomfort, distension, digestive disturbances and weight loss. Ascites is present in the majority of cases {95}.

Macroscopy

The visceral and parietal peritoneum is usually diffusely involved by countless nodules and plaques.

Histopathology

The typical patterns, in order of frequency, are tubular, papillary and solid. Often they co-exist, especially the tubular and papillary types. In contrast to serous tumours of the peritoneum, the papillary pattern is usually less complex and cellular budding from the surface of the papillae is usually inconspicuous. The tumour cells are polygonal, cuboidal or low columnar and have a moderate amount of eosinophilic cytoplasm. Nuclear atypia is usually mild to moderate, although severe atypia may occur in occasional cases. Mitoses are present but may be inconspicuous. It is important to note that minor foci may resemble well differentiated papillary mesothelioma (WDPM) and therefore it may be difficult to distinguish between WDPM and MM in small biopsy specimens {95,650}.

Unusual variants include biphasic, sarcomatoid and deciduoid patterns. Invasion of subperitoneal tissue is usually present, often with dissection into the omental fat. Psammoma bodies are present in about one third of the tumours but are rarely as conspicuous as in serous carcinoma. Baker et al. {95} found necrosis in about one-third of their cases.

Immunohistochemical stains which may be helpful to establish the mesothelial nature of the lesion are discussed in the subsection on WDPM {1435}.

Prognosis and predictive factors

Cerruto et al. {255} found that biphasic tumours had a shorter survival than the epithelioid tumours. Favourable prognostic factors include an age < 60 years, low nuclear grade, low mitotic count, minimal residual disease after cytoreduction and lack of deep invasion. Rare tumours that are localized may also have a better prognosis.

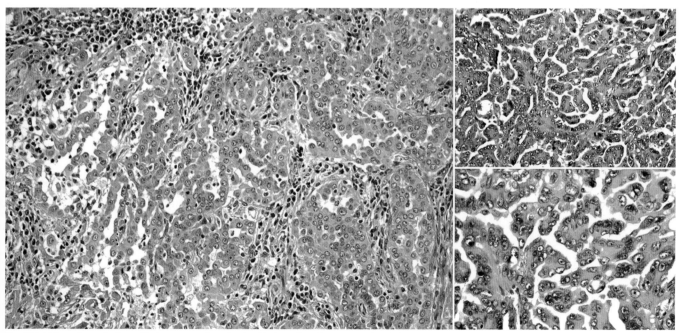

Fig. 2.04 Malignant mesothelioma. Most common pattern showing tubular and papillary pattern with relatively uniform nuclei.

Epithelial tumours of Müllerian type

D. Daya
A.N.Y. Cheung
S. Khunamornpong

K.-R. Kim
J. Prat
R.H. Young

Serous borderline tumour / Atypical proliferative serous tumour

Definition
Serous borderline tumours/atypical proliferative serous tumours (SBT/APSTs) are extra-ovarian neoplasms that resemble ovarian serous borderline/ atypical proliferative tumours.

ICD-O code   8442/1

Epidemiology
The age ranges from 16–67 years with a mean of 32 years.

Clinical features
Infertility and abdominal pain are the most common symptoms but one-third of tumours are incidental findings {124}. At surgery, the peritoneal lesions usually appear as fibrous adhesions or miliary granules that may be mistaken for peritoneal carcinomatosis {124}.

Histopathology
The tumour may resemble either the non-invasive epithelial or desmoplastic subtype of implants of ovarian SBT/APST. Psammoma bodies may be prominent {124}. Endosalpingiosis is commonly present {124}.

Histogenesis
See introduction to serous tumours / pelvic neoplasia, p. 15.

Prognosis and predictive factors
Prognosis is generally excellent although rarely invasive low-grade serous carcinoma of the peritoneum may develop {124}.

Serous carcinoma

Definition
A primary peritoneal tumour that resembles either low- or high-grade serous carcinoma of the ovary. Most are high-grade and are fundamentally different from low-grade serous carcinomas.

ICD-O codes
Low-grade serous carcinoma   8460/3
High-grade serous carcinoma   8461/3

Epidemiology
High-grade peritoneal serous carcinomas (HGPSCs) occur in women with a median age of 62 years. Approximately 15% of common epithelial ovarian cancers are actually "primary" peritoneal carcinomas {1701,1702}. The average age of patients with low-grade peritoneal serous carcinomas (LGPSCs) is 57 years {2017}. See introduction to serous tumours / pelvic neoplasia, p. 15.

Histopathology
LGPSCs are identical to invasive implants from serous borderline tumour/ atypical proliferative serous tumours (SBT/APSTs) but may be much more extensive and are typically characterized by a distinctive pattern of small nests of neoplastic serous cells as typifies low-grade serous carcinoma (LGSC) of the ovary. HGPSCs resemble their ovarian counterparts. Distinction of HGPSC from LGPSC is based primarily on the small, uniform nuclei present in LGPSC. In addition, the nested and papillary patterns with clefts of LGSC of the ovary contrast with the more varied histopathology of high-grade serous carcinoma (HGSC). {1153}. High mitotic activity favours a diagnosis of HGPSC. The distinction from malignant mesothelioma has been previously discussed. *Psammocarcinoma* is a poorly defined entity. It appears to encompass a group of lesions ranging from florid endosalpingiosis with limited epithelial proliferation to LGPSC with psammoma bodies occupying > 75% of the lesion and absent or rare, solid, epithelial proliferation {634,2017}. Because it appears to subsume a wide variety of epithelial proliferations, use of this term is discouraged as it probably represents just the extremely psammomatous end of the spectrum of LGPSC which can have no psammoma bodies and any number of psammoma bodies including the massive amount typical of so-called psammocarcinoma.

To diagnose primary peritoneal carcinoma, both ovaries and fallopian tubes must be grossly and microscopically normal or enlarged only by a benign process. From a practical viewpoint, the

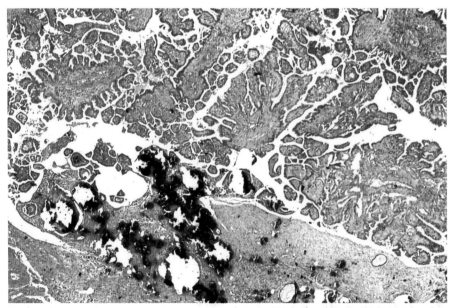

Fig. 2.05 Serous borderline tumour/atypical proliferative serous tumour of the peritoneum. The tumour resembles a mixed epithelial (top) and desmoplastic (bottom) non-invasive peritoneal implant. Psammoma bodies and larger calcified deposits are seen.

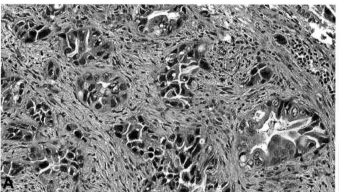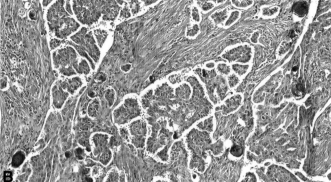

Fig. 2.06 **A** High-grade peritoneal serous carcinoma. The tumour cells show high nuclear-cytoplasmic ratio, nuclear pleomorphism and mitotic activity. **B** Low-grade serous carcinoma. The papillae are lined by tumour cells with small, uniform nuclei. The stroma is hyalinized and psammoma bodies are present. Qualitatively, the tumour resembles an "invasive implant" but quantitatively it is larger. Accordingly, these lesions are one and the same.

distinction of ovarian or tubal carcinoma from peritoneal carcinoma is not critical since the behaviour and treatment are similar (See introduction to serous tumours / pelvic neoplasia, p. 15).

Histogenesis
See introduction to serous tumours / pelvic neoplasia, p. 15.

Genetic profile
TP53 gene mutations and *BRCA* alterations occur commonly in HGPSC but *KRAS* and *BRAF* mutations are very infrequent {1701}. In contrast, LGPSC frequently has *KRAS* and *BRAF* mutations but lacks *TP53* mutations and *BRCA* abnormalities {1788,1789}.

Genetic susceptibility
Germline *BRCA1* mutations occur in HGPSC with a frequency comparable to the *BRCA1* mutation rate in high-grade ovarian serous carcinoma. Peritoneal high-grade serous carcinoma should be considered a phenotype of the familial breast and ovarian cancer syndrome {106}.

Prognosis and predictive factors
The staging, treatment and prognosis are similar to those of ovarian serous carcinoma. Low-grade peritoneal serous carcinomas rarely progress to high-grade tumours. Low-grade peritoneal serous carcinoma is less responsive than high-grade serous carcinoma to chemother-

apy; therefore cytoreduction appears to be more effective treatment. High-grade peritoneal serous carcinoma is treated the same as its ovarian and tubal counterparts.

Others

Endometrioid carcinoma, clear cell carcinoma, mucinous carcinoma, transitional cell carcinoma, squamous cell carcinoma and carcinosarcoma of the peritoneum have been reported but are very rare {1862,1879,2057}. See corresponding sections in chapter on tumours of the ovary.

Smooth muscle tumours

D. Daya
A.N.Y. Cheung
S. Khunamornpong

K.-R. Kim
J. Prat
R.H. Young

Leiomyomatosis peritonealis disseminata

Definition
This is a rare, benign, proliferative lesion, forming multiple nodules of smooth muscle within the peritoneal cavity.

ICD-O Code   8890/1

Synonym
Diffuse peritoneal leiomyomatosis

Epidemiology
The majority of patients are middle-aged, premenopausal women, who are often

pregnant or are in the postpartum period, although exceptional cases have been reported in postmenopausal women {28,1744}.

Etiology
The cause of the disease is unknown, although excessive stimulation by female gonadal steroid hormones, including estrogen and progesterone, seems to have a role, as the disease occurs mostly in women and is commonly associated with pregnancy {578,707}, the use of oral contraceptives and rarely with estrogen-producing ovarian tumours {471,2034}.

Clinical features
Patients are often asymptomatic, although they sometimes present with non-specific symptoms.

Macroscopy
Multiple, discrete, smooth-surfaced and variably sized nodules or masses are scattered over the peritoneum and in the omentum, mimicking peritoneal carcinomatosis. The lesions are small, generally < 1 cm. The cut surface of the lesion is analogous to that of a uterine leiomyoma.

Histopathology
Early lesions show submesothelial

proliferation of smooth muscle, and the proliferation progressively expands to form solid nodules. The nodules consist of histologically bland smooth-muscle cells with little or no mitotic activity. Endosalpingiosis and endometriosis may be in continuity with the nodules. Decidual cells are often admixed with smooth muscle cells in pregnant patients. Nuclear atypia or pleomorphism is usually absent, but a few cases showing malignant transformation have been reported {1027,1744,2066}.

Prognosis and predictive factors

The primary treatment objective is decreasing hormonal stimulation, including cessation of the use of oral contraceptives or hormone replacements, avoidance of pregnancy, the use of a gonadotrophin-releasing hormone analogue or

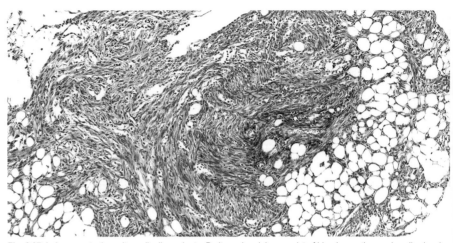

Fig. 2.07 Leiomyomatosis peritonealis disseminata. Peritoneal nodules consist of bland smooth-muscle cells showing a fasciclular arrangement.

an aromatase inhibitor {326,1882}. Surgical excision or removal of the ovaries

should be considered when conservative therapy is ineffective.

Tumours of uncertain origin

D. Daya
A.N.Y. Cheung
S. Khunamornpong
K.-R. Kim
J. Prat
R.H. Young

Desmoplastic small round cell tumour

Definition

Desmoplastic small round cell tumour is a rare, malignant neoplasm showing proliferation of "small round blue cells" that typically involves the abdominal and/or pelvic peritoneum.

ICD-O code   8806/3

Epidemiology

Patients are usually 15–30 years old at the time of presentation; the tumour has a strong male predominance (male-to-female ratio 4:1).

Clinical features

Most of these tumours occur in the abdominopelvic peritoneum, with exceptional cases having been reported in the head and neck region {557,1450}, pancreas {1548}, scrotum and ovary {404,1442,1462}. Patients commonly present with vague abdominal pain and/or distension, a palpable mass, weight loss and other symptoms related to obstruction of the intestinal or urinary tract.

Macroscopy

Tumours are variably sized, firm, white masses often accompanied by necrosis and occasionally by cystic change.

Histopathology

The tumour consists of aggregates of cells sharply surrounded by desmoplastic stroma. The patterns range from sheets to discrete islands, sometimes with a vaguely basaloid appearance, to small clusters and single cells. The tumour cells are uniform, small to medium in size with round,

oval or spindle-shaped hyperchromatic nuclei. There are numerous mitotic figures. The cell borders are indistinct with scanty cytoplasm. Immunohistochemically, the tumour cells are immunoreactive for a wide range of epithelial, mesenchymal and neural markers, including cytokeratin, EMA, desmin, vimentin, WT1 (against c-terminus) and NSE.

Genetic profile

Cytogenetically, this tumour has a unique chromosomal translocation, t(11;22)

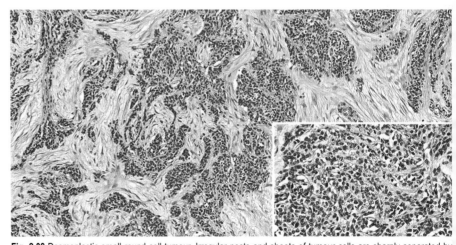

Fig. 2.08 Desmoplastic small round cell tumour. Irregular nests and sheets of tumour cells are sharply separated by desmoplastic stroma. (Inset) Undifferentiated tumour cells show small, round to oval, hyperchromatic nuclei with a scanty amount of cytoplasm.

(p13;q12), that results in the EWS-WT1 fusion protein which can be detected by the reverse transcriptase polymerase chain reaction (RT-PCR) or by fluorescent in situ hybridization (FISH). These molecular hallmarks may help to distinguish it from other small round cell tumours.

Prognosis and predictive factors
Because of the rarity of this tumour and its unusually aggressive presentation, treatment has not been standardized. Complete surgical excision seems to offer the best results, but benefit of postoperative adjuvant chemotherapy and/or radiotherapy has not been established. Two-year event-free survival and overall survival have been reported as 14.4% and 50%, respectively {1500}.

Miscellaneous primary tumours

D. Daya
A.N.Y. Cheung
S. Khunamornpong
K.-R. Kim
J. Prat
R.H. Young

Solitary fibrous tumour

Definition
A mesenchymal tumour of fibroblastic origin with prominent haemangiopericytoma-like vessels.

ICD-O codes
Solitary fibrous tumour   8815/1
Solitary fibrous tumour, malignant 8815/3

Epidemiology
Primary solitary fibrous tumours (SFTs) of the peritoneum (visceral and parietal) are uncommon; only approximately 50 cases have been reported in the English literature {1897,2107}.

Clinical features
Men and women are equally affected. The patient age ranges from 17–78 years (mean 52 years). The most common presentation is an abdominal mass and abdominal pain, followed by weight loss and urinary frequency.

Macroscopy
Most tumours are solid and well circumscribed but they may involve adjacent organs. The tumour typically has a large size (mean size, 12.3 cm; range, 0.6–26 cm).

Histopathology
Histopathological features of primary peritoneal SFTs are the same as those from other sites.

Immunohistochemistry
Immunohistochemically the tumour cells are typically positive for CD34 (90–95% cases). EMA and smooth muscle acting (SMA) immunoreactivity have been reported in 20–25% of cases.

Histogenesis
They presumably have a fibroblastic origin.

Prognosis and prognostic factors
Most primary peritoneal SFTs are benign. In the reported series, tumour size did not predict behaviour. The histological features used for diagnosing malignant SFTs in the peritoneum were similar to those applied for other sites {1897}.

Pelvic fibromatosis

Definition
Fibromatosis is a locally aggressive, myofibroblastic/fibroblastic tumour without potential to metastasize.

ICD-O code   8822/1

Synonym
Desmoid tumour

Clinical Features
Pelvic fibromatosis is less common than mesenteric fibromatosis and occurs almost always in females. Patients with pelvic fibromatosis are typically adults (mean age 30 years, age range 17–62 years) and about one-quarter of these tumours are diagnosed during pregnancy {1166}. Patients with mesenteric tumours often present with an asymptomatic abdominal mass, but abdominal pain and gastrointestinal bleeding or acute abdomen may also be present. The main presenting symptom in patients with pelvic fibromatosis is pain (pelvis, leg, abdomen or vulva) {1166}.

Macroscopy
In contrast to fibromatosis of other sites, mesenteric and pelvic fibromatosis often grow as a solid isolated mass with a relatively circumscribed border {799,1166}. The tumour size is generally 5–14 cm.

Histopathology
Histologically, fibromatosis is characterized by a proliferation of uniform spindle-shaped and stellar shaped cells with a collagenous stroma which contains variably prominent vessels. The tumour cells are usually arranged in long sweeping bundles (parallel to each other) with no cytological atypia. Mitotic activity is variable.

Immunohistochemistry
The tumour cells are variably immunoreactive for muscle specific actin and smooth muscle actin. Desmin, h-caldesmon and S100 are typically negative. Nuclear staining for β-catenin is present in approximately 90% of mesenteric fibromatosis tumours {799}.

Genetic susceptibility
Mesenteric fibromatosis may be familial, in association with Gardner-type familial adenomatous polyposis.

Prognosis and predictive factors
Fibromatosis is likely to recur if incompletely resected; it does not metastasize.

Inflammatory myofibroblastic tumour

Definition
A neoplasm composed of fibroblastic-myofibroblastic cells with an admixture of inflammatory cells including lymphocytes, plasma cells and/or eosinophils.

ICD-O code   8825/1

Epidemiology
The patients are typically children and adolescents but the tumour may occur at any age.

Clinical features
Inflammatory myofibroblastic tumour occurs throughout the body but most frequently in the mesentery, omentum, retroperitoneum and abdominal cavity {356}. The patients typically present with a mass or non-specific symptoms. About 15–30% of patients have constitutional symptoms including weight loss, fever and malaise.

Histopathology
The tumour demonstrates three basic histopathological patterns i.e. myxoid/vascular, compact spindled cell and hypocellular fibrous {356}. These patterns often co-exist in the same tumour.

Immunohistochemistry
The tumour cells are variably immunoreactive for smooth muscle actin, muscle specific actin and desmin. Approximately 50–60% of inflammatory myofibroblastic tumours are immunoreactive for ALK, which correlates with *ALK* gene rearrangement {355}.

Prognosis and prognostic factors
Approximately 25% of extra-pulmonary inflammatory myofibroblastic tumours recur but < 5% of tumours metastasize. No specific histological features have been identified to predict tumour behaviour {647}.

Calcifying fibrous tumour

Definition
A calcifying, fibrous tumour of the peritoneum.

ICD-O code   8817/0

Epidemiology
It is a rare tumour typically involving the visceral peritoneum of the small intestine and stomach as an incidental finding {955}.

Clinical Features
Patients with peritoneal calcifying fibrous tumours are typically adolescents or adults {279,955}.

Macroscopy
On gross examination the tumour is an unencapsulated, well circumscribed mass of variable size.

Histopathology
Histologically it is characterized by paucicellular, collagenous fibrous tissue with prominent lymphoplasmacytic inflammation and calcification, which is either dystrophic or psammomatous.

Immunohistochemistry
The tumour cells are immunoreactive for CD34 in most cases and rare cells may show immunoreactivity for desmin and smooth muscle actin {1334}. ALK and S100 are consistently negative in tumour cells.

Genetic Profile
It may occur in a familial setting {279}.

Prognosis and predictive factors
Calcifying fibrous tumour is clinically benign but local recurrence may be observed.

Extra-gastrointestinal stromal tumour

Definition
A mesenchymal tumour outside the gastrointestinal tract with morphology, immunohistochemical profile and molecular changes similar to gastrointestinal stromal tumours.

ICD-O code   8936/3

Epidemiology
Extra-gastrointestinal stromal tumours are rare and account for approximately 2.5% of all gastrointestinal stromal tumours {1263}. Females are affected more than males {1263,1576,2067,2068}.

Clinical features
Extra-gastrointestinal stromal tumours mainly occur in the omentum, mesentery, retroperitoneum and pelvic cavity {1263,1576,2067,2068}. The most common presentation is an abdominal mass, abdominal discomfort and pain. A small percentage of patients present with symptoms of bowel obstruction and gastrointestinal bleeding. Some tumours are discovered incidentally during surgical operations for other reasons.

Macroscopy
The tumours, can be solitary or multiple, are generally large with a median size > 10 cm (range 21–35 cm) {1263,1576, 2067,2068}. On cut section, they may be solid or cystic. Haemorrhage and necrosis may be prominent. Some of the omental tumours are attached to the stomach or small intestine {1263}.

Histopathology
The histopathological features of extra-gastrointestinal stromal tumours are similar to those of gastrointestinal stromal tumours in the gastrointestinal tract. Solitary tumours in the omentum are more likely to show histological features similar to gastrointestinal stromal tumours of gastric type whereas those which are multinodular are more likely to show

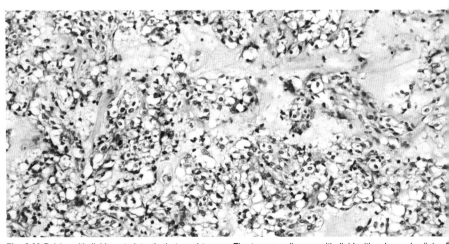

Fig. 2.09 Pelvic epithelioid gastrointestinal stromal tumour. The tumour cells are epithelioid with a loose, hyalinized stroma. The cells are uniform in size and many have a clear cytoplasm.

histological features similar to those of gastrointestinal stromal tumours of small intestine type {1263}.

Immunohistochemistry
More than 90% of tumours are immunoreactive for c-Kit, 50–64% for CD34, 26–31% for smooth muscle actin, 4–8% for desmin and 4–6% for S100 {1263,1576,2067,2068}. A small percentage of extra-gastrointestinal stromal tumours are immunohistochemically negative for c-Kit and most of them (90%) are immunoreactive for DOG1 and protein kinase C theta {2067}. The majority of c-Kit-negative tumours by immunohistochemistry harbour mutations in *PDGFRA* and only a small percentage of such tumours harbour *c-KIT* mutations {2067}.

Genetic profile
Approximately 40–50% of tumours harbour mutations in *c-KIT*. *PDFGRA* mutations are more often seen in tumours with morphology similar to that of gastric type gastrointestinal stromal tumours {1263}.

Prognosis and predictive factors
Multifocality, mitotic activity and necrosis are adverse prognostic factors {442, 1263,1576,2068}. In the omentum, tumours with gastric-type gastrointestinal stromal tumour morphology (more often solitary) do better than those with small intestinal type gastrointestinal stromal tumour morphology (more often multiple). Peritumoral fat infiltration in the omentum is also associated with worse prognosis {1263}.

Endometrioid stromal tumours

Definition
Involvement of the peritoneum by an endometrioid stromal tumour.

ICD-O codes
Low-grade endometrioid
    stromal sarcoma   8931/3
High-grade endometrioid
    stromal sarcoma   8930/3

Etiology
Although endometrioid stromal sarcomas may develop from foci of peritoneal endometriosis, metastasis from a primary uterine tumour is far more common.

Clinical features
Patients may present with abdominal discomfort or a pelvic mass.

Macroscopy
Peritoneal nodules of variable sizes are found.

Histopathology
Tumours resemble their uterine counterparts.

Prognosis and predictive factors
Prognosis is poor for patients with high-grade tumours; low-grade tumours have an indolent course.

Others

Other uncommon tumours and tumour-like lesions include angiosarcoma, epithelioid haemangioendothelioma {869}, granulocytic sarcoma {1269}, clear cell sarcoma {1750}, low-grade myofibroblastic sarcoma {11}, synovial sarcoma {882}, omental-mesenteric myxoid hamartoma {652} and heterotopic mesenchymal ossification {1470}.

Tumour-like lesions

D. Daya
A.N.Y. Cheung
S. Khunamornpong
K.-R. Kim
J. Prat
R.H. Young

Mesothelial hyperplasia

Definition
A non-neoplastic, reactive proliferation of mesothelial cells.

Epidemiology
It is a common incidental finding.

Etiology
Mesothelial hyperplasia is associated with various gynaecological conditions, and is often a response to chronic effusions, inflammation, endometriosis and tumours. Florid mesothelial hyperplasia is most commonly associated with endometriosis {1429}.

Macroscopy
Gross lesions are rare. If present, small nodules may be observed {95}.

Histopathology
The proliferating mesothelial cells may form nodules or sheet-like aggregates, clusters, tubules or papillary structures. The papillae typically contain only scant or no connective tissue cores {1154}. Adjacent reactive fibrosis or inflammation is common. Mild to moderate atypia is not uncommon. Infiltration, invasion or marked nuclear atypia is absent {95,318}. Florid mesothelial hyperplasia should be distinguished from the spread of implants from neoplastic lesions, particularly serous borderline tumour {342} and mesothelioma. Immunohistochemical stains (calretinin +/BerEP4 -) may help confirm the diagnosis {1429}. Uncommon findings include psammoma bodies.

Prognosis and predictive factors
The lesions are benign.

Peritoneal inclusion cysts

Definition
A mesothelial proliferation characterized by cyst formation which may be uni- or multilocular.

ICD-O code   9055/0

Synonyms
Multilocular peritoneal inclusion cysts; benign cystic mesothelioma (not recommended); multicystic mesothelioma (not recommended)

Epidemiology
It is a rare lesion, mostly found in women of reproductive age. In most cases, multilocular peritoneal inclusion cysts are associated with previous surgery, endometriosis or inflammatory disease {330,1239,1629}.

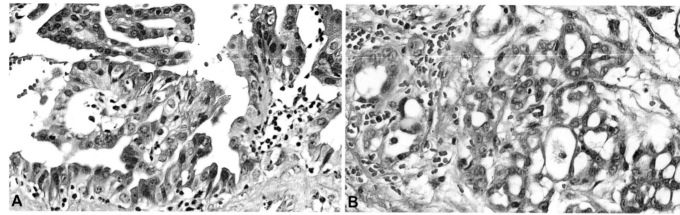

Fig. 2.10 Mesothelial hyperplasia. **A** Tufting and papillary projections. **B** Tubular glands formed by mesothelial cells.

Clinical features

Abdominal pain or mass is the common presentation, often with a history of prior abdominal operation.

Macroscopy

The number and the size of cysts vary considerably. Thin-walled cysts with clear fluid content are attached to pelvic organs or sometimes free-floating. These are often unilocular. Multilocular cysts may be large, up to 20 cm {1629,2018}.

Histopathology

The cyst lining is composed of one to

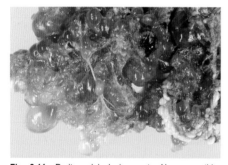

Fig. 2.11 Peritoneal inclusion cysts. Numerous thin-walled cysts involve the omental tissue.

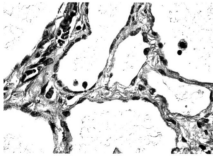

Fig. 2.12 Peritoneal inclusion cysts. Cysts lined by a single layer of mesothelial cells.

several layers of flat to cuboidal mesothelial cells. Mural proliferation of mesothelial cells may be seen. The stroma displays a variable degree of inflammation {1239,1629,2018}.

Histogenesis

Inflammatory processes or hormonal factors may contribute to the pathogenesis of some of these lesions {1629,1954}.

Prognosis and predictive factors

Local recurrences, sometimes multiple, have been reported in up to one-half of cases {1954}. There have been only a few fatal examples of transformation into malignant mesothelioma {653,2018}. In addition to surgical removal, hormonal therapy may have a role in the control of lesions {1383,1954}.

Transitional cell metaplasia

Definition

The presence of benign stratified epithelium on the peritoneal surface that resembles transitional epithelium (urothelium) in the urinary tract.

Clinical features

It is a common incidental finding in the serosa around the fallopian tube, frequently at the tubal-peritoneal junction {1730}.

Histopathology

The epithelium is stratified with oval- to spindle-shaped nuclei, frequently showing longitudinal nuclear grooves or nuclear irregularity, similar to urothelial cells. Circumscribed nests and cysts

lined by transitional epithelium are called Walthard rests.

Histogenesis

It is presumably due to metaplasia of mesothelial cells.

Prognosis and predictive factors

The lesion is benign.

Endometriosis

Definition

The presence of ectopically located endometrial tissue involving the peritoneum.

Epidemiology

Endometriosis is common in women of reproductive age and often leads to infertility {1529}.

Clinical features

Dysmenorrhea and pelvic pain are common presenting symptoms.

Macroscopy

Dark red or bluish nodules or cysts are seen, with dark brown material on the peritoneal surface or in the intra-abdominal organs, often accompanied by adhesions or fibrosis.

Histopathology

The endometrial-type tissue is composed of columnar epithelium of endometrioid- or tubal-type and associated endometrioid-type stroma. In some cases, only stromal cells may be present (stromal endometriosis) {184}. The epithelial cells may show reactive atypia or metaplastic changes {330}.

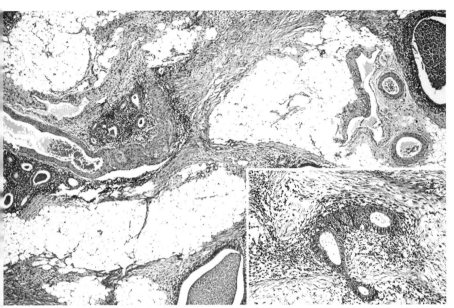

Fig. 2.13 Peritoneal endometriosis. Endometriotic glands between omental fat lobules are surrounded by fibrous tissue. Endometrioid-type glands and associated stromal cells (Inset).

Histogenesis

Implantation of retrograde menstrual endometrium or metaplasia of the peritoneal lining is considered the origin in most cases.

Prognosis and predictive factors

Endometriosis may infrequently be the source of peritoneal or extra-genital neoplasia of Müllerian type, particularly endometrioid or clear cell adenocarcinoma, endometrioid stromal sarcoma or adenosarcoma {133,330,1830}.

Endosalpingiosis

Definition

The presence of benign, tubal-type epithelium almost always forming glands, in the peritoneum or sometimes in the pelvic and retroperitoneal lymph nodes.

Epidemiology

Endosalpingiosis may be found in 7% of women of reproductive-age and is commonly found in association with ovarian serous tumours {460,753,1529}.

Clinical features

This lesion is usually an incidental finding.

Macroscopy

In most cases, there are only small, subserosal nodules or no apparent gross lesion. Formation of a mass is rare {1895}.

Histopathology

Endosalpingiosis usually has a gland- or cyst-like appearance. Blunt papillary projections or minor stratification of the epithelial lining may be present. Endometrial-type stroma is absent.

Histogenesis

It has been proposed that these lesions arise from implanted tubal epithelium {1011,2174}. The histogenesis of endosalpingiosis in lymph nodes is unclear {460}. A report of *KRAS* mutations detected in endosalpingiosis in lymph nodes identical to *KRAS* mutations in the associated ovarian serous borderline tumour/atypical proliferative serous tumours led the investigators to suggest that endosalpingiosis arose from the primary ovarian tumour or developed independently in situ {40}.

Prognosis and predictive factors

Endosalpingiosis may be a rare source of serous tumours in extra-ovarian sites, including lymph nodes {460,463,1235}. Generally endosalpingiosis behaves in a benign fashion; however, progression to low-grade serous carcinoma has been reported {463}.

Histiocytic nodule

Definition

Aggregates of benign histiocytes and reactive mesothelial cells associated with the peritoneal surface.

Synonym

Nodular histiocytic/mesothelial hyperplasia

Epidemiology

This is a rare incidental finding.

Macroscopy

Focal adhesions or small nodules may be seen on the peritoneal surfaces {300}.

Histopathology

Nodules or sheet-like aggregates of a monotonous population of polygonal to

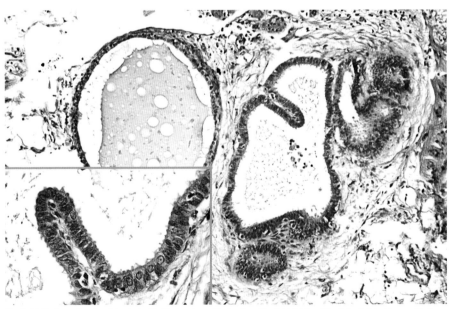

Fig. 2.14 Peritoneal endosalpingiosis. Cystic structure with simple epithelial infolding. The lining is tubal-type epithelium.

oval histiocytes, with a moderate amount of pale, eosinophilic, granular or vacuolated cytoplasm are seen {263,1436}. Nuclear irregularities or grooves may be seen. Rarely, eccentric nuclei and cytoplasmic mucin (so-called muciphages) may mimic to a degree, signet-ring cell carcinoma. A minor component of mesothelial cells may be identified on routine stains or by immunohistochemical stains {263,1436}.

Histogenesis
This is a rare lesion which may result from peritoneal irritation {263}. Cellular aggregation may be mediated through the expression of adhesion molecules by mesothelial cells {1854}.

Prognosis and predictive factors
The lesion is benign.

Ectopic decidua

Definition
Decidualization of submesothelial stromal cells, forming nodule-like aggregations.

Synonym
Deciduosis

Clinical features
This is usually an incidental finding associated with pregnancy or administration of progestins.

Macroscopy
Nodules of soft, white or gelatinous, tan or brown tissue may be visible on the peritoneal surfaces.

Histopathology
Decidualized stromal cells are similar to those in the endometrium associated with pregnancy but may be spindle-shaped and undergo smooth-muscle metaplasia, particularly in pregnant patients. The lesions may raise the differential diagnosis of deciduoid mesothelioma or, in the presence of cytoplasmic vacuolation, metastatic adenocarcinoma {964}.

Histogenesis
Submesothelial stromal cells or stromal endometriosis undergo decidualization due to elevated progesterone levels during pregnancy.

Prognosis and predictive factors
The lesion is benign.

Splenosis

Definition
The presence of benign, splenic tissue in anatomical locations outside the spleen.

Synonym
Autotransplantation of splenic tissue

Epidemiology
This rare condition is associated with a previous, often remote, history of splenic trauma or surgery {911,1482,1905}.

Clinical features
A pelvic or intra-abdominal mass may be incidental or clinically detected.

Macroscopy
Red-brown to bluish-brown nodules or masses, commonly multiple, are present on the serosal surface.

Histopathology
The lesions are composed of benign splenic tissue.

Histogenesis
Splenosis may result from implantation of splenic tissue after spleen disruption {911}.

Prognosis and predictive factors
Splenosis does not require treatment in most cases. Some patients may experience complications that necessitate surgical removal of the lesions, such as bleeding or abdominal pain {1768,1774}.

Others

Other rare tumour-like lesions include nodular peritoneal reaction to foreign material. Material spilled into the peritoneal cavity from a ruptured cystic ovarian teratoma or keratin detached from endometrioid adenosquamous carcinomas from the ovary or endometrium can elicit a foreign body reaction {280,925}. Macroscopically, they appear as nodules which can be mistaken for metastatic carcinoma and microscopically often have the typical appearance of foreign body granulomas. Acellular keratin typifies so-called peritoneal keratin granulomas {280,925}.

Secondary Tumours

D. Daya
A.N.Y. Cheung
S. Khunamornpong
K.-R. Kim
J. Prat
R.H. Young

Metastatic carcinoma

Definition
Disseminated involvement of the peritoneum by metastatic carcinoma.

Epidemiology
In patients with ovarian cancer, peritoneal metastasis is found in about 80% of cases with ascites {352}. For carcinomatosis of non-gynaecological origin, 45% of the primary malignancies are diagnosed during follow-up {313,1661}. Carcinosarcomas often metastasize to the peritoneum.

Etiology
Most originate from the gynaecological or gastrointestinal tract.

Macroscopy
The carcinomas consist of scattered peritoneal and omental nodules. Some display sheet-like growth, covering the peritoneal cavity.

Histopathology
The histological features of peritoneal carcinomatosis often closely reflect those of the primary tumour.

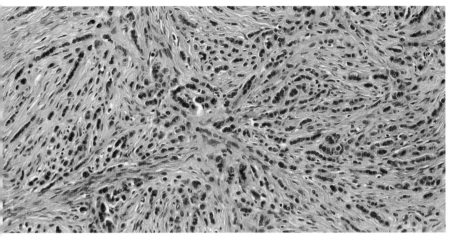

Fig. 2.15 Metastatic lobular carcinoma of the breast. The tumour cells form single files and are set in a desmoplastic stroma.

Prognosis and predictive factors
The prognosis is generally poor and depends on the nature of the primary malignancy.

Low-grade mucinous neoplasm associated with pseudomyxoma peritonei

Definition
Pseudomyxoma peritonei is a clinical term that describes peritoneal involvement by a low-grade, mucinous neoplasm that results in grossly evident mucin in the peritoneal cavity (see secondary tumours of the ovary, p. 83).

Epidemiology
An uncommon condition usually resulting from rupture of a low-grade appendiceal mucinous neoplasm, but potentially originating in other low-grade mucinous neoplasms, including primary ovarian tumours; the latter almost invariably having a teratomatous nature {186,240,1624}.

Macroscopy
The peritoneal cavity is involved, often extensively, by jelly-like mucinous material that may be densely adherent to viscera {2100}.

Histopathology
The histological picture is that of differentiated mucinous epithelium, ranging from that which is morphologically benign, to showing mild to moderate cytological atypia, dissecting in the form of glands and cysts within mucin and often associated with hyaline fibrosis {240,1445,2100}.

Prognosis and predictive factors
The disease typically has a prolonged clinical course, but often leads patient death. The outcome is related to the bulk of the disease, the amount of mucinous epithelium and its degree of atypicality {240,1445,1621}.

Metastatic sarcoma

Most sarcomas are derived from the female reproductive organs, more often from the uterus such as leiomyosarcoma, endometrial stromal sarcoma and carcinosarcoma, but sarcomas originating in extra-genital sites can also involve the peritoneum.

Gliomatosis

Definition
Presence of glial tissue in the peritoneum.

Etiology
Gliomatosis peritonei usually occurs in association with an ovarian teratoma {2092} or rarely with a ventriculoperitoneal shunt {1124}.

Histogenesis
Origin from peritoneal stem cells or glial metaplasia of subjacent mesenchyme has also been postulated {542}.

Clinical features
Ovarian teratomas with gliomatosis are often larger with elevation of the pre-operative CA-125 level {2092}.

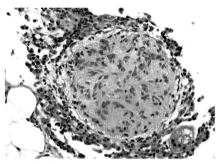

Fig. 2.16 Gliomatosis peritonei. Peritoneal gliomatosis showing a discrete nodule of mature glial tissue.

Macroscopy
Gliomatosis occurs as small peritoneal nodules, which can be extensive (see ovarian teratomas, p. 60).

Histopathology
Sections show mature glial tissue surrounded by fibroadipose tissue of peritoneum.

Prognosis and predictive factors
Gliomatosis peritonei has an excellent outcome.

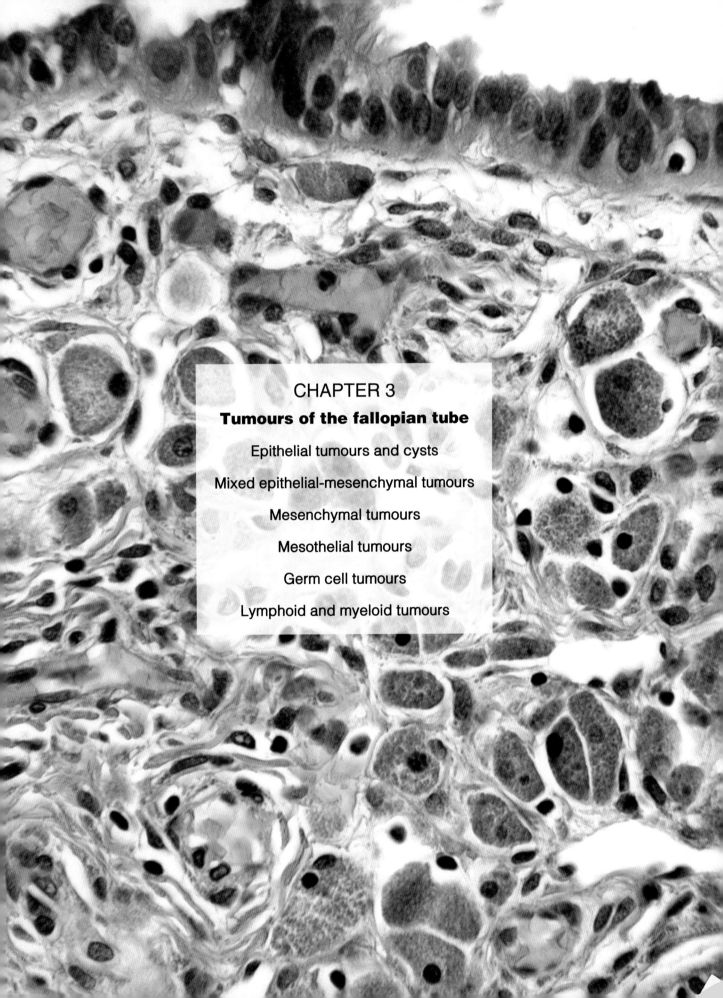

CHAPTER 3

Tumours of the fallopian tube

Epithelial tumours and cysts

Mixed epithelial-mesenchymal tumours

Mesenchymal tumours

Mesothelial tumours

Germ cell tumours

Lymphoid and myeloid tumours

WHO Classification of tumours of the fallopian tube[a,b]

Epithelial tumours and cysts
Hydatid cyst
Benign epithelial tumours
  Papilloma
  Serous adenofibroma   9014/0
Epithelial precursor lesion
  Serous tubal intraepithelial carcinoma   8441/2*
Epithelial borderline tumour
  Serous borderline tumour / Atypical
    proliferative serous tumour   8442/1
Malignant epithelial tumours
  Low-grade serous carcinoma   8460/3
  High-grade serous carcinoma   8461/3
  Endometrioid carcinoma   8380/3
  Undifferentiated carcinoma   8020/3
Others
  Mucinous carcinoma   8480/3
  Transitional cell carcinoma   8120/3
  Clear cell carcinoma   8130/3

Tumour-like lesions
  Tubal hyperplasia
  Tubo-ovarian abscess
  Salpingitis isthmica nodosa
  Metaplastic papillary tumour

Placental site nodule
Mucinous metaplasia
Endometriosis
Endosalpingiosis

Mixed epithelial-mesenchymal tumours
Adenosarcoma   8933/3
Carcinosarcoma   8980/3

Mesenchymal tumours
Leiomyoma   8890/0
Leiomyosarcoma   8890/3
Others

Mesothelial tumours
Adenomatoid tumour   9054/0

Germ cell tumours
Teratoma
  Mature   9080/0
  Immature   9080/3

Lymphoid and myeloid tumours
Lymphomas
Myeloid neoplasms

[a] The morphology codes are from the International Classification of Diseases for Oncology (ICD-O) {575A}. Behaviour is coded /0 for benign tumours, /1 for unspecified, borderline or uncertain behaviour, /2 for carcinoma in situ and grade III intraepithelial neoplasia and /3 for malignant tumours; [b] The classification is modified from the previous WHO classification of tumours {1906A}, taking into account changes in our understanding of these lesions; *These new codes were approved by the IARC/WHO Committee for ICD-O in 2013.

TNM and FIGO classification of tumours of the ovary, fallopian tube and primary peritoneal carcinoma

T - Primary Tumour

TNM	FIGO	
TX		Primary tumour cannot be assessed
T0		No evidence of primary tumour
T1	I	Tumour limited to the ovaries
T1a	IA	Tumour limited to one ovary (capsule intact) or fallopian tube surface; no malignant cells in ascites or peritoneal washings
T1b	IB	Tumour limited to one or both ovaries (capsules intact) or fallopian tubes; no tumour on ovarian or fallopian tube surface; no malignant cells in ascites or peritoneal washings
T1c	IC	Tumour limited to one or both ovaries or fallopian tubes with any of the following:
T1c1	IC1	Surgical spill
T1c2	IC2	Capsule ruptured before surgery or tumour on ovarian or fallopian tube surface
T1c3	IC3	Malignant cells in ascites or peritoneal washings
T2	II	Tumour involves one or both ovaries or fallopian tubes with pelvic extension below pelvic brim or primary peritoneal cancer
T2a	IIA	Extension and/or implants on uterus and/or fallopian tubes and/or ovaries
T2b	IIB	Extension to other pelvic intraperitoneal
T3 and/or N1	III	Tumour involves one or both ovaries or fallopian tubes, or primary peritoneal carcinoma, with cytologically or histologically confirmed spread to the peritoneum outside the pelvis and/or metastasis to the retroperitoneal lymph nodes
N1	IIIA1	Retroperitoneal lymph node metastasis only
N1a	IIIA1i	Lymph node metastasis up to 10 mm in greatest dimension
N1b	IIIA1ii	Lymph node metastasis more than 10 mm in greatest dimension
T3a	IIIA2	Microscopic extrapelvic (above the pelvic brim) peritoneal involvement with or without retroperitoneal lymph node
T3b	IIIB	Macroscopic peritoneal metastasis beyond the pelvis up to 2 cm in greatest dimension with or without retroperitoneal lymph node metastasis
T3c	IIIC	Macroscopic peritoneal metastasis beyond the pelvis more than 2 cm in greatest dimension, with or without retroperitoneal lymph node metastasis (excludes extension of tumour to capsule of liver and spleen without parenchymal involvement of either organ)
M1	IV	Distant metastasis excluding peritoneal metastasis
M1a	IVA	Pleural effusion with positive cytology
M1b	IVB	Parenchymal metastasis and metastasis to extra-abdominal organs (including inguinal lymph nodes and lymph nodes outside the abdominal cavity)

N — Regional Lymph Nodes

NX	Regional lymph nodes cannot be assessed
N0	No regional lymph node metastasis
N1	Regional lymph node metastasis
N1a	Lymph node metastasis up to 10 mm in greatest dimension
N1b	Lymph node metastasis more than 10 mm in greatest dimension

M — Distant Metastasis

M0	No distant metastasis
M1	Distant metastasis
M1a	Pleural effusion with positive cytology
M1b	Parenchymal metastasis and metastasis to extra abdominal organs (including inguinal lymph nodes and lymph nodes outside the abdominal cavity)

pTNM Pathological Classification

The pT and pN categories correspond to the T and N categories.

pM1   Distant metastasis microscopically confirmed

Note: pM0 and pMX are not valid categories.

pN0   Histological examination of a pelvic lymphadenectomy specimen will ordinarily include 10 or more lymph nodes. If the lymph nodes are negative, but the number ordinarily examined is not met, classify as pN0.

Stage Grouping

Stage IA	T1a	N0	M0
Stage IB	T1b	N0	M0
Stage IC1	T1c1	N0	M0
Stage IC2	T1c2	N0	M0
Stage IC3	T1c3	N0	M0
Stage IIA	T2a	N0	M0
Stage IIB	T2b	N0	M0
Stage IIC	T2c	N0	M0
Stage IIIA1	T1/T2	N1	M0
Stage IIIA2	T3a	N0/N1	M0
Stage IIIB	T3b	N0/N1	M0
Stage IIIC	T3c	N0/N1	M0
Stage IV	Any T	Any N	M1

References

American Joint Committee on Cancer (AJCC) Cancer Staging Manual, 7th ed. (2011). Edge SB, Byrd DR, Compton CC, Fritz AG, Greene FL, Trotti III eds. Springer: New York

International Union against Cancer (UICC): TNM Classification of Malignant Tumours, 7th ed. (2009) Sobin LH, Gospodarowicz MK, Wittekind Ch eds. Wiley-Blackwell: Oxford

A help-desk for specific questions about the TNM classification is available at http://www.uicc.org.

Prat J, FIGO Committee on Gynecologic Oncology (2014). Staging classification for cancer of the ovary, fallopian tube, and peritoneum. Int J Gynaecol Obstet 124:1-5.

Epithelial tumours and cysts

C.P. Crum
I. Alvarado-Cabrero
J.G. Bijron
M.L. Carcangiu
J.A. Ferry
V. Parkash
J.M.J. Piek
P. Shaw
R. Soslow
P.J. van Diest
R. Vang

Hydatid cyst

Definition
A paratubal cyst lined by ciliated epithelium.

Synonym
Hydatid of Morgagni

Clinical features
Hydatid cysts may present as an adnexal mass or cyst.

Histopathology
Hydatid cysts are remnants of the Müllerian duct. They are paratubal in location and contain ciliated epithelium identical to that of the fallopian tube. They may rarely be the site of a cystadenoma or borderline/atypical proliferative serous tumour.

Benign epithelial tumours

Papilloma

Papillomas of the fallopian tube are uncommon. They are typically discovered incidentally, but when intraluminal, they may obstruct the tube {641}. The criteria for distinction from papillary tubal hyperplasia are unclear and some authors consider these lesions to be synonymous, although formation of a mass favours a papilloma. They exhibit papillary architecture, the complexity of which exceeds that of the normal plicae. Small, papillary buds fall off delicate, branching, fibrovascular cores lined by bland, serous epithelium. Psammoma bodies may be present {883}.

Serous adenofibroma

Definition
A biphasic tumour in which epithelial cells, resembling those of the fallopian tube, are associated with a fibromatous stroma.

ICD-O code   9014/0

Histopathology
Many fallopian tubes contain localized ovarian stroma beneath serous-type epithelium. The term "serous adenofibroma" has been proposed for these lesions, as well as for mass-forming lesions {176}.

Epithelial precursor lesions

Serous tubal intraepithelial carcinoma

Definition
Serous tubal intraepithelial carcinoma (STIC) is a non-invasive, serous carcinoma in the fallopian tube.

ICD-O code   8441/2

Synonyms
Tubal carcinoma in situ; high-grade tubal intraepithelial neoplasia; tubal intraepithelial carcinoma

Epidemiology
Serous tubal intraepithelial carcinoma (STIC) is the most common malignancy found in risk-reducing salpingo-oophorectomies from women with germ-line *BRCA1* or *BRCA2* mutations, accounting for up to 85% of early cases. It is thought to be the earliest known manifestation of most pelvic serous cancers {631}. STICs are associated with 50–60% of high-grade pelvic serous carcinomas {931,1532,1900}. See also Introduction to serous tumours / pelvic neoplasia, p. 15). STICs are discovered in about 5–10% of asymptomatic *BRCA* mutation carriers with thorough examination of the fallopian tube (Protocol for Sectioning and Extensively Examining the FIMbriated End (SEE-FIM) of the Fallopian Tube) {222, 232,233,362,1504,1517,1577}. The finding of a STIC in women who do not have a *BRCA* mutation or a concomitant high-grade serous cancer is exceedingly rare.

Macroscopy
STIC lesions can be invisible grossly, but when associated with an early carcinoma, a 1–2 mm nodule in the fimbria may be palpated.

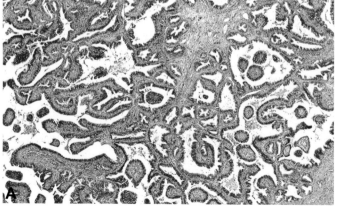
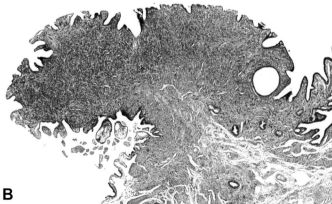

Fig. 3.01 A Fallopian tube papilloma. The tumour consists of papillary structures lined by bland-appearing fallopian tube type epithelium. **B** Serous adenofibroma of the tube. Discrete proliferation of ovarian-like stroma involving fimbria.

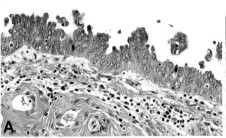
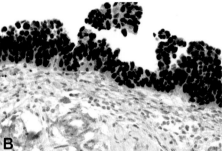
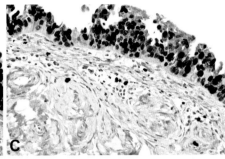

Fig. 3.02 Serous tubal intraepithelial carcinoma. **A** The tubal epithelium is stratified and shows marked cytological atypia and occasional mitotic figures. Cellular discohesion results in shedding of malignant cells into the tubal lumen. **B** Strong nuclear staining for p53 protein is characteristic. **C** Strong nuclear staining for Ki67 protein.

Histopathology

Virtually all STICs (90%) are found in the distal tube, either in the fimbria or the infundibulum. They are characterized by abnormal growth of principally stratified, non-ciliated cells showing marked nuclear pleomorphism, prominent nucleoli, increased nuclear/cytoplasmic ratio and loss of cell polarity. Lack of cellular cohesion is a prominent feature, with shedding of cells into the tubal lumen. Criteria separating an exuberant, non-invasive, high-grade serous carcinoma from a large STIC have yet to be defined. Lesions are usually strongly p53 positive; a minority demonstrates completely absent staining due to nonsense mutations. The Ki-67 index is elevated to at least 15% and can exceed 50% {831,1986}. Lesions with strong p53 staining and less severe cytological atypia have been variously termed "tubal epithelial atypia", "low-grade serous tubal intraepithelial neoplasia", and "serous tubal intraepithelial lesions" {388A,831,1008,1062B,1519}. Strategies for distinguishing these atypias from STIC by histology and biomarkers have been proposed and are still under investigation pending outcome data {1249,1986}. The risk of metastatic disease following excision appears low (about 6%) for localized non-invasive STICs {1519}.

Histogenesis

The precursors of STICs have not been well characterized. It has been proposed that they may arise from an outgrowth of tubal secretory cells {831,1065,1504}. There is mounting evidence that STICs are precursors of ovarian high-grade serous carcinoma {1009} but definitive proof requires additional investigation.
See Introduction to serous tumours / pelvic neoplasia, p. 15.

Genetic profile

92% of STICs contain *TP53* mutations and identical *TP53* mutations are shared with concomitant ovarian high-grade serous carcinomas, supporting a clonal relationship {931,988,1669}.

Genetic susceptibility

BRCA mutation status confers a higher risk of STIC, commensurate with the 10–40% lifetime risk of high-grade serous pelvic carcinoma.

Prognosis and predictive factors

There are limited data but the recurrence rates of pelvic serous carcinoma, following a diagnosis of a localized STIC identified at risk reducing salpingo-oophorectomy, appear to be about 10% {1519}.
The risk imposed by positive peritoneal cytology is unknown. However, the presence of positive washings should prompt a comprehensive examination of the distal fallopian tube {15}.

Epithelial borderline tumours

Serous borderline tumour / Atypical proliferative serous tumour

Definition

Serous borderline tumours/atypical proliferative serous tumours (SBT/APSTs) are fallopian tube neoplasms that resemble their ovarian counterpart.

ICD-O code   8442/1

Epidemiology

Only a few cases have been reported {39A,2167}.

Macroscopy

Usually located in the fimbriae, they appear as a solid and cystic polypoid mass.

Clinical features

Infertility and abdominal pain are the most common symptoms reported.

Histopathology

The tumour resembles ovarian SBT/APST.

Histogenesis

See Introduction to serous tumours, p. 15.

Prognosis and predictive factors

Treatment is conservative and prognosis is excellent.

Malignant epithelial tumours

Serous carcinoma

Definition

Fallopian tube carcinoma (FTC) is an invasive tumour growing in papillary, glandular and solid patterns with high-grade nuclear atypia, identical to other high-grade pelvic serous carcinomas {39B,39C,1335A}.

ICD-O codes

Low-grade serous carcinoma	8460/3
High-grade serous carcinoma	8461/3

Epidemiology

They are the most common histological type of tubal carcinoma, accounting for approximately two-thirds of carcinomas.

Clinical features

Cases with early spread to the peritoneal surfaces present with symptomatology for involvement of these areas. For rare tumours forming a large intraluminal mass, the most common findings are discharge or bleeding, abdominal pain and an abdominal mass {39B,39C,1378}. The classic finding of colicky pain, watery discharge (hydrops tubae profluens) occurs in less than 10% of bulky tubal carcinomas. Positive cytology has been reported in 38–80% of cervical and uterine samplings {1880}.

Histopathology
These tumours are identical to their ovarian counterparts (See Introduction to ovarian serous tumours, p. 15).

Histogenesis
Serous carcinomas of the tube arise from serous tubal intraepithelial carcinomas.

Genetic Profile
See: Ovarian serous tumours

Prognosis and Predictive Factors
The prognosis is similar to the ovarian counterpart (See Introduction to ovarian serous tumours, p. 15).

Endometrioid carcinoma

Definition
A malignant, epithelial tumour resembling endometrioid adenocarcinoma of the uterine corpus.

ICD-O code   8380/3

Epidemiology
Endometrioid carcinomas are the second most common type of tubal carcinoma {39C,1335A}. Rare intraepithelial or invasive endometrioid carcinomas are reported in women with endometrial carcinoma and may signify a second primary site or a metastasis {395}.

Histopathology
Low-grade endometrioid adenocarcinoma is a glandular tumour that can contain areas of squamous or spindle-cell differentiation. High-grade endometrioid carcinomas overlap in appearance with high-grade serous carcinomas and are distinguished by their histology and immunohistochemistry {1335A} (see Introduction to ovarian serous tumours, p. 15). A rare variant is difficult to differentiate from a female adnexal tumour of Wolffian origin (FATWO) {419}. Overall, tumour depth and fimbrial involvement are associated with worse outcome {39B}.

Undifferentiated carcinoma

Definition
A high-grade carcinoma that grows in a solid pattern and shows no evidence of specific differentiation (see p. 40).

ICD-O code   8020/3

Others

Clear cell, mucinous and transitional cell carcinomas of the tube have been reported, but they are very rare {423,825,974,1884}.

ICD-O codes
Mucinous carcinoma   8480/3
Transitional cell carcinoma   8120/3
Clear cell carcinoma   8130/3

Tumour-like lesions

Tubal hyperplasia

Definition
Benign epithelial proliferation.

Epidemiology
It may be associated with hyper-oestrogenic states and gynaecological neoplasia at other sites {2075}. There is no association with *BRCA* mutations {1275}. Pseudoneoplastic hyperplasia is seen with salpingitis {1249}. Tubal hyperplasia may be increased in women with serous tumours {275,1042}. Papillary tubal hyperplasia has been proposed to be a precursor of ovarian SBT/APSTs, noninvasive implants and endosalpingiosis {1011}.

Histopathology
The most common pattern is discrete foci of pseudostratification with minimal loss of nuclear polarity. This pattern is common and present in the majority of tubes examined {1275}. Criteria for the diagnosis are poorly defined and many reflect tangential sectioning. Hyperplasia is often seen in association with inflammation and may mimic carcinoma {1249}. A less common pattern is intraluminal papillary tufting of the tubal epithelium with detached rounded clusters of epithelial cells that are free-floating in the lumen of the tube. At its extreme, such papillary hyperplasia may overlap with entities previously reported as papillomas or even borderline tumours

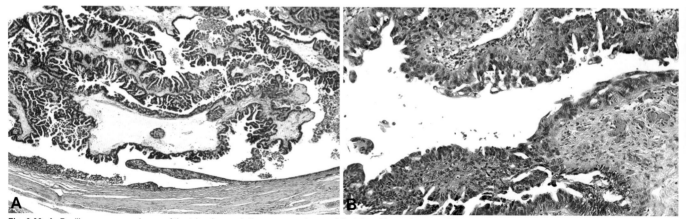

Fig. 3.03 A Papillary serous carcinoma of the tube. An exophytic serous carcinoma of the tube with prominent papillary architecture. **B** High-grade serous carcinoma. Note the marked stratification, papillary growth and exfoliation of malignant cells into the tubal lumen.

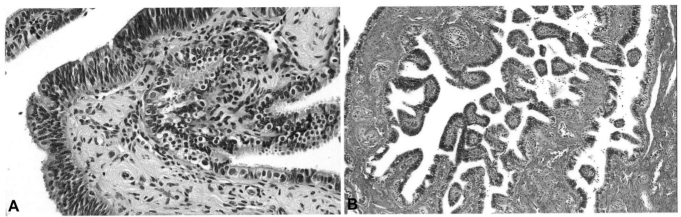

Fig. 3.04 A Tubal hyperplasia. Mild epithelial hyperplasia of the tube with a discrete focus of enhanced pseudostratified epithelium. **B** Papillary tubal hyperplasia. Multiple, small papillae floating in the tubal lumen. This lesion was associated with an ovarian serous borderline tumour/atypical proliferative serous tumour and has been proposed to be a precursor of these tumours {1011}.

of the fallopian tube. In some studies, papillary hyperplasia was associated with serous borderline tumour/atypical proliferative tumours of the ovary {1011,1042}.

Histogenesis

The histogenesis is poorly understood. It possibly arises from epithelial stem cells of the fallopian tube, although these have not been convincingly described.

Tubo-ovarian abscess

Definition

This is a fibro-inflammatory mass, involving the distal fallopian tube and ovary and occasionally other pelvic organs, secondary to pelvic inflammatory disease or other infections {271}.

Histopathology

Histologically, the normal anatomy is markedly distorted, with destructive, acute and chronic inflammation, necrosis, abscess formation and fibrosis involving the fallopian tube and the ovary. Co-existent endometriosis may be present {661}. Sometimes it is associated with an intrauterine device.

Salpingitis isthmica nodosa

Definition

Diverticulosis of the epithelium of the fallopian tube, with associated smooth-muscle hypertrophy and/or hyperplasia.

Epidemiology

There is a strong association with both infertility and ectopic pregnancy {834}.

Macroscopy

The lesion comprises a discrete nodule(s) in the proximal tube.

Histopathology

Histologically, multiple, variably sized, gland-like structures surrounded by hypertrophic and hyperplastic smooth muscle.

Metaplastic papillary tumour

This rare, metaplastic lesion is typically seen in the tubes of postpartum women {1664}. It is characterized by a microscopic, intraluminal, papillary proliferation composed of atypical cells with abundant eosinophilic cytoplasm, resembling a serous borderline tumour/atypical proliferative serous tumour.

Placental site nodule

A small number of placental site nodules have been described. These lesions likely arise from prior ectopic pregnancies and resemble their counterparts in the uterus. To date, the behaviour of all reported lesions has been benign {88}. See section on non-neoplastic gestational trophoblastic disease, p. 162.

Mucinous metaplasia

Mucinous metaplasia in the fallopian tube is probably underreported {2044}. When seen in association with gynaecological, colonic, pancreatobiliary or appendiceal mucinous tumours, a metastasis needs to be considered. It is also seen in the absence of neoplasia, where it is associated with chronic inflammation and other metaplastic changes. Some lesions are associated with multifocal changes

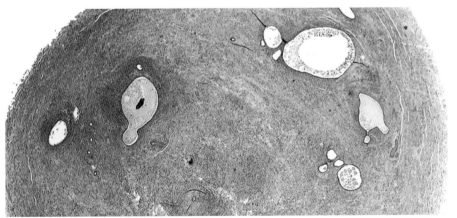

Fig. 3.05 Salpingitis isthmica nodosa. Multiple, variably sized, gland-like structures are surrounded by hypertrophic and hyperplastic smooth muscle.

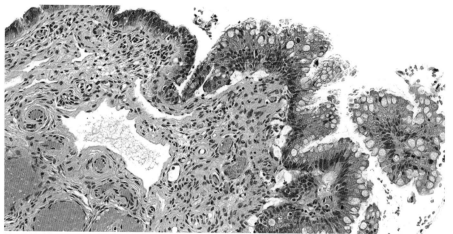
Fig. 3.06 Mucinous metaplasia of the tubal epithelium.

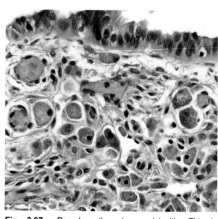
Fig. 3.07 Pseudoxanthomatous salpingitis. This is characterized by numerous pigment-laden macrophages in the lamina propria; often associated with co-existing endometriosis and may represent burnt out endometriosis.

in the endometrium, cervix and ovary, and an association with Peutz-Jeghers syndrome has also been reported {1157}. Neoplastic transformation may occur in this setting {54,1157}.

Endometriosis

Tubal endometriosis is commonly associated with endometriosis at other sites, and the primary symptom is infertility. Typically, this is due to the presence of polypoid lesions causing tubal obstruction at the cornual end {29}. In addition

to forming mass lesions, endometriosis is associated with brown pigmentation of the tube, so-called "pseudoxanthomatous salpingitis" {330}, which is characterized by the presence of a pseudoxanthoma and haemosiderin-laden macrophages. Whether this represents burnt-out endometriosis or an association with endometriosis at other sites remains to be determined. Microscopically, endometriosis may involve the mucosa, myosalpinx or serosa, and varies from resembling normal endometrium in young lesions to fibrotic lesions with scant stroma and epithelium

with haemosiderin-laden macrophages in older lesions. Metaplastic and hyperplastic changes can raise concern for, among other things, intraepithelial carcinoma {887} and, when exuberant and polypoid, adenosarcoma {1463}.

Endosalpingiosis

This lesion is more common in the peritoneum than the fallopian tube. (See chapter 2, p. 99)

Mixed epithelial-mesenchymal tumours

Adenosarcoma

Definition
A biphasic tumour with malignant mesenchymal and benign epithelial components.

ICD-O code   8933/3

Histopathology
The pathology is the same as that of the more common adenosarcomas of the endometrium and ovary {1207}.

Carcinosarcoma

Definition
A biphasic neoplasm composed of high-grade epithelial and mesenchymal elements.

ICD-O code   8980/3

Histopathology
These tumours are identical to carcinosarcomas of the endometrium and ovary {978}.

Mesenchymal tumours

Leiomyoma

Definition
A benign tumour of smooth-muscle cells.

ICD-O code   8890/0

Histopathology
Leiomyomas of the fallopian tube are similar to their counterparts in the uterus. However, if multiple lesions are encountered, the possibility of disseminated leiomyomatosis should be considered.

Leiomyosarcoma

Definition
A malignant tumour of smooth-muscle cells.

ICD-O code   8890/3

Histopathology
See tumours of the uterine corpus, p.139.

Prognosis and predictive factors
These are rare tumours. The few reported cases have typically had an adverse outcome {827,1945}. Similar appearing neoplasms, such as extra-gastrointestinal stromal tumours or PEComas must be excluded {569}.

Others

A variety of other mesenchymal tumours, benign and malignant, may occur in the tube. They are rare and histologically similar to their soft-tissue counterparts. Haemangioma {2041}, chondrosarcoma {1503}, synovial sarcoma {1280} and embryonal rhabdomyosarcoma {206} arising in the tube have been described.

Mesothelial tumours

Adenomatoid tumour

Definition
A benign, subserosal tumour of mesothelial origin.

ICD-O code   9054/0

Histopathology
These tumours are usually discovered incidentally. They measure up to 1–2 cm in size and are located beneath the tubal serosa. They are rarely bilateral {2132}. They consist of variably sized tubules lined by flattened to cuboidal appearing cells {1829}. Immunohistochemistry for mesothelial markers, such as calretinin and D2-40, will confirm the mesothelial origin.

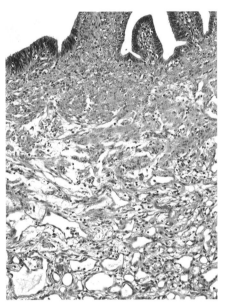

Fig. 3.08 Adenomatoid tumour. Small, irregular spaces lined by mesothelial cells in the wall of the tube.

Germ cell tumours

Teratoma

Definition
A rare tumour composed of mature or immature tissues from more than one germ cell layer.

ICD-O codes
Mature teratoma   9080/0
Immature teratoma   9080/3

Epidemiology
These tumours are extremely rare in the tube. A malignant, mixed germ cell tumour of the tube has been reported {1088}.

Histopathology
Teratomas of the fallopian tube are identical in appearance to ovarian teratomas.

Lymphoid and myeloid tumours

Lymphomas

Definition
Malignant neoplasms composed of lymphoid cells.

Clinical features
Primary tubal lymphomas are exceedingly rare and include an extranodal marginal zone lymphoma associated with salpingitis, low- and high-grade follicular lymphomas and a bilateral peripheral T-cell lymphoma {591,654,1360}. Secondary tubal involvement among patients with lymphoma of the ovaries or sites other than the ovary may occur {1341}. Diffuse large B-cell lymphoma and Burkitt lymphoma are the most common to secondarily involve the tube; follicular lymphoma is also described {1341,1970}.

Histopathology
Histological findings are similar to those seen in other female reproductive organs for the corresponding type of lymphoma (see ovary chapter, p. 79).

Prognosis and predictive factors
Outcome varies widely, depending on the type of neoplasm involving the tube, and on the extent of disease.

Myeloid neoplasms

Definition
Malignant neoplasms of haematopoietic origin, including myeloid leukaemias and myeloid sarcoma, a mass-forming lesion composed of primitive myeloid cells.

Synonyms
Myeloid sarcoma: chloroma, granulocytic sarcoma, extramedullary myeloid tumour

Clinical features
Involvement of the fallopian tube by myeloid neoplasms is rare, although tubal involvement by myeloid sarcoma has been reported. When it occurs, it is generally in conjunction with involvement of the ipsilateral ovary or the uterus {605,920}. Clinical features are similar to those of myeloid sarcoma elsewhere in the female reproductive organs.

Histopathology
Myeloid sarcomas are composed of a diffuse proliferation of primitive myeloid cells with oval, irregular or folded nuclei, fine chromatin, distinct to prominent nucleoli and scant to moderate quantity of cytoplasm. Maturing cells with recognizable myeloid differentiation may be seen.

Genetic profile
Limited data are available, but one granulocytic sarcoma involving the tube and uterus was associated with acute myeloid leukaemia with abnormal eosinophilia, with inv(16)(p13;q32) {605,920}.

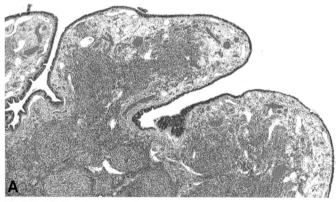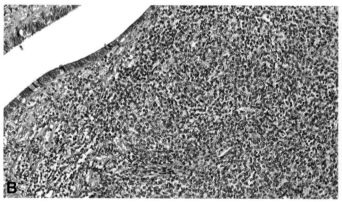

Fig. 3.09 A Follicular lymphoma of the tube. Low power shows multiple, crowded, poorly delineated follicles distorting tubal plicae. **B** Follicular lymphoma of the tube. Higher power image of one neoplastic follicle shows a monotonous population of small to medium-sized cells with oval to slightly irregular nuclei, consistent with centrocytes.

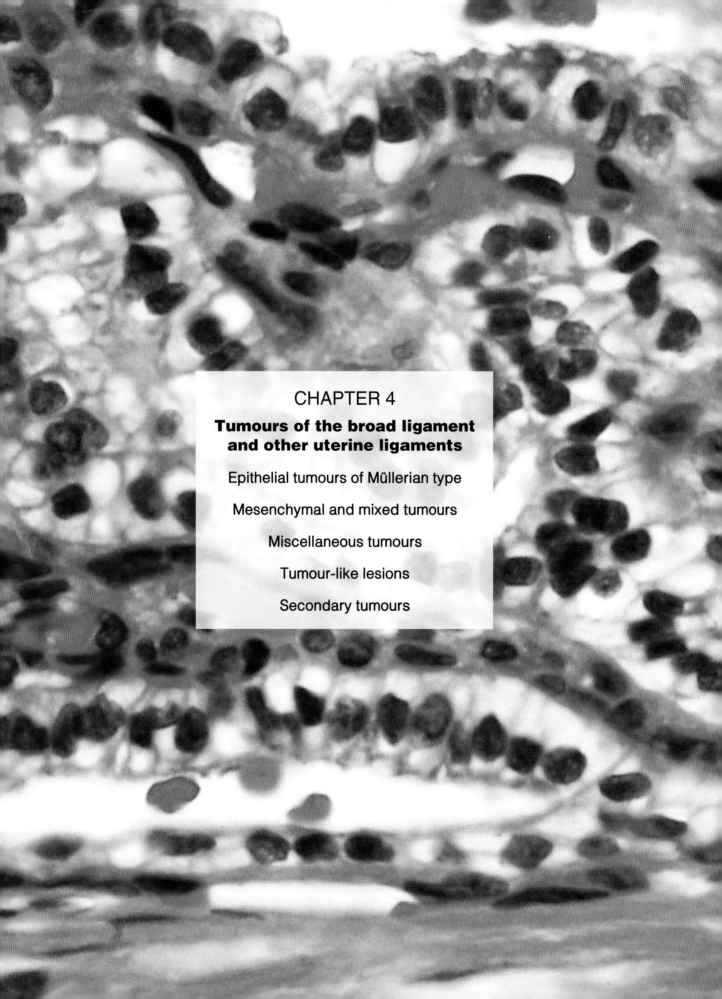

CHAPTER 4
Tumours of the broad ligament and other uterine ligaments

Epithelial tumours of Müllerian type

Mesenchymal and mixed tumours

Miscellaneous tumours

Tumour-like lesions

Secondary tumours

WHO Classification of tumours of the broad ligament and other uterine ligaments[a,b]

Epithelial tumours of Müllerian type

Serous cystadenoma	8440/0
Serous cystadenofibroma / adenofibroma	9013/0
Serous borderline tumour / Atypical proliferative serous tumour	8442/1
Serous carcinoma	
Low-grade serous carcinoma	8460/3
High-grade serous carcinoma	8461/3
Others	
Endometrioid carcinoma	8380/3
Mucinous carcinoma	8480/3
Clear cell carcinoma	8310/3

Mesenchymal and mixed tumours

Leiomyoma	8890/0
Adenomyoma	8932/0
Adenosarcoma	8933/3
Leiomyosarcoma	8890/3
Others	

Miscellaneous tumours

Wolffian tumour	9110/1
Papillary cystadenoma (with von-Hippel-Lindau disease)	8450/0
Ependymoma	9391/3

Tumour-like lesions

Endometriosis
Endosalpingiosis
Adrenal cortical rests

Secondary tumours

---

[a] The morphology codes are from the International Classification of Diseases for Oncology (ICD-O) {575A}. Behaviour is coded /0 for benign tumours, /1 for unspecified, borderline or uncertain behaviour, /2 for carcinoma in situ and grade III intraepithelial neoplasia and /3 for malignant tumours; [b] The classification is modified from the previous WHO classification of tumours {1906A}, taking into account changes in our understanding of these lesions; *These new codes were approved by the IARC/WHO Committee for ICD-O in 2013.

Epithelial tumours of Müllerian type

W.D. Lawrence   J.D. Seidman
I. Alvarado-Cabrero   M. Wells

Serous cystadenoma / Serous cystadenofibroma

Definition
Tumours characterized by epithelial cell types resembling those of the fallopian tube, including ciliated cells. The epithelial component may be associated with a component of stromal cells (cystadenofibroma, adenofibroma) or may lack a stromal component (cystadenoma).

ICD-O codes
Serous cystadenoma   8440/0
Serous cystadenofibroma/
   adenofibroma   9013/0

Epidemiology
Epithelial tumours of Müllerian type are the most common type of epithelial neoplasm of the broad ligament, where tumours of almost every Müllerian cell type have been found {65}. These are one-fifth as common as ovarian tumours, and only 2% are borderline or invasive, compared to 25% in ovarian tumours {66}. Although the literature on serous cystadenomas of the broad ligament is scant, they are said to be the most common type of Müllerian derived epithelial tumour in this location {2102}.

Macroscopy
Most of these tumours are unilateral, unilocular cysts ranging up to 13 cm in diameter {65,66}.

Histopathology
These tumours differ from non-neoplastic cysts of serous type by the presence in the former of a thick wall, composed of cellular stroma resembling ovarian stroma and the absence of folds or plicae.

Histogenesis
See Introduction to serous tumours / pelvic neoplasia, p.15.

Prognosis and predictive factors
These lesions are benign.

Serous borderline tumour / Atypical proliferative serous tumour

Definition
Serous borderline tumour/atypical proliferative serous tumours (SBT/APSTs) are non-invasive tumours that display greater epithelial proliferation and cytological atypia than benign serous tumours but less than low-grade serous carcinoma (LGSC).

ICD-O code   8442/1

Epidemiology
Approximately 36 cases of SBT/APST of the broad ligament have been reported in women 19–67 years of age (mean, 33 years), and all have been unilateral, without evidence of spread {65,1125}.

Macroscopy
All the reported cases have been confined within the leaves of the broad ligament, with the adjacent fallopian tube usually stretched over them. Grossly, they have smooth external surfaces, are thin-walled and unilocular and range from 1–13 cm (average, 6.4 cm) in greatest dimension.

Histology
They have microscopic features similar to those of their ovarian counterparts {65,1125,2102}.

Histogenesis
See Introduction to serous tumours / pelvic neoplasia, p.15.

Prognosis and predictive factors
Prognosis and predictive factors are similar to those of their ovarian counterparts (see ovary chapter, p.15).

Serous carcinoma

Definition
Serous carcinomas involving the broad ligament resemble their ovarian counterparts. See Introduction to serous tumours / pelvic neoplasia, p.15.

ICD-O codes
Low-grade serous carcinoma   8460/3
High-grade serous carcinoma   8461/3

Epidemiology
Primary carcinoma of the broad ligament is extremely rare; about 20 cases have been reported {66,1310,1919} with serous carcinoma being the most frequent. The mean age of patients with these neoplasms is 46 years (range, 29–70 years) {736}.

Clinical features
The most common presenting manifestations are pelvic discomfort, pain and an adnexal mass {736,2102}.

Macroscopy
The tumours are solid or cystic or both and range from 4.5–13cm in greatest dimension; all have been unilateral.

Histopathology
They are similar to their ovarian counterparts.

Histogenesis
See Introduction to serous tumours / pelvic neoplasia, p.15.

Prognosis and predictive factors
Prognosis and predictive factors are similar to those of their ovarian counterparts. See Introduction to serous tumours / pelvic neoplasia, p.15.

Others

Endometrioid, clear cell, transitional and mucinous carcinomas of the broad ligament have been described {1310,1919}.

ICD-O codes
Endometrioid carcinoma	8380/3
Mucinous carcinoma	8480/3
Clear cell carcinoma	8310/3

Histopathology
They are similar to their ovarian counterparts.

Prognosis and predictive factors
Prognosis and predictive factors are similar to those of their ovarian counterparts. See Introduction to serous tumours / pelvic neoplasia, p.15.

Mesenchymal and mixed tumours

W.D. Lawrence   J.D. Seidman
I. Alvarado-Cabrero   M. Wells

Leiomyoma

This is the most common neoplasm occurring in the uterine ligaments and is diagnosed when it is clearly separate from the uterus. Five reported inguinal leiomyomas of the round ligament with a median tumour size of 5 cm have been reported in women with a median age of 52 years {1471}. Leiomyomas in the broad ligament are identical to those occurring in the uterus. Nearly all ligamentous smooth muscle neoplasms are benign. Rare atypical leiomyomas have been reported {1188}.

ICD-O Code   8890/0

Adenomyoma

Definition
Endometriosis with prominent smooth-muscle metaplasia forming a discrete mass is classified as an adenomyoma. One review reports four extra-uterine adenomyomas (two in the mesovarium {1792}), but these are certainly more common because most cases are unreported.

ICD-O code   8932/0

Synonyms
Adenomyomas with uterine-like features; endomyometriosis; uterus-like mass

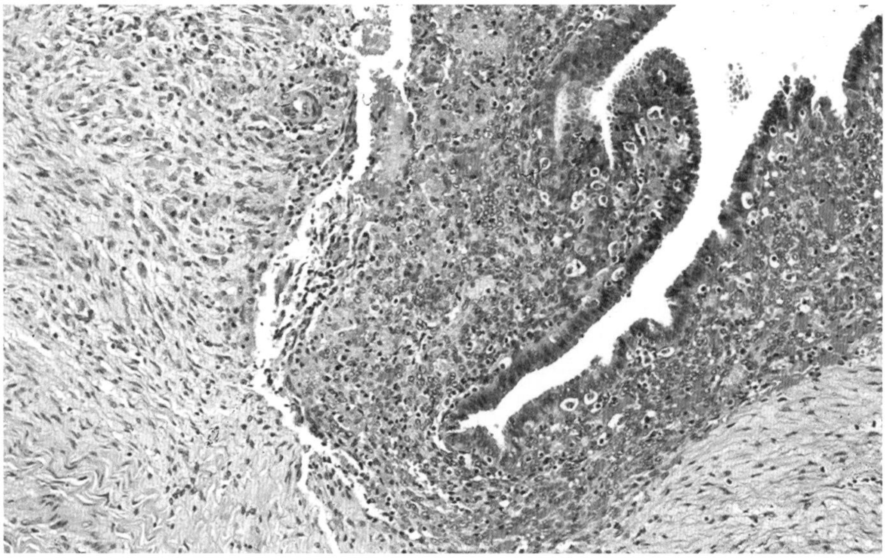

Clinical features
Patients with an adenomyoma (uterus-like mass) vary in age, from 11–59 years {1769}. Most patients present with a pelvic mass, lower abdominal pain or vaginal bleeding {1881}.

Macroscopy
On gross examination, adenomyomas appear as a pear-shaped mass. They can develop within the myometrium or involve the ovary and rarely the uterosacral and broad ligaments. They range in size from 3.5–14 cm.

Histopathology
Histologically, the inner cystic cavity is lined by a mucosa that may reproduce any type of eutopic endometrium {859,1565}. The thickened wall surrounding the ectopic endometrium is composed of normal, organized, myometrial-type smooth muscle. The differential diagnosis includes endometrioma, which may have some degree of subepithelial smooth-muscle metaplasia and extra-uterine leiomyoma with entrapped endometrial-type glands and stroma {1565}.

Histogenesis
For extra-uterine lesions (uterus-like mass) the histogenesis is unknown. Theories include an anomaly of the secondary Müllerian system {1565}, an embryological malformation or a response to hormonal stimulation of multipotential subcoelomic tissues resulting in a supernumerary Müllerian structure like a uterus {1187,1565}. Endometriosis, a phenomenon characterized by smooth-muscle metaplasia in a focus of

Fig. 4.01 Adenomyoma. Cavity lined by endometrial glandular epithelium and stroma overlying hypertrophied smooth muscle that mimics myometrium.

endometriosis {1534}, should also be considered.

Genetic profile
A clonal chromosome deletion 2p21 was reported in endomyometriosis {1982}.

Prognosis and predictive factors
Although a benign, tumour-like mass, it still has the potential for developing into a *bona fide* tumour, identical to those that arise in the uterine corpus. The proven hormone sensitivity to estrogen supports that supposition, as does the one report of a uterus-like mass contiguous with an endometrial adenocarcinoma {1555}.

Adenosarcoma

These biphasic tumours contain epithelial and stromal components identical to those in the uterus. The epithelium is morphologically benign, usually endometrioid or tubal-type and lines leaf-like processes of stroma or occurs as scattered glands within a sarcomatous stroma. The stromal component is a low-grade sarcoma. The presence of high-grade sarcoma should be classified *as adenosarcoma with sarcomatous overgrowth*. Heterologous elements may be present. One case arising in the round ligament, one para-ovarian tumour and three extra-uterine pelvic tumours have been reported {335,873,1270}. Most have arisen in endometriosis.

ICD-O code   8933/3

Leiomyosarcoma

These tumours are identical to those in the uterus. Seventeen cases have been reported in the broad ligament {324,937,962,1451} and only rarely in the round ligament {941}. Although data are scant, criteria for malignancy are the same as those used for the uterus {129}.

ICD-O code   8890/3

Others

Rarely reported tumours include angioleiomyoma {287}, lipoleiomyoma {2004}, lipoma {496}, angiomyolipoma {308} and miscellaneous soft tissue-type sarcomas {178}.

Miscellaneous tumours

W.D. Lawrence   J.D. Seidman
I. Alvarado-Cabrero   M. Wells

Wolffian tumour

Definition
This is a rare, but distinctive, epithelial tumour of Wolffian (mesonephric) origin, characterized by a wide variety of histological patterns that may simulate other pelvic tumours.

ICD-O code   9110/1

Synonyms
Wolffian adenoma; retiform Wolffian adenoma; Wolffian adnexal tumour; female adnexal tumour of probable Wolffian origin (FATWO)

Clinical features
Patients range in age from their mid-teens to > 80 years but the median age is 50 {1557,2120}. They are incidental findings in over one-half the cases {1557}.

Macroscopy
Tumours may be solid, or solid and cystic, and frequently exhibit a lobulated or bosselated configuration {1557}. They range in size from < 1 cm – > 25 cm in maximum dimension. Cut section reveals them to be relatively well encapsulated

{104,1084} and solid or spongy with cystification. Larger tumours in particular, may exhibit haemorrhage and necrosis {1557}.

Histopathology
Microscopic examination typically shows both epithelioid and spindled cells growing in (i) a prominent and distinctive 'sieve-like' pattern, (ii) trabecular patterns comprised of well-formed hollow to solid tubules (iii) diffuse solid patterns or (iv) variable combinations thereof {1557}. Microscopically, Wolffian tumours may mimic sex cord-stromal tumours including Sertoli and Sertoli-Leydig cell tumours as well as granulosa cell tumours {1557} and surface epithelial ovarian cancers, primarily serous and endometrioid carcinomas. The retiform pattern may

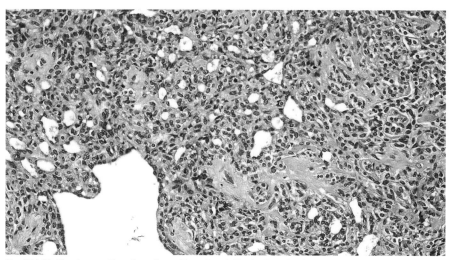

Fig. 4.02 Wolffian tumour. Sieve-like pattern with small, variably-sized but often flattened microcystic spaces punctuate a cellular background with linear anastomosing cords.

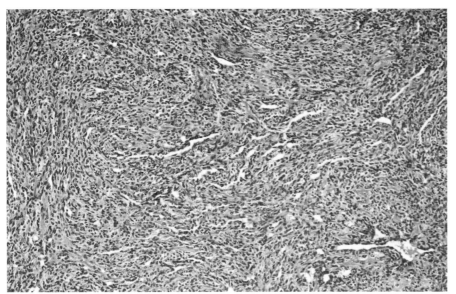

Fig. 4.03 Wolffian tumour. The tumour is composed almost entirely of a solid, highly cellular, spindle-cell component with slit-like spaces.

be mistaken for serous carcinoma but the lack of nuclear atypia and mitotic activity exclude that possibility. The presence of squamous differentiation in endometrioid carcinomas and its absence in Wolffian tumours is also helpful. Although resembling pure Sertoli cell tumours, they lack the interglandular Leydig cells of a Sertoli-Leydig cell tumour. In well sampled tumours, typical histological features of both Sertoli cell tumours and granulosa cell tumours can confirm the diagnosis.

Immunohistochemistry
Immunohistochemically, most Wolffian tumours are positive for inhibin, calretinin, vimentin, CD10, cytokeratins, (specifically, CK 7 and 19), and the melanoma marker A103 {1925}. Estrogen and progesterone receptors vary from strong to absent {2120}. Wolffian tumours are almost universally immunonegative for EMA {1557}.

Histogenesis
A Wolffian origin is suggested by its tendency to arise along the path of the regressing Wolffian ductal system i.e. beginning with the ovarian hilum, passing through the mesosalpinx and lateral uterine walls and ending in the outer one-third of the vagina. Their frequent origin in the leaves of the broad ligament supports their mesonephric nature.

Genetic profile
One group reported Wolffian tumours to be strongly immunopositive for c-Kit.

However, polymerase chain reaction amplification of c-Kit genes located on exons 9, 11, 13, and 17 and of the *PDGFR* gene on exons 12 and 18 found no mutational changes in them {705A}.

Prognosis and predictive factors
Over 70 cases have been described in the literature and most have been benign. However, since approximately 10% of them have pursued an aggressive course, they are generally regarded to be at least of low malignant potential {1557}. Thus far, there have been eight reported cases that exhibited aggressive clinical behaviour manifested mainly by recurrence but rarely by metastasis to the liver and lungs {416, 1869}. Adverse prognostic factors include large size, capsular invasion with rupture and tumour implants. Microscopic features associated with an adverse outcome include hypercellularity, nuclear pleomorphism, and increased mitotic activity {432,730,2120}.

Papillary cystadenoma (with von Hippel-Lindau disease)

Definition
A rare, benign, cystic tumour thought to be of mesonephric origin and characteristically seen in patients with von Hippel-Lindau (VHL) disease.

ICD-O code   8450/0

Synonym
Adnexal papillary tumour of probable mesonephric origin (APMO) {592}

Clinical features
The female homologue to the well-recognized male epididymal cyst in VHL patients was not reported until 1988 {625}; the age range in the few reported cases is from 24–36 {1369}. Virtually all of the reported cases have been unilateral.

Macroscopy
Tumours are usually small, measuring < 0.5 cm in diameter. The inner lining of the cyst wall exhibits fine, papillary protrusions.

Histopathology
The histopathological features are identical to the homologous epididymal cysts in males, notably complex papillary glands with delicate hyalinized and fibrous cores that project into a cyst, containing deeply eosinophilic 'colloid-like' material. Other foci may exhibit solid and tubular patterns. Cuboidal, clear to oxyphilic cells line the papillae and have an immunotype similar to the relatively recently described clear cell papillary renal cell carcinoma {1369}. Indeed, the differential diagnosis includes a clear cell papillary cystadenoma and metastatic papillary clear cell renal carcinoma. The distinction between the two may be aided by immunohistochemical studies {78}.

Histogenesis
Both von Hippel-Lindau (VHL)-associated female and male papillary cystadenomas have been postulated to arise from embryologically-related portions of the urogenital tract {625}. Most investigators have favoured a mesonephric derivation, a fact which has been supported by immunohistochemical studies {187}.

Genetic susceptibility
VHL disease is one of the unusual autosomal dominant disorders where two copies of the VHL gene must be altered to trigger the characteristic manifestations. The latter includes renal cell carcinoma, haemangioblastomas of the central nervous system and retina and various other congenital anomalies. The presence of one of these tumours should raise suspicion for the diagnosis of VHL.

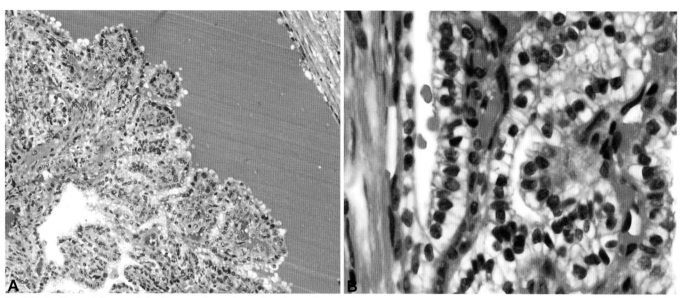

Fig. 4.04 Papillary cystadenoma. **A** Papillary cystadenoma in a patient with von Hippel-Lindau disease. The fibrous cyst wall gives rise to multiple branching papillae lined by cells with clear cytoplasm. The lumen contains a deeply eosinophilic, "colloid-like" material. **B** Papillae are lined by cuboidal to columnar epithelium with bland nuclei and prominent clear cytoplasmic vacuoles above and below the nuclei, resembling day 16-17 secretory endometrium.

Prognosis and predictive factors

Although papillary cystadenomas are benign, they may be the first manifestation of VHL disease. In a recent report, all VHL disease-associated clear cell type papillary cystadenomas exhibited benign behaviour but a sporadic non-VHL case in a 52 year-old woman presented with peritoneal metastases {1369}.

Ependymoma

Definition

A rare, primary, neuroepithelial tumour occurring in the female genital tract and outside of the central nervous system (extramedullary).

ICD-O code 9391/3

Clinical features

Patients range in age from 13–48 years of age. The tumours may be discovered incidentally at surgery or may present with a pelvic mass.

Macroscopy

Ependymomas involving the female reproductive organs, particularly those that are incidental findings, tend to be small. Haemorrhagic necrosis, pseudocystification and myxoid change are frequent in larger examples and may portend malignancy.

Histopathology

Broad ligament ependymomas exhibit the same microscopic and ultrastructural distinctive features of central nervous system ependymomas. They may mimic a serous carcinoma of the Müllerian tract, especially because of the papillary architecture and the occasional finding of psammoma bodies. Being aware of its occurrence in the adnexal structures should raise the question of a neuroepithelial neoplasm and consequent examination of immunostains such as glial fibrillary acidic protein (GFAP). Tumour cells show immunopositivity for GFAP, as well as cytokeratin and vimentin.

Prognosis and predictive factors

As in extra-genital sites, ependymomas are regarded as malignant neoplasms. In the first report of a genital (broad ligament) ependymoma, metastases occurred in both cases {126}. Given the reports of late recurrences in some tumours, the patient should undergo careful long-term surveillance.

Tumour-like lesions

Endometriosis

The presence of ectopically located, endometrial tissue involving the broad ligaments (see chapter 2, p. 98).

Endosalpingiosis

The presence of benign, tubal-type epithelium in the broad ligaments (see chapter 2, p. 99).

Adrenal cortical rests

Definition
The occurrence of adrenal cortical-type tissue in the broad ligament.

Synonym
Adrenal rests

Clinical features
Adrenal cortical rests are most commonly an incidental finding.

Macroscopy
Adrenal cortical rests usually measure no more than several millimetres in size and have a yellowish outer and cut surface {9}.

Histopathology
These lesions are most commonly encountered as spherical, unencapsulated nodules composed of pale, lipid-rich cells. Adrenal cortical rests may be the origin of rarely described cases of steroid cell tumour of the broad ligament, which are usually benign {1632,1685}.

Histogenesis
It remains uncertain whether adrenal cortical rests in the broad ligament represent embryological remnants due to the close proximity of the anlage of the adrenal cortex to the gonadal ridge or a secondary development of coelomic epithelial metaplasia {9}.

Secondary tumours

Metastatic tumours to the broad ligament are often associated with other evidence of adnexal involvement. Metastatic tumours are most often derived from other female reproductive sites. In the case of ovarian epithelial tumours, the broad ligament lesion(s) may show borderline/atypical proliferative or invasive features {771}. Other ovarian tumours, including granulosa cell tumour, may metastasize to the broad ligament. Other tumours involving the broad ligament secondarily include low-grade mucinous neoplasms associated with pseudomyxoma peritonei, uterine or peritoneal leiomyomatosis {1642} and endometrial-type stromal sarcoma of uterine or extra-uterine origin. A wide range of malignant tumours not arising in the female reproductive organs may also metastasize to the broad or round ligaments and present as a primary tumour {505,505,1650}. Prognosis is based on the extent of disease.

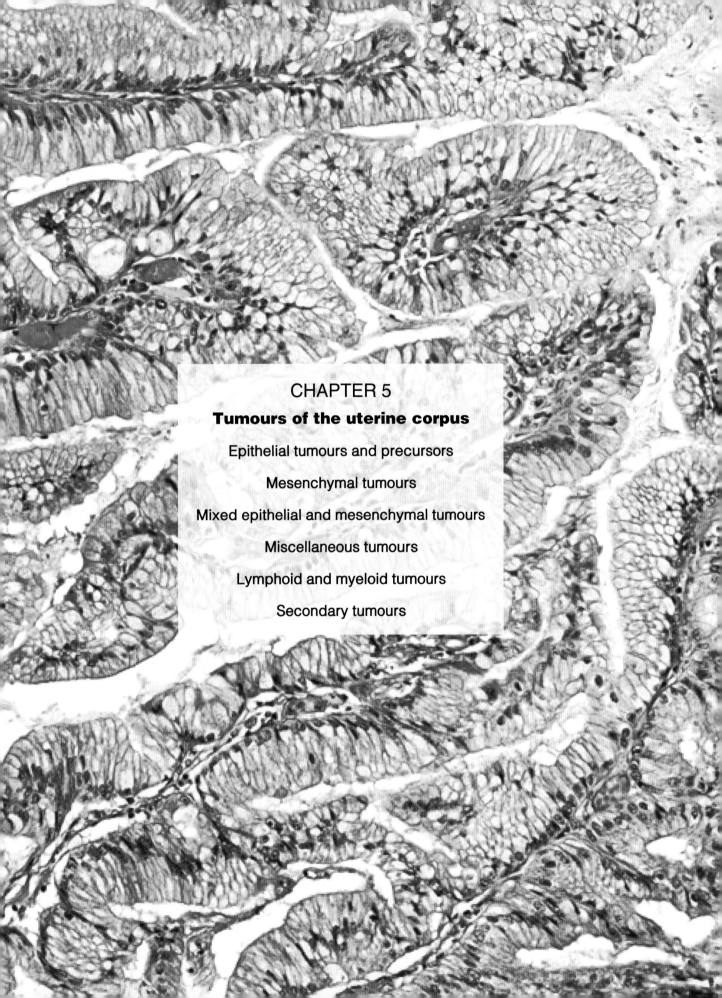

CHAPTER 5

Tumours of the uterine corpus

Epithelial tumours and precursors

Mesenchymal tumours

Mixed epithelial and mesenchymal tumours

Miscellaneous tumours

Lymphoid and myeloid tumours

Secondary tumours

WHO Classification of tumours of the uterine corpus[a,b]

Epithelial tumours and precursors
Precursors
  Hyperplasia without atypia
  Atypical hyperplasia / Endometrioid
    intraepithelial neoplasia   8380/2*
Endometrial carcinomas
  Endometrioid carcinoma   8380/3
    Squamous differentiation   8570/3
    Villoglandular   8263/3
    Secretory   8382/3
  Mucinous carcinoma   8480/3
  Serous endometrial intraepithelial carcinoma   8441/2*
  Serous carcinoma   8441/3
  Clear cell carcinoma   8310/3
  Neuroendocrine tumours
    Low-grade neuroendocrine tumour
      Carcinoid tumour   8240/3
    High-grade neuroendocrine carcinoma
      Small cell neuroendocrine carcinoma   8041/3
      Large cell neuroendocrine carcinoma   8013/3
  Mixed cell adenocarcinoma   8323/3
  Undifferentiated carcinoma   8020/3
  Dedifferentiated carcinoma

Tumour-like lesions
  Polyp
  Metaplasias
  Arias-Stella reaction
  Lymphoma-like lesion

Mesenchymal tumours
Leiomyoma   8890/0
  Cellular leiomyoma   8892/0
  Leiomyoma with bizarre nuclei   8893/0
  Mitotically active leiomyoma   8890/0
  Hydropic leiomyoma   8890/0
  Apoplectic leiomyoma   8890/0
  Lipomatous leiomyoma (lipoleiomyoma)   8890/0
  Epithelioid leiomyoma   8891/0
  Myxoid leiomyoma   8896/0*

  Dissecting (cotyledonoid) leiomyoma   8890/0
  Diffuse leiomyomatosis   8890/1
  Intravenous leiomyomatosis   8890/1
  Metastasizing leiomyoma   8898/1
Smooth muscle tumour of uncertain malignant
  potential   8897/1
Leiomyosarcoma   8890/3
  Epithelioid leiomyosarcoma   8891/3
  Myxoid leiomyosarcoma   8896/3
Endometrial stromal and related tumours
  Endometrial stromal nodule   8930/0
  Low-grade endometrial stromal sarcoma   8931/3
  High-grade endometrial stromal sarcoma   8930/3
  Undifferentiated uterine sarcoma   8805/3
  Uterine tumour resembling ovarian sex cord
    tumour   8590/1*
Miscellaneous mesenchymal tumours
  Rhabdomyosarcoma   8900/3
  Perivascular epithelioid cell tumour
    Benign   8714/0*
    Malignant   8714/3*
Others

Mixed epithelial and mesenchymal tumours
Adenomyoma   8932/0
Atypical polypoid adenomyoma   8932/0
Adenofibroma   9013/0
Adenosarcoma   8933/3
Carcinosarcoma   8980/3

Miscellaneous tumours
Adenomatoid tumour   9054/0
Neuroectodermal tumours
Germ cell tumours

Lymphoid and myeloid tumours
Lymphomas
Myeloid neoplasms

Secondary tumours

---

[a] The morphology codes are from the International Classification of Diseases for Oncology (ICD-O) {575A}. Behaviour is coded /0 for benign tumours, /1 for unspecified, borderline or uncertain behaviour, /2 for carcinoma in situ and grade III intraepithelial neoplasia and /3 for malignant tumours; [b] The classification is modified from the previous WHO classification of tumours {1906A}, taking into account changes in our understanding of these lesions; *These new codes were approved by the IARC/WHO Committee for ICD-O in 2013.

TNM and FIGO classification of carcinomas of the uterine endometrium

T – Primary tumour

TNM	FIGO	
TX		Primary tumour cannot be assessed
T0		No evidence of primary tumour
Tis		Carcinoma in situ (preinvasive carcinoma)
T1	I[a]	Tumour confined to the corpus uteri[a]
T1a	IA[a]	Tumour limited to endometrium or invading less than half of myometrium
T1b	IB	Tumour invades one half or more of myometrium
T2	II	Tumour invades cervical stroma, but does not extend beyond the uterus
T3 and /or N1	III	Local and/or regional spread as specified below:
T3a	IIIA	Tumour invades the serosa of the corpus uteri or adnexae (direct extension or metastasis)
T3b	IIIB	Vaginal or parametrial involvement (direct extension or metastasis)
N1	IIIC	Metastasis to pelvic or para-aortic lymph nodes[b]
	IIIC1	Metastasis to pelvic lymph nodes
N2	IIIC2	Metastasis to para-aortic lymph nodes with or without metastasis to pelvic lymph nodes
T4	IVA	Tumour invades bladder/bowel mucosa[c]
M1	IVB	Distant metastasis (excludes metastasis to vagina, pelvic serosa or adnexae)

Notes: [a] Endocervical glandular involvement only should now be considered as Stage I. [b] Positive cytology has to be reported separately without changing the stage. [c] The presence of bullous oedema is not sufficient evidence to classify as T4. This lesion should be confirmed by biopsy.

N – Regional Lymph Nodes

NX	Regional lymph nodes cannot be assessed
N0	No regional lymph node metastasis
N1	Regional lymph node metastasis

M – Distant Metastasis

M0	No distant metastasis
M1	Distant metastasis (excluding metastasis to vagina, pelvic serosa, or adnexae, including metastasis to inguinal lymph nodes other than para-aortic or pelvic nodes)

Stage grouping

Stage IA	T1a	N0	M0
Stage IB	T1b	N0	M0
Stage II	T2	N0	M0
Stage IIIA	T3a	N0	M0
Stage IIIB	T3b	N0	M0
Stage IIIC	T1, T2, T3	N1, N2	M0
Stage IIIC1	T1, T2, T3	N1	M0
Stage IIIC2	T1, T2, T3	N2	M0
Stage IVA	T4	Any N	M0
Stage IVB	Any T	Any N	M1

References

American Joint Committee on Cancer (AJCC) Cancer Staging Manual, 7th ed. (2011) Edge SB, Byrd DR, Compton CC, Fritz AG, Greene FL, Trotti III eds. Springer: New York

International Union against Cancer (UICC): TNM Classification of Malignant Tumours, 7th ed. (2009) Sobin LH, Gospodarowicz MK, Wittekind Ch eds. Wiley-Blackwell: Oxford

A help-desk for specific questions about the TNM classification is available at http://www.uicc.org.

TNM and FIGO classification of uterine sarcomas

Leiomyosarcoma, Endometrial stromal sarcoma
T – Primary tumour

TNM	FIGO	
T1	I	Tumour limited to the uterus
T1a	IA	Tumour 5cm or less in greatest dimension
T1b	IB	Tumour more than 5cm in greatest dimension
T2	II	Tumour extends beyond the uterus, within the pelvis
T2a	IIA	Tumour involves adnexa
T2b	IIB	Tumour involves other pelvic tissues
T3	III	Tumour involves abdominal tissues
T3a	IIIA	One site
T3b	IIIB	More than one site
N1	IIIC	Metastasis to regional lymph nodes
T4	IVA	Tumour invades bladder or rectal mucosa
M1	IVB	Distant metastasis

Note: Simultaneous tumours of the uterine corpus and ovary/pelvis in association with ovarian/pelvic endometriosis should be classified as independent primary tumours.

Adenosarcoma
T – Primary tumour

TNM	FIGO	
T1	I	Tumour limited to the uterus
T1a	IA	Tumour limited to the endometrium/endocervix
T1b	IB	Tumour invades less than half the myometrium
T1c	IC	Tumour invades one half or more of the myometrium
T2	II	Tumour extends beyond the uterus, within the pelvis
T2a	IIA	Tumour involves adnexa
T2b	IIB	Tumour involves other pelvic tissues
T3	III	Tumour involves abdominal tissues
T3a	IIIA	One site
T3b	IIIB	More than one site
N1	IIIC	Metastasis to regional lymph nodes
T4	IVA	Tumour invades bladder or rectal mucosa

M1	IVB	Distant metastasis

Note: Simultaneous tumours of the uterine corpus and ovary/pelvis in association with ovarian/pelvic endometriosis should be classified as independent primary tumours

N – Regional Lymph Nodes

NX	Regional lymph nodes cannot be assessed
N0	No regional lymph node metastasis
N1	Regional lymph node metastasis

M – Distant Metastasis

M0	No distant metastasis
M1	Distant metastasis (excluding adnexa, pelvic and abdominal tissues)

Stage grouping (Uterine sarcomas)

Stage I	T1	N0	M0
Stage IA	T1a	N0	M0
Stage IB	T1b	N0	M0
Stage IC*	T1c	N0	M0
Stage II	T2	N0	M0
Stage IIA	T2a	N0	M0
Stage IIB	T2 b	N0	M0
Stage IIIA	T3a	N0	M0
Stage IIIB	T3b	N0	M0
Stage IIIC	T1, T2, T3	N1	M0
Stage IVA	T4	Any N	M0
Stage IVB	Any T	Any N	M1

Note: *Stage IC does not apply for leiomyosarcoma and endometrial stromal sarcoma

References

American Joint Committee on Cancer (AJCC) Cancer Staging Manual, 7th ed. (2011) Edge SB, Byrd DR, Compton CC, Fritz AG, Greene FL, Trotti III eds. Springer: New York

International Union against Cancer (UICC): TNM Classification of Malignant Tumours, 7th ed. (2009) Sobin LH, Gospodarowicz MK, Wittekind Ch eds. Wiley-Blackwell: Oxford

A help-desk for specific questions about the TNM classification is available at http://www.uicc.org.

Epithelial tumours and precursors

R. Zaino
S.G. Carinelli
L.H. Ellenson
C. Eng
H. Katabuchi
I. Konishi
S. Lax

X. Matias-Guiu
G.L. Mutter
W.A. Peters III
M.E. Sherman
I.-M. Shih
R. Soslow
C.J.R. Stewart

Precursors

Hyperplasia without atypia

Definition

Endometrial hyperplasia without atypia is an exaggerated proliferation of glands of irregular size and shape, with an associated increase in the gland to stroma ratio compared with proliferative endometrium, but without significant cytological atypia.

Synonyms

Benign endometrial hyperplasia; simple non-atypical endometrial hyperplasia; complex non-atypical endometrial hyperplasia; simple endometrial hyperplasia without atypia; complex endometrial hyperplasia without atypia

Epidemiology

Rates of endometrial hyperplasia without atypia are several-fold higher than for carcinoma {1019,1566}. Risk-factor associations include obesity, polycystic ovarian syndrome and diabetes {504}.

Clinical features

Hyperplasia without atypia results from prolonged oestrogen exposure unopposed by progesterone or progestational agents. It is most commonly diagnosed in the perimenopause, with symptoms of abnormal, non-cyclical vaginal bleeding.

Macroscopy

The endometrium varies from the uniform, 5 mm thick, tan appearance of late proliferative phase to highly thickened, sometimes polypoid or spongy with cysts.

Histopathology

A spectrum of changes is typical. Glands vary in size and shape and may be separated by varying amounts of stroma including back-to-back crowding with little intervening stroma. As this lesion is due to unopposed oestrogenic stimulation, the duration and dose of oestrogen exposure affects the overall appearance {998,1321}. Glands are irregularly distributed, creating a variable density of glands to stroma. While some glands may have normal coiled architecture, others branch or are cystically dilated. The epithelium is of stratified columnar type, with frequent mitotic figures. Focal haemorrhage and stromal breakdown are common.

Proliferation of glands displaying no cytological atypia that exceeds that of normal proliferative endometrium but falls short of the crowding seen in hyperplasia has been termed *"disordered proliferative phase"*.

Histogenesis

Hyperplasia without atypia is the result of unopposed oestrogenic stimulation.

Genetic profile

Hyperplasia without atypia harbours low levels of somatic mutations in scattered histologically unremarkable glands {1322}.

Prognosis and predictive factors

Women exposed to unopposed oestrogen have a 3–4-fold increased endometrial carcinoma risk, rising to 10-fold after a duration of a decade {1455}. Progression to well-differentiated endometrial carcinoma occurs in 1–3% of women with hyperplasia without atypia {998}.

Atypical hyperplasia / Endometrioid intraepithelial neoplasia

Definition

Cytological atypia superimposed on endometrial hyperplasia defines atypical hyperplasia (AH)/endometrioid intraepithelial neoplasia (EIN).

ICD-O code   8380/2

Synonyms

Complex atypical endometrial hyperplasia; simple atypical endometrial hyperplasia; endometrial intraepithelial neoplasia, EIN

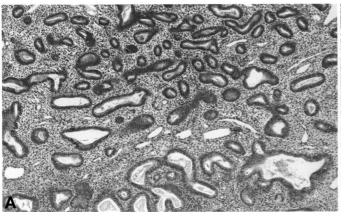
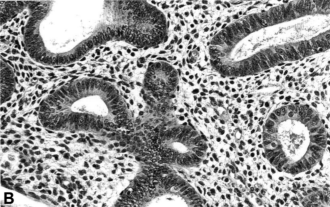

Fig. 5.01 Hyperplasia, without atypia. **A** Architectural changes include glandular branching, dilatation and crowding. **B** Cells lining the glands are columnar with cigar-shaped nuclei and are perpendicular to the basement membrane.

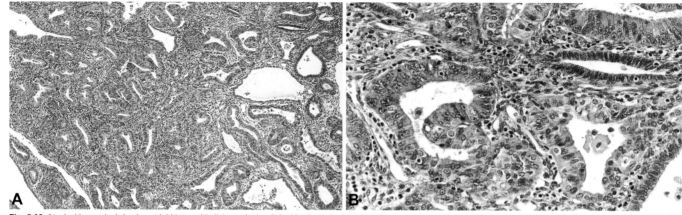

Fig. 5.02 Atypical hyperplasia/endometrioid intraepithelial neoplasia. **A** Architectural changes including aggregates of glands that exceed the volume of stroma. Glandular crowding is visible at low magnification. **B** The cytology of the affected glands (right and left mid field) differs from that of background glands and includes nuclear enlargement, rounding, loss of polarity, pleomorphism and prominent nucleoli.

Epidemiology

The average patient age at presentation is 53 years {1588,1732}. Endogenous or exogenous hyperoestrinism is a risk factor {1917}.

Clinical features

Postmenopausal bleeding or abnormal vaginal bleeding in perimenopausal women is the most common presenting symptom. AH/EIN coexists with carcinoma in approximately 25–40% of women {81,1004,1323,1931}.

Macroscopy

The gross appearance is variable. The endometrium may be diffusely thickened up to 1 cm and may present as a visible focal thickening resembling a polyp. Many lesions, however, have no distinguishing macroscopic features {1556}. The gross appearance is often obscured by hyperplasia without atypia, endometrial polyp or carcinoma, each of which is present in about one-third of cases {237,1323}.

Histopathology

AH/EIN is composed of crowded aggregates of cytologically altered tubular or branching glands. Within the geographic confines of the lesion, the area of glands exceeds that of stroma, resulting in glandular crowding with little intervening stroma.

The distinction between endometrial hyperplasia without atypia and AH/EIN is based on nuclear atypia which may include enlargement, pleomorphism, rounding, loss of polarity and nucleoli {82,998}. Nuclear atypia is variable, both qualitatively and quantitatively. As

these features are somewhat subjective, intraobserver and interobserver variability remains problematic. AH/EIN is often accompanied by metaplastic changes which have no bearing on clinical outcome, but as they display nuclear rounding and enlargement, metaplastic changes add to the difficulty in diagnosing nuclear atypia. Accordingly, the diagnosis of atypia is facilitated by comparison of non-metaplastic epithelium to adjoining normal glands when present, or areas of hyperplasia that do not display metaplastic changes.

Histogenesis

Continuous unopposed oestrogenic stimulation leads to progression of hyperplasia without atypia to AH/EIN. Some studies have found that AH/EIN emerges as a clonal process that begins as a localized lesion usually in a background of hyperplasia without atypia.

Genetic profile

AH/EIN contains many of the genetic changes seen in endometrioid endometrial carcinoma {1180}. These include microsatellite instability, *PAX2* inactivation and *PTEN, KRAS,* and *CTNNB1* (β-catenin) mutation {856,1179,1290,1301}.

Genetic susceptibility

Hereditary susceptibility for AH/EIN parallels that of heritable syndromes associated with an increased risk for endometrioid endometrial carcinoma. These include Cowden syndrome {501} and Lynch syndrome (hereditary non-polyposis colon cancer) {1255}.

Prognosis and predictive factors

One-quarter to one-third of women with a biopsy of AH/EIN will be diagnosed with cancer at immediate hysterectomy or during the first year of follow-up {81,998,1323,1931}. Longer-term risk elevation estimates vary from 14-fold in classic, early studies of AH {998} to 45-fold in EIN studies {81}.

Endometrial carcinomas

Endometrioid carcinoma

Definition

Endometrioid carcinoma of the usual type is a glandular neoplasm displaying an acinar, papillary or partly solid configuration, but lacking the nuclear features of endometrial serous carcinoma.

ICD-O codes

Endometrioid carcinoma	8380/3
Squamous differentiation	8570/3
Villoglandular	8263/3
Secretory	8382/3

Epidemiology

In 2008, there were 288 000 newly diagnosed uterine corpus cancers worldwide of which about 70–80% were of the endometrioid type {545, 546}. Bokhman proposed that endometrial carcinomas are pathogenetically divisible into type I and type II tumours {164,1752}. Risk factors among type I carcinomas (low-grade endometrioid adenocarcinoma and its variants) are similar. Postmenopausal women with higher total concentrations of oestrogens are at increased endometrial carcinoma risk as are women with polycystic ovary syndrome or oestrogen-producing ovarian tumours {860}, earlier age at menarche, later age at menopause, nulliparity or obesity {72,134,223,269, 301,386,504,521,535,1103,1127,1189, 1237,1567,1695,1833,1918,2079,2147}. A positive family history of endometrial carcinoma, Lynch syndrome {112,136,166}

or Cowden syndrome elevates the risk of endometrial carcinoma {136,1893}. Protective factors include later age at first birth and last birth {468,737, 875,1511,1736}, continuous combined hormone replacement therapy, oral contraceptives (high progestin potency), injectable progestins, intrauterine devices, smoking and tubal ligation {1311,2169}.

Clinical features
The average age at diagnosis is about 63 years {384}. 90% of patients have some form of vaginal discharge, usually bleeding. Patients with cervical stenosis may present with pelvic pain, or malignant glandular cells may be found in cervical cytology {1090,2171}. Women with advanced disease may have abdominal distension, pelvic pressure or pain.

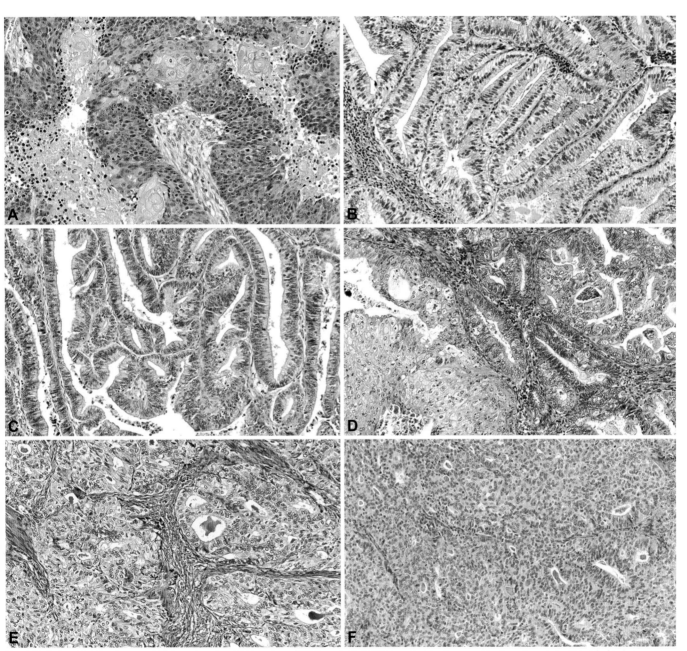

Fig. 5.03 Endometrioid carcinomas. **A** High-grade endometrioid carcinoma (FIGO grade 3). Solid trabeculae of cells with moderate nuclear atypia. Note intermingled squamous differentiation and necrosis. **B** Endometrioid carcinoma with secretory differentiation. Both sub-nuclear and supra-nuclear clear vacuoles are present in the cytoplasm of the stratified columnar cells. **C** Well-differentiated endometrioid carcinoma (FIGO grade 1). Less than 5% of the tumour has a solid growth pattern. **D** Endometrioid carcinoma with squamous differentiation. Squamous differentiation is manifested by sheets of polygonal cells with abundant eosinophilic cytoplasm in the lower left portion of this image, while the remainder of the neoplasm has typical endometrioid glandular differentiation. **E** Moderately differentiated endometrioid carcinoma (FIGO grade 2). Between 6% and 50% of the neoplasm is arranged in solid nests. **F** High-grade, poorly differentiated endometrioid carcinoma (FIGO grade 3). More than 50% of the tumour is arranged as solid sheets of neoplastic cells.

Macroscopy

Tumours can form one or more discrete, tan nodules, while others are diffuse and exophytic. Necrosis and haemorrhage are variable. A subset of tumours arises primarily within the lower uterine segment.

Histopathology

Endometrioid carcinoma typically displays a glandular or villoglandular architecture lined by stratified columnar epithelium with crowded, complex, branching architecture. The lining cells are usually columnar and share a common apical border with adjacent cells, resulting in a smoothly contoured glandular lumen. The cytoplasm of the neoplastic cells is eosinophilic and granular. Nuclear atypia is usually mild to moderate, with inconspicuous nucleoli, except in poorly differentiated carcinomas. The mitotic index is highly variable.

Distinction of well-differentiated endometrioid carcinoma from atypical hyperplasia/endometrioid intraepithelial neoplasia is based on the presence of stromal invasion, defined by loss of intervening stroma (a confluent glandular or cribriform pattern), an altered endometrial stroma (desmoplastic reaction) or a papillary architecture (villoglandular pattern) {1004,1114}.

Grading

Endometrioid carcinomas are primarily graded by their architecture, with those having 5% or less of solid growth considered grade 1, those with between 6 and 50% solid growth considered grade 2, and those with more than 50% solid growth of neoplasm considered grade 3 {382,384}. The presence of grade 3 nuclei involving greater than 50% of the tumour is associated with more aggressive behaviour and therefore justifies upgrading the tumour by one grade {2139}.

Depth of myometrial invasion

Myoinvasion is measured from the endomyometrial junction to the deepest point of invasion. Tumours that involve the lower uterine segment may be of either endometrial or cervical origin.

Endometrioid carcinoma with squamous differentiation

Between 10 and 25% of endometrioid carcinomas contain foci of squamous differentiation {2135} which is recognized by keratin pearl formation, intercellular bridges or solid masses of cells with abundant, polygonally shaped, dense eosinophilic cytoplasm and distinct cell membranes. Squamous differentiation may be at the stromal interface or as morules, bridging adjacent glands. It is important to recognize squamous differentiation since it is not included in the estimation of solid growth for grading endometrioid adenocarcinoma.

Endometrioid carcinoma with secretory differentiation

Less than 2% of architecturally typical endometrioid adenocarcinomas are composed of columnar cells that have single, large, sub or supranuclear vacuoles of glycogen rather than eosinophilic cytoplasm {384,1243}. Consequently, they resemble endometrial glands of the secretory phase. While this occasionally occurs in younger, reproductive-aged women or women treated with progestins, most have been found in non-treated post-menopausal women. Classic endometrioid carcinomas with secretory differentiation are almost always well differentiated.

Less frequent patterns of endometrioid carcinoma include *villoglandular, sertoliform* and *microglandular* types.

Immunohistochemistry

At times distinction between an endocervical and a well differentiated endometrial carcinoma is difficult. Immunohistochemical expression of oestrogen receptor and progesterone receptor favour endometrial origin, while the absence of these hormone receptors, coupled with diffuse reactivity for p16 or positive in situ hybridization for HPV, is consistent with endocervical origin {405,1384}.

Genetic profile

The most frequent alterations include mutation or inactivation of *PTEN* (> 50%) {462,1906}, mutations in *PIK3CA* (30%) {1406,1648}, *PIK3R1* (20–43%) {296,1950}, *ARID1A* (40% of low-grade carcinomas) {675}, *KRAS* (20–26%) {1048} and *TP53* (30% of grade 3 endometrioid carcinomas) {1048}.

About 35% of tumours display microsatellite instability {216,475}. In sporadic endometrioid carcinoma, microsatellite instability is most often due to hypermethylation of the *MLH1* gene promoter {508}. Approximately 10% of tumours have *POLE* mutations resulting in ultra-high frequency of mutations {868}.

Genetic susceptibility

Lynch syndrome (hereditary nonpolyposis colorectal cancer, HNPCC) is due to germline transmission of defective DNA mismatch repair genes (*MSH2, MLH1, MSH6* and *PMS2*) resulting in an autosomal-dominant inheritance pattern. It is the most common cause of familial endometrial carcinoma and is associated also with an increased risk of colon cancer. There is a 25–60% lifetime risk of developing carcinoma {204,2140}. The mean age of onset of Lynch-associated endometrial carcinoma is younger than that of sporadic cancer. Carcinomas in women with Lynch syndrome are relatively more frequent in the lower uterine segment {612}. Cowden syndrome is an autosomal dominant disorder caused by a germline mutation of *PTEN*. The lifetime risk estimate for endometrial carcinoma is 28% {1628}. The median age of diagnosis is in the forties.

Prognosis and predictive factors

FIGO stage, age, histological grade, depth of myometrial invasion and lymphovascular invasion are the most important predictors of lymph node involvement and outcome, and generally apply equally to endometrioid carcinoma and its variants with squamous, secretory or villoglandular differentiation {2135,2140}. The risk of nodal spread and recurrence is related to depth of myometrial invasion. Outer-half myometrial invasion is associated with a significantly diminished survival. Carcinoma confined to adenomyosis, in the absence of invasion of the myometrium, does not alter the prognosis and does not upstage the tumour.

Mucinous carcinoma

Definition

An endometrial carcinoma, in which > 50% of the neoplasm is composed of mucinous cells.

ICD-O code   8480/3

Epidemiology

Mucinous carcinoma accounts for 1–9% of endometrial carcinomas {1628}.

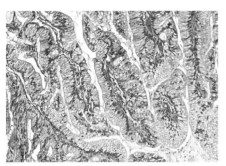

Fig. 5.04 Mucinous carcinoma. The apical portion of the cytoplasm of the neoplastic cells is distended by a pale basophilic secretory product that is characteristic of mucin.

Clinical Features

To judge from the few published cases, the clinical features are similar to the usual type of endometrioid carcinoma. Patients range in age from 47–89 years and present with vaginal bleeding. The tumours are almost always stage I. An association with oestrogen therapy is not unusual.

Macroscopy

Mucinous carcinomas can be suspected by their gelatinous or mucoid texture.

Histopathology

Mucinous carcinoma tends to display a glandular or villoglandular architecture lined by uniform, mucinous, columnar cells with minimal stratification. The mucin is recognized as basophilic globules or slightly pale, granular cytoplasm which is positive for mucicarmine and CEA. Squamous differentiation is frequently present. Nuclear atypia is mild to moderate and mitotic activity is low. Myometrial invasion is typically limited to the inner-half {1251}. Small regions of the tumour that resemble endocervical glands are present in about half of tumours and may cause confusion with endocervical carcinoma. Immunohistochemistry can be helpful in this distinction (see endometrioid carcinoma, p. 126). In endometrial biopsies performed in menopausal and perimenopausal women, proliferative mucinous lesions are often difficult to distinguish from atypical hyperplasia and well differentiated endometrial carcinoma because of lack of associated endometrial stroma. The presence of a confluent or cribriform architecture with even minimal cytological atypia identifies a carcinoma. Proliferations that do not display these features should be classified as atypical mucinous glandular proliferations. These lesions warrant further investigation since they are not infrequently associated with an underlying low-grade carcinoma {1393}.

Genetic profile

There is a high prevalence of somatic *KRAS* mutations in mucinous carcinomas and in papillary mucinous metaplasia {2091}.

Prognosis and predictive factors

Mucinous carcinomas are almost always well differentiated and have a relatively good prognosis {383}.

Serous carcinoma

Definition

Serous carcinoma is characterized by a complex papillary and/or glandular architecture with diffuse, marked nuclear pleomorphism.

ICD-O codes

Serous endometrial
    intraepithelial carcinoma   8441/2
Serous carcinoma   8441/3

Synonyms

Uterine serous carcinoma; serous adenocarcinoma; uterine papillary serous carcinoma (not recommended)

Epidemiology

This is the prototypical type II tumour. Women with serous carcinomas are more often multiparous, current smokers, post tubal ligation, have a history of breast carcinoma and/or tamoxifen use and are less often obese than women with endometrioid carcinomas {194}.

Clinical features

Women are postmenopausal, with a mean age in the late sixties and more often non-Caucasian. Most women present with postmenopausal bleeding. Although many have advanced-stage disease, often it is not apparent by clinical examination since the intra-abdominal disease may be microscopic.

Macroscopy

Since these tumours arise in elderly women, the uterus is usually small, but it may be enlarged by tumour. The uterine cavity may be distended by a tumour mass but the tumour is often inconspicuous, arising on the surface of an endometrial polyp.

Histopathology

Serous endometrial intraepithelial carcinoma (SEIC) frequently develops directly on a polyp or in atrophic endometrium. When the lesion is confined to the epithelium, it is classified as *"Serous intraepithelial carcinoma"*. It is important to recognize that even in the absence of demonstrable invasion, this is a carcinoma that can shed cells and metastasize widely to extra-uterine sites. A complex papillary architecture is characteristic of the pure form of uterine serous carcinoma although a solid growth pattern and glandular architecture may occur. The papillae vary from short, branching and hyalinized, to long, thin and delicate. Each fibrovascular papilla is lined by epithelial cells with large atypical nuclei,

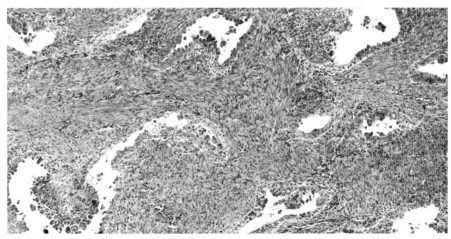

Fig. 5.05 Serous carcinoma, gaping gland pattern. Deeper portions of serous carcinomas are often composed of irregular glands with gaping lumina, rather than papillae. The high-grade nuclei, coupled with the scalloped apical border, help to define the lesion as serous rather than endometrioid.

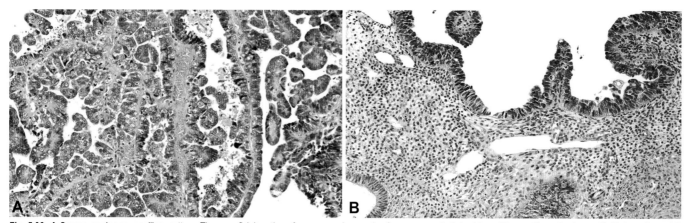

Fig. 5.06 A Serous carcinoma, papillary pattern. The superficial portion of serous carcinomas is often composed of short branching papillary structures with high-grade nuclei, scalloped apical borders to the cytoplasm and sometimes epithelial cell tufting. **B** Serous endometrial intraepithelial carcinoma (SEIC). The lesion (top) is arising in an otherwise atrophic endometrium (bottom) with an atrophic gland on the left.

prominent nucleoli and scant cytoplasm. The luminal surface often appears scalloped or frayed, since a common apical border is often lacking. Mitotic figures are numerous. When the tumour invades the myometrium it frequently displays gaping glands.

There is a subset of high-grade glandular endometrial adenocarcinomas with ambiguous features that could reflect serous or endometrioid differentiation {611}. Immunhistochemical stains for p53 can assist in this situation, as aberrant p53 expression (intense and diffuse staining of at least 75% of the tumour cells or complete absence of p53 immunoreactivity) correlates with a *TP53* mutation and supports the diagnosis of serous carcinoma. In contrast, a p53 stain showing variable intensity in less than 75% of the neoplastic cells correlates with wild type *TP53* and therefore the tumour is more likely a high-grade endometrioid carcinoma, although some high-grade endometrioid carcinomas harbour a *TP53* mutation. A very high Ki-67 labelling index is also more typical of serous carcinoma but, like *TP53* mutations, does not exclude a high-grade endometrioid carcinoma. Some of these tumours may represent an unusual pattern of serous carcinoma and some may represent a true, mixed serous and endometrioid carcinoma. Because of the highly aggressive nature of serous carcinoma, clinicians regard even a relatively minor component of serous carcinoma as tantamount to a pure serous carcinoma.

Histogenesis

Serous endometrial intraepithelial carcinoma (SEIC) is the non-invasive, immedi-

ate precursor of invasive uterine serous carcinoma. SEIC replaces the surface epithelium and/or glands of the endometrium without invading surrounding stroma and is nearly always associated with atrophic endometrium or an endometrial polyp {45}. Both SEIC and uterine serous carcinoma share cytological features; including nuclear enlargement, marked atypia and pleomorphism and a high nuclear to cytoplasm ratio, accompanied by frequent mitotic figures and abnormal mitotic figures. Since the histological distinction of SEIC from early stromal invasion by serous carcinoma is often impossible, it is recommended that these lesions in biopsies be termed *"minimal uterine serous carcinoma"* {2024}.

Genetic profile

The most common somatic mutations in uterine serous carcinoma include *TP53* (80–90%), *PIK3CA* (24–40%), *FBXW7* (20–30%), and *PPP2R1A* (18–28%) {868, 990}. The clonal relationship between SEIC and associated uterine serous carcinoma has been reported {990}, with the same somatic mutations in *PIK3CA, PPP2R1A, FBXW7* and *TP53*.

Genetic susceptibility

Germline *BRCA1/2* mutations may be associated with the development of serous carcinoma {202, 1043, 1044, 1081, 1092,1722}.

Prognosis and predictive factors

A unique feature of SEIC is that, although it does not invade the endometrium, it is frequently associated with disseminated pelvic serous carcinoma {2024,2166}. Serous carcinoma confined to the endo-

metrium has an overall excellent prognosis {643,1738}. Any extra-uterine spread will almost always result in recurrence and death. Comprehensive staging is needed to accurately determine risk of recurrence.

Clear cell carcinoma

Definition

Clear cell carcinoma is a neoplasm composed of polygonal or hobnail-shaped cells with clear or eosinophilic cytoplasm arranged in papillary, tubulocystic or solid patterns, with at least focal high-grade nuclear atypia.

ICD-O code   8310/3

Epidemiology

These uncommon endometrial carcinomas (2%) are considered one of the type II endometrial carcinomas. Multiparity and cigarette smoking are more common, while diabetes mellitus and obesity are less frequent than in women with endometrioid carcinoma {194,312,1049,1502}.

Clinical features

Postmenopausal bleeding is the most frequent presenting symptom, although occasional tumours are diagnosed by identification of malignant cells on Pap smears. The mean age at diagnosis is in the late sixties {3}.

Histopathology

Clear cell carcinoma is characterized by the presence of polygonal or hobnail-shaped cells with clear, or less frequently,

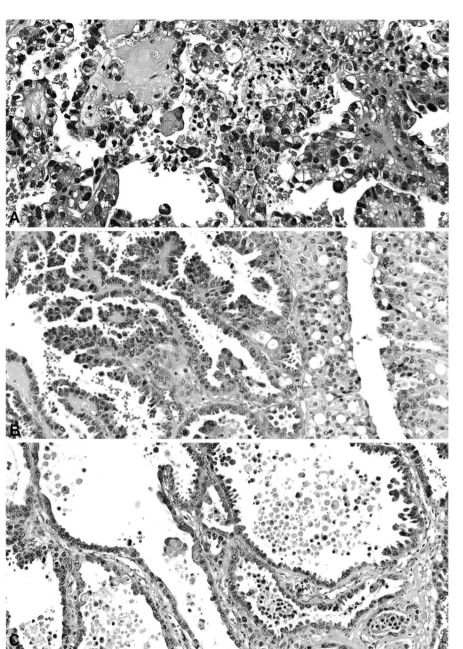

Fig. 5.07 A Clear cell carcinoma. Note the clear cytoplasm with hobnail cells. The papillae have hyalinized cores.
B Clear cell carcinoma, papillary and solid patterns. The papillary pattern of clear cell carcinoma (left) is composed of short branching papillae with hyalinized fibrovascular cores. Cytoplasm may be clear, eosinophilic or of hobnail appearance. The solid pattern (right) contains interspersed cells with clear cytoplasmic vacuoles. **C** Clear cell carcinoma, tubulocystic pattern. Hobnail cells are often seen in the tubulocystic pattern, with protrusion of apical cytoplasm containing nuclei into the lumen.

eosinophilic cytoplasm displaying a tubulocystic, papillary or solid architecture. The papillae are often short and branching, with hyalinized stroma {1007}. Nuclear atypia is prominent, with marked nuclear pleomorphism and variably sized nucleoli. Mitotic figures are usually, but not always, numerous. About two-thirds of clear cell carcinomas contain densely eosinophilic extracellular globules or

hyaline bodies. Clear cell carcinoma usually arises in the background of atrophic endometrium or endometrial polyps. Difficulty in distinguishing clear cell carcinoma from serous or the secretory or squamous variants of endometrioid carcinoma has complicated study of these tumours.

Immunohistochemistry
Clear cell carcinoma is usually ER and PR

negative and rarely overexpresses p53 {1050}. The Ki-67 labelling index is at least 25–30%. In contrast, low-grade endometrioid carcinoma is usually strongly positive for ER and PR and negative for p53, whereas serous carcinoma is negative or weakly positive for ER and PR and diffusely positive for p53 {1049,1050}. Tumour cells express HNF-1B in most cases.

Genetic profile
Somatic mutations in *PTEN* and *TP53* have been reported in 30–40% of cases {48}, mutations in *PIK3CA* in approximately 20%, with a lower frequency of *KRAS* mutations and microsatellite instability in about 10–15% {48,1648}. Loss of expression of BAF250a *(ARID1A)* occurs in 26% of clear cell carcinomas, without mutations in *ARID1A* {2027}.

Prognosis and predictive factors
The overall survival varies greatly, from 21–75%, probably reflecting misclassification of histological mimics; serous and secretory endometrioid carcinoma {3,1502,1658}. Most studies reported a 5-year survival of less than 50% regardless of stage {5,1007,2009}.

Neuroendocrine tumours

Definition
A diverse group of neoplasms that share a morphological neuroendocrine phenotype.

ICD-O codes
Low-grade neuroendocrine tumour
  Carcinoid tumour   8240/3
High-grade neuroendocrine carcinoma
  Small cell neuroendocrine
    carcinoma   8041/3
  Large cell neuroendocrine
    carcinoma   8013/3

Synonyms
For carcinoid: well differentiated endocrine tumour, grade 1;
For small cell neuroendocrine carcinoma: small cell carcinoma; neuroendocrine carcinoma, small cell type, grade 3;
For large cell neuroendocrine carcinoma: neuroendocrine carcinoma, large cell type, grade 3

Epidemiology
Neuroendocrine tumours are rare, representing < 1% of endometrial cancers

and no specific risk factors have been described.

Clinical features
Neuroendocrine tumours usually occur in postmenopausal patients, with an average age at diagnosis of about 60 years for small cell neuroendocrine carcinoma (SCNEC) {795,1959} and 55 years for large cell neuroendocrine carcinoma (LCNEC) {1904}. Post-menopausal bleeding is a common presenting symptom but many women are diagnosed at an advanced stage with a palpable pelvic or vaginal mass or pain {1904,1959}.

Macroscopy
SCNEC usually produces bulky, exophytic, polypoid intraluminal masses with variable myometrial invasion.

Histopathology
Two examples of primary carcinoid tumours of the uterine corpus have been reported {293,651}. SCNEC resembles small cell carcinoma of the lung {795,1959} and is composed of ovoid, poorly cohesive cells, with condensed chromatin and scant cytoplasm. There is frequent nuclear moulding, numerous mitotic figures, necrosis and apoptotic bodies. The growth pattern may be diffuse, trabecular, nested or have rosette-like structures. LCNECs {445} are recognized by their arrangement in well demarcated nests, trabeculae or cords with peripheral palisading. Tumour cells are large, polygonal, with vesicular or hyperchromatic nuclei and a prominent nucleolus. There is high mitotic activity and extensive geographic necrosis (See cervical neuroendocrine tumours, p. 196).

Immunohistochemistry
SCNEC may react for chromogranin A, synaptophysin, CD56, vimentin and cytokeratins (dot-like pattern).
To establish a diagnosis of LCNEC, a neuroendocrine growth pattern should be present in at least part of the tumour, with expression of one or more of the neuroendocrine markers chromogranin, CD56 (the latter is not very specific), synaptophysin in > 10% of the neoplastic cells.

Genetic profile
Hyperploidy for chromosomes 4, 8 and 10 has been demonstrated by FISH analysis in some cases.

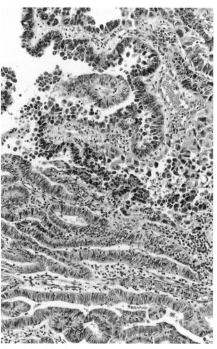

Fig. 5.08 Mixed carcinoma; serous and endometrioid types. Serous carcinoma (top) composed of cells with marked nuclear atypia and a scalloped apical border contrasting with endometrioid carcinoma (bottom) composed of stratified columnar cells with a smooth apical border.

Prognosis and predictive factors
Although the prognosis for SCNEC and LCNEC is poor, there is one report that indicates favourable prognosis when the tumour was confined to an endometrial polyp {170}.

Mixed carcinomas

Definition
A mixed endometrial carcinoma is composed of two or more different histological types of endometrial carcinoma, at least one of which is of the type II category.

ICD-O code
Mixed cell adenocarcinoma   8323/3

Histopathology
At least two histological cell types must be recognizable on H&E-stained sections. The most commonly encountered mixture is endometrioid and serous carcinoma. The minimum percentage of the second component has arbitrarily been set at 5% (see below). Immunohistochemistry may clarify the presence of two distinct cell types. The types present

should be specified in the diagnostic report.

Immunohistochemistry
A combination of PTEN, p53, and p16 helps to discriminate between endometrioid and serous carcinoma {34}, as almost all serous carcinomas display aberrant p53 staining (see ovarian high-grade serous carcinoma, p. 22) and diffuse staining for p16, whereas endometrioid carcinomas display a patchy distribution of p16. PTEN expression is lost in endometrioid carcinoma but generally not in serous carcinoma.

Histogenesis
A mixed endometrioid and serous carcinoma may represent progression from low-grade endometrioid to serous carcinoma {1233}.

Prognosis and predictive factors
The behaviour of these tumours correlates with the highest grade component. A threshold of as little as 5% of a serous component in a mixed carcinoma adversely influences outcome {696,1543}.

Undifferentiated and dedifferentiated carcinomas

Definition
Undifferentiated carcinoma of the endometrium is a malignant epithelial neoplasm with no differentiation. Dedifferentiated carcinoma is composed of undifferentiated carcinoma and a second component of either FIGO grade 1 or 2 endometrioid carcinoma.

ICD-O code
Undifferentiated carcinoma   8020/3

Epidemiology
Undifferentiated carcinomas are uncommon. There is a possible association with Lynch syndrome {196,610,1875}.

Clinical features
The median age in one study was 55 years {1875}. Most patients report postmenopausal bleeding at presentation, with a minority reporting abdominal pain {1875}.

Macroscopy
Most undifferentiated carcinomas form large, polypoid, intraluminal masses

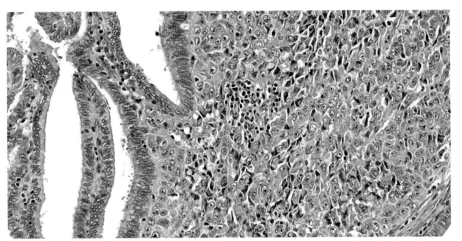

Fig. 5.09 Undifferentiated carcinoma, also designated dedifferentiated carcinoma. A well-differentiated carcinoma on the left abuts an undifferentiated carcinoma on the right.

ranging from 2–15 cm in size {39,1875}. Necrosis is common. Most tumours involve the uterine corpus; however, many involve the lower uterine segment {1875}.

Histopathology

Monomorphic undifferentiated carcinoma
This carcinoma is composed of small to intermediate-sized, dyshesive cells of relatively uniform size arranged in sheets without any obvious nested or trabecular architecture resembling lymphoma, plasmacytoma, "high-grade endometrial stromal sarcoma" or small cell carcinoma {39}. No gland formation is present. The nuclear chromatin is usually condensed. Most cases have > 25 mitotic figures per 10 HPF. Occasional tumours contain pleomorphic nuclei in a monomorphic background. Although the stroma is generally unapparent, some have a myxoid matrix. Tumour-infiltrating lymphocytes are often numerous {1875}.

Dedifferentiated carcinoma
Almost 40% of otherwise monomorphic

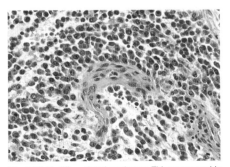

Fig. 5.10 Undifferentiated carcinoma. This monomorphic type has rhabdoid features, with cytoplasm containing eccentrically placed nuclei.

undifferentiated carcinoma contain a second component of either FIGO grade 1 or 2 endometrioid carcinoma {1776,1875}; this phenomenon has been described as "dedifferentiated carcinoma." In these cases, the differentiated endometrioid component usually lines the endometrial cavity, while the undifferentiated component grows beneath it.

Immunohistochemistry
Undifferentiated carcinomas display evidence of epithelial differentiation in only occasional tumour cells, with intense EMA {39,1875} and CK18 {1875} expression in the absence of staining with pan-cytokeratins. Tumour cells express vimentin but not ER, PR or E-cadherin {1875}. Chromogranin and/or synaptophysin staining can be present in a minority of tumour cells {39}.

Histogenesis
Some tumours may arise through a process of dedifferentiation.

Genetic profile
Approximately one-half of tumours display high microsatellite-instability with *MLH1* promoter methylation and loss of expression of MLH1 and PMS2 {610}.

Genetic susceptibility
Rare cases of undifferentiated carcinoma arising in individuals with Lynch syndrome have been described {1875}.

Prognosis and predictive factors
The behaviour of these tumours is highly aggressive, with recurrence or death from tumour in 55–95% of women {39,1875}.

Tumour-like lesions

Polyp

Definition
A localized, disorganized proliferation of benign glandular and stromal elements that is usually elevated above the surface of the adjacent endometrium.

Epidemiology
Endometrial polyps can occur at any age but are most common in the perimenopausal age range {472}. Polyps are present in 2–23% of patients investigated for abnormal uterine bleeding {1195}. There is an increased frequency of polyps in women receiving hormonal replacement or tamoxifen therapy.

Clinical features
Small endometrial polyps may be asymptomatic {450}. Larger polyps are associated with abnormal endometrial bleeding and occasionally with infertility; pedunculated polyps may protrude through the cervical os. Polyps occurring in postmenopausal patients have a higher risk of associated endometrial neoplasia (5% of cases) {1063}.

Macroscopy
Most endometrial polyps are solitary but multiple polyps occur in 10–20% of cases, particularly in patients receiving tamoxifen. Polyps may be pedunculated or sessile; they arise anywhere in the fundus or lower uterine segment. They vary in size from a few millimetres to > 5 cm in diameter {1195}. Polyps typically have a smooth bosselated surface and appear fibrous in cross section, often with small cystic spaces reflecting dilatation of glandular elements.

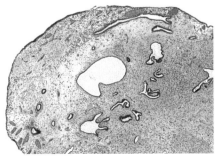

Fig. 5.11 Endometrial polyp. Narrow tubular to cystically dilated glands are scattered in a fibrous stroma.

Histopathology

Both glands and stroma are altered in polyps. The glandular component is composed of tubules that may be simple, branched or cystically dilated, and are lined by inactive or proliferating epithelium, but may occasionally contain foci of hyperplasia or carcinoma {1206}. The stroma may be cellular resembling that of basal endometrium, but often is rich in collagen and contains thick-walled blood vessels, sometimes with haemosiderin deposition {924}. Secretory epithelial changes, if present, are typically poorly developed. Reactive surface changes, including shedding and haemorrhage, are common, as are a range of metaplasias. Endometrial polyps associated with tamoxifen therapy more often show epithelial metaplasias, prominent stromal fibrosis and periglandular stromal cuffing {902}. Polyps with a prominent smooth-muscle component are described as adenomyomatous. Polyps are a disproportionately common site for development of SEIC and small invasive serous carcinomas {1206}.

Histogenesis

Polyps arise as monoclonal overgrowths of genetically altered endometrial stromal cells with secondary induction of polyclonal benign glands. Chromosomal analysis of polyp stroma shows, in the majority of cases, clonal translocations, involving 6p21-p22, 12q13–15, or 7q22 regions 2–5.

Metaplasias

Definition

Endometrial metaplasias reflect a change from one mature histological cell type to another {1303}, and are composed of cells that have cytoplasmic, nuclear and/or architectural differentiation that differ from that of normal endometrioid glands. In the endometrium, metaplasia often represents a cellular alteration that does not result in a mature (normal) cell type.

Synonyms

Papillary syncytial metaplasia; hobnail metaplasia; eosinophilic metaplasia; ciliated cell metaplasia; tubal metaplasia; squamous metaplasia; morular metaplasia; mucinous metaplasia; secretory metaplasia; papillary metaplasia

Histopathology

Metaplastic changes are most often found in abnormal endometria, including hyperplasia, endometritis, shedding, atypical hyperplasia or carcinoma, and are often mixed {149,237,1100}.

Papillary syncytial metaplasia is an exophytic proliferation of eosinophilic cells forming small syncytia or micropapillary processes on the surface of the endometrium or within glands and is often associated with glandular and stromal breakdown {2146}.

Eosinophilic and ciliated cell metaplasias are characterized by epithelial cells with abundant, densely eosinophilic cytoplasm or numerous apical cilia {1303}.

Mucinous metaplasia reflects the presence of pale, basophilic cytoplasm that is either vacuolated or granular {1395}.

Hobnail metaplasia is characterized by

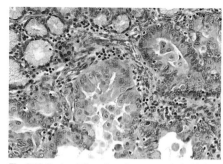

Fig. 5.13 Eosinophilic and mucinous metaplasia. Various types of metaplasias often coexist. Glands displaying mucinous metaplasia (top left) coexist with glands with striking eosinophilic metaplasia (lower left).

glandular cells, often with prominent eosinophilic cytoplasm, and a nucleus, which protrudes into the gland lumen.

Squamous metaplasia is composed of masses of polygonal-shaped cells with dense, eosinophilic cytoplasm and occasionally keratinization, which may occur as either concentrically lamellated, intraglandular elements called squamous morules or bridging adjacent glands.

Secretory metaplasia is characterized by cells containing sub or supranuclear vacuoles, resembling early secretory endometrium.

Papillary proliferation is characterized by fibrovascular stromal cores covered by cytologically bland epithelium {812,1068}. There is a variation from small foci of simple papillae with short non-branching stalks to extensive complex papillae with elongated stalks and branches {812,1068}. The lining epithelium consists of a single layer of cells with bland nuclei and pale eosinophilic or mucinous cytoplasm.

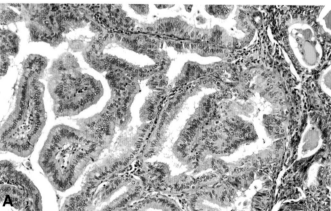
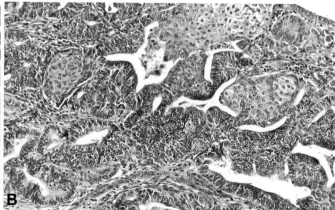

Fig. 5.12 A Mucinous metaplasia. Metaplasias typically occur in abnormal endometrium. This mucinous metaplasia, consisting of cells with abundant apical mucin, is occurring in hyperplastic glands. **B** Squamous metaplasia. Intraglandular squamous morules, characterized by cells with abundant, dense, eosinophilic cytoplasm, most often occur in the setting of hyperplasia without atypia, atypical hyperplasia/endometrioid intraepithelial neoplasia and well-differentiated carcinoma.

Histogenesis

Endometrial metaplasias can be secondary to non-specific endometrial breakdown, chronic inflammation or an abnormal hormonal state.

Prognosis and predictive factors

The metaplastic change is often associated with a variety of endometrial lesions but, in and of itself, has no clinical significance.

Arias-Stella reaction

Definition

Striking cellular and nuclear atypia of cells within endometrial glands, often occurring in association with gestation, gestational trophoblastic disease, treatment with gonadotropins or high doses of progestins {786,1580}.

Synonyms

Arias Stella phenomenon; Arias Stella effect

Clinical features

This change is asymptomatic.

Histopathology

The typical form is seen in the zona spongiosa. The glands are crowded and lined entirely, or in part, by cells with massively abundant, clear, glycogen rich or eosinophilic cytoplasm, and large bulbous nuclei with irregular outlines and smudged

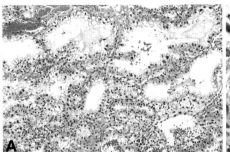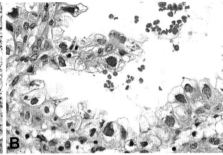

Fig. 5.14 Arias-Stella reaction. **A** Irregularly dilated glands lined by cells with striking nuclear atypia and abundant clear cytoplasm may mimic the tubulocystic pattern of clear cell carcinoma. The young age and history of a gestation would be very unusual for clear cell carcinoma. **B** The striking cytological atypia suggests a high-grade neoplasm, however, the chromatin is smudged, optically clear or degenerated.

or vesicular chromatin. Hobnail cells and intraglandular cellular tufting are common; simple elongated papillary projections may also be seen. Mitotic activity is rarely observed. The lesion must be distinguished from the tubulocystic pattern of clear cell carcinoma {1393}.

Lymphoma-like lesion

Definition

A diffuse infiltration of lymphoid cells that mimics lymphoma or leukaemia {2112}.

Synonyms

Pseudolymphoma; lymphoid hyperplasia

Clinical features

This represents an exaggerated form of endometritis and, usually, women present during the reproductive-age period with vaginal bleeding.

Histopathology

Lymphoma-like lesions are typically superficial and non-mass forming. There is a dense infiltration of the endometrium by lymphoid cells with a predominance of large cells with features of immunoblasts, sometimes in ill-defined aggregates with mitotic activity or with germinal centres. Apoptotic debris and tingible body macrophages may result in a starry-sky pattern. There is typically a background of chronic endometritis, including small lymphocytes, plasma cells and neutrophils. Lymphocytes are usually a mixture of B and T lymphocytes although in different proportions; plasma cells are polytypic {629}.

Mesenchymal tumours

E. Oliva
M.L. Carcangiu
S.G. Carinelli
P. Ip

T. Loening
T.A. Longacre
M.R. Nucci
J. Prat
C.J. Zaloudek

Leiomyoma

Definition

A benign, smooth-muscle tumour that has several variant morphological features.

ICD-O codes

Leiomyoma	8890/0
Cellular leiomyoma	8892/0
Leiomyoma with bizarre nuclei	8893/0
Mitotically active leiomyoma	8890/0
Hydropic leiomyoma	8890/0
Apoplectic leiomyoma	8890/0
Lipomatous leiomyoma (lipoleiomyoma)	8890/0
Epithelioid leiomyoma	8891/0
Myxoid leiomyoma	8896/0
Dissecting (cotyledonoid) leiomyoma	8890/0
Diffuse leiomyomatosis	8890/1
Intravenous leiomyomatosis	8890/1
Metastasizing leiomyoma	8898/1

Synonym

Symplastic leiomyoma (leiomyoma with bizarre nuclei)

Epidemiology

Leiomyomas, including variants, are the most common uterine tumour and usually affect women in their fourth and fifth decades. Variant forms account for approximately 10% of cases. Patients with hereditary leiomyomatosis and renal cancer syndrome present at a younger age. Those with metastasizing leiomyoma usually have a history of prior hysterectomy for leiomyomas.

Clinical features

Most patients are asymptomatic but

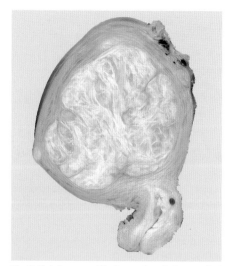

Fig. 5.15 Leiomyoma. The tumour is well circumscribed with a multinodular, whorled and homogeneous white cut surface.

one-third present with menorrhagia, pelvic pain or pressure. Abdominal symptoms occur more frequently in patients receiving progestational therapy or who are pregnant. Symptoms are largely related to the number, size and location of the tumours. Rarely, patients with intravenous leiomyomatosis present with cardiovascular involvement. Patients with benign metastasizing leiomyoma usually present at a median interval of 15 years after hysterectomy {894}. The lungs are the commonest extrauterine location {894} but rarely, other sites can be involved {425,814,1929}. Other less common clinical features include ascites, erythrocytosis secondary to tumour erythropoietin production, coexistent leiomyomatosis peritonealis disseminata, and hereditary leiomyomatosis, an autosomal dominant disorder in which uterine leiomyomas coexist with cutaneous leiomyomas and renal cell carcinomas {1682}.

Macroscopy

Leiomyomas are often multiple (> 75%) and may be intramural, submucosal or subserosal. Submucosal and subserosal tumours may be polypoid or pedunculated; the former may undergo torsion and/or prolapse through the cervical os while the latter may detach from their pedicle and result in a so-called parasitic leiomyoma. Tumours are well circumscribed but non-encapsulated, range widely in size and characteristically have a bulging, firm, whorled, white cut surface. Some tumours, particularly if oedematous, highly cellular or epithelioid, are soft. Highly cellular tumours and those with fat (lipoleiomyoma) are sometimes either focally or diffusely tan to yellow. Infarction, sometimes with haemorrhage, is common, particularly in large tumours and cystic change is occasionally seen, especially in oedematous or myxoid tumours. Leiomyomas in pregnant patients may have a beefy-red appearance ("red degeneration"). Progestational therapy may induce multiple foci of haemorrhagic infarction (apoplectic change) {181}. Occasionally, tumours with hydropic change may project from the serosa as beefy bulbous protrusions (so called cotyledonoid/dissecting leiomyoma). Rarely, numerous ill-defined, often confluent small nodules are present within the myometrium (diffuse leiomyomatosis). Intravenous leiomyomatosis forms worm-like plugs protruding from myometrial or broad ligament veins. Although in most instances only a small number of vessels are involved, occasionally it is extensive {327}.

Histopathology

Most leiomyomas have a well-demarcated border and are composed of spindle cells arranged in intersecting fascicles. Cells have indistinct borders, eosinophilic fibrillary cytoplasm and cigar-shaped nuclei with small nucleoli; mitoses are infrequent. Rarely, nuclear palisading may be seen. Collagen deposition may result in prominent hyalinization. Rarely, calcification may be seen. Infarct-type necrosis, defined by the presence of a band of granulation tissue with or without associated haemorrhage or fibrosis between viable and non-viable tumour, may be seen. The non-viable areas have a "mummified" appearance. In an early stage of infarction, only single or groups of apoptotic cells are seen showing pyknotic nuclei and dense eosinophilic cytoplasm {811,814}.

Cellular leiomyoma

There is significant increased cellularity when compared to the surrounding myometrium and, when highly cellular, mimics an endometrial stromal tumour. In highly cellular tumours, the neoplastic cells are arranged diffusely (often in the centre) or in fascicles (at the periphery). Thick-walled vessels and cleft-like spaces are common. The cells typically have scant cytoplasm, lack nuclear atypia and mitoses are rare {712}. The border is usually irregular and merges with the surrounding myometrium. Foci of normocellular leiomyoma may be present.

Leiomyoma with bizarre nuclei

This tumour (previously termed atypical leiomyoma) contains isolated bizarre cells or, more often, groups of them on

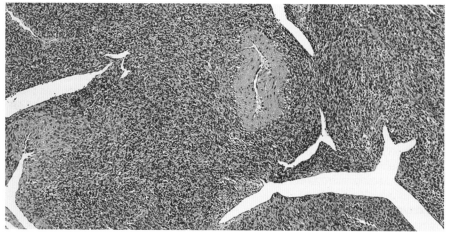

Fig. 5.16 Highly cellular leiomyoma. The tumour is highly cellular resembling an endometrial stromal tumour, however, it shows fascicular growth as well as large and thick-walled blood vessels characteristic of smooth-muscle tumours.

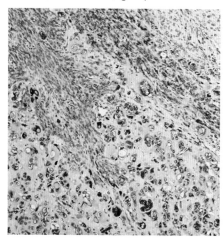

Fig. 5.17 Leiomyoma with bizarre nuclei. The bizarre nuclei alternate with areas of conventional leiomyoma.

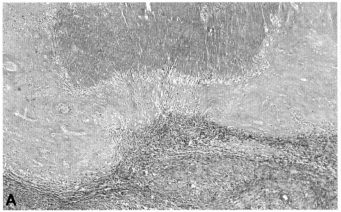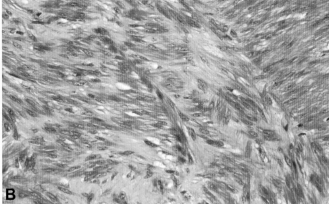

Fig. 5.18 A Leiomyoma with infarct-type necrosis. An area of granulation tissue and hyalinization separates viable from non-viable tumour, the latter (top) showing a mummified appearance. **B** Leiomyoma. Intersecting fascicles of cytologically bland, spindled cells with cigar-shaped nuclei and eosinophilic cytoplasm are present.

a background of an otherwise typical leiomyoma. Typically, it is present focally but rarely this change is extensive, producing confluent zones of atypia. The tumour cells typically have eosinophilic cytoplasm (sometimes appearing globular) {197,1464} and are bizarrely shaped, multilobated or contain multiple, hyperchromatic nuclei; intranuclear cytoplasmic pseudoinclusions may be seen. Nuclear chromatin is often smudged. Mitotic activity is typically low but karyorrhectic nuclei, which may mimic atypical mitotic figures, are common {469,1134}. Tumour cell necrosis is absent but infarct-type necrosis may be seen.

Mitotically active leiomyoma
It often has > 10 mitotic figures per 10 HPF but typically lacks cytological atypia and tumour cell necrosis {129,1400, 1492,1526}. These tumours are usually seen in the reproductive age group, are often submucosal and are sometimes associated with hormone therapy. They may also show hypercellularity and focal bizarre nuclei; in these cases care must be taken to exclude a leiomyosarcoma.

Hydropic leiomyoma
This variant is characterized by conspicuous zonal, watery oedema. Hyalinization may also be seen. The oedema and hyalinization may result in the tumour cells growing in thin delicate cords. The tumours are often vascular and if the hydropic change is extensive, a characteristic nodularity is sometimes noted {348}.

Leiomyoma with apoplectic change.
Progestational therapy typically induces so-called "apoplectic" change characterized by zones of haemorrhagic infarc-

tion surrounded by hypercellular areas often associated with increased mitoses and sometimes myxoid change. If early only single cell apoptosis is seen and late stages may exhibit hyalinization and/or zones of tissue dropout {181}.

Lipoleiomyoma (lipomatous variant)
This is characterized by single or groups of mature adipocytes admixed with the smooth muscle component. Some such tumours may have a chondroid appearance or resemble hibernomas {157,278}. Other heterologous elements such as bone, cartilage, skeletal muscle, haematopoietic or lymphoid cells may rarely be found in leiomyomas {551}.

Epithelioid leiomyoma
It is composed of rounded or polygonal cells with an "epithelial-like" morphology {511,1525}. The tumour cells are arranged in sheets, cords, trabeculae or nests and have appreciable eosinophilic or clear cytoplasm. Tumours with a plexiform growth and < 1 cm are referred to as *plexiform tumourlets*.

Myxoid leiomyoma
is hypocellular with cells widely separated by myxoid acid-mucin stroma (alcian blue positive). The tumour cells show no cytological atypia and have rare to absent mitoses. They lack an infiltrative border.

Cotyledonoid dissecting leiomyoma
This *dissecting variant of leiomyoma* is characterized by irregular dissection of bland smooth muscle cells within the myometrium {1641}. There may be extension outside the uterus, sometimes with conspicuous hydropic change {1642}.

Intravenous leiomyomatosis (IVL)
IVL is characterized by the presence of benign smooth muscle within vascular spaces outside the confines of a leiomyoma, free floating within the lumen or adherent to the vessel wall. The tumour is often prominently vascular and commonly hydropic {853} but it rarely has the appearance of another leiomyoma variant. The cells are usually bland with rare mitoses {346,1379}. Occasionally they contain a minor component of endometrial glands {346} and rarely exhibit cysts that may contain blood. As vascular intrusion occurs occasionally in typical leiomyomas as a focal phenomenon, a diagnosis of IVL is reserved for cases where worm-like growths of smooth muscle are observed, grossly.

Diffuse leiomyomatosis
Innumerable hypercellular tumour nodules that merge imperceptibly with each other and myometrial smooth muscle. Tumour cells lack atypical features. {341,1312}.

Metastasizing leiomyoma
This resembles a typical leiomyoma but it is found in the lungs of women with a history of typical uterine leiomyomas. Entrapment of bronchioalveolar epithelium is often seen within the lesions {579,894}.

Leiomyomatosis and renal cancer syndrome
This autosomal dominant disorder is associated with a germline mutation in the fumarate hydratase (*FH*) gene. It is characterized by multiple leiomyomas that frequently have increased cellularity, multinucleated and atypical nuclei with prominent red to orange nucleoli

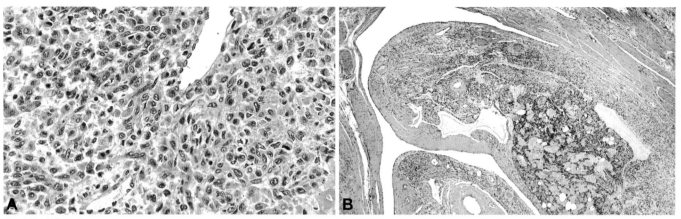

Fig. 5.19 A Epithelioid leiomyoma. A fascicular growth is absent and the tumour cells are not spindle-shaped. The cells show rounded nuclei and have eosinophilic cytoplasm. **B** Intravenous leiomyomatosis. This benign, smooth-muscle proliferation grows within vascular spaces. It has large, thick-walled blood vessels and cleft-like spaces.

surrounded by a clear halo, as well as haemangiopericytoma-like vessels {1682}.

Others
Histological changes associated with GnRH-agonists include irregular border, increased cellularity, focal infarction, hyalinization, massive lymphoid infiltrate, decrease in blood vessel number and calibre and other vascular changes {357,365,387,865,1574}. Uterine artery embolization usually results in infarct-type necrosis and marked acute inflammation {366,1149,2012}. Anti-fibrinolytic agents such as tranexamic acid, used in the treatment of menorrhagia and/or leiomyomas, can also produce thrombosis and infarction {813}.

Immunohistochemistry
Leiomyomas express desmin and h-caldesmon, smooth muscle actin, histone deacetylase 8 {428}, smooth muscle myosin heavy chain {14,1349,2006}, oxytocin receptor {1112} ER, PR and WT1 {244,1055}. CD10 is expressed in up to 40% of highly cellular leiomyomas {428,1112,1422}. p53 and p16 are often positive in leiomyomas with bizarre nuclei but not helpful in the differential diagnosis of leiomyosarcoma {281}.

Histogenesis
Occurrence of non-random X chromosome inactivation is indicative of clonal origin of leiomyomas {717,1111,1175,1541}. Individual nodules in diffuse leiomyomatosis have been shown to be of different clonal origin, as shown by the presence of non-random X-chromosome inactivation involving different alleles in different tumours {114}. Some metastasizing leiomyomas have been postulated to

represent hormone-mediated multifocal hyperplastic or neoplastic smooth muscle proliferations {306,320,967} although several of them are the result of vascular or lymphatic dissemination from uterine leiomyomas {64, 162, 228, 1056, 1314}. Pulmonary and uterine lesions have been shown to have identical patterns of androgen receptor allelic inactivation and X-chromosome inactivation, indicating that these are indeed clonal {1474,1922}.

Genetic profile
Approximately 40% of leiomyomas have chromosomal abberations (i.e. rearrangements of the HMGA locus) such as t(12;14) (q15;q23–24) involving the short arm of chromosome-6, and interstitial deletions of the long arm of chromosome 7 {1111,1541,1813}. *MED12* mutations are often seen in leiomyomas but they are uncommon in leiomyomas with bizarre nuclei {1148}.

Genetic susceptibility
Patients with leiomyomas associated with hereditary leiomyomatosis and renal cancer syndrome have germline, heterozygous loss-of-function mutation of the fumarate hydratase gene (1q43) {1682}. A distinctive cytogenetic profile of metastasizing leiomyoma has also been found in a subset (3%) of uterine leiomyomas but not in other types of benign or malignant smooth-muscle tumours {1385}.

Prognosis and predictive factors
Conventional leiomyoma and its variants are usually associated with a benign course, although experience with some of these variants is limited {129,811,814}. Diffuse leiomyomatosis is associated with a good outcome {1606}. Intravenous

leiomyomatosis can recur (< 5%) up to 15 years after hysterectomy {327}. In approximately 70% of patients, recurrence is related to inferior vena cava and cardiac involvement {110,1456}. Patients with metastasizing leiomyoma have an indolent clinical course but tumours may continue to grow and eventually result in respiratory failure {894}. The majority of epithelioid leiomyomas behave in a benign fashion but some, even with relatively low mitotic activity and cytological atypia, may recur locally {1002}.

Smooth muscle tumour of uncertain malignant potential

Definition
Smooth muscle tumour of uncertain malignant potential (STUMP) is a smooth-muscle tumour with features that preclude an unequivocal diagnosis of leiomyosarcoma, but that do not fulfill the criteria for leiomyoma, or its variants, and raise concern that the neoplasm may behave in a malignant fashion {129}.

ICD-O code   8897/1

Synonym
Atypical smooth muscle neoplasm

Histopathology
In general, the reasons why an unequivocal benign or malignant diagnosis cannot be made are related to a combination of features (Table 5.1). For example, when mitotic indices are higher than in the usual leiomyoma but lower than in most leiomyosarcomas, or when the type of necrosis cannot be determined with certainty, or when some other

Table 5.1 Uterine smooth-muscle tumours with spindle-cell differentiation of uncertain malignant potential.

Tumour cell necrosis	Moderate-to-severe atypia	Mitotic count (per 10 HPF)	Mean mitotic count in tumours with recurrence (per 10 HPF)	Cases with recurrence
Absent	Focal/multifocal	< 10	4 (range 3–5)	13.6% (3 of 22 cases) {68 ,811}
	Diffuse	< 10	4.3 (range 2–9)	10.4% (7 of 67 cases) {129,145,1865,1981}*
Present	None	< 10	2.8 (range 1–4)	26.7% (4 of 15 cases) {41,68,129}
Absent	None	≥ 15	Not applicable	0% (0 of 39† cases) {129,811}

*One of the four tumours also had epithelioid cells
†Three had ≥ 20 mitotic figures per 10 HPF; an unknown proportion also had counts between 10 and 14 {129}.

problematic finding such as epithelioid or myxoid change is present {41,68, 129,145,644,811,1865,1981}. The frequency of recurrence of such tumours, based on a variety of histological features shown, is relatively low (Table 5.1). Since the majority of these tumours do not recur {1134}, some pathologists do not wish to include the term malignancy in the diagnosis. To acknowledge their inability to establish a definitive diagnosis for these problematic neoplasms, they prefer the diagnostic term *"atypical smooth-muscle neoplasm"* appended with a note describing the features that preclude an unequivocal benign or malignant diagnosis. It should be emphasized that this is a diagnosis that should only rarely be made.

Immunohistochemistry
Cell-cycle regulatory protein immunoexpression (p16, p21, p27 and p53) to distinguish uterine leiomyosarcoma from leiomyoma variants has not been useful {1273}.

Prognosis and predictive factors
See Table 5.1 {41,68,129,145,811,1865, 1981}

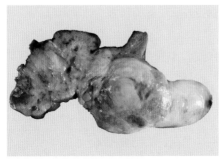

Fig. 5.20 Leiomyosarcoma. Large tumour with a variegated cut surface and areas of necrosis and hemorrhage.

Leiomyosarcoma

Definition
A malignant smooth-muscle tumour, most commonly displaying spindle cell morphology but occasionally showing epithelioid or myxoid features.

ICD-O codes
Leiomyosarcoma	8890/3
Epithelioid leiomyosarcoma	8891/3
Myxoid leiomyosarcoma	8896/3

Epidemiology
Leiomyosarcoma is the most common uterine sarcoma accounting for 1–2% of all uterine malignancies {4} with an incidence of 0.3–0.4/100 000 women per year {708} that increases in women on tamoxifen therapy for breast cancer {198}. The majority occur in patients > 50 years of age {590,1147}.

Clinical features
The most common symptoms include abnormal vaginal bleeding (56%), palpable pelvic mass (54%) and pelvic pain (22%). Occasionally, the presenting manifestations are related to tumour rupture (haemoperitoneum), extra uterine extension (up to one-half), or metastases. As symptoms and signs greatly overlap with those seen in leiomyomas, malignancy should be suspected when tumour growth is detected in menopausal women who are not on hormonal replacement therapy {1465,1490}. Leiomyosarcoma may spread locally or regionally and may be associated with gastrointestinal or urinary- tract symptoms. Haematogenous dissemination is most often to the lungs.

Macroscopy
Leiomyosarcomas are either single masses or, when associated with leiomyomas, the largest mass. They are typically large with a mean diameter of 10 cm (only 25% are < 5 cm). About two-thirds are intramural, one-fifth submucosal and one-tenth subserosal, while only 5% arise in the cervix. The cut surface is typically soft, bulging, fleshy, necrotic and haemorrhagic with irregular margins. The rare myxoid tumours are typically gelatinous and may be deceptively circumscribed {933}.

Histopathology
Spindle cell leiomyosarcomas
These are cytologically high-grade and composed of spindle and/or pleomorphic cells with eosinophilic cytoplasm often forming interlacing but disorganized fascicles. Pleomorphism is usually overt but, in a minority of tumours, is not striking. The utility of grading is controversial, and no universally accepted grading system

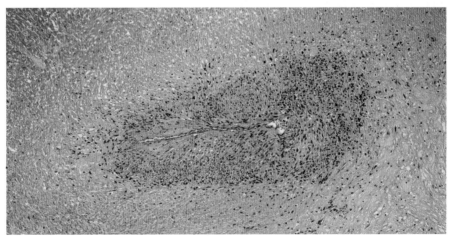

Fig. 5.21 Leiomyosarcoma. Viable tumour in a perivascular arrangement with abrupt transition to tumour cell necrosis. Atypical neoplastic cells are present in the viable tissue.

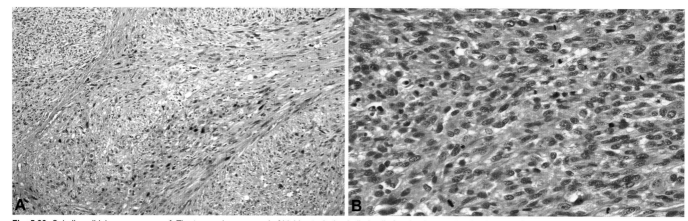

Fig. 5.22 Spindle cell leiomyosarcoma. **A** The tumour is composed of highly atypical spindled cells forming intersecting fascicles. **B** The spindled cells show nuclear atypia and brisk mitotic activity.

exists. Multinucleated tumour cells are found in 50% of cases and osteoclast-like cells are rarely seen {1169}. The mitotic index is usually high {1484}. Tumour cell necrosis occurs in about one-third and it is characterized by an abrupt transition from viable to non-viable areas, the former typically having a perivascular distribution. Within the necrotic zones, atypical cells can still be seen. Both cytological atypia and mitotic activity should usually be present to diagnose leiomyosarcoma, because of difficulty in the reliable distinction between infarct-type and tumour cell necrosis {129,1095}. Vascular space invasion is identified in up to 10–20% of cases and often an infiltrative border is present.

Epithelioid leiomyosarcomas
are composed predominantly or entirely of round or polygonal cells with eosinophilic, or much less commonly, clear cytoplasm {1525}. Tumour cells grow diffusely or in nests and/or cords. Although nuclear pleomorphism is usually mild,

some tumours show moderate to marked nuclear atypia. The mitotic index is generally > 3 per 10 high-power fields {1525}.

Myxoid leiomyosarcomas
have abundant myxoid stroma and commonly show irregular myometrial and sometimes, vascular invasion, and are often at least focally hypocellular with relatively bland cytological features and infrequent mitoses {211,1479}. Well sampled tumours usually exhibit cellular pleomorphism and appreciable mitotic activity, at least focally.

Immunohistochemistry
Desmin, h-caldesmon, smooth muscle actin, and histone deacetylase 8 (HDAC8) are positive in most tumours {428} but may be lost or weak if poorly differentiated, epithelioid or myxoid. They are often immunoreactive for CD10 {1422} and cytokeratins and EMA (the latter most often in epithelioid tumours). Conventional leiomyosarcomas express ER and PR and androgen receptors in

about 30–40% of the cases. Although some express c-Kit (CD117) and DOG1, no c-Kit mutations have been identified {1562,1666}. Recent studies have shown statistically significant higher Ki-67 levels in leiomyosarcomas compared to leiomyomas {23,281,832,1287,1402}. p53 overexpression and mutations have been described in a minority of tumours (25–47%) {23,281,832}. Strong and diffuse p16 immunoreaction {23,832,1402}, especially when accompanied by p53 strong positivity, favours leiomyosarcoma (with the exception of leiomyomas with bizarre nuclei) {68}.

Genetic profile
Leiomyosarcomas have both complex numerical and structural chromosomal aberrations {562,1672} and it is suggested that genomic instability is a hallmark of malignancy in uterine smooth muscle tumours {562}. In particular, frequent losses of 10q and 13q as well as occasional gain of 17p and losses of 2p and 16q have been observed {782,1542}. At least

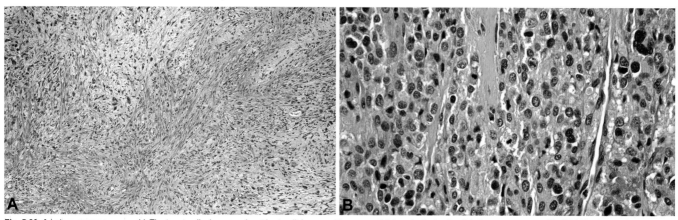

Fig. 5.23 A Leiomyosarcoma, myxoid. The tumour displays prominent hypocellular, myxoid areas containing atypical cells. **B** Leiomyosarcoma, epithelioid. The tumour has a nested appearance and the cells are rounded, with abundant eosinophilic cytoplasm and atypical nuclei. There are numerous mitotic figures.

some tumours have X inactivation that differs from their accompanying leiomyomas, suggesting that leiomyosarcoma occurs de novo. Malignant transformation of leiomyomas (e.g. bizarre leiomyoma) is anecdotal and remains to be proven. MED12 mutations are uncommon in these tumours and HMGA2 related translocations are not seen {1148,1167}.

Genetic susceptibility
Overexpression of the c-MYC proto-oncogene occurs in about 50% of leiomyomas and leiomyosarcomas {833}. The MDM2 protein is overexpressed in some leiomyosarcomas but not in leiomyomas {691} while KRAS is not expressed in leiomyosarcomas (in contrast to a small minority of leiomyomas) {691}. Lack of γ-smooth-muscle isoactin gene appears to highly correlate with a histological diagnosis of leiomyosarcoma {1933}. Abnormalities of the retinoblastoma-cyclin D pathway are found in about 90% of tumours {436} as the gene is deleted in about three-quarters of leiomyosarcomas {782}. Recently, p16, also known as INK4 or cyclin-dependent kinase inhibitor 2A (CDKN2A), has been implicated in the genesis of leiomyosarcoma {163,888}. p16 protein binds the CDK4–cyclin D complex and acts as a negative cell-cycle regulator. Consequently, p16 deletion results in a loss of tumour suppression.

Prognosis and predictive factors
Leiomyosarcoma is associated with poor prognosis even when confined to the uterus at time of initial diagnosis {4,403,1147,1411}. Overall 5-year survival rates range from 15–25% {1035,1484} while the 5-year survival rate is 40–70% for stage I and II tumours {159,590,

1191,1375,1376,1475,2043}. Stage is the most powerful prognostic factor. For tumours confined to the corpus, size is an important prognostic factor {511,645,848,1376} with tumours < 5 cm in diameter being associated with better survival rates {400,645}. Several series have found mitotic index to be of prognostic significance {4,400,590}, whereas others have not {511,2003}. Premenopausal women have a more favourable outcome in some series {590,2043} but not in others. In spindle cell leiomyosarcomas, most recurrences are detected within two years, while myxoid and epithelioid variants often recur late (up to ten years).

Endometrial stromal and related tumours

Endometrial stromal nodule

Definition
A benign endometrial stromal tumour that has a well-circumscribed margin and is composed of cells that resemble proliferative-phase endometrial stroma. Finger-like projections or immediately adjacent nests of tumour cells (measuring < 3 mm in greatest extent from the main mass) and < 3 in number are acceptable. Lymphovascular invasion excludes the diagnosis.

ICD-O code   8930/0

Epidemiology
This is a rare neoplasm. Patients range in age from 23–86 (mean, 53) years {266,457,1910}.

Clinical features
Patients often present with abnormal uterine bleeding or abdominal pain. The uterus may be enlarged or there may be a pelvic mass {266,457,1910}.

Macroscopy
Tumours are commonly submucosal or intramural and only rarely, subserosal; if submucosal, they are typically polypoid. They range in size up to 22 (mean 7) cm and are well circumscribed. Their cut surface is solid yellow to tan; cyst formation may occur, but predominantly cystic tumours are rare. Areas of necrosis and haemorrhage may be present {266,457,1910}.

Histopathology
They generally have a well demarcated border but may show very limited infiltration. Most tumours are densely cellular and characterized by a diffuse growth of uniform small cells with scant cytoplasm, round to oval nuclei and inconspicuous nucleoli. Mitotic activity is variable (generally low but may be brisk) without atypical forms. Whorling of tumour cells around arterioles is typical. Generally, the tumour contains small-sized vessels but sometimes large vessels, typically located at the periphery of the tumour, are present. Collagen bands, foamy histiocytes and cholesterol clefts may be present; the latter two often in the vicinity of areas of necrosis. Unusual variants include tumours with smooth- or skeletal-muscle differentiation (rare), fibromyxoid change, sex cord-like differentiation, endometrioid-type glands and rhabdoid or epithelioid morphology {266,457,1910} (see section on low-grade endometrial sarcoma, p. 142). The immunoprofile for endometrial stromal nodule is identical to that of endometrial stromal sarcoma.

Histogenesis
The lesion is of endometrial stromal derivation.

Genetic profile
Most tumours harbour t(7;17)(p21;q15), which results in a fusion between JAZF1 and SUZ12 {969,1390,1418}. This rearrangement is more commonly seen in tumours with conventional morphology, but can also occur in those with smooth muscle, fibroblastic/myxoid and sex cord-like differentiation {298}. Rearrangements of EPC1, PHF1, and MEAF6 have not been

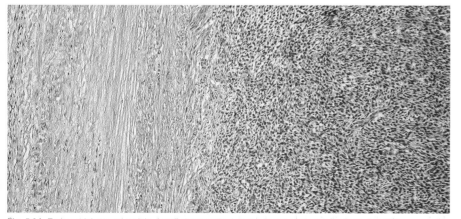

Fig. 5.24 Endometrial stromal nodule. A well-circumscribed margin is seen between the tumour and the surrounding myometrium.

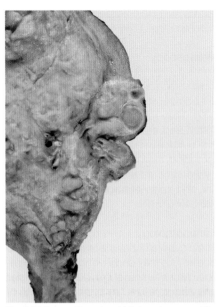

Fig. 5.25 Low-grade endometrial stromal sarcoma. The tumour forms coalescent white to tan masses that are associated with prominent "worm-like plugs" permeating the uterine wall and myometrial veins.

found in endometrial stromal nodules to date.

Prognosis and predictive factors

Patients have an excellent outcome. It is important to extensively sample the tumour-myometrial interface to exclude conspicuous, permeative growth or lymphovascular invasion diagnostic of stromal sarcoma.

Low-grade endometrial stromal sarcoma

Definition

Low-grade endometrial stromal sarcoma (LGESS) is a malignant tumour composed of cells resembling stromal cells of proliferative-phase endometrium, displaying permeative, infiltrative growth into the myometrium and/or lymphovascular spaces. High mitotic activity does not exclude the diagnosis.

ICD-O code   8931/3

Synonym

Endolymphatic stromal myosis (not recommended)

Epidemiology

Low-grade endometrial stromal sarcoma represents < 1% of all uterine malignancies, but is the second most common uterine malignant mesenchymal tumour {4,708}. It occurs over a wide age range with a mean of 52 years {261}, but patients tend to be younger than those with other uterine sarcomas.

Clinical features

Patients typically present with abnormal uterine bleeding or abdominal pain. Less commonly, they are asymptomatic; occasionally metastasis (most commonly ovary or lung) may be the initial presentation. The uterus may be enlarged or there may be a pelvic mass. The frequency of adnexal involvement and lymph node metastasis is approximately 10% and up to 30% respectively {466}. An association with prolonged oestrogenic stimulation, including tamoxifen, or history of pelvic radiation has been reported.

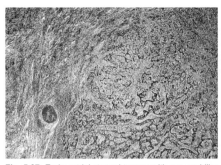

Fig. 5.27 Endometrial stromal tumour with sex cord-like differentiation. Inter-anastomosing cords and islands with an epithelial-like morphology are present in a background of endometrial stromal neoplasia.

Macroscopy

These tumours may present as an intracavitary polypoid or intramural mass often with ill-defined borders and overt permeative myometrial infiltration and/or intravascular, worm-like plugs of tumour protruding from intramyometrial or parametrial veins. Some tumours may be deceptively well circumscribed. Size is variable but most range from 5–10 cm {261}. They typically have a yellow to tan, fleshy cut surface with haemorrhage and necrosis occasionally seen {266}.

Histopathology

Irregularly sized and shaped islands of tumour cells typically extensively permeating the myometrium ("tongue-like" growth) without an associated stromal response are seen; lymphovascular invasion may be apparent. The tumour cells grow in sheets and are typically small with scant cytoplasm and uniform, oval to fusiform nuclei. They show minimal to no cytological atypia and low-mitotic activity (usually < 5 per 10 HPF) although higher counts occur. A delicate network of arterioles is common

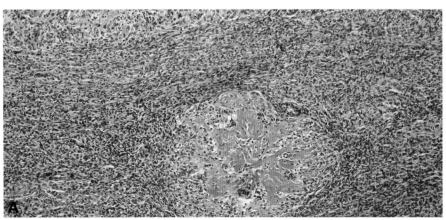

Fig. 5.26 Endometrial stromal sarcoma with focal smooth muscle differentiation. **A** Conventional endometrial stromal neoplasia is juxtaposed to areas with smooth muscle differentiation displaying a starburst morphology (bottom). **B** The focal smooth-muscle differentiation shows typical expression of desmin.

and hyaline plaques, foamy histiocytes, cystic change, haemorrhage and necrosis can be seen {266,1380}. Both endometrial stromal nodules and low-grade endometrial stromal sarcomas can display the following variant morphology which can be admixed: i) smooth muscle differentiation which is most often seen as nodules with central hyalinization and radiating collagen bands that at the periphery encircle rounded cells ("starburst" pattern) that merge with small and immature bundles of smooth muscle {909,1417,2087}; ii) fibromyxoid change characteristically imparts a hypocellular appearance; however, the typical permeative growth pattern, tumour cytomorphology and vascular network are present {1423,2087}; iii) sex cord-like differentiation, which recapitulates the appearance of sex cord-stromal (most commonly granulosa and Sertoli cell) tumours of the ovary {334}; iv) endometrioid-type glands, typically with a "proliferative" appearance {339,1213,1215}. Skeletal muscle differentiation, rhabdoid, epithelioid, clear cell change, focal bizarre nuclei (if sarcoma), adipocytic differentiation, pseudopapillary appearance and multinucleated giant cells are rarely seen {94,517,573,1110,1214, 1231,1415, 1416}.

Immunohistochemistry
The tumour cells are typically but not always diffusely and strongly positive for CD10, often positive for smooth-muscle actin and occasionally for desmin, but they are negative for h-caldesmon and HDAC8. Desmin and h-caldesmon are typically positive in areas showing smooth-muscle differentiation and often positive in areas of sex cord-like differentiation. Androgen receptor and pan-cytokeratin (AE1/AE3)

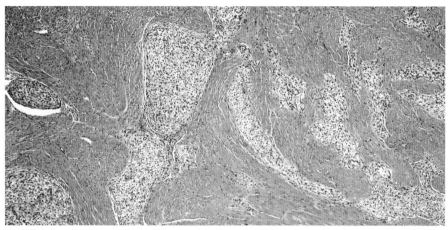

Fig. 5.28 Low-grade endometrial stromal sarcoma. Irregular nests of "blue" cells permeate the myometrium without an associated stromal reaction. Note the presence of lymphovascular invasion (left).

may be positive in the neoplastic stromal cells and areas of sex cord-like and epithelial differentiation. ER (only α isoform), PR and WT-1 are typically positive. Inhibin, calretinin, melan-A and CD99 can be positive in areas of sex cord-like differentiation {94,96,100,314,428,816,1284, 1415,1422,1860}. Tumours of endometrial stromal derivation may express aromatase {1571} and c-Kit (CD117) but do not harbour *c-KIT* mutations {1651}.

Histogenesis
The tumours are of endometrial stromal derivation.

Genetic profile
Most endometrial stromal sarcomas harbour t(7;17)(p21;q15) which results in a fusion between *JAZF1* and *SUZ12 (JJAZ1)* {298,573,690,780,828,969,1259}. This aberration can be seen in tumours with conventional morphology and those with smooth muscle and sex cord-like

differentiation, fibromyxoid change and benign epithelioid cells {783,969,997, 1259,1418}. The t(7;17)(p21;q15) appears to be the most common rearrangement being present in approximately 50% of endometrial stromal sarcomas tested. Other rearrangements described include t(6;7)(p21;p15), t(6;10;10)(p21;q22;p11), and t(1;6)(p34;p21) which result in *PHF1-JAZF1, EPC1-PHF1* and *MEAF6-PHF1* rearrangements. Of these, the *EPC1-PHF1* is the next most common and rearrangements involving 6p21 are more commonly seen in tumours with sex cord-like differentiation {399,1256}. These translocations involve members of the polycomb gene family suggesting a shared pathogenetic mechanism {334}.

Prognosis and predictive factors
Stage is the most important prognostic factor. Five-year disease specific survival for stages I and II is 90% compared to 50% for stages III and IV {4}.

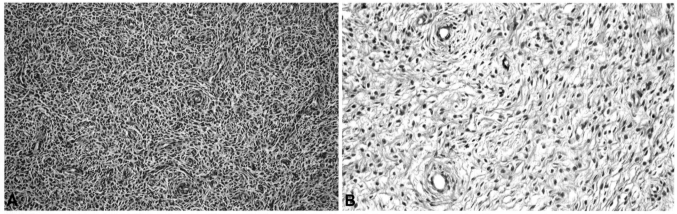

Fig. 5.29 A Low-grade endometrioid stromal sarcoma. The tumour cells resemble the stromal cells in proliferative endometrium. They are uniformly small, with scant cytoplasm, oval nuclei and often whorl around arteriole-type vessels. **B** Endometrial stromal tumour with fibroblastic appearance. The tumour is hypocellular but it shows the characteristic arterioles as well as the uniform oval cells of a typical endometrial stromal neoplasm.

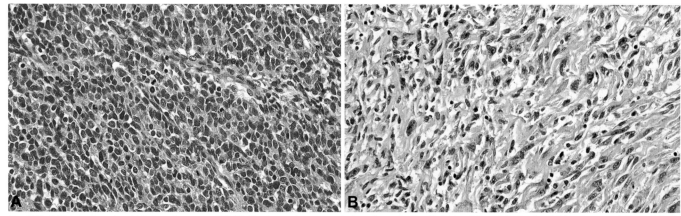

Fig. 5.30 A High-grade endometrial stromal sarcoma, t(10;17). The tumour is composed of small round cells with brisk mitotic activity forming tight nests separated by a delicate vasculature. **B** Undifferentiated uterine sarcoma. Highly atypical neoplastic cells showing no specific differentiation. The tumour cells do not resemble proliferative-phase endometrium.

High-grade endometrial stromal sarcoma

Definition
A malignant tumour of endometrial stromal derivation with high-grade, round-cell morphology sometimes associated with a low-grade spindle cell component that is most commonly fibromyxoid.

ICD-O code   8930/3

Epidemiology
This is a rare tumour whose true frequency is unknown, as tumours previously considered undifferentiated uterine sarcoma may belong to this category {44,997,1054}.

Clinical features
Patients range in age from 28–67 (mean, 50) years. Patients most often present with abnormal vaginal bleeding (menorrhagia or peri/postmenopausal bleeding) and can present with an enlarged uterus or a pelvic mass {1054}.

Macroscopy
The tumours may be seen as intracavitary polypoid and/or mural mass(es) with or without obvious myometrial invasion. They typically range in size up to 9 (median, 7.5) cm and often show extra-uterine extension at the time of diagnosis. Sectioning shows a tan to yellow, fleshy cut surface; haemorrhage and necrosis may be seen {1054}.

Histopathology
On low-power examination, this tumour may have the typical infiltrative growth and vasculature of its low-grade counter-part, however, it commonly shows confluent permeative and destructive growth, often with invasion into the outer-half of the myometrium {1054}. There is a variable mixture of closely juxtaposed high-grade round cell (usually predominant) and low-grade spindle cell components. The round cell areas are hypercellular and the cells are arranged in vague to well defined nests and separated by a delicate capillary network. The round cells have a modest amount of eosinophilic to granular cytoplasm, irregular nuclear contours and granular to often vesicular chromatin, with variably distinct nucleoli. Occasionally, the round cells are non-cohesive imparting a pseudo-papillary/glandular appearance or have focal rhabdoid morphology. Rarely, primitive neuroectodermal differentiation in the form of Flexner-Wintersteiner rosettes or Homer-Wright pseudorosettes may be seen {44}. Mitotic activity is typically > 10 per 10 HPF and is typically very striking. Necrosis is usually present. The spindle cell component usually has fibromyxoid features. Lymphovascular invasion is typically present {1995}. Rarely, a high-grade sarcoma is seen in association with areas that have the appearance of conventional low-grade endometrial stromal sarcoma and also can be diagnosed as high-grade endometrial stromal sarcoma.

The high-grade component of tumours with t(10;17) is CD10, ER and PR negative but shows strong diffuse cyclin D1 positivity (> 70% nuclei); the low-grade spindle cell component is typically strongly and diffusely CD10, ER and PR positive and shows variable, heterogeneous cyclin D1 expression (< 50%) {1053}. The high-grade component is also c-Kit positive but DOG1 negative.

Histogenesis
The tumour is of endometrial stromal derivation.

Genetic profile
High-grade endometrial stromal sarcoma typically harbours the *YWHAE-FAM22* genetic fusion as a result of t(10;17) (q22;p13) {1054}.

Prognosis and predictive factors
In comparison to low-grade endometrial stromal sarcomas, patients have earlier and more frequent recurrences (often < 1 year) and are more likely to die of disease. They appear to have a prognosis that is intermediate between low-grade endometrial stromal sarcoma and undifferentiated uterine sarcoma {1054}.

Undifferentiated uterine sarcoma

Definition
A tumour arising in the endometrium or myometrium, lacking any resemblance to proliferative-phase endometrial stroma, with high-grade cytological features and with no specific type of differentiation.

ICD-O code   8805/3

Synonym
Undifferentiated endometrial sarcoma (not recommended)

Epidemiology
This tumour is rare. Patients are typically

postmenopausal. The mean age is 60 years.

Clinical features
Approximately two-thirds of patients present with high-stage disease (stage III/IV). They typically have postmenopausal bleeding or signs/symptoms secondary to extrauterine spread {997,1902}.

Macroscopy
They are often intraluminal polypoid masses, usually > 10 cm, with a fleshy cut surface and areas of necrosis and/or haemorrhage.

Histopathology
On low-power magnification, margins are poorly defined with destructive invasion of the myometrium. The tumour cells typically grow in sheets, have a storiform or herringbone pattern and show marked cytological atypia. Rhabdoid morphology or myxoid background may be seen. Brisk mitotic activity, including atypical forms and lymphovascular invasion are common. Rarely, some tumours show a sharp transition to low-grade endometrial stromal neoplasia, which may suggest an endometrial stromal origin in some tumours ("dedifferentiated low-grade endometrial stromal sarcoma").

Immunohistochemistry
These tumours are variably CD10 positive and ER and PR weakly positive or negative. Cyclin D1 can be diffusely positive but in those cases the tumours are also typically positive for CD10 (which excludes *YWHAE-FAM22* sarcomas). Focal smooth muscle actin, desmin, EMA or keratin positivity may be seen {997}.

Histogenesis
The histogenesis is unknown; however, rare tumours may be of endometrial stromal derivation as has been suggested by microRNA studies.

Genetic profile
These tumours can have complex chromosomal changes, including gains of 2q, 4q, 6q, 7p, 9q, 20q and losses of 3q, 10p, 14q {690}.

Prognosis and predictive factors
Most patients present with high-stage disease (> 60%). Even patients with stage I tumours usually die within two years {997,1902}. Adjuvant therapy does not appear to improve prognosis {1902}.

Uterine tumour resembling ovarian sex cord tumour

Definition
Neoplasms that resemble ovarian sex cord tumours, without a component of recognizable endometrial stroma {334,1415}.

ICD-O code　　　　　　　　8590/1

Epidemiology
They typically occur in middle-aged women (mean, 50 years) {397}.

Clinical features
Patients may present with abnormal bleeding or pelvic pain, but a subset is found incidentally {397}.

Macroscopy
They may be intramural, submucosal or polypoid, intracavitary masses. They have a well-defined or slightly irregular margin, average 6 cm and are yellow or tan with a variably soft to firm consistency.

Histopathology
Uterine tumours resembling ovarian sex cord tumours (UTROSCT) are well circumscribed but may have a pseudo-infiltrative appearance due to incorporated smooth-muscle bundles {816,1820}; rarely, true myometrial invasion can occur. They grow in sheets, cords, nests, trabeculae or tubules and sometimes have a retiform or glomeruloid appearance. Most tumour cells have scant cytoplasm but some may display abundant eosinophilic or foamy cytoplasm {816,1374}. Cytological atypia is minimal and mitoses are rare in most tumours. Vascular invasion, heterologous elements (mucinous epithelium) and necrosis may be seen occasionally.

Immunohistochemistry
The tumour cells are usually immunoreactive for cytokeratin and WT-1, frequently for smooth muscle actin or desmin and less commonly for sex cord markers (calretinin, inhibin, CD99, Melan-A, CD56) {100,427,796,816,985}. ER and PR are often positive {985}.

Genetic profile
The tumours do not have the *JAZF1-SUZ12* fusion that characterizes endometrial stromal tumours {1820}, indicating that they are unlikely to be of endometrial stromal derivation.

Prognosis and predictive factors
Most tumours have a benign clinical course {756}.

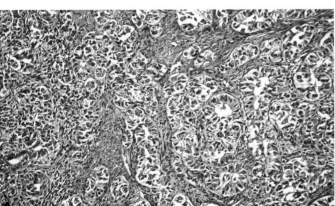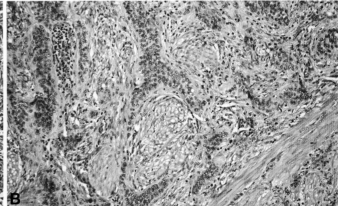

Fig. 5.31 Uterine tumour resembling an ovarian sex cord tumour. **A** Hollow and solid tubules lined by columnar cells with abundant cytoplasm are seen, reminiscent of a Sertoli cell tumour of the ovary. **B** Bland-appearing cells forming anastomosing cords are reminiscent of an adult granulosa cell tumour, and are dissecting muscle bundles.

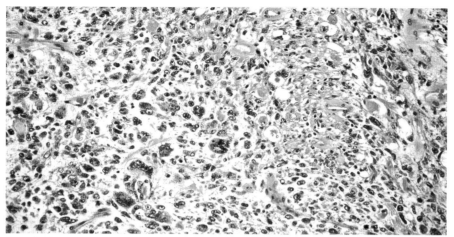

Fig. 5.32 Pleomorphic rhabdomyosarcoma. Many tumour cells have abundant eosinophilic cytoplasm and large, sometimes multinucleated, atypical nuclei.

Miscellaneous mesenchymal tumours

Rhabdomyosarcoma

Definition
A malignant, heterologous, mesenchymal tumour showing evidence of skeletal-muscle differentiation.

ICD-O code   8900/3

Epidemiology
The tumour is rare, but it is the most common heterologous sarcoma of the uterus. The uterine corpus is the second most common site for this tumour following the cervix in the female reproductive organs in adults {543}. Pleomorphic and embryonal subtypes are most frequent; spindled and alveolar variants are exceedingly rare. Embryonal rhabdomyosarcoma usually affects reproductive age patients while those with pleomorphic rhabdomyosarcoma are typically postmenopausal {515}.

Clinical features
Patients commonly present with vaginal bleeding. Half of those with pleomorphic rhabdomyosarcoma have extra-uterine disease at the time of diagnosis {516,1087,1289,1432}.

Macroscopy
Tumours are frequently bulky. Embryonal rhabdomyosarcoma may form multiple polypoid projections into the endometrial cavity, and both embryonal and pleomorphic rhabdomyosarcoma may form poorly defined polypoid, submucosal or intramural masses. On sectioning, they are fleshy, soft and white to grey and extensive areas of necrosis or haemorrhage may be seen {516,1087,1289,1432}.

Histopathology
Pleomorphic rhabdomyosarcoma shows a variable admixture of highly atypical spindled and polygonal cells, some with brightly eosinophilic cytoplasm and eccentrically located nuclei, sometimes with cross-striations, forming poorly defined non-cohesive clusters. The neoplastic cells show marked cytological atypia and giant cells; strap cells may also be seen {516,1432}. Embryonal rhabdomyosarcoma is characterized by a proliferation of small primitive cells with scant cytoplasm and oval nuclei. The cells tend to condense under the surface epithelium and around entrapped endometrial glands ("cambium layer"). There are often alternating hypo- and hypercellular areas. The former typically have an oedematous or myxoid background while the latter typically are formed by small aggregates of cells that may show focal rhabdomyoblastic differentiation with cross-striations {1087,1289}. Spindle-cell rhabdomyosarcoma is composed of fascicles of spindled cells, some containing bright eosinophilic cytoplasm and cross-striations {1220} while in alveolar rhabdomyosarcoma the cells are disposed in loose alveoli that contain non-cohesive, variably sized, rounded cells with eosinophilic cytoplasm {580}. Brisk mitotic activity is typically seen.

Immunohistochemistry
Rhabdomyosarcomas are typically positive for muscle-specific actin, desmin, myogenin and MyoD1, myoglobin and myosin but negative for smooth muscle actin {1087}.

Histogenesis
The tumour may originate from mesenchymal cells or may represent stromal overgrowth of a malignant mixed Müllerian tumour {1432}.

Prognosis and predictive factors
Pleomorphic and alveolar subtypes are associated with worse outcome than embryonal rhabdomyosarcoma, probably because they more frequently invade the myometrium and lymphovascular channels. Older age (> 20 years) and advanced stage are also reported to be independent poor prognostic factors {543}.

Perivascular epithelioid cell tumour

Definition
A perivascular epithelioid cell tumour (PEComa) is a mesenchymal tumour, typically containing epithelioid cells with clear to eosinophilic, granular cytoplasm demonstrating melanocytic and smooth-muscle differentiation, thought to be derived from the so-called perivascular epithelioid cell.

ICD-O codes
Benign perivascular epithelioid
    cell tumour   8714/0
Malignant perivascular epithelioid
    cell tumour   8714/3

Epidemiology
Most tumours occur in perimenopausal women (mean 51 years) {563}. Some are seen in patients with the tuberous sclerosis complex, although less commonly than in tumours arising outside the gynaecological tract {1096,1116,1969}.

Clinical features
Patients present with a pelvic mass or abnormal bleeding.

Macroscopy
Tumours range in size from 0.5–13 (mean, 3.5) cm and most are solitary {563}.

Histopathology
They may have a well circumscribed or

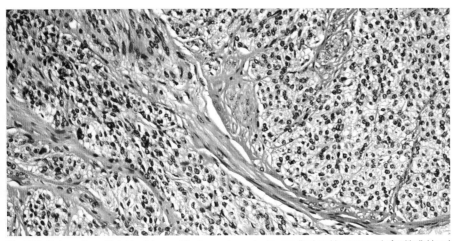

Fig. 5.33 Perivascular epithelioid cell tumour. The tumour is poorly circumscribed and is composed of epithelioid and spindle cells with clear cytoplasm. Notice the presence of scant intracytoplasmic melanin pigment (upper left).

an infiltrative border, the latter sometimes having a "tongue-like" appearance. There is a variable admixture of epithelioid and spindled cells. The epithelioid cells are arranged in nested or diffuse patterns while the spindled cells are arranged in short fascicles and nests. A prominent and delicate vascular network may be conspicuous. Sclerosis may be present {775,1096}. The cytoplasm is clear to slightly eosinophilic and granular and the nuclei are typically oval to round and normochromic with small nucleoli. Occasionally, nuclear atypia is present. Some tumours contain scattered, multinucleated cells or giant cells with a central eosinophilic zone, surrounded by a peripheral clear zone (so-called "spider cells") {563}. Mitotic activity is variable, but often low.

Immunohistochemistry
Tumours express HMB-45 (92%), Melan-A (72%), and MiTF (50%) {563}. Up to 80% stain positive for smooth muscle actin; desmin and h-caldesmon expression is less common. Tumours frequently express hormone receptors. In some patients, additional perivascular aggregates of HMB-45-positive epithelioid cells are seen in the adjacent myometrium, ovary, pelvic soft tissues and lymph nodes ("PEComatosis") {519}.

Genetic profile
Most sporadic and syndromic tumours demonstrate inactivation of the *TSC1* or *TSC2* genes with subsequent activation of the mammalian target of rapamycin (mTOR) pathway {1170}. Mutation and loss of heterozygosity of *TSC2* with loss of expression of tuberin, the protein encoded by *TSC2*, is found in most of these tumours. *TFE3* gene rearrangement, with no apparent inactivation of the *TSC1* or *TSC2* genes is rare {1150}.

Genetic susceptibility
Rare tumours arise in association with lymphangioleiomyomatosis and the tuberous sclerosis complex {1116}.

Prognosis and predictive factors
Parameters that impact prognosis include size (> 5 cm), infiltrative margins, high-grade nuclear atypia, cellularity, mitotic index (> 1/50 HPF), necrosis and vascular invasion. PEComa with nuclear pleomorphism and/or multinucleated giant cells only or size > 5 cm are classi-

fied as "of uncertain malignant potential," while tumours with two or more worrisome features are considered to be at high-risk for aggressive behaviour {173,563}. Clinically aggressive tumours spread to the lungs, although local recurrences, bone metastases and, rarely, lymph node metastases occur. Tumours with inactivation of the *TSC1* or *TSC2* genes may respond to mTOR inhibitor therapy {454,1992}.

Others

Inflammatory myofibroblastic tumour is a rare tumour that typically occurs in children and young women {1552}. Patients present with vaginal bleeding, abdominal pain or, rarely, with weight loss and fever {1552}. Tumours are usually polypoid and/or intramural masses with a fleshy or gelatinous, grey-white cut surface {636,1552}. On microscopic examination, they show an expansile or ill-defined border {1552}. The spindle, polygonal or stellate cells grow in intersecting fascicles or are set in a hypocellular (myxoid) or hyalinized background. Some cells may have a ganglion-like appearance. Focal moderate cytological atypia occurs and mitoses are low (< 5/10 HPF). A lymphoplasmacytic infiltrate is common {1552}. Tumour cells are ALK1 positive while smooth muscle actin and desmin are usually negative or only weakly positive {1552}. These tumours appear to have a benign course.
A variety of other mesenchymal tumours, benign and malignant, may occur in the uterus. They are rare and histologically similar to their soft-tissue counterparts. Benign tumours include lipoma, haemangioma and lymphangioma {292,451}. Malignant tumours include angiosarcoma {1252,1691,1891}, liposarcoma {1238}, osteosarcoma {500,706}, chondrosarcoma {958}, alveolar soft part sarcoma {1350} and rhabdoid tumour {781}.

Mixed epithelial
and mesenchymal tumours

M. Wells
E. Oliva
J. Palacios
J. Prat

Adenomyoma

Definition
A benign tumour composed of a variable number of endometrial glands and endometrial-type stroma surrounded by smooth muscle, the latter being most prominent.

ICD-O code   8932/0

Epidemiology
Adenomyomas are much more common in the corpus than the cervix {635,1876}.

Clinical features
They predominantly affect premenopausal women that present with menstrual disturbances and/or abnormal vaginal bleeding.

Macroscopy
They are generally circumscribed and range from polypoid intracavitary to serosal-based masses but most are mural. They

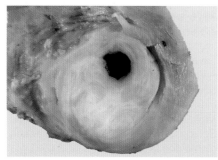

Fig. 5.34 Adenomyoma. The gross cut surface shows a whitish, fairly well circumscribed solid mass with focal haemorrhage.

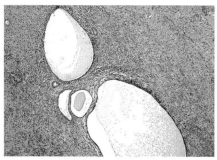

Fig. 5.35 Adenomyoma, typical type. Endometrioid glands are surrounded by endometrial stroma which in turn is surrounded by myomatous tissue.

have a firm, whorled-white cut surface and a variable number of cysts may be seen but are usually absent or inconspicuous.

Histopathology
Typical adenomyomas are composed of glands that may be cystically dilated, lined by endometrial-type epithelium and surrounded by endometrial stroma which in turn is surrounded by fascicles of smooth muscle which is typically the predominant component. Squamous, tubal and mucinous metaplasia may be seen. The smooth muscle component may show the range of changes seen in leiomyomas, including bizarre nuclei {635,1876}.

Atypical polypoid adenomyoma

Definition
A polypoid lesion composed of glands showing cytologic atypia and usually architectural complexity set in a fibromuscular stroma.

ICD-O Code   8932/0

Macroscopy
Atypical polypoid adenomyomas are often centred in the lower uterine segment; they average about 2 cm in diameter but can be up to 6 cm and have a rubbery consistency {1115,1182,1193,2129}.

Histopathology
Atypical polypoid adenomyoma shows architectural complexity of the glandular component with associated cytological atypia. There is often prominent squamous metaplasia in the form of squamous morules that may show central necrosis. The glandular component may have a lobulated architecture. The glands are surrounded by a cellular but benign stromal component that may be myomatous or myofibroblastic {1115,1182,1193,1815,2129}.

Genetic profile
These tumours may be associated with *MLH-1* promoter hypermethylation (ap-

proximately 40%) and microsatellite instability, as seen in complex atypical hyperplasia and endometrioid adenocarcinoma {1441}.

Genetic susceptibility
Three cases of atypical polypoid adenomyoma have been associated with Turner syndrome {340}.

Prognosis and predictive factors
Progression to, or association with atypical hyperplasia or endometrioid adenocarcinoma within the lesion and in the adjacent endometrium has been described {583,729,1193}. There is about a 10% risk of endometrial carcinoma in women with atypical polypoid adenomyoma, which is considerably higher than the overall risk of < 1% in women with endometrial polyps {729,2155}.

Adenofibroma

Definition
A tumour composed of an admixture of Müllerian epithelium and stroma, both components being benign. The stroma is derived from endometrial stroma, which it may resemble, but it is more often fibroblastic.

ICD-O code   9013/0

Synonyms
Müllerian adenofibroma; papillary adenofibroma

Epidemiology
These usually occur in postmenopausal women and are rare {12,147,2145}.

Clinical features
Most patients present with abnormal vaginal bleeding, discharge or a prolapsing mass. Rare cases have been associated with tamoxifen therapy {722,1437}.

Macroscopy
They are typically polypoid masses within the endometrial cavity, but may involve the lower uterine segment. Rarely,

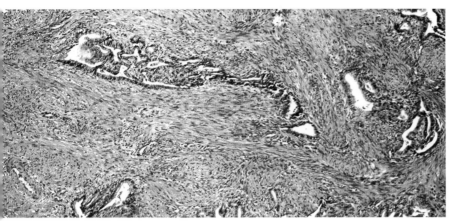

Fig. 5.36 Atypical polypoid adenomyoma. Complex atypical endometrial glands with squamous differentiation are present in a background of cellular smooth muscle.

adenofibromas may be mural or serosal. They are usually solid but a minor cystic component may be seen.

Histopathology

Typically benign, endometrial-type epithelium covers broad papillary fronds of stroma which project intraluminally or form small tubular glands, which are present in a more abundant stroma. The mesenchymal component shows benign-appearing cells with an endometrial stromal or fibroblastic morphology. In contrast to adenosarcomas there is no periglandular stromal condensation, atypia or mitotic activity.

Prognosis and predictive factors

If strictly defined, these lesions are benign. The rare reported cases of myometrial or pelvic vein invasion are probably examples of low-grade adenosarcoma {337,598,1731}.

Adenosarcoma

Definition

A mixed epithelial and mesenchymal tumour, in which the epithelial component is benign or atypical and the stromal component is low-grade malignant. When at least 25% of the tumour contains a high-grade sarcomatous component it is classified as an "adenosarcoma with sarcomatous overgrowth."

ICD-O code   8933/3

Synonym

Müllerian adenosarcoma

Clinical features

The majority occur in postmenopausal women but about 30% are found in premenopausal patients, including adolescents {333,338,398,864}. The usual presenting symptoms are abnormal vaginal bleeding but there may also be discharge or a mass protruding into the vagina. As-

sociations with previous pelvic radiotherapy, long-term unopposed oestrogen therapy, in particular tamoxifen therapy, have been reported {63,161,243,332, 837}. There may be a history of uterine polyp(s) which, on review, may be reinterpreted as adenosarcoma {905}.

Macroscopy

These tumours are typically polypoid, and rarely mural or serosal. They have a mean diameter of 6.5 cm and may fill most of or the entire uterine cavity. The cut surface is firm with small cysts containing watery or mucoid fluid. If there is sarcomatous overgrowth, there is more likely to be myometrial invasion and the tumours tend to be larger with a fleshy, haemorrhagic and necrotic cut surface {328,692,928,987,1325,2088}.

Histopathology

On low power, papillary to polypoid projections of cellular stroma typically protrude into cystically dilated gland lumens. Some glands may be elongated and compressed, imparting a phyllodes-like architecture. The stroma is typically more cellular and condensed ("collaring") around the glands. The epithelium is usually endometrioid but often shows mucinous, squamous or tubal metaplasia. The stroma typically resembles neoplastic endometrial stroma but it is often fibroblastic, particularly away from the glands {333,338,398,864}. It may show heterologous elements (including immature cartilage and skeletal muscle) and sex cord-like differentiation {277,323,1947,2058}. The stromal component shows variable mitotic activity but even a minimal degree, in the presence of cellularity and typical architectural features, warrants a

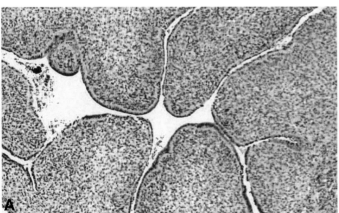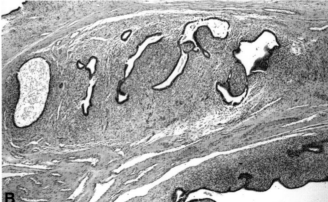

Fig. 5.37 Adenosarcoma. **A** Polypoid fronds composed of cellular stroma are conspicuous, imparting a leaf-like appearance. **B** Prominent periglandular condensation of cellular stroma around benign-appearing glands.

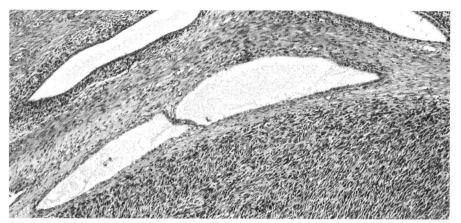

Fig. 5.38 Adenosarcoma with sarcomatous overgrowth. A minor component of typical adenosarcoma is adjacent to high-grade sarcoma which has overgrown the underlying neoplasm.

diagnosis of adenosarcoma. The amount of stroma almost always exceeds the epithelial component.

Adenosarcoma with sarcomatous overgrowth is an adenosarcoma in which the stromal component is a high-grade sarcoma. It is seen in approximately 10% of adenosarcomas and often exhibits myometrial and vascular invasion. The areas of sarcomatous overgrowth show greater nuclear pleomorphism and mitotic activity than the adenosarcomatous areas and more often show heterologous elements, including malignant cartilage, skeletal muscle or liposarcoma.

Immunohistochemistry
The mesenchymal component of adenosarcomas typically expresses CD10, ER and PR {13,42,43,1814}. These markers are often lost in areas of sarcomatous overgrowth, which also typically show strong immunoreactivity for Ki-67 and p53 {13,1814}.

Prognosis and predictive factors
Uterine adenosarcomas can recur locally in up to 30% of cases, particularly in the vagina; recurrences can be early or late. The presence of deep myometrial invasion is a risk factor for recurrence. Metastatic disease is usually associated with tumours exhibiting sarcomatous overgrowth {62}. Outcome for these patients is poor {987}.

Carcinosarcoma

Definition
A biphasic tumour composed of high-grade carcinomatous and sarcomatous elements.

ICD-O code   8980/3

Synonym
Malignant mixed Müllerian tumour

Epidemiology
These tumours account for < 5% of all uterine malignancies. There is an association with tamoxifen therapy or long-term unopposed estrogen usage {461,512,785,947,1209}. They may also occur as a long-term complication of pelvic radiotherapy {1440}. The mean time-interval from irradiation to the development of tumour is between 10 and 20 years {1440}. Patients with carcinosarcoma share the same predisposing risk factors as for endometrial carcinoma.

Clinical features
These tumours typically occur in postmenopausal women who usually present with vaginal bleeding. Approximately one-third have evidence of extra-uterine spread at the time of diagnosis. On clinical examination, there is often uterine enlargement or a pelvic mass. The tumour prolapses through the cervix in about one-half of patients {402,422,1120,1784}.

Macroscopy
The tumour is characteristically large and polypoid, filling the entire uterine cavity and often protruding through the cervical os. It is typically soft, with areas of haemorrhage, necrosis and cystic degeneration on cut section. There is frequent myometrial invasion and sometimes cervical involvement.

Histopathology
There is typically an intimate admixture of high-grade epithelium and mesenchyme; one or the other may predominate. The two components are usually distinct and sharply demarcated but merging can be observed. The epithelium is most often of endometrioid or serous types but other Müllerian cell types may be encountered. The mesenchymal component is, for the

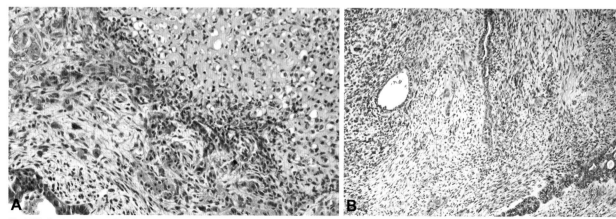

Fig. 5.39 Carcinosarcoma. **A** Malignant cartilage as well as rhabdomyoblasts are seen as the heterologous mesenchymal component. The malignant epithelial component is present in the extreme lower left corner. **B** Two distinct components, a high-grade carcinoma and sarcoma, are closely admixed but do not merge.

most part, a high-grade, non-specific sarcoma, but heterologous elements including rhabdomyosarcoma, chondrosarcoma and, rarely, osteosarcoma are seen in 50% of cases {1440}. Neuroectodermal differentiation may rarely occur {509}. These tumours commonly exhibit deep myometrial and lymphovascular invasion.

Histogenesis
These tumours are thought to be of epithelial derivation, exemplifying epithelial-mesenchymal transition {374,1724, 1817,2097}.

Genetic profile
Several genetic and molecular studies have confirmed their clonal origin and have shown them to have a similar molecular profile to high-grade endometrial carcinomas, with *TP53* mutation being the most common molecular alteration {1871,1912}. Nearly 50% of these tumours carry mutations of the PI3K/AKT and/or RAS/RAF pathways, the most frequent being those affecting *PIK3CA*, seen in around 20% of tumours {154,673}. A variety of other molecular defects have been recently reported in carcinosarcomas affecting and including *VEGFA* {499}, *HMGA2* {1616}, *HPRT1* {982} and dysregulation of microRNA in a single small imprinted region of chromosome 14q32 {449}. Changes in the Akt/β-catenin pathway and transcriptional repression of E-cadherin seem to be essential for the establishment of the phenotypic characteristics of carcinosarcoma {248,1662}.

Prognosis and predictive factors
These tumours are associated with a poor outcome and have a pattern of spread similar to high-grade endometrial carcinoma {544,1377,2065}. A high proportion of patients with apparently clinically stage I disease have evidence of extrauterine spread at the time of diagnosis. Metastatic spread is typically to pelvic and para-aortic lymph nodes, sometimes with distant haematogenous metastases to lung, brain and bone. However, most patients die as a consequence of local pelvic/abdominal recurrence. The risk of advanced stage disease and of metastasis is closely related to the depth of myometrial invasion. Serous and clear cell carcinomatous elements are associated with a higher frequency of other adverse prognostic features. The presence of heterologous elements is a statistically significant poor prognostic factor in stage I patients {544}; the presence of a rhabdomyosarcomatous component has the worst prognosis.

Miscellaneous tumours

J. Prat
E. Oliva
J. Palacios
M. Wells

Adenomatoid tumour

Definition
A benign tumour of mesothelial origin {1370}.

ICD-O code
9054/0

Clinical features
Patients range widely in age (average, 45 years). Most of the tumours are incidental findings {1370}. Multifocal/diffuse tumours have been reported in immunosuppressed patients {8}.

Macroscopy
Most tumours are located in the outer myometrium. They are usually solitary, small (often < 4 cm) and solid but rarely can be diffuse, multifocal, large (> 10 cm) or predominantly cystic {8,702,1370,1446}. They have relatively ill-defined borders (when compared to leiomyomas) with a nodular, grey-white, firm cut surface {1370}.

Histopathology
Inter-anastomosing pseudo glands or pseudo vascular spaces (most common), variably sized tubules (if small, signet ring-like appearance), cysts and diffuse and, less commonly, papillary growths or combination thereof can be seen. Cells are flattened to cuboidal with scant pale to eosinophilic cytoplasm that may contain vacuoles and round nuclei with small nucleoli. Cytological atypia and mitotic activity are inconspicuous. Striking smooth-muscle hypertrophy is often present as well as variable lymphoid infiltrate, including germinal centres {1370}. Alcian-blue positive material is seen within lumens and vacuoles {1370}.

Immunohistochemistry
Tumour cells express AE1/AE3, CAM 5.2, CK7, CK18 and 19, calretinin, WT-1, D2-40 and HMBE-1 {1370,1705}.

Histogenesis
They are of mesothelial derivation {1370,1829}.

Prognosis and predictive factors
This tumour is benign.

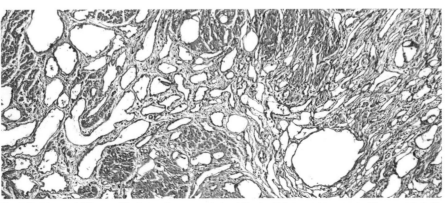

Fig. 5.40 Adenomatoid tumour. The tumour is composed of variably sized tubules and some cysts. It is associated with prominent smooth muscle hypertrophy.

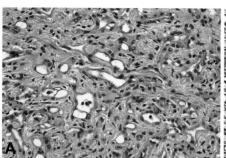
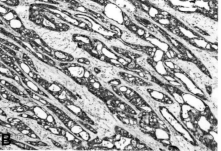
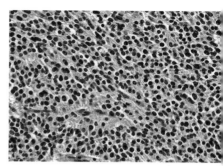

Fig. 5.41 Adenomatoid tumour. **A** Interanastomosing pseudovascular and pseudoglandular spaces are lined by flat innocuous cells, some with a signet ring-like appearance, and admixed with scattered lymphocytes. **B** The tumour cells show a strong immunoreactivity for calretinin.

Fig. 5.43 Central-type PNET. The small tumour cells lie on a delicate fibrillary background indicative of neural differentiation.

Neuroectodermal tumours

Definition
A malignant tumour of peripheral or central neuroectodermal derivation {509}.

Synonyms
Peripheral-type primitive neuroectodermal tumour; extraskeletal Ewing sarcoma; PNET; Central-type primitive neuroectodermal tumour; medulloblastoma; neuroblastoma; ependymoblastoma

Epidemiology
These tumours are rare {509}.

Clinical features
They occur in postmenopausal women (> 50 years) who present with vaginal bleeding and/or mass and often (around 50%) have extra-uterine disease at diagnosis {417,509}.

Macroscopy
They are typically large (up to 20 cm, mean 6 cm) and fleshy with a white to tan, friable cut surface showing haemorrhage and necrosis {509}.

Histopathology
Tumours can be divided into those either resembling their central nervous system counterparts or peripheral PNET/Ewing sarcomas. Most tumours are composed of a monotonous population of small to medium-sized round primitive cells that grow in sheets, nests and cords. They display high nuclear to cytoplasmic ratio and brisk mitotic activity. Neural, glial, ependymal or medulloepithelial cells, with or without rosettes, may be seen in central-type tumours {417,509}. Homer-Wright rosettes can be seen in both. Association with endometrial adenocarcinoma, adenosarcoma, malignant mixed Müllerian tumour or high-grade sarcoma can occur.

Immunohistochemistry
Both subtypes are Fli-1 positive. They often express CD99, synaptophysin, NSE, CD56, neurofilaments and S-100, while GFAP (supporting a central origin) and AE1/AE3 are less frequently positive {509}.

Genetic profile
Peripheral PNETs are characterized by a recurrent t(11,22)(q24;q12) translocation resulting in *EWS/FLI-1* fusion product {254,509,1476}.

Prognosis and predictive factors
Central-type and peripheral PNETs are highly malignant tumours associated with short survival rates (usually < 3 years) despite aggressive treatment, especially if high-stage {417,509}.

Germ cell tumours

Germ cell tumours such as teratomas and yolk sac tumours can develop in the endometrium, either in pure form or associated with endometrioid carcinoma {1373}, which may be overgrown by the germ cell tumour {1646}. In its pure form, it is speculated that these tumours result from aberrant migration of primordial germ cells.

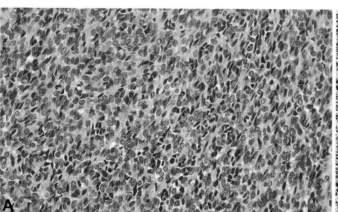
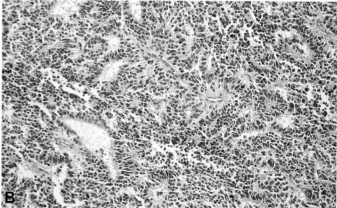

Fig. 5.42 A Ewing sarcoma/Peripheral PNET. The tumour is composed of sheets of small blue round cells that have scant cytoplasm and round to oval nuclei with inconspicuous nucleoli. **B** Central-type PNET. The tumour cells form tubular structures as well as perivascular and ependymal rosettes indicative of ependymal differentiation.

Lymphoid and myeloid tumours

J. Prat
J.A. Ferry

E. Oliva
J. Palacios
M. Wells

Lymphomas

Definition
Malignant neoplasms composed of lymphoid cells.

Clinical features
Lymphomas rarely arise in the uterine corpus; more commonly, the corpus is secondarily involved by a lymphoma arising in another site. Adult women over a wide age-range are affected. They often present with vaginal bleeding, and less often with pelvic or abdominal pain {1971}.

Macroscopy
The tumours are typically soft and fleshy and often poorly demarcated.

Histopathology
The most common type of primary lymphoma is diffuse large B-cell lymphoma. Less common types include Burkitt lymphoma, follicular lymphoma and extranodal marginal zone lymphoma {731,824,972,1955}. Rare B- and T-lineage lymphoblastic lymphoma {972,1894}, peripheral T-cell lymphoma {939} and primary endometrial NK/T-cell lymphoma, nasal-type, have been reported {1248,2011}. A similar variety of lymphomas can involve the corpus secondarily, although with less of a striking predominance of diffuse large B-cell lym-

phoma (see Table 1.3, p. 80) {972,1971} The tumour cells often grow between residual endometrial glands and percolate between myometrial muscle bundles, but diffuse effacement can be seen. Sclerosis is inconspicuous in contrast with cervical lymphomas.

Prognosis and predictive factors
Patients with primary uterine lymphoma with localized disease appear to have a good prognosis. Endometrial marginal zone lymphoma has a very good prognosis {1955}. Patients with widespread disease or with secondary uterine involvement have a poor prognosis {710}.

Myeloid neoplasms

Definition
Malignant neoplasms of haematopoietic origin, including myeloid leukaemias and myeloid sarcoma, a mass-forming lesion composed of primitive myeloid cells.

Synonyms
Myeloid sarcoma is also known as chloroma, granulocytic sarcoma or extramedullary myeloid tumour.

Clinical features
Females of any age can be affected. When there is involvement of the female reproductive tract by myeloid leukaemia,

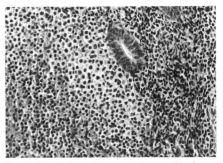

Fig. 5.45 Endometrial marginal zone lymphoma. High power shows a monotonous population of small lymphoid cells with oval nuclei, smooth dark chromatin and moderately abundant pale cytoplasm consistent with marginal zone cells, surrounding an endometrial gland.

involvement of the corpus is common and may be clinically silent {1128,1419}. Rarely, patients have myeloid sarcoma involving the uterine corpus and may have vaginal bleeding or pain. Myeloid sarcoma sometimes represents the first presentation of myeloid neoplasia; in other cases it is concurrent with acute myeloid leukaemia in the bone marrow.

Histopathology
Neoplasms are composed of a diffuse proliferation of primitive myeloid cells with oval, irregular or folded nuclei, fine chromatin, distinct to prominent nucleoli and scant to moderate quantity of cytoplasm. Maturing cells with recognizable myeloid differentiation may be seen.

Histogenesis
A rare occurrence of a therapy-related myeloid neoplasm has been reported, following chemotherapy for breast cancer {1536}.

Prognosis and predictive factors
Prognosis appears better with localized disease; it varies depending on type of underlying genetic abnormality.

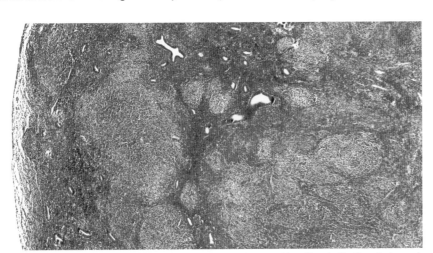

Fig. 5.44 Endometrial marginal zone lymphoma. Low power shows confluent nodules of lymphoid cells replacing much of endometrium and invading the myometrium.

Secondary tumours

J. Prat
J.A. Ferry
E. Oliva
J. Palacios
M. Wells

Definition
Tumours of the uterine corpus that originate from a primary extrauterine tumour.

Clinical features
The mean age of patients is 60 years and they may present with abnormal uterine bleeding.

Macroscopy
Solitary or multiple tumours may occur. They range from incidental microscopic findings to large bulky masses, as in cases of direct spread from cervical carcinoma.

Site of origin
In most cases the primary tumour is known. Rarely, a tumour diagnosed in curettage or hysterectomy represents the first sign of an extrauterine primary tumour. Secondary tumours of the uterine corpus can be divided into two major groups; tumours of genital and tumours of extragenital organs. Neoplasms of neighbouring organs such as cervix, fallopian tubes, ovaries, bladder and rectum can metastasize to the uterine corpus via lymphatics or blood vessels but mostly represent direct extension.

Haematogenous or lymphatic uterine metastases from any extragenital primary tumour may occur but are extremely rare. Reported primary tumours include carcinomas of the breast, stomach, colon, pancreas, gallbladder, lung, urinary bladder and thyroid and melanoma {880,1785,1896,1936}. Mammary lobular carcinoma, gastric signet-ring cell carcinoma and colonic carcinoma are the most frequently reported extragenital primary tumours {524,1936}.

Histopathology
Metastatic carcinoma in the corpus should be suspected if one or more of the following features are present: i) an unusual histological pattern for primary endometrial carcinoma; ii) Diffuse replacement of endometrial stroma with sparing of pre-existing glands; iii) Lack of premalignant changes in endometrial glands; iv) disproportionate involvement of the serosa and outer myometrium. Immunohistochemical studies are often required.

Prognosis and predictive factors
Patients typically have a poor prognosis as there is usually widely disseminated disease.

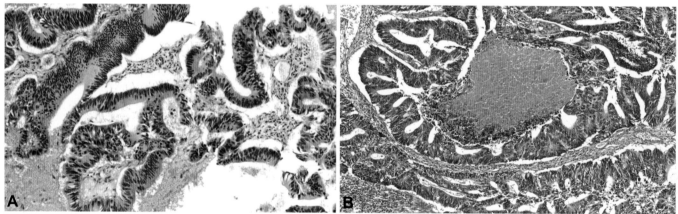

Fig. 5.46 Metastatic colon carcinoma to the endometrium. **A** The tumour mimics endometrioid adenocarcinoma. **B** Dirty necrosis and "garland appearance".

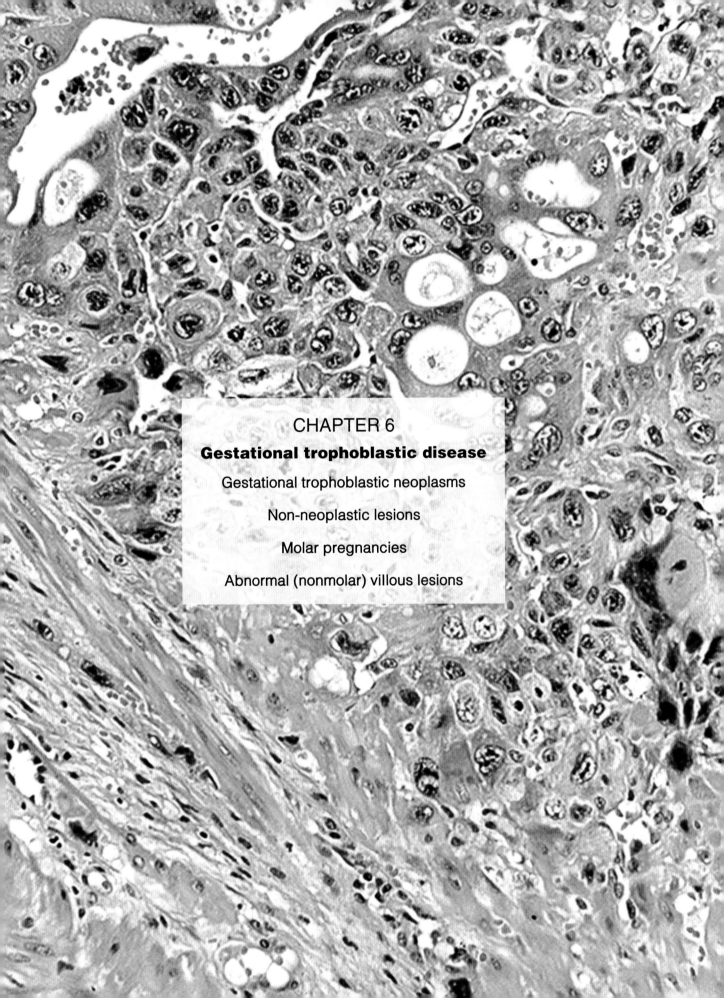

CHAPTER 6

Gestational trophoblastic disease

Gestational trophoblastic neoplasms

Non-neoplastic lesions

Molar pregnancies

Abnormal (nonmolar) villous lesions

WHO Classification of gestational trophoblastic disease[a,b]

Neoplasms

Choriocarcinoma	9100/3
Placental site trophoblastic tumour	9104/1
Epithelioid trophoblastic tumour	9105/3

Non-neoplastic lesions

Exaggerated placental site
Placental site nodule and plaque

Molar pregnancies

Hydatidiform mole	9100/0
Complete	9100/0
Partial	9103/0
Invasive	9100/1

Abnormal (nonmolar) villous lesions

[a] The morphology codes are from the International Classification of Diseases for Oncology (ICD-O) {575A}. Behaviour is coded /0 for benign tumours, /1 for unspecified, borderline or uncertain behaviour, /2 for carcinoma in situ and grade III intraepithelial neoplasia and /3 for malignant tumours; [b] The classification is modified from the previous WHO classification of tumours {1906A}, taking into account changes in our understanding of these lesions; *These new codes were approved by the IARC/WHO Committee for ICD-O in 2013.

TNM and FIGO classification of gestational trophoblastic tumours

T – Primary tumour

TNM	FIGO[a]	
TX		Primary tumour cannot be assessed
T0		No evidence of primary tumour
T1	I	Tumour confined to uterus
T2	II	Tumour extends to other genital structures: vagina, ovary, and broad ligament, fallopian tube by metastasis or direct extension
M1a	III	Metastasis to lung(s)
M1b	IV	Other distant metastasis

Note: [a]Stages I–IV are subdivided into A and B according to the prognostic score.

M – Distant metastasis

M0	No distant metastasis
M1	Distant metastasis
M1a	Metastasis to lung(s)
M1b	Other distant metastasis

Note: Genital metastasis (vagina, ovary, broad ligament, fallopian tube) is classified T2. Any involvement of non-genital structures, whether by direct invasion or metastasis is described using the M classification.

Prognostic grouping

Group	T	M	Risk category
I	T1	M0	Unknown
IA	T1	M0	Low
IB	T1	M0	High
II	T2	M0	Unknown
IIA	T2	M0	Low
IIB	T2	M0	High
III	Any T	M1a	Unknown
IIIA	Any T	M1a	Low
IIIB	Any T	M1a	High
IV	Any T	M1b	Unknown
IVA	Any T	M1b	Low
IVB	Any T	M1b	High

Prognostic factor	Prognostic score			
	0	1	2	4
Age	< 40	≥ 40		
Antecedent pregnancy	Hydatidiform mole	Abortion	Term pregnancy	
Months from index pregnancy	< 4	4–6	7–12	> 12
Pretreatment serum beta-hCG (IU/ml)	$< 10^3$	$10^3 - < 10^4$	$10^4 - < 10^5$	$\geq 10^5$
Largest tumour size including uterus	< 3 cm	3–5 cm	> 5 cm	
Sites of metastasis	Lung	Spleen, kidney	Gastrointestinal tract	Liver, brain
Number of metastases		1–4	5–8	> 8
Previous failed chemotherapy			Single drug	Two or more drugs

Risk categories: Total prognostic score, ≤ 6 = low risk; ≥ 7 = high risk

References

American Joint Committee on Cancer (AJCC) Cancer Staging Manual, 7th ed. (2011) Edge SB, Byrd DR, Compton CC, Fritz AG, Greene FL, Trotti III eds. Springer: New York

International Union against Cancer (UICC): TNM Classification of Malignant Tumours, 7th ed. (2009) Sobin LH, Gospodarowicz MK, Wittekind Ch eds. Wiley-Blackwell: Oxford

A help-desk for specific questions about the TNM classification is available at http://www.uicc.org.

Gestational trophoblastic neoplasms

P. Hui
R. Baergen
A.N.Y. Cheung
M. Fukunaga

D. Gersell
J.M. Lage
B.M. Ronnett
N.J. Sebire
M. Wells

Choriocarcinoma

Definition
A malignant, trophoblastic tumour consisting of a trimorphic proliferation of intermediate trophoblastic cells, syncytiotrophoblast and cytotrophoblast, in the absence of chorionic villi.

ICD-O code   9100/3

Epidemiology
In the US and Europe, the incidence of choriocarcinoma is 0.02–0.05/1000 pregnancies {193,1346,1592,1801,1812}, but it can be as high as 0.4–2/1000 pregnancies in South-eastern Asian countries {207,1512}. The risk of developing choriocarcinoma is 2–3% following a complete hydatidiform mole and < 0.5% after a partial hydatidiform mole {140,1132,1181,1718}.

Etiology
Complete hydatidiform moles progress to choriocarcinoma in 2–3% of cases if untreated and partial hydatidiform moles do so in less than 0.5% of cases {140,1132,1181,1718}. Choriocarcinoma may also develop after a normal or an ectopic pregnancy. Rare intraplacental or in situ choriocarcinoma have been encountered in full term placentas {1717}

and some patients may present with concurrent metastatic disease {2148}.

Clinical features
Choriocarcinoma typically occurs in women of reproductive age (average 29–31 years), with rare cases reported in girls in their teens and postmenopausal patients {1404}. Vaginal bleeding and/or extra-uterine haemorrhage are the most common symptoms. Before the introduction of chemotherapy, 50% of choriocarcinomas developed after a complete hydatidiform mole, 25% followed an abortion and 25% occurred after a term pregnancy {91}. With modern surveillance programs, histological diagnosis of postmolar choriocarcinoma has become less common as treatment is often administered based on serological and imaging studies only. As a result, 50% of the tumours are currently diagnosed following a term pregnancy and 25% are diagnosed after a recognized hydatidiform mole {1812}. Although the latency varies from weeks to many years, the histological diagnosis is made at an average of 13 months after a complete hydatidiform mole, and 1–3 months after a term pregnancy {1404}. Marked elevation of serum hCG is invariably present {142,1404,1803}.

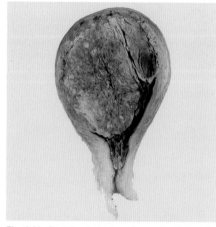

Fig. 6.01 Gestational choriocarcinoma. Sagittal section demonstrates a bulky, destructive, hemmorrhagic and necrotic mass involving the uterine corpus with extension into the cervical canal.

Macroscopy
The tumour is generally bulky and destructive with single to multiple dark-red masses with extensive central haemorrhage and variable amounts of necrosis. The tumour may arise in extra-uterine sites involved by an ectopic pregnancy (fallopian tube, ovary, etc.) {260,1405}.

Histopathology
Choriocarcinoma presents either as diffusely infiltrative or solid masses of cohesive sheets of trimorphic malignant trophoblast,

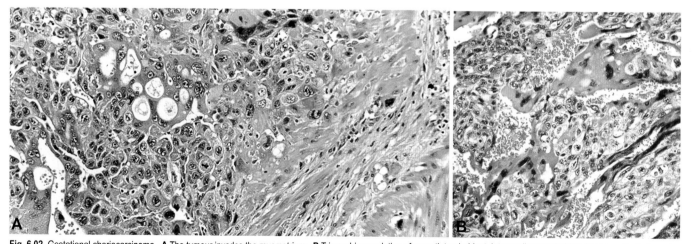

Fig. 6.02 Gestational choriocarcinoma. **A** The tumour invades the myometrium. **B** Trimorphic population of syncytiotrophoblast, intermediate trophoblast (masses of cells in centre and lower left with clear cytoplasm and variably sized nuclei) and cytotrophoblast (mass of cells in upper left containing smaller more uniform sized nuclei).

Table 6.1 Diagnostic features of gestational trophoblastic tumours

Diagnostic features	Choriocarcinoma	PSTT	ETT
Age	Reproductive years (average 29–31 years)	20 to 63 years (average 30–32 years)	15–48 years (average 36 years)
Antecedent pregnancy	Term pregnancy, Complete hydatidiform mole	Term pregnancy	Term pregnancy
Interval time from index gestation	A few months to 14 years (average 2 months after term pregnancy and 13 months after complete mole)	2 weeks to 17 years (median 12 to 18 months)	1 to 25 years (average 6.2 years)
Clinical presentation	Vaginal bleeding Persistent GTD	Missed abortion, amenorrhea	Vaginal bleeding
Pretreatment hCG (mIU/ml)	$> 10 \times 10^3$	$< 1 \times 10^3$	$< 3 \times 10^3$
Gross appearance	Circumscribed or Invasive haemorrhagic masses	Expansile to infiltrative solid mass	Expansile solid mass
Tumour location	Corpus	Corpus	Cervix, Lower uterine segment, Corpus
Tumour border	Infiltrative	Infiltrative	Pushing
Tumour growth pattern	Trimorphic pattern consisting of all three types of trophoblast Extensive haemorrhage and necrosis	Large masses of tumour cells replacing vascular wall Tumour cells split myometrial smooth muscle fibres at tumour periphery	Sheets, nests and cords, Geographic necrosis, Deposition of hyaline-like material, Colonizing mucosal surface epithelium
Tumour cells	Villous intermediate trophoblast, syncytiotrophoblast and cytotrophoblast	Implantation site type intermediate trophoblast	Chorionic type intermediate trophoblast
Cytological atypia	Marked	Moderate to marked	Mild to moderate
Stroma	No intrinsic tumour stroma or vasculature Ki-67 labelling index of > 90%	Intimately infiltrates myometrial muscle fibres	Presence of nearby decidualized stromal cells
Immunohistochemistry	Diffuse positivity for hCG, hPL and HSD3B1 in syncytiotrophoblast	Diffuse positivity for hPL and Mel-CAM Scattered multinuclear cells positive for hCG Ki-67 labelling index of 5–10%	Diffuse positivity for p63, Rare individual cells positive for hPL and Mel-CAM Ki-67 labelling index of > 10%

PSTT, placental site trophoblastic tumour; ETT, epithelioid trophoblastic tumour; hCG, human chorionic gonadotropin; hPL, human placental lactogen

consisting of intermediate trophoblast and cytotrophoblast, rimmed with syncytiotrophoblast. Haemorrhage and necrosis are invariably present and lymphovascular invasion is common. Cytological atypia is generally striking and mitotic figures are numerous {180,1404,1803}. The tumour does not have intrinsic stromal and vascular elements. Differential diagnoses include other trophoblastic tumours (see Table 6.1), non-gestational choriocarcinoma and poorly differentiated carcinoma with trophoblastic differentiation. Complete hydatidiform mole when hydropic villi are not present, immature trophoblast in early gestation and exaggerated placental site can also simulate choriocarcinoma in curettings.

Immunohistochemistry
All tumour cells express cytokeratin AE1/AE3 and a high Ki-67 labelling index (> 90%) is typically observed. The tumour characteristically exhibits strong and diffuse immunoreactivity with hCG and HSD3B1 in syncytiotrophoblast and also in a variable number of mononucleate trophoblastic cells. The intermediate trophoblastic cells express Mel-CAM, HLA-G and MUC-4 {1164}.

Genetic profile
Highly complex karyotypes {1610,1751} with recurrent 7p amplification and 8p deletion have been reported irrespective of the type of the antecedent gestation {17}. An XX sex chromosome composition is present in the majority of choriocarcinomas {2080}.

Prognosis and predictive factors
If untreated, choriocarcinoma metastasizes in > 50% of cases; frequently to the vagina, lung, liver, brain and kidney {378,1302,1404}. Metastasis is, however, rarely seen currently as a result of close patient follow-up by the gestational trophoblastic disease surveillance program. Over 90% of patients are cured by various combined or sequential chemotherapy regimens {1342,1720}. See Table 6.2 {959,1344}, p. 161, for parameters of clinical risk assessment.

Placental site trophoblastic tumour

Definition
A trophoblastic tumour consisting of neoplastic implantation site-type intermediate trophoblast.

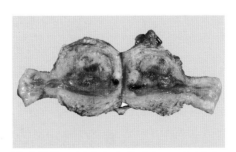

Fig. 6.03 Placental site trophoblastic tumour. A white-tan solid mass lesion involves the endomyometrium.

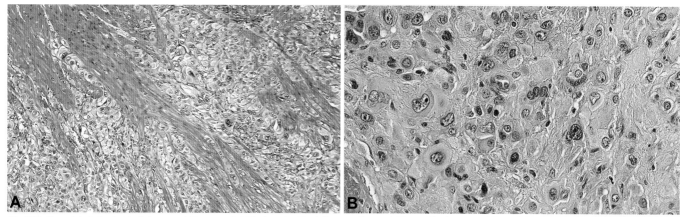

Fig. 6.04 Placental site trophoblastic tumour. **A** Tumour cells infiltrate and split existing smooth muscle fibres at the tumour periphery. **B** Tumour cells have abundant eosinophilic cytoplasm and marked cytological atypia with frequent large convoluted nuclei.

ICD-O code   9104/1

Clinical features

Placental site trophoblastic tumour (PSTT) occurs in women ranging in age from 20–63 years (mean 30 years) {89,270,1709,2123}. Two-thirds of the cases follow a full-term pregnancy with a median latency of 12–18 months {89,270}. Vaginal bleeding is the most common presentation. Less common symptoms include amenorrhea and abdominal pain. Mild to moderate elevation of serum hCG of < 1000 mIU/ml (average 680 mIU/ml) is detectable in 80% of the cases {539,719,1452}. At presentation, over 80% of the cases are FIGO stage I tumours {89}. FIGO stage II disease commonly involves adnexa, pelvic lymph nodes and parametrium.

Macroscopy

PSTT generally involves the endomyometrium as nodular, solid masses of 1–10 cm in size. Deep myometrial invasion is seen in 50% of the cases. The cut surface of the tumour is usually solid and fleshy with a white-tan to light yellow colour. Focal haemorrhage and necrosis are present in nearly half of the cases {89,2123}.

Histopathology

The tumour has an infiltrative growth of aggregates to sheets of large, polyhedral to round, predominately mononucleate placental site intermediate trophoblast. Scattered multinucleated cells are common. At the periphery, the tumour cells typically infiltrate and separate myometrial smooth-muscle fibres. Cytologically, the cells have abundant amphophilic, eosinophilc or clear cytoplasm, and nuclear atypia is generally pronounced with frequent, large, convoluted nuclei and marked hyperchromasia. Most tumours have a low mitotic count ranging from 2–4 per 10 HPF {89,1761,2123}. Characteristically, the tumour cells may completely replace the vascular wall of myometrial vessels. The differential diagnoses include other trophoblastic tumours (epithelioid trophoblastic tumour and choriocarcinoma; see Table 6.1, p. 159), poorly differentiated carcinoma, epithelioid leiomyoma or leiomyosarcoma, and most commonly an exaggerated placental site.

Immunohistochemistry

Tumour cells diffusely express hPL, MUC-4, HSD3B1, HLA-G and Mel-CAM (CD146). Expression of hCG and inhibin is more limited. The proliferation index is generally modestly increased, with Ki-67 expressed in 10–30% of cells {89,1764}.

Histogenesis

PSTT arises from trophoblast with differentiation towards implantation-site intermediate trophoblast {1764}.

Genetic profile

PSTT shows rare genetic imbalances

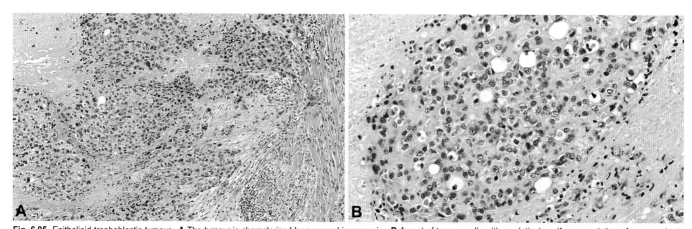

Fig. 6.05 Epithelioid trophoblastic tumour. **A** The tumour is characterized by geographic necrosis. **B** A nest of tumour cells with a relatively uniform population of mononucleate intermediate trophoblastic cells surrounded by necrotic debris.

Table 6.2 FIGO/WHO scoring system of prognostic and predictive parameters for trophoblastic tumours {959,1344}

Prognostic Factor	0	1	2	4
Age	< 40	≥ 40		
Antecedent pregnancy	Mole	Abortion	Term Pregnancy	
Interval, months from index gestation	< 4	4–6	7–12	> 12
Pretreatment hCG (mIU/ml)	< 10^3	10^3–10^4	10^4–10^5	> 10^6
Largest tumour size, including uterus	< 3cm	3–5cm	> 5cm	
Site of metastases	Lung	Spleen, kidney	GI tract	Brain, liver
Number of metastases		1–4	5–8	> 8
Previous failed chemotherapy			Single agent	Two or more agents
Total score				
Low-risk, score ≤ 6; high-risk, score ≥ 7; hCG, human chorionic gonadotropin				

analysed by comparative genomic hybridization {790,2062}. There is also a preferential requirement of paternal X chromosome in the tumour genome {789,791,2080}.

Prognosis and predictive factors
Most patients are cured by simple hysterectomy. However, 25–30% of patients may develop recurrent disease and about a half of those may die of the tumour {539,558,1452}. Histological parameters that correlate with prognosis include tumour cells with clear cytoplasm, depth of invasion, tumour size, necrosis and high mitotic count (> 5 per 10 HPF). However, only advanced FIGO stage, antecedent pregnancy of 48 months or more and the presence of tumour cells with clear cytoplasm are independent predictors of worse prognosis {89,1697}.

Epithelioid trophoblastic tumour

Definition
A trophoblastic tumour consisting of neoplastic chorionic-type intermediate trophoblast.

ICD-O code   9105/3

Clinical features
Epithelioid trophoblastic tumour (ETT) oc-
curs in women ranging in age from 15–48 years (mean of 36.1 years) {518,1759}. Vaginal bleeding or menometrorrhagia are the most common symptoms. Antecedent gestations include term pregnancy in 67%, spontaneous abortion in 16% and hydatidiform mole in 16% of cases {697,993,1759}. The latency ranges from 1–15 years with an average of 6.2 years {518,1332}. Mild to moderate elevation of serum hCG of < 2500 mIU/ml is detectable in 80% of the cases {518,1447}.

Macroscopy
The tumour generally forms discrete nodules or cystic haemorrhagic masses deeply invading surrounding structures. Nearly half of the cases arise in the cervix or lower uterine segment. The cut surface of the tumour is white-tan to brown, with varying amounts of haemorrhage and necrosis. Ulceration and fistula formation are not uncommon {518,1254,1759}.

Histopathology
ETT is characterized by nodular growth of medium-sized tumour cells arranged in nests or cords to large masses. The cells are relatively uniform with a moderate amount of finely granular, eosinophilic to clear cytoplasm, distinct cell membranes and round nuclei with distinct small nucleoli. Nuclear atypia is generally moderate and the mitotic count
ranges from 0–9 per 10 HPF. Deposition of eosinophilic hyaline-like material is characteristically present in the centre of tumour nests or between tumour cells {295,518,1759,1761}. Extensive or "geographic" necrosis is often present. Decidualized stromal cells may be found at the tumour periphery {518}. When the cervix is involved, tumour cells may colonize the mucosal epithelium simulating high-grade squamous intraepithelial lesion {518}. Differential diagnoses include other trophoblastic tumours (Table 6.1) and cervical squamous cell carcinoma. ETT may coexist with other trophoblastic neoplasms {1747}.

Immunohistochemistry
The tumour cells diffusely express H3D3B1, HLA-G, p63, cyclin E and inhibin-α. Mel-CAM and hPL are expressed in a small percentage of cells and the Ki-67 labelling index is > 10% {1764}.

Histogenesis
ETT arises from trophoblast with differentiation towards chorionic-type intermediate trophoblast {1759,1761,1763}. Possible malignant transformation from a placental site nodule to ETT has been reported {1934}.

Genetic profile
A recent study found an absence of Y chromosome complement in the majority of tumours {2080}. A comparative genomic hybridization study showed an undisturbed genome in three tumours {2060}.

Prognosis and predictive factors
The prognosis of ETT is similar to that of PSTT with metastasis occuring in 25% of cases and 10% of patients dying of disease {1759}. The survival is nearly 100% for non-metastatic cases but decreases to 50–60% in patients with metastasis. Among the histological features, only high mitotic count (> 6 per 10 HPF) was found to be an unfavourable factor {1131}.

Non-neoplastic lesions

P. Hui
R. Baergen
A.N.Y. Cheung
M. Fukunaga

D. Gersell
J.M. Lage
B.M. Ronnett
N.J. Sebire
M. Wells

Exaggerated placental site

Definition
An exaggerated placental site represents part of the spectrum of normal implantation-site change.

Synonyms
Exaggerated implantation site; syncytial endometritis (not recommended)

Clinical features
The lesion is associated with normal gestation or hydatidiform mole and has no specific clinical symptoms {1911,2114}.

Histopathology
The lesion consists of an exuberant infiltration of mononucleate implantation-site intermediate trophoblast, typically accompanied by multinucleate giant cells. It does not alter the overall endomyometrial anatomy. Nuclear atypia can resemble that in PSTT but mitotic figures are absent {2114}. Lack of a mass lesion and low Ki-67 labelling index (< 1%) separate exaggerated placental site (EPS) from placental site trophoblastic tumours {1760,1761,1764}. Molar-associated exaggerated placental sites have greater atypia than their non-molar counterparts and the proliferation index is slightly increased (approximately 5–10%).

Histogenesis
EPS has the morphological and immunohistochemical features of intermediate trophoblast at the implantation site {1761}.

Placental site nodule and plaque

Definition
A benign, well circumscribed nodule or plaque with abundant hyalinized stroma containing chorionic-type intermediate trophoblast.

Clinical features
Placental site nodule (PSN) is generally an incidental finding in endometrial or endocervical curettings {2115}. It is sometimes detected in a woman being evaluated for abnormal cervical cytology.

Macroscopy
The lesion is nodular, ranging in size from 4–10 mm {787,2115}.

Histopathology
The lesion consists of single to multiple well circumscribed nodules or plaques of hyalinized extracelluar matrix, in which chorionic-type intermediate trophoblast is haphazardly distributed as single cells, clusters or cords {787,2115}. PSNs can have central necrosis. Cytological atypia, manifested as enlarged nuclei with hyperchromatic but often smudgy chromatin, is typically present focally. At times, cytological atypia and proliferation exceed what is observed in a PSN but falls short of that seen in ETT. These lesions have been referred to as atypical PSNs {1165,1934}. The clinical significance of these lesions is not known as they have not been studied in detail. PSN is distinguished from epithelioid trophoblastic tumour (ETT) by its microscopic size, mucosal location, extensive hyalinization, lower cellularity, and lack of geographic necrosis. Mitotic figures are only rarely encountered.

Immunohistochemistry
The trophoblastic cells generally have a low Ki-67 labelling index (< 8%) {1764}. They express p63 but unlike ETT, lack cyclin E expression {1165}.

Histogenesis
PSN has the morphological and immunohistochemical features of chorionic-type intermediate trophoblast {1761,1762}. It has been suggested that progression of PSN to ETT may be possible, with atypical PSN being an intermediate step {1165,1934}.

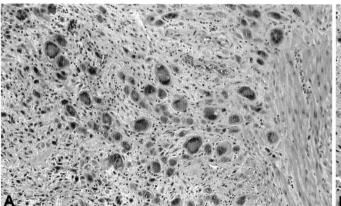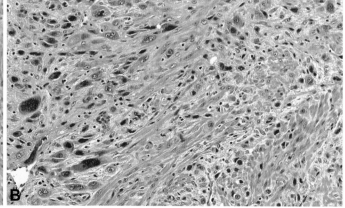

Fig. 6.06 Exaggerated placental site. **A** Exuberant infiltration of implantation-site intermediate trophoblast involving endometrium and underlying myometrium. Numerous multinucleated intermediate trophoblastic cells are present. **B** Infiltration of implantation site intermediate trophoblast involving superficial myometrium. Several cells are spindle shaped simulating smooth muscle.

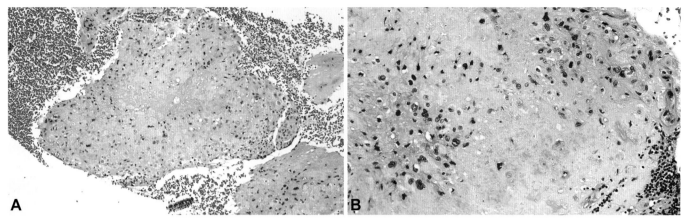

Fig. 6.07 Placental site nodule. **A** Well-circumscribed nodule with hyalinized centre surrounded by chorionic-type intermediate trophoblastic cells. **B** The lesion consists of hyalinized nodules with embedded small to medium-sized chorionic intermediate trophoblastic cells as single cells or clusters.

Molar pregnancies

P. Hui
R. Baergen
A.N.Y. Cheung
M. Fukunaga
D. Gersell
J.M. Lage
B.M. Ronnett
N.J. Sebire
M. Wells

Hydatidiform mole

Definition
An abnormal placenta with variable degrees of trophoblastic hyperplasia and villous hydrops. The presence of excessive paternal genome is the fundamental genetic etiology.

ICD-O code   9100/0

Synonym
Molar pregnancy

Epidemiology
The prevalence of gestational trophoblastic disease (GTD) varies markedly by country, with the highest incidence of hydatidiform mole in South-eastern Asia (3.8–13/1000 pregnancies) and the lowest incidence in the US and Europe (0.5–1.84/1000 pregnancies) {70,90,207,723}. Significant risk-factors include maternal age < 15 years and > 40 years {90,723,1017,1716}, previous hydatidiform mole {90}, Asian ethnicity and genetics {1184,1797}. Possible risk factors include diet and socioeconomic status {1171}. Gravidity, oral contraceptive use, parity, smoking, herbicides, paternal age and blood type are not significant risk factors {185,1448}.

Complete hydatidiform mole

Definition
A non-neoplastic, proliferative disorder of the placenta, resulting in villous hydrops and trophoblastic hyperplasia without embryonic development. Androgenetic diploidy (diploid paternal-only genome) is the fundamental genetic etiology in the majority of cases.

ICD-O code   9100/0

Synonyms
Complete molar pregnancy; complete mole

Clinical features
Vaginal bleeding in the second trimester, excessive uterine size, marked elevation of serum hCG, and both absence of fetal

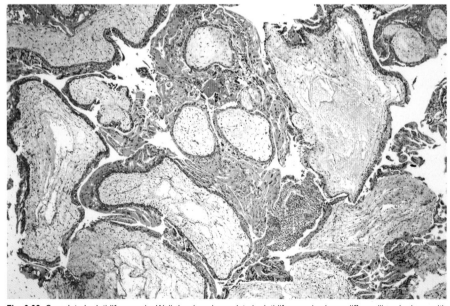

Fig. 6.08 Complete hydatidiform mole. Well-developed complete hydatidiform mole shows diffuse villous hydrops with frequent cistern formation.

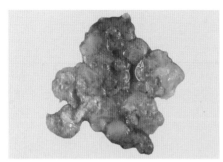

Fig. 6.09 Complete hydatidiform mole. Marked hydropic change transforms all chorionic villi into grape-like vesicles of variable sizes.

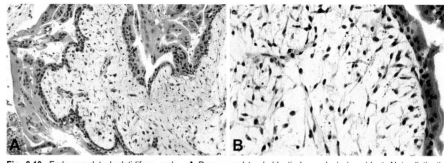

Fig. 6.10 Early complete hydatidiform mole. **A** Pronounced trophoblastic hyperplasia is evident. Note distinctive polypoid appearance of this villus. **B** The villous stroma of early complete hydatidiform mole consists of cellular, bluish myxoid stroma. There is prominent karyorrhexis.

heart tones and a "snow storm" pattern by ultrasonography are characteristic findings for a well-developed complete hydatidiform mole {140}. Other rare symptoms include hyperemesis, hyperthyroidism, pre-eclampsia, pulmonary embolism and ovarian theca lutein cysts {1872}. In countries with routine prenatal care, the typical clinical presentation is an abnormal ultrasound or as vaginal bleeding or a missed abortion {141,570}.

Macroscopy
Well-developed complete hydatidiform mole (CHM) consists of bulky, bloody tissue with hydropic changes uniformly transforming all villi into semi-transparent vesicles of variable sizes. Normal placental structures or fetal parts are absent, although very rare exceptions exist {87}. Early complete hydatidiform moles have minimal or no gross evidence of abnormal villi {899}.

Histopathology
Well-developed complete hydatidiform moles present with diffuse villous enlargement, marked hydropic changes, frequent cistern formation and pronounced trophoblastic hyperplasia. Significant cytological atypia is almost always present and mitotic figures are common. There are no fetal or non-villous placental tissues present, although rare exceptions exist {87}. An exaggerated placental site is nearly always present. The villi of a very early complete hydatidiform mole (evacuated during the first trimester) may not be enlarged but have a distinct polypoid appearance {899,1715}. Although the hydropic change may be minimal, the villous stroma is abnormally cellular and myxoid with prominent karyorrhexis. Mild to moderate trophoblastic hyperplasia is generally present in a circumferential or random fashion. Occasional cases may show marked trophoblastic proliferation and significant cytological atypia indistinguishable from those of choriocarcinoma. Differential diagnoses include partial hydatidiform mole (Table 6.3), hydropic abortion and early non-molar gestation with some degree of trophoblastic hyperplasia. Absence of p57 nuclear staining in cytotrophoblast and villous stromal cells is confirmatory {1234}, see below, and if available, DNA genotyping offers precise diagnosis of the disease {151,1106,1617}.

Immunohistochemistry
p57 is a cyclin dependent kinase inhibitor encoded by the paternally imprinted and maternally expressed gene *CDKN1C* on chromosome 11p15.5. Without the maternal genome, complete moles, including early forms, have absent p57 nuclear staining in cytotrophoblast and villous stromal cells. In contrast, partial mole and non-molar abnormal gestations (i.e. hydropic abortions, trisomies, digynic triploidy, placental mesenchymal dysplasia) contain the maternal genetic complement and therefore have strong nuclear p57 staining in these cell types. Accordingly, such differential p57 expression is very useful in the distinction of complete mole from partial mole and abnormal villous lesions associated Beckwith-Wiedemann syndrome. (see Table 6.3).

Histogenesis
Complete hydatidiform moles have proliferating cells recapitulating chorionic villous trophoblast {1758}. Its precise histogenesis is not known.

Genetic profile
Complete hydatidiform moles have a diploid androgenic-only genome in the majority of cases, with two paternal haploid chromosome sets of either monospermic/homozygous (80–90%) or dispermic/heterozygous (10–20%) origin {863,1106}. Also, they all inherit a maternal-only mitochondrial DNA {1996}. Rare tetraploid, complete moles may exist with four paternal haploid sets in the genome {582}.

Genetic susceptibility
A subset of recurrent, familial, biparental, complete hydatidiform moles develop as a result of abnormal imprinting and overexpression of the paternal genome due to maternal mutations of *NALP7/NLRP7* on chromosome 19q13.4 {1319}.

Prognosis and predictive factors
The prevalence of persistent gestational trophoblastic disease (GTD) is 15–29% after CHM and 2–3% of the patients develop choriocarcinoma {1344}. The risk of persistent GTD may be higher for heterozygous complete hydatidiform mole than for homozygous ones {86}. The risk of subsequent CHM is 1–1.8% after one prior and 10–18% after two consecutive hydatidiform moles {617,1714}.

Partial hydatidiform mole

Definition
A hydatidiform mole with a spectrum of villous populations ranging from normal size to substantial hydrops with mild, focal trophoblastic hyperplasia. Diandric-monogynic triploid genome is the fundamental genetic etiology in most cases.

ICD-O code   9103/0

Synonyms
Partial molar pregnancy; partial mole

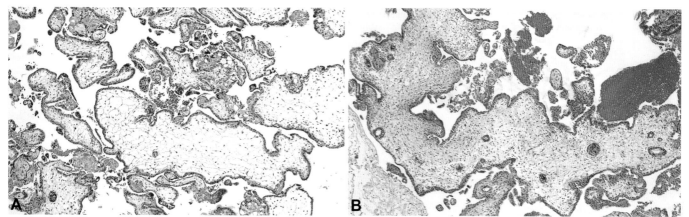

Fig. 6.11 Partial hydatidiform mole. **A** Two intermixed populations of villi are present along with scalloped villous contours and round trophoblastic pseudo-inclusions. **B** Trophoblastic pseudo-inclusions in a partial hydatidiform mole. Note their round to oval shape.

Clinical features

Patients present with vaginal bleeding or missed or incomplete abortion in the late first or early second trimester, normal or mildly elevated serum hCG {141} and a focally cystic placenta on ultrasound. A fetus may be detectable {556}. The majority of cases are not suspected as molar until routine histological examination is performed.

Macroscopy

Normal sized villi admixed with hydropic vesicles are characteristic. A gestational sac, fetal parts or intact fetus may be evident {622}. Specimens from the first trimester usually show no macroscopic abnormalities.

Histopathology

Partial hydatidiform moles (PHM) typically demonstrate two intermixed villous populations, consisting of enlarged hydropic villi and normal-sized but fibrotic ones although these may represent a spectrum rather than distinct bimodal populations. Central cistern formation, scalloped villous contours, and round to oval trophoblastic pseudo-inclusions are characteristic. Mild to moderate trophoblastic hyperplasia may be present in circumferential distribution or in the form of surface syncytiotrophoblast "knuckles" with intracytoplasmic lacunae. Fetal blood vessels and nucleated red blood cells are often present {622,1715}. Differential diagnoses include complete hydatidiform mole, early complete hydatidiform mole (Table 6.3), hydropic abortions, gestations with chromosomal abnormalities, placental mesenchymal dysplasia and twin gestations with complete hydatidiform mole

Table 6.3 Diagnostic features of hydatidiform moles

Diagnostic feature	CHM	VECHM	PHM
Clinical presentation	Vaginal bleeding in second trimester (average 16 weeks) Excessive uterine size Hyperemesis, toxaemia, preeclampsia or hyperthyroidism	Missed abortion (6.5–12 weeks of gestation)	Vaginal bleeding, missed or incomplete abortion in late first or early second trimester
Pretreatment hCG (mIU/ml)	Elevated (> 100 × 10³ in > 43% of cases)	Normal or elevated (< 100 × 10³)	Normal or elevated (< 100 × 10³ in > 93% of cases)
Ultrasound	Snow storm pattern without foetus formation	-	Focal cystic change with foetus formation
Macroscopy	Bulky specimen with hydropic change involving all villi Absence of gestational sac and foetal development	Frequently no gross abnormality	Hydropic change involving some villi Gestational sac and foetal tissue may be present
Chorionic villi	Diffuse enlargement Round to oval shapes	Normal size, polypoid or cauliflower shapes	Mild, with syncytiotrophoblast knuckles
Trophoblastic hyperplasia	Marked, often circumferential with intervillous trophoblast bridging	Mild, often on villous tips	Mild, with syncytiotrophoblast knuckles
Cytological atypia	Marked	Mild to moderate	Limited to mild
Villous stroma	Marked oedema with frequent cistern formation and trophoblastic inclusions Absence of vasculature and nucleated RBCs	Cellular and myxoid with prominent karyorrhexis Foetal capillaries may be present	Occasional cistern formation Round to oval trophoblastic pseudo-inclusions Presence of vasculature and nucleated RBCs (not always evident)
p57 immunostain	Absence of nuclear staining in cytotrophoblast and villous stromal cells	Absence of nuclear staining in cytotrophoblast and villous stromal cells	Presence of nuclear staining in cytotrophoblast and villous stromal cells
DNA genotyping	Diploid diandric (paternal-only) genome	Diploid diandric (paternal-only) genome	Triploid diandric-monogynic genome
CHM, complete hydatidiform mole; VECHM, very early complete hydatidiform mole; PHM, partial hydatidiform mole; hCG, human chorionic gonadotropin			

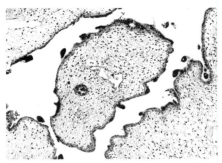

Fig. 6.12 Partial hydatidiform mole. Trophoblastic hyperplasia is mild in the form of syncytiotrophoblast "knuckles" (sprouts).

and coexisting normal fetus {218}. Triploidy on flow cytometry is consistent with but is not diagnostic of PHM {622}. If available, DNA genotyping offers precise diagnosis of the disease {788,1617}.

Histogenesis
Partial hydatidiform mole has proliferating cytotrophoblast and syncytiotrophoblast recapitulating chorionic villous trophoblast {1758}. Its precise histogenesis is not known.

Genetic profile
With one extra paternal haploid, partial hydatidiform moles have a triploid karyotype of 69XXY (70%), 69XXX (27%) and 69XYY (3%) {826,1046}. Rare tetraploid cases with two extra paternal haploid chromosomal complements exist {1320}.

Prognosis and predictive factors
Persistent gestational trophoblastic disease (GTD), mostly invasive hydatidiform mole, occurs in approximately 0.5–5% of PHM {1585}. The risk of developing choriocarcinoma is < 0.5% {1181,1718}. In contrast to complete hydatidiform mole, maternal age > 40 years and prior molar pregnancy have not been reported to be risk factors for persistent GTD {140,540}.

Invasive hydatidiform mole

Definition
A hydatidiform mole, complete or partial, that invades the myometrium and/or uterine vasculature.

ICD-O code   9100/1

Synonym
Chorioadenoma destruens (not recommended)

Clinical features
Vaginal bleeding with persistent elevation of serum hCG after primary evacuation of a hydatidiform mole is characteristic {589}.

Macroscopy
The lesion consists of invasive molar tissue extending from the endometrium into the myometrium. Hydropic villi may be visible and uterine perforation may occur {589}.

Histopathology
Most invasive hydatidiform moles are sequalae of complete hydatidiform mole that retain their histological characteristics and demonstrates myometrial and/or vascular invasion.

Histogenesis
Both complete and partial hydatidiform moles may develop into invasive hydatidiform mole.

Prognosis and predictive factors
Chemotherapy is highly effective with a cure rate over 80% depending on the extent of the disease {140}.

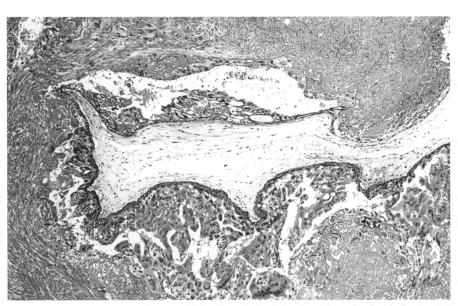

Fig. 6.13 Invasive complete hydatidiform mole. Molar villi invade deeply into the uterine wall and are in direct contact with smooth-muscle fibres without intervening decidua.

Abnormal (nonmolar) villous lesions

P. Hui
R. Baergen
A.N.Y. Cheung
M. Fukunaga

D. Gersell
J.M. Lage
B.M. Ronnett
N.J. Sebire
M. Wells

Definition

Various non-molar, villous lesions with histological features simulating a partial hydatidiform mole.

Clinical features

Missed abortion or incomplete abortion {622}

Macroscopy

They vary from normal gross findings to discernible vesicle formation.

Histopathology

Chorionic villi often display some degree of irregularity in size and shape, with focal, mild, trophoblastic hyperplasia (sometimes manifested as syncytiotrophoblastic "snouts") and occasional trophoblastic inclusions, thus having a partial spectrum of the histological alterations seen in a partial hydatidiform mole. Entities include hydropic abortions, chromosomal trisomy syndromes, digynic triploid conceptions, and placental mesenchymal dysplasia/Beckwith-Wiedemann syndrome (BWS) {218,622}. DNA genotyping analysis effectively separates these lesions from a partial hydatidiform mole {1106}. p57 immunostain does not distinguish partial hydatidiform mole from all above (with the exception of BWS) as the marker is expressed in cytotrophoblast and villous stromal cells in all these conditions.

Histogenesis

They have diverse origins related to the specific diagnosis causing the abnormal villous morphology.

Genetic profile

Diverse chromosomal or genetic alterations may be found.

Prognosis and predictive factors

These are non-molar entities and thus have the same low-risk of persistent gestational trophoblastic disease (GTD) as any other morphologically unremarkable non-molar conception.

CHAPTER 7

Tumours of the uterine cervix

Squamous cell tumours and precursors

Glandular tumours and precursors

Benign glandular tumours and tumour-like lesions

Other epithelial tumours

Neuroendocrine tumours

Mesenchymal tumours and tumour-like lesions

Mixed epithelial and mesenchymal tumours

Melanocytic tumours

Germ cell, lymphoid and myeloid tumours

Secondary tumours

WHO Classification of tumours of the uterine cervix[a,b]

Epithelial tumours
Squamous cell tumours and precursors
  Squamous intraepithelial lesions
    Low-grade squamous intraepithelial lesion 8077/0
    High-grade squamous intraepithelial lesion 8077/2
  Squamous cell carcinoma, NOS 8070/3
    Keratinizing 8071/3
    Non-keratinizing 8072/3
    Papillary 8052/3
    Basaloid 8083/3
    Warty 8051/3
    Verrucous 8051/3
    Squamotransitional 8120/3
    Lymphoepithelioma-like 8082/3
  Benign squamous cell lesions
    Squamous metaplasia
    Condyloma acuminatum
    Squamous papilloma 8052/0
    Transitional metaplasia
Glandular tumours and precursors
  Adenocarcinoma in situ 8140/2
  Adenocarcinoma 8140/3
    Endocervical adenocarcinoma, usual type 8140/3
    Mucinous carcinoma, NOS 8480/3
      Gastric type 8482/3
      Intestinal type 8144/3
      Signet-ring cell type 8490/3
    Villoglandular carcinoma 8263/3
    Endometrioid carcinoma 8380/3
    Clear cell carcinoma 8310/3
    Serous carcinoma 8441/3
    Mesonephric carcinoma 9110/3
    Adenocarcinoma admixed with
      neuroendocrine carcinoma 8574/3
Benign glandular tumours and tumour-like lesions
  Endocervical polyp
  Müllerian papilloma
  Nabothian cyst
  Tunnel clusters
  Microglandular hyperplasia
  Lobular endocervical glandular hyperplasia
  Diffuse laminar endocervical hyperplasia
  Mesonephric remnants and hyperplasia
  Arias Stella reaction
  Endocervicosis
  Endometriosis
  Tuboendometrioid metaplasia
  Ectopic prostate tissue

Other epithelial tumours
  Adenosquamous carcinoma 8560/3
    Glassy cell carcinoma 8015/3
  Adenoid basal carcinoma 8098/3
  Adenoid cystic carcinoma 8200/3
  Undifferentiated carcinoma 8020/3
Neuroendocrine tumours
  Low-grade neuroendocrine tumour
    Carcinoid tumour 8240/3
    Atypical carcinoid tumour 8249/3
  High-grade neuroendocrine carcinoma
    Small cell neuroendocrine carcinoma 8041/3
    Large cell neuroendocrine carcinoma 8013/3

Mesenchymal tumours and tumour-like lesions
Benign
  Leiomyoma 8890/0
  Rhabdomyoma 8905/0
  Others
Malignant
  Leiomyosarcoma 8890/3
  Rhabdomyosarcoma 8910/3
  Alveolar soft-part sarcoma 9581/3
  Angiosarcoma 9120/3
  Malignant peripheral nerve sheath tumour 9540/3
  Other sarcomas
    Liposarcoma 8850/3
    Undifferentiated endocervical sarcoma 8805/3
    Ewing sarcoma 9364/3
Tumour-like lesions
  Postoperative spindle-cell nodule
  Lymphoma-like lesion

Mixed epithelial and mesenchymal tumours
Adenomyoma 8932/0
Adenosarcoma 8933/3
Carcinosarcoma 8980/3

Melanocytic tumours
Blue naevus 8780/0
Malignant melanoma 8720/3

Germ cell tumours
Yolk sac tumour

Lymphoid and myeloid tumours
Lymphomas
Myeloid neoplasms

Secondary tumours

---

[a] The morphology codes are from the International Classification of Diseases for Oncology (ICD-O) {575A}. Behaviour is coded /0 for benign tumours, /1 for unspecified, borderline or uncertain behaviour, /2 for carcinoma in situ and grade III intraepithelial neoplasia and /3 for malignant tumours; [b] The classification is modified from the previous WHO classification of tumours {1906A}, taking into account changes in our understanding of these lesions; *These new codes were approved by the IARC/WHO Committee for ICD-O in 2013.

TNM and FIGO classification of carcinomas of the uterine cervix

T – Primary tumour

TNM	FIGO	
TX		Primary tumour cannot be assessed
T0		No evidence of primary tumour
Tis[a]		Carcinoma in situ (preinvasive carcinoma)
T1	I	Tumour confined to the cervix (extension to corpus should be disregarded)
T1a[b]	IA	Invasive carcinoma diagnosed only by microscopy. Stromal invasion with a maximal depth of 5.0 mm measured from the base of the epithelium and a horizontal spread of 7.0 mm or less[c]
T1a1	IA1	Measured stromal invasion 3.0 mm or less in depth and 7.0 mm or less in horizontal spread
T1a2	IA2	Measured stromal invasion more than 3.0 mm and not more than 5.0 mm with a horizontal spread of 7.0 mm or less

Note: The depth of invasion should be taken from the base of the epithelium, either surface or glandular, from which it originates. The depth of invasion is defined as the measurement of the tumour from the epithelial–stromal junction of the adjacent most superficial papillae to the deepest point of invasion. Vascular space involvement, venous or lymphatic, does not affect classification.

T1b	IB	Clinically visible lesion confined to the cervix or microscopic lesion greater than T1a/IA2
T1b1	IB1	Clinically visible lesion 4.0 cm or less in greatest dimension
T1b2	IB2	Clinically visible lesion more than 4.0 cm in greatest dimension
T2	II	Tumour invades beyond uterus but not to pelvic wall or to lower third of vagina
T2a	IIA	Tumour without parametrial invasion
T2a1	IIA1	Clinically visible lesion 4.0 cm or less in greatest dimension
T2a2	IIA2	Clinically visible lesion more than 4.0 cm in greatest dimension
T2b	IIB	Tumour with parametrial invasion
T3	III	Tumour extends to pelvic wall, involves lower one-third of vagina, causes hydronephrosis or nonfunctioning kidney
T3a	IIIA	Tumour involves lower one-third of vagina
T3b	IIIB	Tumour extends to pelvic wall, causes hydronephrosis or nonfunctioning kidney
T4	IVA	Tumour invades mucosa of the bladder or rectum, or extends beyond true pelvis[d,e]

Notes: [a] FIGO no longer includes Stage 0 (Tis). [b] All macroscopically visible lesions even with superficial invasion are T1b/IB. [c] Vascular space involvement, venous or lymphatic, does not affect classification. [d] Bullous oedema is not sufficient to classify a tumour as T4. [e] Invasion of bladder or rectal mucosa should be biopsy proven according to FIGO.

N – Regional Lymph Nodes

NX	Regional lymph nodes cannot be assessed
N0	No regional lymph node metastasis
N1	Regional lymph node metastasis

M – Distant Metastasis

M0	No distant metastasis
M1	Distant metastasis (includes inguinal lymph nodes and intraperitoneal disease except metastasis to pelvic serosa). It excludes metastasis to vagina, pelvic serosa, and adnexa

Stage grouping

Stage	T	N	M
Stage 0*	Tis	N0	M0
Stage I	T1	N0	M0
Stage IA	T1a	N0	M0
Stage IA1	T1a1	N0	M0
Stage IA2	T1a2	N0	M0
Stage IB	T1b	N0	M0
Stage IB1	T1b1	N0	M0
Stage IB2	T1b2	N0	M0
Stage II	T2	N0	M0
Stage IIA	T2a	N0	M0
Stage IIA1	T2a1	N0	M0
Stage IIA2	T2a2	N0	M0
Stage IIB	T2b	N0	M0
Stage III	T3	N0	M0
Stage IIIA	T3a	N0	M0
Stage IIIB	T3b	Any N	M0
	T1, T2, T3	N1	M0
Stage IVA	T4	Any N	M0
Stage IVB	Any T	Any N	M1

Notes: *FIGO no longer includes stage 0 (Tis)

References

American Joint Committee on Cancer (AJCC) Cancer Staging Manual, 7th ed. (2011) Edge SB, Byrd DR, Compton CC, Fritz AG, Greene FL, Trotti III eds. Springer: New York

International Union against Cancer (UICC): TNM Classification of Malignant Tumours, 7th ed. (2009) Sobin LH, Gospodarowicz MK, Wittekind Ch eds. Wiley-Blackwell: Oxford

A help-desk for specific questions about the TNM classification is available at http://www.uicc.org.

Squamous cell tumours and precursors

M. Stoler
C. Bergeron
T.J. Colgan
A.S. Ferenczy
C.S. Herrington

K.-R. Kim
T. Loening
A. Schneider
M.E. Sherman
D.C. Wilbur
T. Wright

Low-grade squamous intraepithelial lesion

Definition

An intraepithelial lesion of squamous epithelium that represents the clinical and morphological manifestation of a productive HPV infection. Low-grade refers to the associated low risk of concurrent or future cancer.

ICD-O code   8077/0

Synonyms

Cervical intraepithelial neoplasia, grade 1 (CIN 1); mild squamous dysplasia; flat condyloma; koilocytotic atypia; koilocytosis

Epidemiology

The epidemiology of low-grade squamous intraepithelial lesion (LSIL) follows the epidemiology of HPV infections {57, 59,249,325,980,1916}. HPV infections are very common, affecting up to 80% of women in their early 20s, but being detectable in only 5% in their 50s {1627} More than 40 HPV types infect the cervix, although 13–15 high-risk (HR) and 4–6 low-risk (LR) types account for the majority of infections and most clinically valid HPV tests only test for 13–14 HR types {981,1122,1916}.

Clinical features

LSILs are asymptomatic lesions and are

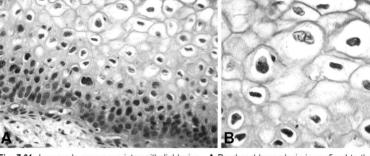

Fig. 7.01 Low-grade squamous intraepithelial lesion. **A** Parabasal hyperplasia is confined to the lower third of the epithelium. The upper layers exhibit differentiation and koilocytotic atypia. **B** High-power view demonstrates koilocytotic atypia as defined in the text.

identified through cytological screening and colposcopy.

Macroscopy

Cervical HPV lesions are not usually visible to the naked eye, except for exophytic or papillary lesions that are most often equivalent to a condyloma acuminatum. Condylomata acuminata are also LSILs {160,388,412,465}. Colposcopy does not reliably segregate LSIL from high-grade squamous intraepithelial lesion (HSIL) and both may co-exist in the cervix, not only in the same quadrant or area of acetowhitening, but in separate areas or quadrants {1177}. Two distinct areas may be due to infection by two different HPVs or by the same HPV {1546}. Sophisticated molecular microdissection studies support the concept of "one lesion, one virus" {1546}.

Histopathology

A two tier system of low- and high-grade intraepithelial lesions is more biologically relevant and histologically more reproducible than the three-tier CIN 1, CIN 2 and CIN 3 terminology used in the prior edition and is therefore recommended {412,1840}.

LSIL (koilocytosis or flat condyloma or CIN 1) is the morphological manifestation of the differentiation-dependent expression of an HPV virion production program on the host squamous cells {465,1838, 1839}. There is no way to predict HPV type by morphology, although some data suggest that HPV 16 and HPV 18 produce more rapidly growing and larger lesions {84,249,251,836,1845,2176}. The inherent difficulty in distinguishing pure HPV infection from CIN 1 in histologically flat epithelium (sometimes referred to as flat condyloma) is understandable since, by the above definition, they are biologically the same {465,1250,1537}. Some pathologists attempt to make this distinction and subdivide LSILs into lesions showing koilocytosis without atypia, flat condylomata and CIN 1. The Lower Anogenital Squamous Terminology Standardization (LAST) project did not support this approach, recommending that all of these lesions be designated LSILs, reflecting their common biology.

LSIL is characterized by a proliferation of basal/parabasal-like cells that may be minimal but at most extends no more than one-third of the way up the epithelium {1005,1586,2032}. Mitotic activity is

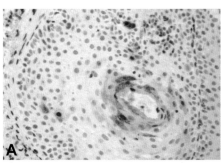
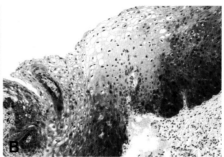

Fig. 7.02 Patterns of p16 expression in low-grade squamous intraepithelial lesion (LSIL). Immunostaining for p16 in LSIL may be totally negative, show patchy positivity not involving the basement membrane (**A**) or be truly positive (in approximately one-third of cases). Note that only "block-type" positivity, as shown in **B**, should be considered truly positive.

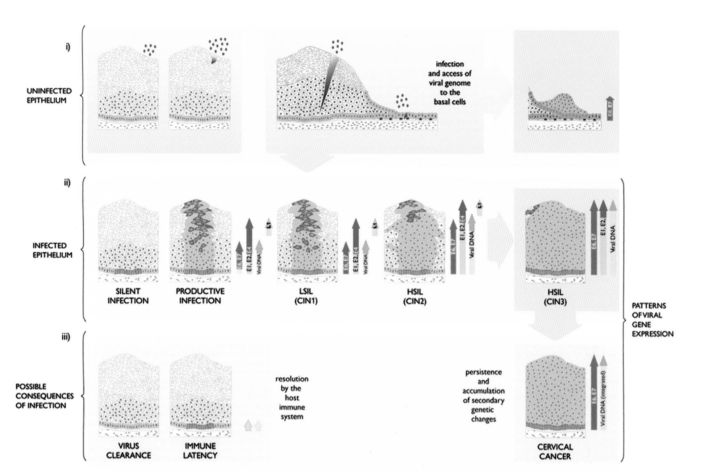

Fig. 7.03 High-Risk HPV Infection and its possible consequences. **(i)** The detection of HPV DNA in a tissue biopsy may indicate productive (LSIL) or (HSIL) infection; the presence of virus particles at the epithelial surface without infection (e.g. from recent transmission); or a latent or silent infection. Infection requires the entry of HPV virions into the mitotically active epithelial cells of the basal layer, which in stratified epithelium is thought to require a microwound. In the columnar cell layers, infection is thought to be facilitated by the proximity of the target cell to the epithelial surface, which may allow the virus to access a cell type that is unable to support the full productive life cycle (right). The significance of infection of different cell types remains to be properly assessed.

(ii) Following infection (shown in (i)), expression from the viral genome can sometimes be suppressed (e.g. by genome methylation), leading to a "silent" infection in which the viral genomes are retained in the basal layer without apparent disease. Infection may alternatively lead to an ordered pattern of viral gene expression leading to virus synthesis and release from the upper epithelial layers (productive infection or LSIL), or to deregulated viral gene expression and high-grade intraepithelial neoplasia (HSIL). Persistent high-grade disease is associated with an increasing risk of genome integration into the host cell chromosome and progression to cancer. Cells in cycle are indicated by the presence of red nuclei. Cells expressing E4 are shown in green, while those expressing L1 are shown in yellow. The brown shading identifies all the cells (differentiated and undifferentiated) that contain viral genomes.

(iii) In most cases, HPV infections are resolved as a result of a cell-mediated immune response (left). This may lead to viral clearance or to viral latency and the persistence of viral episomes in the epithelial basal layer without life-cycle completion. Viral gene expression patterns during latency are not well characterized. Persistent deregulated gene expression, as occurs in CIN 3 and following viral genome integration, can lead to the accumulation of secondary genetic changes in the infected host cell and development of cancer. This is facilitated by over-expression of the high-risk E6 and E7 proteins. Cells in cycle are shown by red nuclei. Brown shading in the immune latency state indicates cells harbouring viral episomes. In cervical cancer, the viral genome is often integrated with loss of expression of full-length E1, E2, E4 and E5, and the L1 and L2 capsid proteins, and with de-regulated expression of E6 and E7.

confined to this zone and for most LSILs the mitoses are not abnormal. In the upper three-quarters to two-thirds of the epithelium, the cells differentiate and gain cytoplasm; however, nuclear enlargement persists such that the nucleo-cytoplasmic ratio is increased. In addition there is usually nuclear hyperchromasia, nuclear membrane irregularities and often development of a well-defined halo-like vacuole around the nucleus. The latter cytoplasmic change, together with the nuclear abnormalities, has been termed

koilocytosis, koilocytotic atypia or HPV cytopathic effect {976,1250}. Koilocytosis is usually most prominent in the upper third of the epithelium. The surface cells may exhibit parakeratosis or hyperkeratosis. While most LSILs exhibit koilocytosis, not all do. Other findings include bi- or multinucleation. Importantly, all SILs have histocytological abnormalities in all layers of the epithelium. The finding of markedly atypical single cells in the basal third of the epithelium, or abnormal mitotic figures, should not be interpreted

as LSIL, as these features correlate with DNA instability and aneuploidy and therefore represent HSIL {56,388}. Besides HSIL, LSIL must be distinguished from mimics of LSIL due to a variety of infectious or inflammatory processes that are unrelated to HPV infection {249,379,412, 679,1297,1754,2051}. Approximately one-third of histological LSIL show diffuse (so-called "block-positive") p16 immunostaining involving the basal and parabasal cell layers {139,595,897,1676,2020}. Accordingly, this finding should not be interpreted

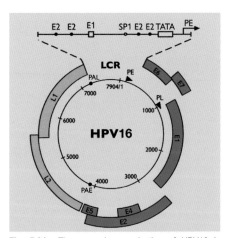

Fig. 7.04 The genomic organization of HPV16 is typical of the high-risk alpha-papillomaviruses (including HPV18), and comprises a long control region (LCR) and eight genes that are necessary for different stages of the virus life cycle. These genes encode a larger number of gene products as a result of mRNA splicing. The LCR contains binding sites for cellular transcription factors as well as for the viral E1 and E2 proteins that control viral replication and gene expression. Reprinted from {465}.

as absolutely indicative of HSIL. The diagnosis rests on the appearance of the lesion on H&E stains.

Histogenesis

Most cervical LSILs (80–85%) are due to infection with HR HPV types {57,59,1916}. The remainder of true LSILs are caused by LR HPV types. HPV negative LSIL should be viewed as a histological mimic or technical failure of the HPV assay.

Genetic profile

Little is known to be clinically useful regarding host genetic changes in LSIL. From a viral standpoint, any HPV type capable of infecting the cervical mucosa may produce LSIL morphology. LSILs are generally DNA stable and their enlarged nuclei are usually euploid or polyploid {465}.

Genetic susceptibility

HPV infections are ubiquitous in human populations. Immunosuppression seems to favour HPV lesion persistence or emergence of rarer HPV types. Once acquisition of HPV as a risk factor is controlled for, clinical testing for familial/genetic susceptibility factors yields little if any information regarding risk of progression to HSIL or carcinoma {980,1994}.

Prognosis and predictive factors

The outcome for a patient with biopsy proven LSIL is excellent as regression is expected on average within approximately one year. HPV type is highly correlated with risk of concomitant or progression to HSIL or worse and the majority of that risk is associated with HPV type 16. Other factors associated with the development of HSIL and carcinoma include older age, immunosuppression and smoking. In a few limited studies, positive p16 immunohistochemistry is suggestive of increased risk of progression {1339,1444,1937,2020}. However, issues of histological interpretive variability and completeness of disease ascertainment confound such studies {412}. No single or combination of biomarkers has been found to predict definitively whether a given lesion will persist, progress or regress. Further, the potential therapeutic impact of biopsy on natural history, by removing or inducing regression in one-quarter to one-third of cases, confounds the development of any such marker for clinical use {1845}. In addition, a patient with a post-colposcopic histopathological diagnosis of LSIL still has an approximately 10% chance of harbouring an HSIL due to the biopsy missing the most severe lesion {250,379,678,1916}.

High-grade squamous intraepithelial lesion

Definition

A squamous intraepithelial lesion that carries a significant risk of invasive cancer development if not treated {412,1586}.

ICD-O code   8077/2

Synonyms

Cervical intraepithelial neoplasia, grade 2 (CIN 2); cervical intraepithelial neoplasia, grade 3 (CIN 3); moderate squamous dysplasia; severe squamous dysplasia; squamous carcinoma in situ (CIS)

Epidemiology

Detection of high-grade squamous intraepithelial lesion (HSIL) tends to occur two decades earlier than invasive carcinoma, but epidemiological risk factors are generally similar {980}. The detection of large, single foci of HSIL (CIN 3) may be related to older age, longer history of sexual activity and less frequent screening {2077}. Limited data suggest that approximately one-third of inadequately

treated HSIL (CIN 3) will progress to carcinoma over 30 years {1236} with risks potentially related to larger lesion size {1921}. In general, HSIL occurs at an older age than LSIL although there is broad overlap and HSIL has been demonstrated to develop within a year or two of HPV infection in adolescents {809,810,979,980}. The cross-sectional prevalence of HSIL in Western screened population is 0.5–1% {2052}. The risk of progression of untreated HSIL to cancer is estimated to be 0.5–1% per year {1236}. Estimates of regression to LSIL or normal vary from 30–50% depending on age, lesion size and HPV type but are confounded by the potential therapeutic impact of biopsy, which may be as large as 30% {1438,1845,1948,2021}. HPV-16 and 18 together account for approximately 50% of HSILs, a fraction that will be dramatically decreased in vaccinated populations {351,2023}.

Clinical features

HSILs are asymptomatic lesions detected by cytology and colposcopy.

Macroscopy

Unless exophytic (papillary), HSILs are usually not visible on routine clinical examination. Visible lesions, especially those associated with an HSIL Pap smear, or with clinical bleeding or ulceration, should raise concern for carcinoma {214,548,1177}. In recent clinical trials, one-quarter to one-third of prevalent HSILs may be in quadrants that, to some colposcopists, appear non-conspicuous {1847}. Hence biopsy protocols are evolving to increase the number of biopsies and sample the worst part of the lesion {593,2021}.

Histopathology

Our improved understanding of HPV biology supports the grouping of CIN 2 with CIN 3 under the HSIL designation {412}. CIN 2 has the poorest interobserver reproducibility of any cervical biopsy diagnosis {596}. More than half of CIN 2 biopsies on follow up excision have CIN 3 as a final diagnosis {1845}. No biomarker defines a distinct intermediate state of CIN 2 and the emerging consensus is that CIN 2 is a mix of biological CIN 1 and CIN 3, the true nature of which is confounded by issues of colposcopic biopsy sampling and pathological interpretive variability {412}. However, in women who

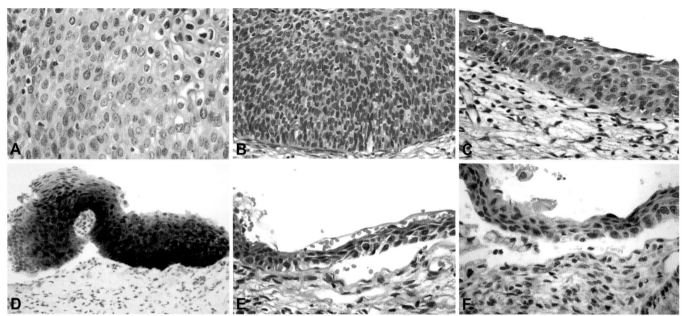

Fig. 7.05 A High-grade squamous intraepithelial lesion (CIN 2). Some HSILs may still have overlying koilocytosis, but the degree of proliferation in the parabasal zone exceeds the criteria for LSIL. **B** High-grade squamous intraepithelial lesion (CIN 3). This lesion is classically characterized by full thickness immaturity, irregular polarity and numerous mitotic figures. **C** Atypical squamous metaplasia versus high-grade squamous intraepithelial lesion. In problematic cases, the differential diagnosis may not be resolvable by H&E alone. **D** Atypical squamous metaplasia (ASM) versus high-grade squamous intraepithelial lesion (p16 staining). As an adjunctive stain when the differential diagnosis is between ASM and HSIL, a positive p16 strongly favours an HSIL interpretation for management purposes. **E** Differential diagnosis of thin metaplasia *versus* high-grade squamous intraepithelial lesion. **F** The negative p16 staining of the lesion shown in E is good evidence against a diagnosis of HSIL. Patchy p16 staining as shown should not be interpreted as a positive result.

want to maintain their fertility, clinicians may request that pathologists try as hard as possible to distinguish HSIL (CIN 2) from HSIL (CIN 3) to allow for the possibility of regression of HSIL (CIN 2), thereby potentially sparing young women of childbearing age the complications that may arise from cervical excision {272}.

Under H&E microscopy, there is a proliferation of squamous cells most frequently in the zone of metaplasia and near the current squamocolumnar junction. The cells have abnormal nuclear features including increased nuclear size, irregular nuclear membranes, and increased nucleo-cytoplasmic ratios accompanied by mitotic figures. There is less cytoplasmic differentiation than in LSIL as the proliferating cell compartment extends up into the middle third (HSIL (CIN 2)) or superficial third (HSIL (CIN 3)) of the epithelium {1005,1586}. Mitotic figures are more abundant than in LSIL and are not necessarily confined to the lower third of the epithelium; rather they are frequently found in the middle and/or superficial thirds of the epithelium. Abnormal mitotic figures are commonly present and, when present in lesions lacking parabasal proliferation into the middle third of the epithelium, favour HSIL over LSIL. The presence of distinct and/or large nucleoli in

HSIL is unusual and raises the differential diagnoses of both inadequately sampled carcinoma and reparative or inflammatory mimics of HSIL. The latter are typically p16 negative {412}.

Variants of HSIL {412,1005}
Thin HSIL is a high-grade intraepithelial lesion that is usually < 10 cells thick. If there is doubt about the nature of the proliferation (e.g. immature metaplasia versus SIL) then p16 staining can be used as described below {623,897}.
In *keratinising HSIL*, there is an abnormal keratinizing layer on the surface and the epithelium typically contains dyskeratotic cells with markedly atypical, often pleomorphic nuclei. The histology is more like the HPV-associated HSILs seen in cutaneous sites with keratinizing epithelium such as vulva or perianus. Such lesions may more often be seen in ectocervical locations {1005}.
Lesions that are clinically *condylomatous* can histologically harbour HSIL. Such changes may be focal, but the HSIL area dictates prognosis and treatment.
Papillary squamous carcinoma in situ, or non-invasive papillary squamo-transitional carcinoma is a papillary lesion with fine and less acuminate papillations that histologically is completely covered

by epithelium that shows the features of HSIL and may resemble urothelial neoplasia. This diagnosis should only be made if the lesion has been completely excised and stromal invasion excluded {192,957,1626}.

Immunohistochemistry
p16 immunohistochemistry can be extremely helpful in the assessment of HSILs, particularly in the evaluation of lesions considered morphologically to represent HSIL (CIN 2) and in the distinction between HSIL and its mimics, such as immature squamous metaplasia and atrophy. A full discussion of the use of p16 immunostaining is contained in the recommendations of the LAST project {412}.

Histogenesis
High-risk (HR) HPVs are found in over 90% of cervical HSILs. Whether HSILs develop from LSILs or evolve independently is controversial {465,980,1546}. Attempts to study this are confounded by issues of interpretive variation and sampling {1948}. Biologically, an HSIL can be thought of as a clonal expansion of cells that are driven to proliferate by the abnormal expression of HPV E6 and HPV E7 in cells still capable of cell division {465,1838}.

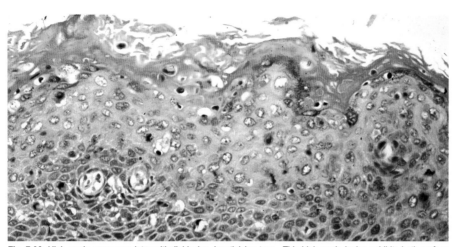

Fig. 7.06 High-grade squamous intraepithelial lesion, keratinizing type. This high-grade lesion exhibits both surface and individual cell keratinization analogous to what is more often seen on the vulva.

Genetic profile

HSILs are monoclonal in most of cases if microdissected and they exhibit aneuploidy more frequently than polyploidy, a reflection of genetic instability {316,502,683}. In addition, they show relatively more frequent HPV DNA integration compared to LSIL {1155,1985}. Chromosomal abnormalities shared more frequently with cancer than LSIL include abnormalities of 1p and 3q {906, 938,1034}.

Genetic susceptibility

There is weak evidence at best for HLA variation or other genetic susceptibility markers such as *TP53* codon 72 polymorphism {949,1014,1674}.

Prognosis and predictive factors

No biomarkers are yet proven to be clinically reliable for segregating the HSIL that needs treatment from the HSIL that can be safely followed without also considering the clinical and colposcopic characteristics of the lesion and the patient as a whole.

Most patients are cured by treatment and meta-analyses of subjects who underwent cryotherapy, laser ablation, loop electro-surgical excision procedure (LEEP) or surgical conization for the treatment of SIL (CIN) of any grade reveal no substantial differences in outcome. The size of the lesion, which correlates with the completeness of the excision/ablation, and whether HSIL reaches the margins, predict recurrence. Recent data demonstrate that testing for HPV DNA at 12 months post therapy is the best predictor of recurrent or residual disease {60,61}.

Squamous cell carcinoma

Definition

An invasive epithelial tumour composed of squamous cells of varying degrees of differentiation.

ICD-O codes

Squamous cell carcinoma, NOS	8070/3
Keratinizing	8071/3
Non-keratinizing	8072/3
Papillary	8052/3
Basaloid	8083/3
Warty	8051/3
Verrucous	8051/3
Squamotransitional	8120/3
Lymphoepithelioma-like	8082/3

Epidemiology

Cervical cancer is the second or third most common cancer in women with approximately 0.5 million cases worldwide {58,546}. Cervical cancers worldwide increased from an estimated 378 000 in 1980 to 500,000 per year in recent years {545,546}, reflecting an average annual increase of 0.6% {568}. Approximately 76% of recent cases occur in low-resource nations, with numbers increasing in all but high-income countries {546,568}. The median age at death in wealthier nations is 55 years {568}. In the US and elsewhere, cervical cancer rates fell during the first half of the twentieth century, presumably secondary to improved public health measures and changes in lifestyle factors, and then dropped again in the latter half of the century with implementation of Pap smear screening. The large disparities in incidence and mortality between heavily affected nations in Africa and Asia and lower rates in wealthier North American and European countries is largely attributable to effective programs to detect cancer precursors coupled with infrastructure to clinically manage precursor lesions {545}. Within high-income nations, cervical cancer disproportionately afflicts disadvantaged women who have not received adequate screening and follow-up {1505}. The incidence varies from as high as 100/100,000 in unscreened populations to 1–5/100,000 in highly screened Western populations.

Etiology

Nearly all cervical cancers are caused by persistent infections with one of around 15 carcinogenic types of human

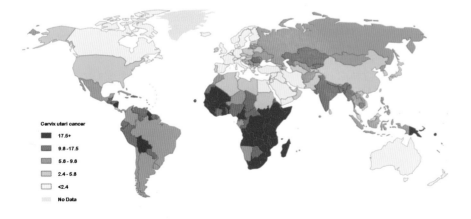

Cervix uteri cancer
- 17.5+
- 9.8-17.5
- 5.8-9.8
- 2.4-5.8
- <2.4
- No Data

Fig. 7.07 Worldwide distribution of cervical cancer mortality. From: Globocan 2012 {546}

papillomaviruses (HPV) {172,1005,1693} and the proportion with squamous histology is approximately 70%. The ratio of squamous to non-squamous histology is most related to screening which is demonstrably more effective at identifying the proximate precursor of squamous cell carcinoma, high-grade squamous intraepithelial lesion (HSIL), for treatment {1686,1734}.

HPV-16 and 18 demonstrate the strongest carcinogenic potency, accounting for approximately 70% of cancers, with HPV-16 the major causal agent of squamous cell carcinoma and HPV-18 contributing approximately equally to adenocarcinoma. The development of HPV vaccines that are highly effective in preventing HPV-16/18 infections (and the anticipated expansion of coverage to additional HPV types) will dramatically change the epidemiology of HPV infection and cervical neoplasia {199,1694}. However, administering the vaccine is challenging {1505}, and may not alter the course of HPV infections among women who are already infected {1694}.

The etiology of cervical cancer can be divided into multiple phases such as HPV acquisition, HPV persistence and progression to cervical cancer precursors (corresponding approximately to HSIL (CIN 3), and progression to invasion {1693}. Sexual activity, especially numbers of sexual partners, is a strong risk factor for HPV acquisition; however, single contacts with high-risk men may result in infection and risk plateaus with many contacts {430,943}. The incidence of HPV infections spikes at ages of sexual initiation and cumulative prevalence is extremely high among adolescents and young women; however, most infections spontaneously regress, as assessed by molecular HPV DNA testing {572,764}. Thus, persistent infection with carcinogenic HPVs is necessary for carcinogenesis, but not sufficient, and the sojourn time from acquisition through persistence, and thence to development of a cancer precursor, and finally to progression to invasion generally requires decades. Data suggest that the final step, progression from HSIL (CIN 3) to invasion, is slowest, though variable among women. Factors associated with greater risk of HPV persistence include HPV type (especially HPV-16), immunodeficiency, smoking, multiparity, long-term oral contraceptive use, possibly chronic inflammation and/or

Genus + Species	Type	Invasive Cervical Cancer	IARC Category	Squamous Cell Carcinoma	Adeno Carcinoma	Tropism
Alpha 1	HPV32		3			mucosal
	HPV42					
Alpha 2	HPV3					
	HPV10					
	HPV28		3			
	HPV29		3			cutaneous
	HPV77		3			
	HPV94					
	HPV117					
	HPV125					
Alpha 3	HPV61	0.01	3			
	HPV62		3			
	HPV72		3			
	HPV81		3	0.4		
	HPV83		3	0.4		
	HPV84		3			mucosal
	HPV86		3			
	HPV87		3			
	HPV89		3			
	HPV102					
	HPV114					
Alpha 4	HPV2		3			
	HPV27		3			cutaneous
	HPV57		3			
Alpha 5	HPV26	0.37	2B	0.22		
	HPV51	1.25	1	0.75	0.54	
	HPV69	0.08	2B			
	HPV82	0.07	2B	0.26		
Alpha 6	HPV30	0.37	2B			
	HPV53	0.26	2B	0.04		
	HPV56	0.84	1	1.09		
	HPV66	0.08	2B	0.19		
Alpha 7	HPV18	10.28	1	11.27	37.3	mucosal
	HPV39	1.67	1	0.82	0.54	
	HPV45	5.68	1	5.21	5.95	
	HPV59	1.08	1	1.05	2.16	
	HPV68	1.04	2A	0.37		
	HPV70	0.11	2B			
	HPV85		2B			
	HPV97					
Alpha 8	HPV7		3		41.62	cutaneous (mucosal)
	HPV40		3		1.08	
	HPV43				0.54	
	HPV91	0.01	3		1.08	
Alpha 9	HPV16	61.35	1	54.38		
	HPV31	3.65	1	3.82	0.54	
	HPV33	3.83	1	2.06		
	HPV35	1.94	1	1.27		mucosal
	HPV52	2.71	1	2.25		
	HPV58	2.22	1	1.72		
	HPV67	0.31	2B			
Alpha 10	HPV6	0.11	3	0.07		
	HPV11	0.02	3	0.07		
	HPV13		3			mucosal
	HPV44	0.01	3			
	HPV74	0.01	3			
Alpha 11	HPV34	0.07				mucosal
	HPV73	0.52	2B	0.49		
Alpha 12						
Alpha 13	HPV54					
Alpha 14	HPV71					mucosal
	HPV90		3			
	HPV106		3			

Fig. 7.08 Disease Association of the Alpha HPVs. The high-risk Alpha types of IARC category 1 and 2A HPV types are classified (respectively) as carcinogenic and possibly-carcinogenic. Despite limited epidemiological data, the 2B classification is proposed for types that are probably carcinogenic because of their close phylogenetic relationship with the established carcinogenic types. HPV types in category 3 are considered non-carcinogenic. The remaining types have not yet been classified because of insufficient data. Types that are closely related evolutionarily (e.g., HPV16 and 31) can exhibit different degrees of cancer risk, which is thought to be related to different protein functions and patterns of gene expression. Reprinted from {465}.

concurrent sexually transmitted diseases, such as chlamydia, and positive family history {247,430,575,642,1317,1804}. Notably, co-morbidities such as human immunodeficiency virus (HIV) infection, transplantation and medications may reduce cell-mediated immunity, leading to higher risk of HPV persistence.

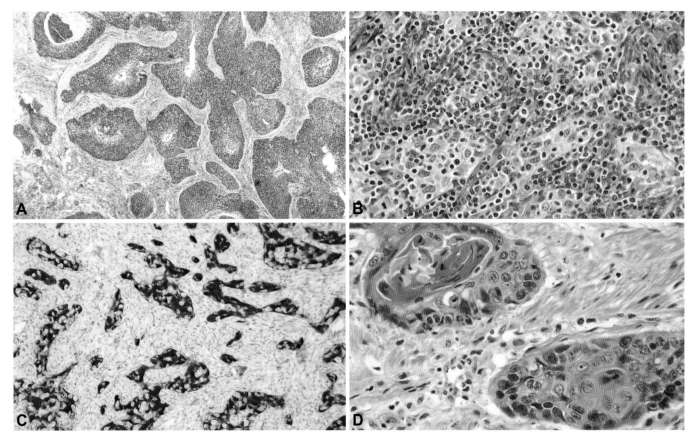

Fig. 7.09 A Squamous cell carcinoma, usual type. This tumour is characterized by infiltrative sheets and nest of cells without overt keratinization. **B** Lymphoepithelioma-like carcinoma. These tumours can have such a dense lymphoid infiltrate that their true nature as a poorly differentiated squamous carcinoma is obscured. **C** Lymphoepithelioma-like carcinoma. The epithelial component not only marks with keratin but, like most cervical carcinomas, is strongly p16 positive as shown here. **D** Squamous cell carcinoma. This tumour exhibits overt keratinization either as keratin pearls or as individual densely keratinized cells.

Circumcision may lower HPV infection rates among men and reduce risks among their partners {246}. Cervical adenocarcinomas comprise approximately 10–25% of cervical cancers (see section on glandular tumours and precursors, p. 183). Like squamous cell carcinomas, nearly all of these cancers are caused by HPV infection, but the type spectrum is narrower, and HPV-18 is proportionately more important {1005,1734}. Limited data suggest that HPV-18 is underrepresented among lower grades of squamous cell precursors, is over-represented among cancers judged as "early onset" or "rapidly developing" {755} and is associated with frequent integration of HPV DNA into the human genome of cancer cells {1985}. Historically, cytological detection of adenocarcinoma, and its immediate precursor, adenocarcinoma in situ (high-grade cervical glandular intraepithelial neoplasia (CGIN)), has been considered insensitive compared with detection of the more common squamous precursor lesions {1686}. However, successful

adoption of HPV DNA testing for screening and implementation of prophylactic vaccination could eradicate this disparity because the range of HPV types in endocervical neoplasia is covered by these approaches {935}.

Clinical features

Patients with small tumours may be asymptomatic. Abnormal vaginal bleeding and contact bleeding, discharge and pain are correlated with larger tumour size, necrosis and extra-cervical extension. With lateral growth into the parametrium, ureteral obstruction may lead to anuria and uraemia. Pelvic sidewall involvement can cause sciatic pain and, less commonly, lymphoedema of the lower extremities. Anterior tumour growth in advanced stage of disease causes urinary frequency, bladder pain and haematuria. Direct extension into the bladder may cause urinary retention from bladder outlet obstruction and eventually a vesicovaginal fistula. Posterior extension leads to low back pain, tenesmus

and rectovaginal fistula. A large proportion of carcinomas are now detected at a pre-clinical stage in countries with screening programs. Staging is still primarily performed by clinical examination of tumour size and extent, and the FIGO staging system is used most commonly {361,669}. With the success of screening and vaccination programs, an increasing proportion of invasive squamous cell carcinomas present at a microscopic stage that requires the precise application of histopathological criteria. Such tumours may be termed superficially invasive squamous cell carcinomas {412}.

Macroscopy

On visual inspection, cervical cancer may appear as a red, friable, exophytic or ulcerated lesion. Palpation can detect induration or nodularity of the cervix or the parametria in advanced lesions. Squamous cell carcinoma may be predominantly exophytic, papillary or polypoid, or else it may be mainly endophytic, such that it infiltrates into the surrounding structures. Endophytic tumours covered by normal epithelium, or tumours arising in the portion of the cervical canal that are not visible or accessible to sampling, may be clinically occult for some considerable period of time.

Histopathology

Invasive squamous cell carcinomas of the cervix vary in their pattern of growth, cell type and degree of differentiation. While some variant patterns are described below, few of these variations impact therapy or prognosis once stage and grade are accounted for {440,973,1825,2133}. The majority of carcinomas are of the usual type and, unlike carcinomas of the vulva or other lower anogenital sites where tumours that are not associated with HPV are more common or may even be in the majority, virtually all the variations of cervical squamous cell carcinoma are of an HPV-driven etiology {429,1994}. It seems to be a characteristic of HPV-16/18 associated carcinomas of the cervix and at other anatomical sites (vulva, oropharynx/tonsils) that most of them are immature non-keratinizing, basaloid neoplasms {1005,1010,1841,1842}.

Most carcinomas exhibit sheet-like growth and infiltrate as networks of anastomosing bands or single cells with an intervening desmoplastic or inflammatory stroma. Superficial stromal invasion may be associated with stromal loosening, desmoplasia and/or increased epithelial cell cytoplasmic eosinophilia. When invasion cannot be excluded on biopsy because neoplastic squamous epithelium shows overlapping features of HSIL but underlying stroma is not present, the phrase "at least HSIL, invasive carcinoma cannot be excluded" is suggested {412}. Grading based on the degree of nuclear pleomorphism, size of nucleoli, mitotic

frequency and necrosis, all of which correlate with growth rate, may convey some degree of prognostic information related to tumour sensitivity to chemotherapy or radiation therapy. Based on the extent of squamous differentiation, tumours may be graded as well, moderately or poorly differentiated, or perhaps more reliably into low-grade and high-grade. Not all keratinizing carcinomas are low-grade or well differentiated since the nuclear features noted above apply {1005,1010, 1841,1842}.

Keratinizing and non-keratinizing squamous cell carcinoma

Squamous cell carcinoma of the usual type may be non-keratinizing or keratinizing. However, the extent of keratinization required to diagnose a keratinizing squamous cell carcinoma is not clearly defined.

Non-keratinizing tumours are composed of polygonal squamous cells growing in sheets or nests that may have intercellular bridges, but keratin pearls are not present {1841}. Cellular and nuclear pleomorphism is more obvious in higher grade tumours and mitotic figures are usually numerous. The nuclei are relatively large with unevenly distributed, coarsely granular chromatin and nucleoli are readily discernible and may be irregular or multiple. Tumours composed of smaller cells with a very high nuclear to cytoplasmic ratio and less prominent nucleolation may overlap on H&E with 'small cell carcinomas' of the cervix. The latter term should be reserved for tumours that are neuroendocrine in nature (see cervical neuroendocrine tumours, p. 196) and behave clinically like their very aggressive pulmonary counterpart. Rarely squamous carcinoma may be mixed with true small cell neuroendocrine

carcinoma and discerning this may require immunohistochemistry {665,1843}. Statistically however, in the presence of a small cell neuroendocrine component, adenocarcinoma is the more likely partner in a histologically mixed tumour, possibly because both components are associated with HPV-18. The high-grade neuroendocrine component may well govern the patient's prognosis.

Keratinizing tumours contain keratin pearls, abundant keratohyaline granules or display dense cytoplasmic keratinization, and may be of any grade. The nuclei are usually large and hyperchromatic with coarse chromatin and may appear more smudgy and lack the easily seen nucleoli of the non-keratinizing carcinomas. Keratinizing carcinoma may have some correlation with keratinizing SIL as a precursor and may in very early stages be more likely to be ectocervical in location. They also may be masked in cytological preparations by cytological overlap with HSIL and associated keratotic reactions on the surface {1560}.

Basaloid squamous cell carcinoma

This under-recognized variant of squamous cell carcinoma is an aggressive tumour wherever in the body it has been described and hence the tumour is considered high-grade {392,665,1010,1826, 1928}. Basaloid squamous cell carcinoma is composed of nests of immature, basal-type squamous cells with scanty cytoplasm that resemble closely the cells of HSIL (CIN 3) of the cervix. Some individual cell keratinization may be present but keratin pearls are rarely seen. The nuclei may be quite pleomorphic, and high mitotic counts and "geographical" or "comedo-like" necrosis are frequent co-variables. This tumour, along with

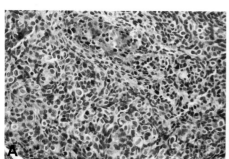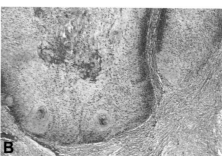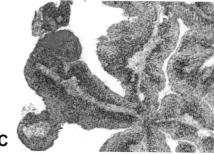

Fig. 7.10 A Basaloid squamous cell carcinoma. These high-grade tumours are composed of cells with a high nucleo-cytoplasmic ratio and typically show evidence of rapid cell growth, with frequent mitoses and/or apoptosis. **B** Verrucous carcinoma. At low power these very well-differentiated tumours exhibit bulbous papillae and a broad pushing growth front. **C** Papillary squamous cell carcinoma. Superficial biopsies exhibit frond-like growth with the papillae lined by relatively undifferentiated high-grade epithelium. Note that the invasive component is not visible in this image.

adenoid cystic carcinoma, occupies the aggressive end of the spectrum of basaloid tumours of the cervix, as they correlate with higher stage presentations and poorer outcomes. At the opposite end are low-grade lesions such as adenoid basal carcinoma or basal cell epithelioma (see other cervical epithelial tumours, p. 194). Distinction may be difficult on small biopsy. Basaloid tumours are typically associated with high-risk HPV infection {665}.

Verrucous carcinoma

Verrucous carcinoma, a tumour that is much more common on the vulva, is a highly differentiated squamous cell carcinoma that has a hyperkeratotic, undulating, warty surface and invades the underlying stroma in the form of bulbous epithelial pegs with a pushing border {1176,1842}. Because these tumours may have very thick epithelium, superficial biopsy or cytology may underestimate the severity of the disease process. The tumour cells have abundant cytoplasm, and their nuclei show minimal atypia. HPV cytopathic effect (koilocytosis) is specifically not found. Verrucous carcinomas have a tendency to recur locally after excision but do not metastasize. They are distinguished from condylomata acuminata by their broad papillae that lack fibrovascular cores and the absence of koilocytosis. Verrucous carcinoma is distinguished from the more common types of squamous cell carcinoma in that it shows no more than minimal nuclear atypia and does not exhibit infiltrative growth.

Warty/condylomatous squamous cell carcinoma

This lesion is defined as a squamous cell carcinoma with a warty surface and low-power architecture analogous to a condyloma or Bowenoid lesion of the vulva. In early invasive lesions the epithelium may be keratinizing {171,470,1010, 1928,2032}. Cells displaying changes analogous to koilocythic atypia characterize the tumour.

Papillary squamous cell carcinoma

This is a tumour in which thin or broad papillae with connective tissue stroma are covered by epithelium showing the features of HSIL. A superficial biopsy may not reveal evidence of invasion but complete excision of the clinically visible lesion reveals an underlying invasive tumour of the usual type. Papillary squamous cell carcinoma differs from warty squamous carcinoma by the lack of Bowenoid morphology, and from transitional cell carcinoma by its more overt squamous differentiation, although mixed squamotransitional forms have been described {26,171,192,957,1626}.

Squamotransitional carcinoma

Rare transitional cell carcinomas of the cervix have been described that are indistinguishable from their counterparts in the urinary bladder. They may occur in a pure form or may contain malignant squamous elements {26,171,192,957,1626}. Such tumours demonstrate papillary architecture with fibrovascular cores, lined by a multilayered, atypical epithelium resembling HSIL (CIN 3). There is no evidence that this tumour is related to transitional cell metaplasia, an infrequently occurring benign reaction that is related to atrophy and may mimic HSIL {412,2016}.

Lymphoepithelioma-like carcinoma

This is a rare tumour in the cervix. Histologically, it is strikingly similar to the nasopharyngeal tumour of the same name. It is composed of poorly defined islands of undifferentiated squamous cells in a background intensely infiltrated by lymphocytes. The tumour cells have uniform, vesicular nuclei with prominent nucleoli and moderate amounts of slightly eosinophilic cytoplasm. The cell borders are indistinct, often imparting a syncytial-like appearance to the groups.

The tumours of the cervix are most likely HPV-related as are all cervical cancers {1121,1935,2013}, and are therefore p16 positive. Convincing evidence that Epstein-Barr virus (EBV) plays a role in the genesis of cervical lymphoepithelioma-like carcinoma is lacking {93,960,1121, 1173,1361,1878,2013}.

Histogenesis

Virtually all cervical squamous cell carcinomas are thought to arise from a precancerous intraepithelial lesion (HSIL). The histological variation in the appearance of carcinomas is perhaps partially related to both the location of the precancer in the cervix, the variation in HSIL histology and the patterns of genes activated in the progression from precancerous to invasive disease. However, the details and precise genes underlying this variability remain largely unknown.

Genetic profile

A worldwide study of over 10 000 cancers has shown that virtually all cervical squamous cell carcinomas are high-risk HPV positive {429}. Immunohistochemistry for p16 captures the HPV E7 (and by implication E6) oncogene activation that drives most carcinomas (at least in the early stage). Hence, a very high fraction of cervical carcinomas are p16 positive by IHC, unless genetic loss or inactivation by, for example, methylation of the p16 locus turns off the gene, a tendency more common in invasive tumours than in HSIL (CIN 3). *TP53* mutations are relatively rare, except in advanced cases. Loss of heterozygosity (LOH) has been detected in multiple chromosomal regions in invasive carcinoma (1q, 3p, 3q, 6p, 6q, 11q, 17p, 18q) and many of these are also seen not only in HSIL (CIN 2/3) but also in advanced disease. Some of these chromosomal abnormalities are being tested as potential biomarkers of progression risk {700,907,1034,1130}. However, a recent systematic review of biomarker utility does not find sufficient evidence for any of these (except p16) to be used currently in routine clinical practice {412,1937}.

Genetic susceptibility

Few studies have addressed familial clustering in cervical carcinoma and, as for SIL, the attributable risk profile for cancer development is dominated by HPV, all other factors being of relatively small magnitude {480,738,1305,1498}. For example, the relative risk (RR) when a mother or a daughter is affected by cervical cancer is only 2 compared to a RR of > 50–100 for HPV-16. An aggregation of tobacco-related cancers and cancers linked with HPV and immunosuppression was found in such families. Thus, familial predisposition for cervical cancer is likely to implicate genes that modulate immune response, e.g. human leukocyte antigen (HLA) haplotypes and/or shared sexual or lifestyle factors in family members {1674}. The suggestion that the *TP53* codon 72 polymorphism is associated with cervical cancer risk was not substantiated in a large pooled analysis {949}.

Prognosis and predictive factors

The clinical factors that influence prognosis in invasive cervical squamous carcinoma are stage of disease, age of the patient and, within FIGO stages IB and

IIA, depth of invasion, volume of disease and lymphatic or vascular invasion, all of which are correlates of the risk of lymph node metastasis and systemic spread {213,361,440,444,522,618,973,1625, 1675,1825}. In a large series of cervical cancer patients treated by radiation therapy, the frequency of distant metastases (most frequently to the lung, abdominal cavity, liver and gastrointestinal tract) was shown to increase with increasing stage of disease. A combination of external radiotherapy, intracavitary radiation and platinum based chemotherapy (chemoradiation) versus surgery produce similar results for stages IB and IIA invasive cancer. More advanced tumours are usually treated with chemoradiation {1625}.

Among histopathological variables not included in the staging system for cervical cancer, the histological subtype of squamous cell carcinoma or grade of tumour do not seem to be strong independent predictive factors, except perhaps at the extremes, e.g. verrucous carcinoma. Many pathway related markers that can be tested by molecular or immunohistochemical assays on tissue such as p53, c-myc, HER2, EGFR, VEGF and more comprehensive multigene array platforms, etc. have been evaluated in a preliminary fashion, but outside of a clinical trial setting none are considered a routine part of current practice {441,793,929,1025,1327,1345, 1808,1868,2035}.

Benign squamous lesions

Squamous metaplasia

Definition
The process whereby cervical glandular epithelium is replaced with squamous epithelium.

Synonyms
May be qualified by descriptors such as mature, immature or atypical.

Epidemiology
Squamous metaplasia is ubiquitous and physiological.

Clinical features
Squamous metaplasia manifests clinically primarily on colposcopy and may ap-

pear on cytology and histology reports to aid in correlation. All forms of squamous metaplasia as a diagnosis imply that the lesion is not a form of squamous intraepithelial lesion (SIL) or one that carries neoplastic risk {220,623,897,1458}.

Histopathology
Prior to puberty the original squamocolumnar junction is distinct, joining the prepubescent, native, squamous mucosa with the endocervix and there is little if any squamous metaplasia. At puberty, hormonal and other biochemical factors are thought to induce changes such that there is eversion of the columnar epithelium, which then undergoes squamous metaplasia through a microscopic sequence of reserve cell hyperplasia, immature squamous metaplasia and mature squamous metaplasia, with the formation of a new squamocolumnar junction {1841}. Eventually, the metaplastic epithelium may be histologically indistinguishable from the native squamous epithelium except for the fact that the former is covering endocervical glands. The cervical transformation zone is defined histologically as the zone between the original and current squamocolumnar junction and the area around that junction where the epithelium is thinnest and particularly susceptible to oncogenic stimuli like HPV infection, the initial step of which requires basement membrane attachment. Most recently, a unique population of junction-zone immature metaplastic squamous cells has been described that may be even more uniquely susceptible to high-risk HPV infection {747}. p16 immunostaining is negative in squamous metaplasia; this can be useful for distinguishing between immature squamous metaplasia and high-grade SIL in problematic cases {220,623,897,1458}.

Condyloma acuminatum

Definition
A benign proliferation characterized by papillary fronds containing fibrovascular cores and lined by stratified squamous epithelium with definite evidence of HPV infection. The lesion is a grossly evident morphological variant of low-grade squamous intraepithelial lesion (LSIL).

Synonyms
LSIL (condylomatous variant); CIN 1

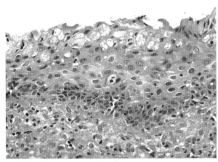

Fig. 7.11 Immature squamous metaplasia. In the early phase of squamous metaplasia the overlying columnar epithelium may be evident. The relative immaturity of the squamous cells may cause confusion with high-grade squamous intraepithelial lesion.

(condylomatous variant); genital wart of the cervix

Epidemiology
LSILs architecturally resembling condylomata acuminata are much more common in external genital sites than in the cervix. Condylomata acuminata are associated most strongly with low-risk HPV types, particularly HPV types 6 and 11, but not entirely specifically {388,1846,2029}

Clinical features
The lesion may present as a visible wart-like process on the cervix or as an abnormal Pap smear, which will be interpreted as LSIL since the architecture cannot be determined cytologically. The HPV type and grade of SIL in lesions architecturally consistent with a cervical condyloma dictate the clinical outcome.

Macroscopy
The lesion looks like a genital wart on a mucosal surface if large enough to see. Colposcopy enhances visualization.

Histopathology
The squamous epithelium covering the knuckle-like fronds of the lesion exhibits acanthosis, papillomatosis and koilocytosis as defined in the section on LSIL. A less mature variant with a metaplastic appearance (immature papillary squamous metaplasia) has been described {2005}.

Histogenesis
See low-grade squamous intraepithelial lesion, p. 172.

Genetic profile
See low-grade squamous intraepithelial lesion, p. 172.

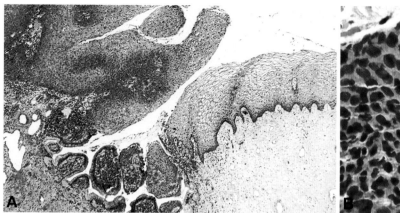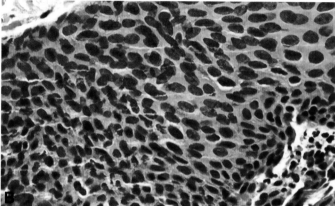

Fig. 7.12 A Condyloma acuminatum. This lesion has the low-power architectural features of a condyloma. Condyloma acuminatum is an exophytic variant of low-grade squamous intraepithelial lesion. This pattern is more frequently, but not specifically, associated with low-risk HPV types. **B** Transitional metaplasia. The full thickness of the epithelium is replaced by immature appearing cells; there is no pleomorphism and no mitotic activity.

Genetic susceptibility
See low-grade squamous intraepithelial lesion, p. 172.

Prognosis and predictive factors
See low-grade squamous intraepithelial lesion, p. 172.

Squamous papilloma

Definition
A benign exophytic lesion composed of a papillary frond(s) with an internal fibrovascular core covered by mature squamous epithelium without atypia. The lesion is specifically not an HPV-associated process.

ICD-O code   8052/0

Synonyms
Benign papilloma; squamous polyp; fibroepithelial polyp

Epidemiology
The lesion is common, albeit rarer in the cervix than in the vulva or vagina.

Clinical features
Most often misdiagnosed as a condyloma or low-grade squamous intraepithelial lesion (LSIL). In the vagina, so-called micropapillomas or micropapillomatosis is now proven not to be HPV-associat-

ed and should lack the koilocytosis described in LSIL {137,624}.

Histopathology
The epithelial cytology is the key diagnostic feature. The differential diagnosis includes squamous metaplasia and papillary immature squamous metaplasia. In the latter, the epithelium is metaplastic with mild atypia due to abnormal nuclear maturation but koilocytosis is lacking. However, this lesion may be HPV-associated as noted above {1458,2005}. Papillary immature squamous metaplasia maybe associated with HPV infection, as noted above.

Transitional metaplasia

Definition
A form of metaplasia in which the cervical squamous epithelium resembles benign urothelium due to a lack of cellular maturation.

Synonym
Urothelial metaplasia

Epidemiology
It is an incidental microscopic finding in uterine, cervical and vaginal samples from perimenopausal and postmenopausal women.

Clinical features
Many cases diagnosed as transitional metaplasia on biopsy are really high-grade squamous intraepithelial lesions (HSIL). Correlation of cytology and histology with additional testing can aide in excluding HSIL.

Histopathology
Transitional cell metaplasia is characterized by a normal or moderately thickened squamous epithelium, lack of cell maturation, spindled and streaming nuclei with frequent longitudinal nuclear grooves, a low nucleo-cytoplasmic ratio, and rare or absent mitotic figures. It may be misdiagnosed as HSIL because of an apparent lack of cellular maturation at lower magnifications, especially when the lesion involves endocervical glands, displays isolated nuclear atypia or koilocytosis, or involves the resection margin of LEEP conization specimens with HSIL {709,2016}. HPV is not present and p16 immunohistochemistry is negative.

Histogenesis
The lesion is a variant form of squamous metaplasia in the transformation zone.

Prognosis and predictive factors
Accurately diagnosed, the prognosis is no different from normal.

Glandular tumours and precursors

D.C. Wilbur
T.J. Colgan
A.S. Ferenczy
L. Hirschowitz
T. Loening
W.G. McCluggage

Y. Mikami
K.J. Park
B.M. Ronnett
A. Schneider
R. Soslow
M. Wells
T. Wright

Adenocarcinoma in situ

Definition
An intraepithelial lesion containing malignant-appearing glandular epithelium that carries a significant risk of invasive adenocarcinoma if not treated.

ICD-O code
8140/2

Synonym
High-grade cervical glandular intraepithelial neoplasia (HG-CGIN)

Clinical features
The mean age of presentation is in the fourth decade, 10–15 years before the mean age for invasive endocervical adenocarcinoma. The most common presentation of adenocarcinoma in situ (AIS) /HG-CGIN is abnormal cervical cytology that shows atypical endocervical glandular cells {1278}. AIS/HG-CGIN is of-ten found in association with high-grade squamous intraepithelial lesions (HSIL) {2136}.

Macroscopy
AIS/HG-CGIN may be seen colposcopically but can be difficult to see if the lesion is high in the endocervical canal. Occasional cases are multifocal. A clinically visible lesion may represent concurrent HSIL.

Histopathology
Neoplastic epithelium replaces normal epithelium on the endocervical surface and in endocervical glands. The lesion is confined to the pre-existing normal endocervical epithelium and therefore the normal lobular architecture is retained. The neoplastic epithelium has a pseudostratified columnar arrangement with relative depletion of intracytoplasmic mucin, although appreciable intracytoplasmic mucin remains in some cases. In the most common "usual"/endocervical-type AIS, nuclei are enlarged, fusiform, and hyperchromatic, with irregular, coarse chromatin and occasionally with prominent nucleoli. Mitotic figures and apoptotic bodies are virtually always present. The lesion may show intestinal differentiation with goblet cells, or "endometrioid" features with smaller, dense nuclei and very little mucinous/apical cytoplasm. Rarely, neuroendocrine and Paneth cells are present. Intestinal differentiation in endocervical glands almost always indicates a premalignant or malignant lesion, although the nuclear features of malignancy may be subtle. Lesional epithelium is strongly and diffusely positive for p16 and ProEx™C (aberrant S-phase induction) and shows an increased proliferation index with Ki-67. Characteristically there is loss of estrogen, and more specifically, progesterone receptor expression {1203}.

There is a variant pattern of AIS referred to as *"stratified mucin-producing intraepithelial lesion (SMILE)"*. This lesion consists of stratified epithelium with cells containing mucin in the form of discrete vacuoles or as cytoplasmic clearing throughout all cell layers. Nuclear atypia, hyperchromasia, mitoses and apoptotic bodies are usually present. p16 immunohistochemistry is positive and there is a high Ki-67 proliferation index. SMILE often occurs in association with HSIL and/or AIS/HG-CGIN but may rarely appear as an isolated finding {1459}.

Lesions with cytological atypia that is less than AIS/HG-CGIN have sometimes been referred to as endocervical glandular dysplasia (EGD) or low-grade cervical glandular intraepithelial neoplasia (LG-CGIN). This is a poorly reproducible diagnosis for which criteria are not well defined. Minimal nuclear atypia with hyperchromasia and slightly increased mitoses or apoptotic bodies are sometimes cited as criteria. Ancillary studies are helpful in further clarifying these atypias, as diffuse, strong p16 reactivity, high Ki-67 proliferation index, and lack

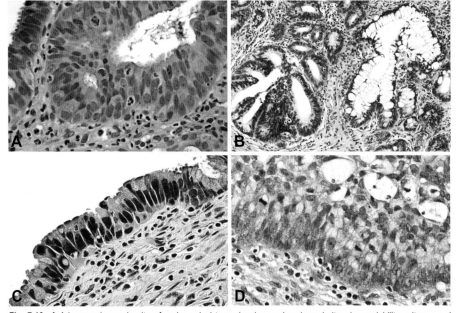

Fig. 7.13 **A** Adenocarcinoma in situ of endocervical type showing nuclear irregularity, size variability, mitoses and apoptosis. **B** Adenocarcinoma in situ. There is atypical epithelium characterized by pseudostratified nuclei and hyperchromasia (left). The gland on the right shows prominent intestinalization of the epithelium. **C** Adenocarcinoma in situ with minimal stratification. The endocervical lining mucosa is abnormal, with mild nuclear pseudostratification, hyperchromasia, and enlargement. Although atypical, the features fall short of an outright diagnosis of adenocarcinoma in situ. However, p16 immunohistochemistry was strongly positive, warranting a final interpretation of adenocarcinoma in situ. **D** Stratified mucin-producing intraepithelial lesion (SMILE). The stratified epithelium contains cells with mucin vacuoles in all cell layers. Nuclear atypia, hyperchromasia and mitotic figures are present.

of hormone receptor expression support interpretation as poorly sampled or morphologically incomplete AIS/HG-CGIN. Lesions showing these immunohistochemical characteristics should be classified as AIS/HG-CGIN for management purposes {1208}.

Histogenesis
AIS/HG-CGIN is virtually always associated with high-risk HPV, most commonly types 16 and 18 {1545}.

Prognosis and predictive factors
In most instances, AIS/HG-CGIN, including SMILE, can be successfully treated with loop excision and close cytological follow up. Hysterectomy may be preferred if childbearing is not an issue. If conservatively managed, close follow-up by colposcopic, cytological and HPV testing are essential.

Adenocarcinoma, NOS

Definition
An invasive epithelial tumour showing glandular differentiation.

ICD-O code   8140/3

Epidemiology
Adenocarcinoma currently comprises 10–25% of all cervical carcinomas in developed countries, compared to 5–10% three decades ago {2106}. This increase has resulted from a decline in squamous carcinomas secondary to screening programs and better identification of glandular lesions in cervical cytology samples. A potential association with long-term oral contraceptive use, particularly with progestational agents and with unopposed estrogen use, has been postulated but not proven. The mean age at presentation is about 50 years {1018}.

Etiology
The majority (94%) of cervical adenocarcinomas are associated with high-risk HPV (with exceptions noted below), most commonly types 18, 16 and 45. Some, but not all, studies suggest that type 18 and its variants are more common than type 16, which is the opposite of squamous carcinoma {47,215,421,1545}.

Clinical features
Abnormal uterine bleeding and a mass lesion are present in about 80% of cases.

Macroscopy
Approximately 50% of tumours show exophytic growth patterns. A smaller percentage show surface ulceration or diffuse infiltration of the cervical wall, leading to a barrel-shaped cervix.

Histopathology
Each of the variants has in common glands with cytoarchitectural atypia that infiltrate the cervical stroma. A surface component with a papillary architecture may also be prominent. In some adenocarcinomas, particularly those that are high-grade, non-specific patterns such as nests, clusters and individual cells are seen. The histopathology for each of the variant forms of adenocarcinoma is described in the following sections. Lesions with only minimal stromal invasion may be referred to as early invasive adenocarcinoma. Criteria for early invasion include frankly infiltrating glands or tumour cells nests, extension of atypical glands beyond the depth of the normal endocervical glands, neoplastic endocervical glands that are too complex to be adenocarcinoma in situ or with stromal reaction in the form of oedema, chronic inflammation or desmoplasia. Occasional cases may show groups of cells with abundant eosinophilic (or differentiated) cytoplasm. Measuring the extent of the lesion is important in assigning FIGO stage and risk of spread/survival but an exact measurement of this type of lesion may be difficult because of lack of a specifically defined basement membrane separating glands from stroma, as is commonly noted in squamous lesions.

Prognosis and predictive factors
Five year survival has been reported to be nearly identical to that for squamous cell carcinoma by stage; 77% (all stages), 100% (IA1), 93% (IA2), 89% (IB1), 83% (IB2), 49% (II), 34% (III), and 3% (IV) {83,283}. There is little evidence for prognostic differences between the histological variants with the exception of details noted in the following sections.

Endocervical adenocarcinoma, usual type

Definition
The most common form of endocervical adenocarcinoma, with relative mucin depletion.

ICD-O code   8140/3

Epidemiology
The usual type of endocervical adenocarcinoma constitutes about 90% of all adenocarcinomas of the cervix.

Clinical features
Abnormal uterine bleeding and a mass lesion are present in about 80% of cases.

Macroscopy
Approximately 50% of tumours show an exophytic growth pattern. A smaller percentage show surface ulceration or diffuse infiltration of the cervical wall leading to a barrel-shaped cervix.

Histopathology
Most often, the tumours are well- to moderately differentiated, having complex architectural patterns composed of round to oval mucin-poor glands that exhibit cribriform or papillary structures. Patterns resembling microglandular hyperplasia of the cervix or microcysts may be seen, as may single-cell patterns. Large pools of mucin may occasionally be present within the stroma. The neoplastic epithelium shows a characteristic pseudostratified architecture with enlarged, elongated and hyperchromatic nuclei. The latter appearance is evident at higher magnification

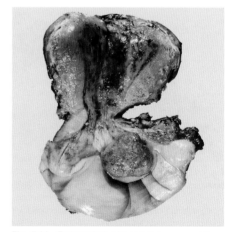

Fig. 7.14 Endocervical adenocarcinoma, usual type. These tumours often present as large exophytic polypoid masses.

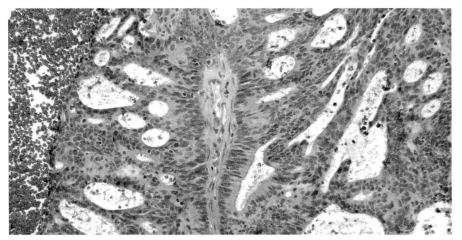

Fig. 7.15 Endocervical adenocarcinoma, usual type. The presence of large, confluent cribriform glands favours the diagnosis of an invasive carcinoma. The usual type of adenocarcinoma shows apical mucin depletion, pseudostratification and necrotic debris within gland spaces.

and is attributable to the apical zone of amphophilic to eosinophilic cytoplasm, where mitotic figures are characteristically situated ("floating mitotic figures"). Prominent macronucleoli and apoptotic bodies are frequently seen. Tumours are always strongly and diffusely p16 and ProEx™C immunoreactive and show increased proliferation indices with Ki-67 {2173}.

Histogenesis
Usual types of endocervical adenocarcinomas are virtually always associated with high-risk HPV {47}.

Mucinous carcinoma, NOS

Definition
A mucinous adenocarcinoma that cannot be classified as any of the specific types of cervical adenocarcinoma.

ICD-O code   8480/3

Histopathology
This tumour is an invasive adenocarcinoma that shows evidence of mucinous differentiation but does not show the specific features of usual type, gastric type, intestinal type or signet-ring-cell type adenocarcinoma.

Mucinous carcinoma, gastric type

Definition
A mucinous adenocarcinoma that shows gastric type differentiation {1268}.

ICD-O code   8482/3

Synonyms
Minimal deviation adenocarcinoma (if extremely well differentiated); adenoma malignum (if extremely well differentiated)

Epidemiology
In Japanese studies, this category may represent as many as 25% of cervical adenocarcinomas {961,1013}. The extremely well differentiated form (minimal deviation adenocarcinoma/adenoma malignum) accounts for about 1% of all adenocarcinomas of the cervix. The mean age at presentation is about 42 years {637,758}. An association with Peutz-Jeghers syndrome has been noted {996}.

Clinical features
The typical presentation is with vaginal bleeding or mucoid discharge. Presentation with metastases to the ovary can be seen.

Macroscopy
Tumours typically present as firm and indurated masses, often with a "barrel-shaped" cervical expansion. The cut surface may be haemorrhagic, friable, or mucoid, with a tan to yellow colour.

Histopathology
The tumour consists of mucinous epithelium invading the endocervical stroma in variably-sized simple, and often angulated, cystic glands, with some solid areas and infolded papillae. The atypical glands extend below the normal level expected for benign endocervical glands. The glands are characteristically irregular and dilated, but may also be fused or show a cribriform pattern {961,1013}. The surrounding stroma may show desmoplasia but in some regions this is absent or minimal. These tumours are composed

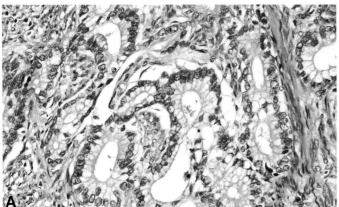
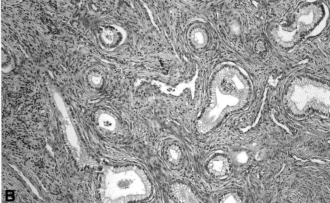

Fig. 7.16 A Mucinous carcinoma, gastric type. This neoplasm shows gastric type differentiation with abundant clear to eosinophilic cytoplasm and obvious nuclear atypia. There are cribriform glands present. The cells have been shown to stain with markers of pyloric gland mucin. **B** Adenoma malignum (minimal deviation adenocarcinoma). The cytoplasm shows gastric differentiation, but nuclei are bland and little, if any, stromal reaction is present.

of cells with abundant clear or pale, eosinophilic cytoplasm and distinct cell borders. Typically, nuclei are enlarged, irregular and hyperchromatic. Mitotic figures are present, but may be rare.

Minimal deviation adenocarcinoma / adenoma malignum mostly shows gastric differentiation and thus can conceptually be included in the spectrum of gastric type adenocarcinoma as an extremely well differentiated form {1217}. If the tumour shows non-well differentiated areas, it should be classified as gastric type adenocarcinoma.

Histogenesis
Gastric type adenocarcinomas, including minimal deviation adenocarcinoma/ adenoma malignum, are most often not associated with high-risk HPV {1013, 1460} and are hence negative or only focally positive for p16 {961,1460}. Its genesis more closely resembles gastric carcinogenesis. These tumours may be associated with lobular endocervical glandular hyperplasia, the latter possibly representing a precursor lesion. Immunohistochemical studies are positive for markers of pyloric gland mucins (MUC6 and HIK1083), CK7, p53 and CEA, while CK20 may be only focally positive {1208}. *TP53* mutations, which are uncommon in HPV-associated tumours, are often found in these tumours {1460}.

Genetic profile
Mutations in the *STK11* tumour suppressor gene on chromosome 19p (associated with Peutz-Jeghers syndrome) have been noted in about half of the minimal deviation variant {996,1057}.

Prognosis and predictive factors
Gastric type adenocarcinomas are thought to have a worse prognosis compared to the usual types. They may behave more aggressively and are associated with more frequent peritoneal and abdominal spread. A 5-year disease-free survival of 30% has been shown compared to 74% for the usual type {961}. Despite its extremely well differentiated appearance, this also applies to minimal deviation adenocarcinoma (adenoma malignum), which has a less favourable prognosis than the usual type endocervical adenocarcinoma, perhaps because it presents at a higher stage, secondary to lack of cytology/molecular screening sensitivity. 20–30% of patients at any stage, and 50% with stage 1 disease survive beyond 2 years {1460}.

Mucinous carcinoma, intestinal type

Definition
A mucinous adenocarcinoma that shows areas of intestinal type differentiation.

ICD-O code   8144/3

Histopathology
These tumours recapitulate adenocarcinomas of the intestine, and show the focal presence of goblet, argentaffin and Paneth cells. The intestinal differentiation may be focal in lesions which otherwise show typical mucinous-type epithelium.

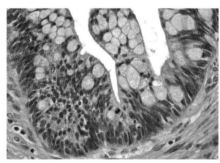

Fig. 7.17 Mucinous carcinoma, intestinal type. This neoplasm shows abundant goblet cell differentiation.

Histogenesis
High-risk HPV has been detected in the intestinal variant {47}.

Mucinous carcinoma, signet-ring cell type

Definition
A rare adenocarcinoma that shows focal or diffuse signet-ring cell differentiation.

ICD-O code   8490/3

Histopathology
There are many cells with abundant mucin in distended cytoplasmic vacuoles which displace the nuclei (signet-ring cells). p16 may be positive or negative depending on the HPV status of the individual tumour.

Histogenesis
Signet-ring cell adenocarcinomas may or may not be associated with high-risk HPV, depending on whether their underlying histogenesis is of usual type or gastric type, respectively {105,640}.

Villoglandular carcinoma

Definition
A variant of endocervical adenocarcinoma which shows a distinct exophytic, villous-papillary growth.

ICD-O code   8263/3

Synonyms
Well-differentiated villoglandular adenocarcinoma

Clinical features
This carcinoma typically occurs in a younger age population as compared to the usual type (average about 35 years) {2125}.

Macroscopy
This variant typically presents as an exophytic mass.

Histopathology
The lesions are by definition architecturally well differentiated. Cytological atypia is mild or moderate at most. The exophytic portion of the tumour shows villous fronds of variable thickness, that are covered by tall, endocervical-type columnar cells with limited or no mucin. Mitotic figures and pseudostratification are present. These tumours have a distinctive cellular, fibrous stroma with a prominent spindled component. Polymorphonuclear leukocytes may permeate the stroma of the exophytic papillae. Invasion is typically superficial but some cases may exhibit deep stromal invasion.

Histogenesis
HPV types 16, 18 or 45 are the main causative genotypes identified {47,849}.

Prognosis and predictive factors
When superficially invasive, this variant is only rarely associated with lymph node metastasis and has an excellent prognosis. However, some recent reports suggest that these tumours can be aggressive. Therefore, conservative management has been suggested as appropriate only in superficial lesions of pure villoglandular morphology, without high-grade atypia and with no lymphovascular invasion {1951}. Management decisions should be

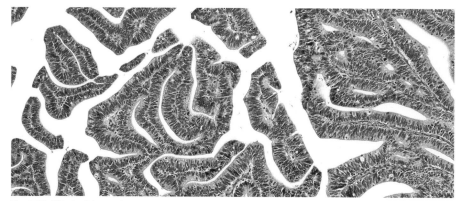

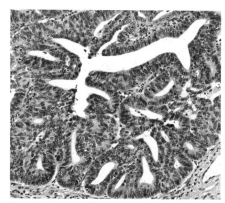

Fig. 7.18 Villoglandular carcinoma. A complex branching exophytic neoplasm with fronds lined by well-differentiated neoplastic cells. Mitotic activity tends to be low but clearly evident.

Fig. 7.19 Endometrioid carcinoma, closely resembling endometrioid carcinoma of the uterine corpus.

based on complete excisions, including conization, rather than biopsies {520}.

Endometrioid carcinoma

Definition
An adenocarcinoma arising in the cervix that has endometrioid morphological features.

ICD-O code   8380/3

Epidemiology
These tumours are rare and account for no more than 5% of all endocervical adenocarcinomas. Usual type adenocarcinomas have similar morphological features which has caused erroneously high prevalence figures in some studies.

Etiology
When these tumours are morphological variants of usual type adenocarcinomas they are associated with high-risk HPV. Rare tumours thought to arise from cervical endometriosis are not associated with high-risk HPV.

Clinical features
They are similar to usual type endocervical adenocarcinoma.

Macroscopy
They are similar to usual type endocervical adenocarcinoma.

Histopathology
These tumours are morphologically similar to endometrioid adenocarcinomas arising in the uterine corpus. The most important differential diagnosis is with endometrial adenocarcinomas of endometrioid type extending from the uterine corpus. Endometrioid endocervical adenocarcinomas are typically diffusely and strongly p16 positive in contrast to tumours of endometrial origin, which most often have a patchy pattern of p16 expression. In endometrial carcinomas, this staining can be somewhat extensive, with up to 80% of tumour cells positive in some cases, but with only rare/occasional tumours having diffuse expression {839}. Rare variants may be extremely well-differentiated and have been termed

minimal deviation endometrioid adenocarcinoma {2127}.

Prognosis and predictive factors
Some studies have suggested a better prognosis when compared to usual and mucinous types {375}.

Clear cell carcinoma

Definition
An adenocarcinoma composed predominantly of clear or hobnail cells whose architectural patterns are solid, tubulocystic and/or papillary.

ICD-O code   8310/3

Epidemiology
Clear cell adenocarcinomas of the cervix are rare and have arisen in two distinct populations; in association with *in utero* diethylstilbestrol (DES) exposure {742} and sporadically {867}. DES-exposed patients are rarely seen now and have been younger with an average age of 19

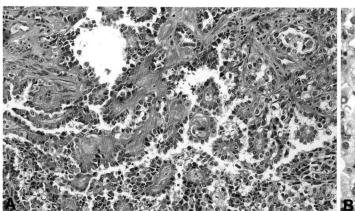

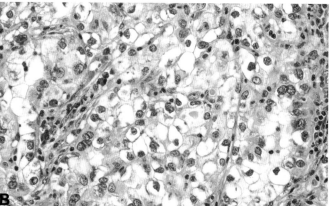

Fig. 7.20 Clear cell carcinoma. **A** This tumour displays a papillary architecture and contains cells with clear or eosinophilic cytoplasm showing high-grade nuclear atypia. **B** This tumour shows a solid pattern.

years as compared to an average of 47 years for sporadic tumours.

Etiology
Similar to other rare variants, these tumours may be associated with high-risk HPV {47}.

Clinical features
Tumours arising in the setting of DES-exposure are typically ectocervical. Sporadic tumours arise in the endocervix and have presentations similar to the usual type of endocervical adenocarcinoma.

Histopathology
The most common pattern is tubulocystic with lining cells composed of hobnail, flat or clear cells. Papillary tumours also occur. Solid tumours typically contain abundant glycogen-rich cytoplasm and sometimes eosinophilic intracytoplasmic hyaline globules. High-grade nuclear atypia is seen at least focally in most cases.

Prognosis and predictive factors
The prognosis is not known to be different from other variants of endocervical adenocarcinoma {1572}.

Serous carcinoma

Definition
A rare adenocarcinoma of the cervix with an identical histological appearance to endometrial or adnexal serous carcinoma.

ICD-O code   8441/3

Epidemiology
Serous carcinoma of the cervix is exceedingly rare. Tumours with this morphology that occur in young patients are most often associated with HPV and represent "serous-like" usual type adenocarcinomas {778}, while older patients have tumours with mutant p53 expression akin to their endometrial and adnexal counterparts {1362}.

Clinical features
These tumours present with abnormal vaginal bleeding, watery discharge, and abnormal cervical cytology.

Macroscopy
The macroscopy is similar to other endocervical adenocarcinomas.

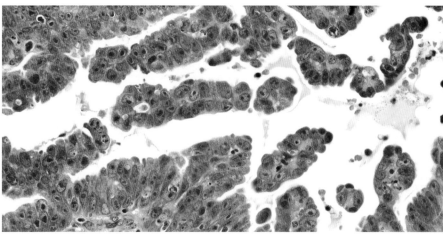

Fig. 7.21 Serous carcinoma. These tumours show prominent tufted papillae lined by hobnail cells with high-grade nuclear features.

Histopathology
The tumours display a complex papillary architecture with cellular budding and frequent psammoma body formation. Glandular areas may also be seen. Nuclear atypia is generally high-grade. Cervical involvement by the far more common endometrial and adnexal serous carcinomas must be excluded.

Prognosis and predictive factors
In a single series, poor prognosis was associated with older age, higher stage, tumours greater than 2 cm, invasion greater than 1 cm, lymph node metastasis, and elevated serum CA125 {2170}.

Mesonephric carcinoma

Definition
An adenocarcinoma arising from mesonephric remnants.

ICD-O code   9110/3

Etiology
These tumours are not associated with high-risk HPV {903}.

Clinical features
Mesonephric adenocarcinoma is a rare adenocarcinoma variant. It has a wide age of presentation with a mean of about 50 years {344,1782}.

Macroscopy
These tumours commonly arise in the lateral to posterior cervical wall and may be deeply invasive and bulky or exophytic. They more commonly involve the lower uterine segment than do other cervical adenocarcinomas.

Histopathology
Characteristically, there are a variety of architectural patterns, including tubular glands lined by mucin-free cuboidal epithelium containing eosinophilic, hyaline secretion within their lumina. Other patterns include branching, slit-like spaces with intraluminal fibrous papillae (retiform), solid, papillary, ductal, and spindle cell patterns. Distinction from benign mesonephric hyperplasia (which is often found in association) is based on architectural gland crowding, haphazard infiltrative growth, elevated mitotic activity, intraluminal cellular debris and nuclear atypia (which can be variable). Mesonephric adenocarcinomas are uniformly reactive for cytokeratin and epithelial membrane antigen, and often express calretinin, vimentin and CD10 (apical and luminal). They are typically negative for estrogen and progesterone receptors and CEA. They may express PAX8, TTF1 and p16 focally {903}.

Prognosis and predictive factors
There have been too few series reported to ascertain whether, stage for stage, the prognosis differs from other variants of cervical adenocarcinoma. However, it has been suggested that, although these neoplasms may be indolent, they have a propensity for late recurrence and metastasis {1782}.

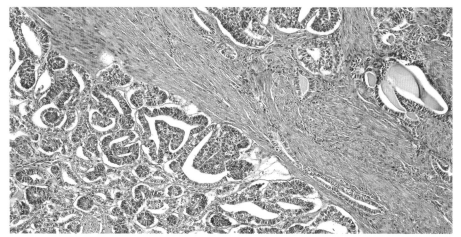

Fig. 7.22 Mesonephric adenocarcinoma. These tumours show a variety of architectural patterns but have in common glandular structures lined by mucin-free cuboidal epithelium and containing eosinophilic, hyaline secretion within their lumina.

Adenocarcinoma admixed with neuroendocrine carcinoma

Definition
Tumours showing neuroendocrine differentiation in association with variants of cervical adenocarcinoma.

ICD-O code   8574/3

Epidemiology
Tumours showing features of low-grade neuroendocrine tumour (typical or atypical carcinoid tumours) are rare in the cervix. High-grade neuroendocrine carcinomas with small cell neuroendocrine differentiation are more common than the large cell variants. Both types arise over a wide age range.

Etiology
All small cell variants have been reported to be positive for HPV {238}.

Clinical features
Tumours with components of small and large cell neuroendocrine carcinoma present with vaginal bleeding, a cervical mass, and/or an abnormal cervical cytology. Small cell variants may produce hormones such as ACTH, serotonin, and ADH leading to associated clinical syndromes.

Macroscopy
Small cell variants of adenocarcinoma usually present as large, bulky and ulcerated tumours which can completely encompass the cervix and invade contiguous organs.

Histopathology
Adenocarcinoma may represent only a small component of these tumours and may be in situ or invasive. The small cell component shows scant cytoplasm with hyperchromatic, moulded nuclei, finely granular chromatin and indistinct nucleoli. The cells can be arranged in solid sheets, nests or trabeculae. Large cell components show medium to large cells with moderate to abundant cytoplasm and large atypical nuclei with prominent macronucleoli. Eosinophilic cytoplasmic inclusions are helpful clues to the diagnosis and are present in about 70% of cases. Mitoses and apoptotic debris are frequently seen in both small and large cell variants. Positivity with pan-neuroendocrine markers including chromogranin A, synaptophysin and CD56 is consistent with neuroendocrine differentiation (see cervical neuroendocrine tumours, p. 196).

Prognosis and predictive factors
Small and large cell variants are highly aggressive and have a poor prognosis.

Benign glandular tumours and tumour-like lesions

Endocervical polyp

Definition
An exophytic lesion lined by benign endocervical epithelium covering a fibrovascular core.

Epidemiology
Endocervical polyps are common lesions that may occur at any age, but are more common after 40 years of age.

Clinical features
Most are asymptomatic but they may be associated with vaginal bleeding (especially post-coital) and/or discharge.

Macroscopy
The majority of polyps measure less than 1 cm and are single.

Histopathology
Endocervical polyps consist of fibroepithelial structures covered by benign cuboidal to columnar endocervical type epithelium, with glands permeating the central stroma. The mucosa often exhibits squamous metaplasia or microglandular hyperplasia (see following sections) and can also show cystic glands filled with mucus. Rarely, surface papillary proliferation or stromal decidual change may occur in polyps. The surface of polyps may be inflamed or eroded and associated reactive/reparative changes of both epithelium and stroma may be present. These changes may lead to interpretations of "atypical glandular cells" in cervical cytology specimens.

Prognosis and predictive factors
Endocervical polyps are benign lesions, although rarely they can be involved by in situ or invasive carcinomas, either solely or as part of more generalized cervical involvement.

Müllerian papilloma

Definition
A rare, benign papillary tumour of childhood which arises in the upper vagina and cervix. It is considered to be of Müllerian origin {1032}.

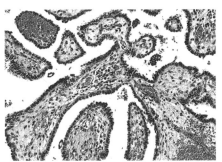

Fig. 7.23 Müllerian papilloma. These benign proliferations of childhood show finely branched fibrous papillae lined by a single layer of bland cuboidal to columnar epithelium and no mitotic activity.

Epidemiology
This lesion arises almost exclusively in children, typically between the ages of 2 and 5 years (range 1–9 years).

Clinical features
Presentation is with vaginal bleeding or discharge.

Macroscopy
Typically, it is a single or multifocal friable polypoid cervical lesion, generally < 2 cm in greatest dimension.

Histopathology
The lesion consists of finely branched fibrous papillae lined by a single layer of benign cuboidal to columnar epithelium. The epithelium may show squamous metaplasia or hobnail-type cells which can mimic clear cell carcinoma; however the nuclear morphology is bland, without atypia or mitotic activity.

Prognosis and predictive factors
The follow up is benign; however local recurrence has been reported which is probably secondary to incomplete excision.

Nabothian cyst

Definition
Cystic structures in the endocervical wall lined by normal, but often attenuated, endocervical epithelium and filled with mucus.

Epidemiology
Nabothian cysts are a common finding, especially in multiparous women.

Etiology
Nabothian cysts are caused by a blockage of the endocervical gland neck with resultant entrapment of mucus and cystic expansion.

Clinical features
Most lesions are asymptomatic, but they can be associated with chronic cervicitis and mucous discharge. In cases of deep wall Nabothian cysts, the cervix can become enlarged and clinically suspicious of a malignant process.

Macroscopy
The cysts may be single or multiple, are filled with mucus and usually range from 2 – 10 cm in diameter. They are generally located near the surface of the endocervical canal but can occasionally be found deep in the endocervical wall.

Histopathology
Cystic spaces are round to slightly irregular and are lined by a single layer of non-atypical cuboidal, columnar or attenuated endocervical epithelium. There may sometimes be tubal metaplasia. No associated stromal reaction is noted.

Prognosis and predictive factors
These are benign lesions.

Tunnel clusters

Definition
Rounded, lobular aggregates of benign, endocervical glands in the cervical wall.

Epidemiology
Tunnel clusters are usually an incidental pathologic finding that affects approximately 10% of adult women who are generally multiparous.

Clinical features
Tunnel clusters are most often asymptomatic but can occasionally cause a mucoid discharge.

Macroscopy
About 40% of cases of the cystic variety will show a grossly visible, lobular mass lesion. They are multiple in 80% of cases.

Histopathology
Tunnel clusters consist of rounded, lobular aggregates of oval to round, closely packed endocervical-lined tubules of varying size. Non-cystic tunnel clusters show predominantly small glands,

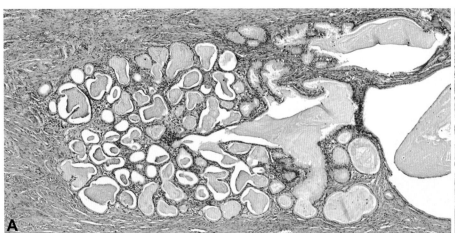
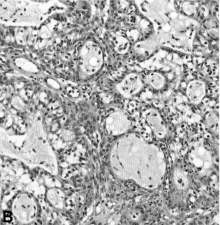

Fig. 7.24 A Tunnel cluster. The lesion shows a well-circumscribed lobular aggregate of closely packed rounded, cystic glands lined by bland endocervical type epithelium containing mucin. The lack of a stromal reaction or infiltrative growth pattern helps to differentiate tunnel clusters from endocervical adenocarcinoma. **B** Microglandular hyperplasia. Closely packed endocervical glands of variable size are permeated by polymorphonuclear leukocytes, and lined by columnar to cuboidal cells with subnuclear mucin vacuoles. There is reserve cell hyperplasia at the periphery of some of the glands. The nuclei show mild variability in size but no significant pleomorphism. No mitotic figures are seen in this example.

while cystic tunnel clusters show dilated glands. The lining is a single layer of flattened cuboidal or columnar cells. Atypia and mitotic activity are generally absent.

Histogenesis
The association with multiparity suggests that tunnel clusters may represent involutional change within endocervical glandular hyperplasia. Some tunnel clusters may contain gastric type mucins {966}.

Prognosis and predictive factors
Tunnel clusters are benign lesions with no risk of recurrence or malignant transformation.

Microglandular hyperplasia

Definition
A benign, endocervical gland proliferation with a characteristic pattern of subnuclear vacuolation, usually with a component of closely packed small glands, with epithelial tufting.

Epidemiology
Microglandular hyperplasia (MGH) is most common in the reproductive years and is commonly associated with progestins or pregnancy.

Clinical features
MGH is usually asymptomatic, but can be associated with bleeding and is often found within an endocervical polyp.

Macroscopy
MGH is usually a microscopic finding but may form a friable mass.

Histopathology
MGH shows closely packed glands, often with associated reserve cell hyperplasia. The glands are composed of columnar to cuboidal cells with mucin vacuoles, most often subnuclear, which may result in a signet-ring appearance to the cells. Nuclei are small and regular and the mitotic index is low. The stroma is often infiltrated by acute and chronic inflammatory cells, and stromal hyalinization may be seen. Variant patterns include solid, reticular, and trabecular. The major differential diagnosis in florid cases is with clear cell carcinoma which will have significant cytological atypia, an infiltrative growth pattern and most often presents with a mass lesion.

Histogenesis
MGH is most commonly associated with hormonal stimulation and may arise from reserve cell proliferation {2039}.

Prognosis and predictive factors
MGH is a benign lesion with no malignant potential.

Lobular endocervical glandular hyperplasia

Definition
A distinct, lobular proliferation of benign-appearing endocervical glands often centred on a larger central gland that commonly exhibits gastric/pyloric differentiation.

Synonym
Pyloric gland metaplasia

Clinical features
Lobular endocervical glandular hyperplasia (LEGH) may occur in reproductive age or postmenopausal women. It may be an incidental microscopic finding or it can be associated with a watery or mucoid vaginal discharge. In some cases, a mass lesion may have been discovered on radiological examination.

Macroscopy
LEGH may be mass-forming and associated with a grossly identifiable cystic lesion in some cases.

Histopathology
This lesion consists of lobular proliferations of small to moderate sized endocervical glands, some with cystic change, often centred on a larger central gland, and usually confined to the inner half of the cervical stroma. The glands are lined by benign-appearing, columnar, mucinous epithelium with minimal atypia and rare mitotic figures. The cells have been shown to contain pyloric gland-type mucin (HIK 1083, MUC6 positive) {1266}.

Histogenesis
This condition represents a metaplastic process showing features of gastric pyloric glands. HPV is not detected {2059}.

Genetic profile
Cases with atypical features show gains of chromosome 3p and loss of 1p which are abnormalities shared by minimal deviation adenocarcinoma.

Genetic susceptibility
This may occur in patients with Peutz-Jeghers syndrome.

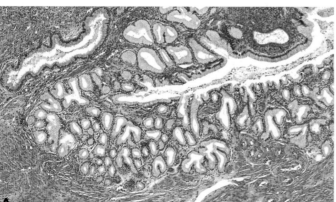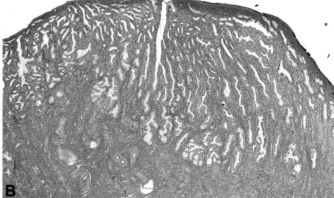

Fig. 7.25 A Lobular endocervical glandular hyperplasia. A lobulated proliferation of benign-appearing endocervical epithelium centred on a larger gland. These lesions can show minimal cytological atypia and have a gastric-type immunophenotype. **B** Diffuse laminar endocervical hyperplasia. This proliferation consists of a band-like proliferation of tightly packed endocervical glands that is sharply demarcated from the underlying stroma.

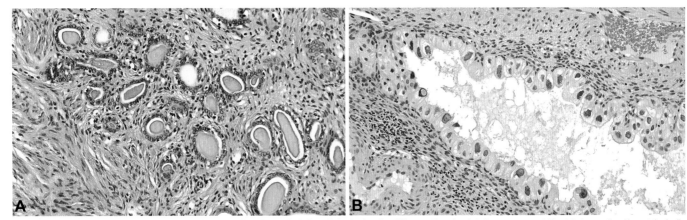

Fig. 7.26 A Mesonephric remnants. The lesion is composed of small, round tubules with luminal eosinophilic secretions in a lobular arrangement. The tubules are lined by cytologically bland, non-stratified cuboidal cells. Mitotic figures are not seen. **B** Arias-Stella reaction. Note the typical nuclear pleomorphism, smudged chromatin and atypia.

Prognosis and predictive factors

Some cases of LEGH have been shown to be associated with adenocarcinoma in situ/high-grade cervical glandular intraepithelial neoplasia (AIS/HG-CGIN) and/or minimal deviation/gastric type adenocarcinomas, including adenoma malignum suggesting that it is a potential precursor lesion {1268,1330}.

Diffuse laminar endocervical hyperplasia

Definition

A band-like proliferation of closely packed, benign endocervical glands below the surface of the endocervical canal.

Clinical features

Diffuse laminar endocervical hyperplasia (DLEH) typically presents in premenopausal women as an incidental finding.

Histopathology

DLEH consists of a band-like proliferation of tightly packed small to medium-sized endocervical glands below the surface of the endocervical canal and is sharply demarcated from the underlying cervical stroma. The cells can have mild reactive atypia. Differentiation from neoplasia can be problematic and relies on the sharp border, lack of malignant cytological features, and lack of invasive stromal desmoplastic changes {844}.

Prognosis and predictive factors

DLEH is a benign lesion.

Mesonephric remnants and hyperplasia

Definition

Embryonic remnants of mesonephric ducts and their benign proliferations.

Epidemiology

Mesonephric remnants are found in 10–20% of adult cervices and up to 40% of cervices in newborns and children. Mesonephric hyperplasia is most common in the reproductive and postmenopausal age groups and is nearly always an incidental finding in a hysterectomy or cone biopsy specimen {552}.

Clinical features

Remnants are most commonly an incidental finding, while hyperplasia may be either incidental or may rarely present with abnormal cervical cytology.

Histopathology

Mesonephric remnants consist of small, lobular, well-circumscribed aggregates of tubules lined by cuboidal cells with minimal nuclear atypia and containing luminal eosinophilic secretions. The tubules typically surround a central duct. Mesonephric hyperplasia may be lobular (most common) or diffuse and consists of a proliferation of remnant glands and ducts with cellular morphology similar to that described above, with some columnar cells present. There is no strict size cut-off between "normal" mesonephric remnants and mesonephric hyperplasia but a size of 6 mm has been suggested. Occasional ductal proliferations may show pseudostratified columnar cells with papillary tufts or bridging. Occasional mitotic activity may be present but atypia is generally minimal. No stromal response is present. Cells typically are immunoreactive for CD10 (luminal pattern) and can show focal immunostaining for p16. Ki-67 immunohistochemistry shows a low proliferation index (1–2%) which can be useful in differentiating this lesion from adenoma malignum {1224}.

Prognosis and predictive factors

Mesonephric remnants and hyperplasias are benign lesions. Rare mesonephric adenocarcinomas arise from mesonephric remnants/hyperplasia.

Arias Stella reaction

Definition

An incidental, usually pregnancy-related, glandular epithelial cell change similar to Arias-Stella change of the endometrium.

Etiology

Arias-Stella reaction is found in pregnant patients or occasionally in non-pregnant patients using hormonal agents and patients with gestational trophoblastic disease.

Clinical features

Arias-Stella reaction is an incidental microscopic finding.

Histopathology

Arias-Stella reaction consists of enlarged glandular cells with vacuolated clear or oxyphilic cytoplasm, hyperchromatic but often smudgy nuclei with hobnail features and occasional intraglandular tufting or papillae. Mitotic activity is rare. The process may involve the lining of a single or small group of endocervical glands, but can rarely become confluent. It can occur within an endocervical polyp. The major differential diagnosis is with clear cell adenocarcinoma or endocervical adenocarcinoma in situ, particularly in small biopsies.

Prognosis and predictive factors
Arias-Stella reaction is a benign lesion with no malignant potential.

Endocervicosis

Definition
Benign endocervical-type glands that typically involve the outer half of the cervical wall {2105}.

Clinical features
In one series, the patients ranged in age from 29–45 years, and they most commonly presented with pelvic pain.

Macroscopy
The lesion usually presents as a nodular mass or cysts involving the anterior cervical wall; size ranges from 1–2.5 cm.

Histopathology
The lesion is composed of variably sized and shaped glands, including cystically dilated glands, involving the outer cervical wall. The glands are lined by banal appearing endocervical type epithelium, with either a columnar or flattened appearance. Mitotic activity is rare to absent. Stromal reaction may be seen with mucin extravasation. Other sites, such as the bladder wall, can be involved.

Histogenesis
Patients with cervical endocervicosis often have a history of Caesarean section, which suggests that prior surgery may cause displacement of endocervical epithelium into the outer cervical wall.

Prognosis and predictive factors
This is a benign process.

Endometriosis

Definition
Endometrial-type glands and stroma occurring within the cervix.

Epidemiology
Endometriosis develops in premenopausal women with a wide age range (third to sixth decades).

Clinical features
It is typically an incidental finding in the cervix, but may be associated with abnormal cervical cytology.

Macroscopy
It may present as thickened, granular or haemorrhagic mucosa or as blood-filled cysts.

Histopathology
There are two types of cervical endometriosis; superficial and deep. The former is more common and is not associated with pelvic endometriosis. The latter is associated with pelvic endometriosis and occurs in the outer aspects of the cervix. Superficial endometriosis is located within the inner one-third of the cervical wall, just below the normal endocervical glands. The endometriotic glands are round to oval and may be cystic. They are lined by pseudostratified epithelium resembling normal or weakly proliferative endometrium with some mitotic figures. A stromal component is generally present surrounding the glands, but may be minimal. There is often stromal haemorrhage or haemosiderin pigment. The endometriotic glands can be positive for p16 but the pattern of expression is almost always patchy to some degree, with more diffuse expression present focally in glands with prominent or extensive tubal metaplasia; this latter phenomenon can create difficulty in differentiation from endocervical adenocarcinoma in situ in small biopsies. Bcl2 is usually diffusely positive but focal or patchy staining may occur in adenocarcinoma in situ {492}. Deep endometriosis has a similar mor-

phological appearance and staining pattern. A variant, composed of endometrial stroma without glands, is referred to as stromal endometriosis.

Histogenesis
Superficial endometriosis may be localized to areas of prior surgical procedures, suggesting a metaplastic process or more uncommonly implantation. Deep endometriosis is secondary to extension of pelvic endometriosis from the cul-de-sac.

Prognosis and predictive factors
Endometriosis is a benign lesion; however malignancies can rarely arise in these foci.

Tuboendometrioid metaplasia

Definition
Replacement of the typical endocervical-type epithelium by tuboendometrioid epithelium.

Synonyms
Tubal metaplasia; endometrioid metaplasia

Epidemiology
Tuboendometrioid metaplasia is most commonly an incidental finding during the reproductive years.

Etiology
The various types of metaplasia are most commonly reparative lesions secondary to a prior procedure to the cervix, most commonly loop excision.

Clinical features
It can present with abnormal cervical cytology, but generally has no specific associated symptoms.

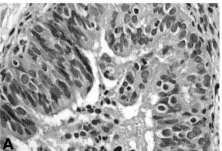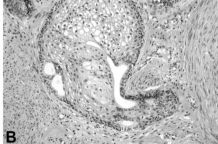

Fig. 7.27 A Tuboendometrioid metaplasia. This metaplasia can mimic adenocarcinoma in situ because of its pseudostratified nature and because it can be mitotically active. **B** Ectopic prostate tissue. The nest consists of cells recapitulating normal prostatic epithelium with prominent areas of squamous metaplasia.

Histopathology

The lesion shows tubal or endometrioid differentiation with ciliated, columnar and intercalated (peg) cells in the former (identical to fallopian tube epithelium) and non-ciliated pseudostratified epithelium (identical to endometrial epithelium) in the latter. Mixtures of these two forms commonly occur and typically express Bcl2. Although p16 immunohistochemistry can show focal reactivity in these metaplasias, diffuse positivity as occurs in true endocervical HPV-associated neoplasias is lacking. Oxyphilic meta-plasia shows abundant eosinophilic cytoplasm with enlarged irregular nuclei, but without mitotic activity. The major diagnostic issue with metaplasias is differentiation from neoplastic glandular lesions, particularly in cervical cytology specimens. Lack of malignant nuclear features and mitotic activity are the most reliable discriminators in excluding a neoplastic process {1414}.

Prognosis and predictive factors

Metaplasias are benign incidental findings with no malignant potential.

Ectopic prostate tissue

Ectopic prostate tissue is characterized by replacement of endocervical epithelium with typical benign-appearing prostatic glands containing basal cells and showing variable degrees of squamous differentiation.

Other epithelial tumours

T.J. Colgan
L. Hirschowitz
K.-R. Kim
W.G. McCluggage

Adenosquamous carcinoma

Definition

A malignant epithelial tumour comprising both adenocarcinoma and squamous cell carcinoma.

ICD-O code   8560/3

Histopathology

There should be sufficient differentiation of the adenocarcinomatous component to include histologically recognizable glands. Scattered mucin-producing cells may occur in a squamous cell carcinoma {1671} and such tumours should not be labelled as adenosquamous carcinomas. Since the presence of mucin within squamous carcinomas has not been shown to have any prognostic or predictive value, routine staining for mucin in squamous carcinomas is not recommended. Carcinomas which lack evidence of squamous differentiation (intercellular bridges, keratinization) but have abundant mucin-producing cells should be diagnosed as poorly differentiated adenocarcinomas.

A clear cell variant of adenosquamous carcinoma, characterized by cytoplasmic clearing of the squamous component due to extensive glycogen, has been described {614}.

Very rarely, a carcinoma displays three cell types (epidermoid, mucin-producing, and intermediate). These tumours can be labelled "mucoepidermoid carcinomas" and may represent a distinctive entity as has been shown for salivary gland tumours.

Histogenesis

Both squamous intraepithelial lesion (SIL) and adenocarcinoma in situ (AIS) are precursor lesions for adenosquamous carcinomas. HPV-18, followed by HPV-16, are the most prevalent HPV types {2096}. Expression of ARID1A (the adenine, thymine-rich interactive domain 1A) is frequently lost in adenosquamous carcinomas {884}.

Genetic profile

The chromosomal translocation t(11;19)-associated *CRTC1-MAML2* gene fusion is identified in cervical mucoepidermoid, but not adenosquamous carcinomas {537,1074}. This translocation is also found in salivary mucoepidermoid carcinomas and suggests that cervical mucoepidermoid carcinoma represents an entity distinct from adenosquamous carcinoma.

Prognosis and predictive factors

Although some studies have found that adenosquamous differentiation is an independent prognostic parameter indicating a poorer outcome {784,1051,1119}, the balance of evidence suggests that, stage for stage, adenosquamous carcinoma has a similar behaviour and prognosis to squamous and adenocarcinomas {31,670,1137,1767}. However, it has been suggested that adenosquamous differentiation may be a predictor of poorer outcome in carcinomas of a more advanced stage {531}. In one study, HPV negativity in an adenosquamous carcinoma was an indicator of poor prognosis {1024}.

Glassy cell carcinoma

Definition

A poorly differentiated variant of adenosquamous carcinoma.

ICD-O code   8015/3

Clinical features

Glassy cell carcinomas are rare, comprising only 1–2% of cervical carcinomas, and typically occur in young women. They grow rapidly and may have distant metastases at presentation.

Etiology

HPV-18 has been identified in glassy cell carcinomas {885}.

Macroscopy

Glassy cell carcinomas may present with a barrel shaped cervix.

Histopathology

Glassy cell carcinoma is a poorly differentiated variant of adenosquamous carcinoma characterized by cells with sharp cytoplasmic margins, "ground glass" appearing eosinophilic cytoplasm, and large round to ovoid nuclei with prominent nucleoli {1107}. Unlike non-keratinizing squamous carcinomas, glassy cell carcinoma often shows a prominent eosinophil infiltrate in the stroma surrounding the nest of neoplastic epithelium {1123}. Usually a pre-invasive component is not seen. Glassy cell carcinomas produce intestinal-type mucin and express MUC2 {885}. Similar to most cervical carcinomas, the tumour cells do not express oestrogen and progesterone receptors {69}. There is likely to be significant inter-observer variability in the diagnosis of this tumour type.

Prognosis and predictive factors

Glassy cell carcinomas were reported to have a poor prognosis and worse outcome than other cervical carcinomas {1107}, but recent studies have not confirmed this initial impression {664,772}. Tumours may have a poor response to radiotherapy, although chemotherapy shows some effect {1123,1185,1265}.

Adenoid basal carcinoma

Definition

An epithelial tumour composed of small, well differentiated, rounded nests of basaloid cells.

ICD-O code   8098/3

Synonym

Adenoid basal epithelioma

Etiology

In contrast to other carcinomas, it is postulated that ABC has its origin from a reserve cell {667,1733}. Adenoid cystic carcinoma (ACC) is another tumour within this morphological spectrum. High-risk HPV (types 16, 33) has been identified in ABC {666,846,1468}.

Clinical features

This tumour usually occurs in women older than 50 years. Patients are generally asymptomatic; the tumour is usually discovered as an incidental microscopic finding {188}.

Macroscopy

Usually no gross abnormality unless another subtype of carcinoma is also present.

Histopathology

Adenoid basal carcinoma (ABC) is an epithelial tumour composed solely of small, well-differentiated, rounded nests of basaloid cells that have scanty cytoplasm and which resemble basal cell carcinomas in the skin. The tumour cells form rounded nests or cords which infiltrate the superficial cervical stroma. The nests of tumour cells may contain central cystic spaces that are filled with necrotic debris and there may also be focal glandular or squamous differentiation in the centre of the nests. The small cells are p16 positive {1468}. A definitive diagnosis of ABC requires evaluation of the entire tumour {1468,1652}. ABC is often associated with squamous intraepithelial lesion or another carcinoma subtype {188,550}. The presence of any invasive carcinoma subtype with ABC should be reported as a 'mixed carcinoma'. 'Adenoid basal

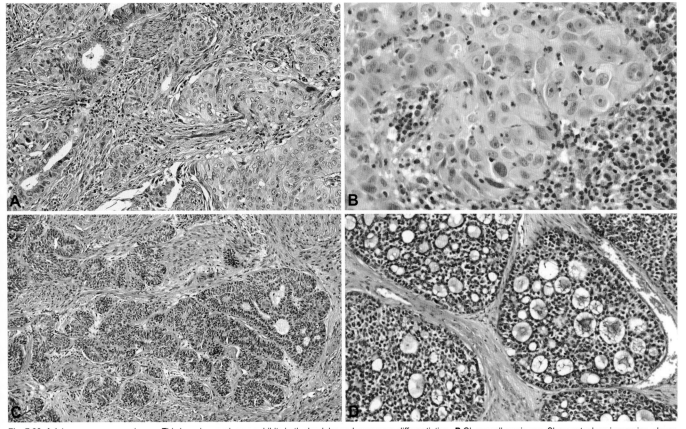

Fig. 7.28 **A** Adenosquamous carcinoma. This invasive carcinoma exhibits both glandular and squamous differentiation. **B** Glassy cell carcinoma. Sharp cytoplasmic margins, glassy, "ground glass" eosinophilic cytoplasm and large round-to-oval nuclei with prominent nucleoli characterize this tumour. **C** Adenoid basal carcinoma. The tumour is characterized by well-differentiated cords and nests of basaloid cells with scanty cytoplasm and focal gland formation. **D** Adenoid cystic carcinoma of the cervix. The tumour is composed of islands of basaloid cells with punched-out spaces containing basophilic material.

hyperplasia' has been described, and may be distinguished from ABC. Adenoid basal hyperplasia is characterized by a similar proliferation of small basaloid nests extending less than 1 mm from the basement membrane {904}. The differential diagnosis of ABC includes other basaloid carcinomas, such as adenoid cystic carcinoma (ACC), basaloid squamous cell carcinoma, and neuroendocrine carcinomas {665}. ABC and ACC share many immunohistochemical similarities {667}. ACC is often CD117 positive, in contrast to adenoid basal carcinoma {285}.

Prognosis and predictive factors
Pure ABC is a low-grade tumour with an excellent prognosis and rarely metastasizes {188}. Although the alternate term "adenoid basal epithelioma" has been suggested to reflect this good outcome, ABC is an established term and should be retained {188}. The outcome of mixed carcinomas and ABC is largely dependent upon prognostic features of the non-ABC component. In view of this altered prognosis a diagnosis of ABC should be restricted to cases that consist entirely of ABC {1652}.

Adenoid cystic carcinoma

Definition
A tumour that resembles adenoid cystic carcinoma of the salivary glands.

ICD-O code   8200/3

Histopathology
This tumour shows pseudoglandular, cribriform-like and tubular patterns containing basement membrane-like material. Cytologically, the nuclei are angulated and hyperchromatic, without prominent nucleoli. There may be two tumours demonstrating this morphological pattern, one being a true adenoid cystic carcinoma (ACC) and the other being an ACC-like basaloid squamous cell carcinoma {667}. Immunohistochemistry and molecular analysis can be used to distinguish these tumours, including myoepithelial markers (p63, CD10, calponin, smooth muscle actin) and the *myb-NFIB* gene fusion {191} which are positive in true salivary gland type tumours. Papilloma virus HPV-16 has been reported in some cases {1468}.

Undifferentiated carcinoma

Definition
A carcinoma lacking any specific differentiation.

ICD-O code   8020/3

Histopathology
These are carcinomas composed of sheets of cells with no evidence of squamous or glandular differentiation. They are extremely rare tumours in the cervix. Immunohistochemistry may help in establishing a specific tumour type, for example p63 immunoreactivity suggesting a squamous carcinoma or neuroendocrine marker positivity a neuroendocrine carcinoma. p16 immunohistochemical stains and HPV in situ hybridization can be of use in differentiating metastatic from primary tumours {1660}.

Neuroendocrine tumours

T.J. Colgan   I. Kim
L. Hirschowitz   W.G. McCluggage

Low-grade neuroendocrine tumour

Definition
The recommended terminology for neuroendocrine tumours arising in the cervix is similar to that used for gastro-entero-pancreatic neuroendocrine tumours {174}. Low-grade, neuroendocrine tumours exhibit neuroendocrine and organoid differentiation {169,1850}. This category includes both grade 1 and grade 2 tumours.

ICD-O codes
Low-grade neuroendocrine tumour
    Carcinoid tumour   8240/3
Low-grade neuroendocrine tumour
    Atypical carcinoid tumour   8249/3

Synonyms
For carcinoid tumour: Low-grade neuroendocrine tumour, grade 1

For atypical carcinoid tumour: Low-grade neuroendocrine tumour, grade 2

Etiology
High-risk HPV can be identified in most cervical NETs {1161,1843,2038}.

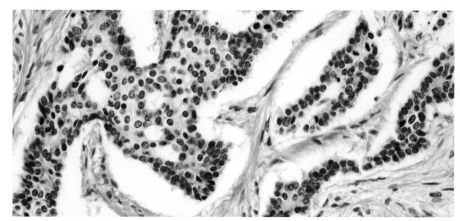

Fig. 7.29 Low-grade neuroendocrine tumour. Islands and ribbons of uniform epithelial cells with granular cytoplasm and small, round, uniform nuclei indicate a grade 1 tumour. Retraction artifact is present around the tumour islands.

Clinical features
The presentation and macroscopy of neuroendocrine tumours (NETs) are similar to other cervical carcinomas, with vaginal bleeding/discharge and/or detection of a cervical mass {1457}. NETs are only infrequently detected by

cytology {1306,2001}. The macroscopic appearance of NETs is not distinctive. NETs (especially of low-grade) may produce a variety of peptides such as calcitonin, gastrin, serotonin, substance P, vasoactive intestinal peptide, pancreatic polypeptide, somatostatin, and adrenocorticotrophic hormone {2,1719}, but only in rare cases do patients present with symptoms or biochemical evidence of ectopic hormone production, or subsequently develop carcinoid syndrome as a result of metastatic disease {954}.

Histopathology

Cervical low-grade NETs are extremely rare and are primarily defined by the same architectural and cytological features used at other sites. Grade 1 tumours are characterized by abundant cytoplasm, characteristic granular chromatin and visible to prominent nucleoli. Growth patterns can be organoid, spindled, nested, islands or trabecular. Grade 2 tumours are distinguished from grade 1 tumours by their greater degree of nuclear atypia and mitotic activity, as well as rare areas of necrosis. There is no specific evidence for the formulaic use of Ki-67 labelling index and mitotic count for the grading of cervical neuroendocrine tumours, as is recommended for gastro-entero-pancreatic tumours.

Immunohistochemistry
Immunohistochemistry for synaptophysin, chromogranin, CD56 and neuron-specific enolase can facilitate the histological diagnosis (see high-grade neuroendocrine carcinoma).

Histogenesis

Neuroendocrine differentiation occurs within neoplasms arising from the cervical epithelium. Cells that express neuroendocrine markers are present in some cases of cervical adenocarcinoma in situ and could be the precursor of cervical neuroendocrine tumours {1064,1219}. Both preinvasive and invasive squamous and glandular neoplasia may be found in association with cervical NETs but glandular lesions are proportionately commoner.

Genetic profile

The most frequent allelic loss in NETs is localized 3p deletion {1161,2038}. Occasional 9p21 deletions have also been identified {2038}.

Prognosis and predictive factors

Grade 1 neuroendocrine tumours generally follow an indolent course; however, they retain the potential for metastatic spread. Grade 2 neuroendocrine tumours are more aggressive neoplasms, although few cases have been reported with available follow-up {2098}. Their behaviour may be similar to large cell neuroendocrine carcinomas {1806}. Quantitative Ki-67 immunohistochemistry has been shown to be prognostically important in non-gynaecological sites {948,1016}.

High-grade neuroendocrine carcinoma

Definition

The recommended terminology for neuroendocrine tumours arising in the cervix is similar to that used for gastro-entero-pancreatic neuroendocrine tumours {174}. High-grade neuroendocrine carcinomas are composed of high-grade malignant cells and may be of either small cell or large cell type. Both types are considered grade 3.

ICD-O codes

Small cell neuroendocrine
   carcinoma   8041/3
Large cell neuroendocrine
   carcinoma   8013/3

Synonyms

For small cell neuroendocrine carcinoma: small cell carcinoma; neuroendocrine carcinoma, small cell type, grade 3;
For large cell neuroendocrine carcinoma: neuroendocrine carcinoma, large cell type, grade 3

Clinical features

See low-grade neuroendocrine tumour in the previous section. In addition, high-grade neuroendocrine carcinoma of small cell type (SCNEC) is by far the most common of these tumours. Like their pulmonary counterparts, they are extremely aggressive, even at low stage.

Macroscopy

See low-grade neuroendocrine tumour.

Histopathology

High-grade neuroendocrine carcinoma (NEC) of small cell type (SCNEC) is characterized by the presence of a monotonous population of small cells with ovoid hyperchromatic nuclei, often exhibiting

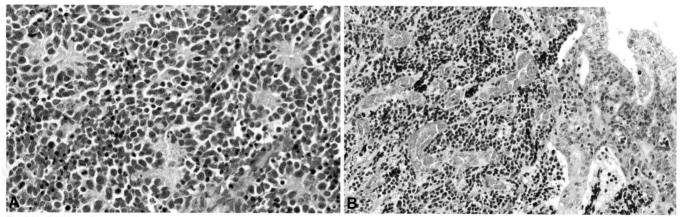

Fig. 7.30 A High-grade neuroendocrine carcinoma, small cell type. The small cells have ovoid to angulated nuclei with moulding, and scanty cytoplasm. Rosette-like structures and abundant apoptotic activity are present. **B** High-grade neuroendocrine carcinoma, small cell type, with adenocarcinoma in situ (high-grade cervical glandular intraepithelial neoplasia). This small cell neuroendocrine carcinoma shows a monotonous population of small cells with hyperchromatic nuclei and an associated adenocarcinoma in situ with nuclear stratification (right).

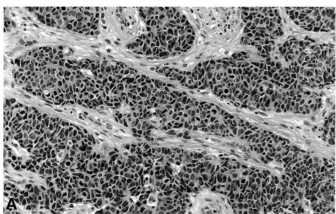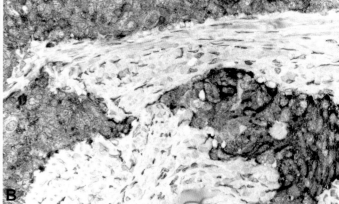

Fig. 7.31 A Large cell neuroendocrine carcinoma. Islands of large cells with pleomorphic, moulded nuclei, a high mitotic index and notable eosinophilic cytoplasm. **B** Large cell neuroendocrine carcinoma. Immunohistochemistry for synaptophysin is positive.

moulding, and scanty cytoplasm. There is usually abundant mitotic and apoptotic activity with extensive necrosis, lymphovascular and perineural invasion. SCNEC may be accompanied by in situ or invasive squamous or adenocarcinoma {143,532,1161,1491}. High-grade neuroendocrine carcinoma (NEC) of large cell type (LCNEC) has a diffuse, organoid, trabecular, or cord-like pattern and is composed of neoplastic cells with abundant cytoplasm, large nuclei, prominent nucleoli, and a high mitotic rate. Focal glandular differentiation may be present {394,986,1579}. The differential diagnosis includes cervical carcinomas of both squamous and glandular type.

Immunohistochemistry
Immunohistochemical staining for neuroendocrine markers (chromogranin, synaptophysin, CD56) may provide support for a diagnosis of SCNEC, but a proportion of these neoplasms may not express any neuroendocrine markers {1219}. TTF1 is not uncommonly positive and this finding is of no value in the distinction from a pulmonary primary {1086,1219}. SCNEC must be distinguished from lymphoma and a squamous cell carcinoma with small cells. Diffuse p63 nuclear immunoreactivity is typical of squamous cell carcinoma. SCNEC may occasionally fail to express cytokeratins. CD56 and synaptophysin are the most sensitive markers for SCNEC; chromogranin and PGP9.5 are less so. However, CD56 staining can be present in non-neuroendocrine carcinomas {1219}.

A definitive diagnosis of LCNEC requires immunohistochemical stains for neuroendocrine markers. LCNECs may be p63 positive {1219}. Isolated neuroendocrine cells may be found in cervical squamous cell carcinomas and adenocarcinomas and, without the typical morphological features, these should not be diagnosed as LCNECs.

Histogenesis
Cervical SCNEC is reliably associated with high-risk HPV. HPV-18 is identified more frequently than in cervical squamous cell carcinoma {748}.

Genetic factors
Amplification of chromosome 3q has been identified in neuroendocrine tumours {891}.

Prognosis and predictive factors
High-grade neuroendocrine carcinomas are highly aggressive tumours and frequently present at an advanced stage {639,1457}. Five-year survival for SCNEC of all stages is reported to be 14–39%, with poorer survival in higher stage disease {2,143,1161,1850}. The management of high-grade neuroendocrine carcinoma may include specific neuroendocrine-based systemic chemotherapy and radiation therapy including axial sites.

Mesenchymal tumours and tumour-like lesions

M.R. Nucci
M.L. Carcangiu
G.P. Nielsen
E. Oliva
B. Quade

Benign tumours

Leiomyoma

Definition
A benign tumour showing smooth-muscle differentiation and containing a variable amount of collagen-rich extracellular matrix.

ICD-O code   8890/0

Synonyms
Fibroid; myoma

Epidemiology
In contrast to the uterine corpus, cervical leiomyomas are very uncommon; their frequency has been estimated to be 0.6% in hysterectomy specimens {1924}.

Clinical features
Symptoms most commonly include bleeding, dyspareunia or those referable to mass effect. Although uncommon in pregnancy, large or polypoid tumours may complicate pregnancy. Tumours at this site are less amenable to uterine artery embolization than those of the corpus {926,1514}.

Macroscopy
Leiomyomas form spheroidal masses that have white, light pink or tan, whorled or trabecular incised surfaces, similar to those seen in the uterine corpus. Although non-infiltrative, the interface

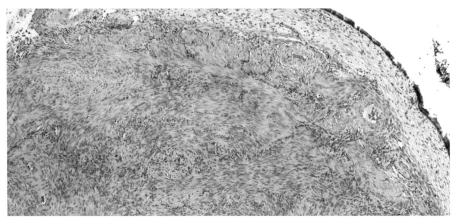

Fig. 7.32 Leiomyoma. These tumours are typically well circumscribed and composed of intersecting fascicles of spindle shaped cells, similar in appearance to their uterine corpus counterpart.

between cervical leiomyomas and their surrounding collagenous stroma may appear less defined compared to that of uterine leiomyomas.

Histopathology
They closely resemble their counterparts in the myometrium (see uterus chapter, p. 135–138 for images). The histological parameters used to determine malignancy are the same as those used in the uterus. Histological variants have not been well described in the cervix.

Histogenesis
Benign cervical smooth muscle tumours most likely arise from scattered smooth muscle cells in normal cervical stroma, which presumably accounts for their rarity relative to the uterine corpus.

Genetic profile
The genetic profile is presumably similar to that of leiomyoma of the uterine corpus.

Prognosis and predictive factors
These are benign neoplasms.

Rhabdomyoma

Definition
A rare, benign tumour of the lower female genital tract showing skeletal muscle differentiation, composed of mature, neoplastic rhabdomyoblasts separated by varying amounts of fibrous or oedematous stroma {329,705}.

ICD-O code   8905/0

Epidemiology
This is a rare, benign tumour of the lower female genital tract.

Clinical features
It affects adult patients and more commonly occurs in the vagina.

Macroscopy
It usually appears as a solitary, nodular or sometimes polypoid proliferation, usually less than 3 cm.

Histopathology
Rhabdomyomas are composed of haphazardly arranged, interlacing, mature, bland-appearing rhabdomyoblasts with an oval or tubular shape. Cytoplasmic cross-striations are numerous and easily detectable. Mitoses and necrosis are absent. The stroma can be fibrous or oedematous. Immunohistochemically, the tumour cells are reactive for desmin, skeletal muscle actin, myogenin and MyoD1. Ultrastructurally, the cytoplasm appears packed with myofibrils, and Z-bands are easily recognizable {329} (see vagina chapter, p. 218).

Prognosis and predictive factors
This is a benign, non-recurring tumour.

Other benign tumours

Rarely, the cervix may be the site of other benign neoplasms, including lipoleiomyoma {2004}, spindle cell lipoma {2134}, neurofibroma {1039,2010} and schwannoma {1877}.

Malignant tumours

Leiomyosarcoma

Definition
A malignant tumour showing smooth muscle differentiation.

ICD-O code   8890/3

Epidemiology
Primary sarcomas account for less than 1% of malignant cervical tumours {910} and leiomyosarcoma is the most common type.

Clinical features
These tumours present as masses that expand or replace the cervix.

Macroscopy
Tumours may form polypoid masses that project into the endocervical and vaginal canal, and may ulcerate through normal mucosa. Sectioned surfaces are typically flat, white or grey, and soft or "fleshy." Myxoid variants often appear gelatinous. The border with the adjacent cervical stroma may be poorly defined or show overt infiltration.

Histopathology
Tumours are typically composed of spindle-shaped neoplastic cells; variants include those with prominent myxoid matrix or epithelioid cytology. Although not extensively studied owing to its rarity, it has been inferred that criteria for malignancy are similar to tumours in the uterine corpus. Atypical mitoses can be seen, correlating with the high level of genomic instability detectable by cytogenetic and molecular methods {562,1542,1668,2002}. Immunohistochemistry with smooth muscle markers such as smooth muscle actin, desmin and h-caldesmon may facilitate tumour histotyping {1392}.

Histogenesis
These tumours most likely arise from scattered smooth muscle cells in normal cervical stroma, which presumably accounts for their rarity relative to the uterine corpus.

Prognosis and predictive factors
Prognostic factors for cervical leiomyosarcoma have not been well studied.

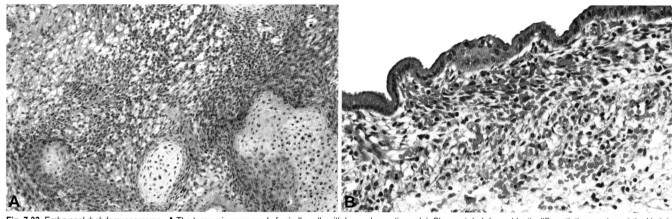

Fig. 7.33 Embryonal rhabdomyosarcoma. **A** The tumour is composed of spindle cells with hyperchromatic nuclei. Clear-cut rhabdomyoblastic differentiation can be subtle. Nodules of cartilage occur in up to 50% of tumours. **B** A typical collection of tumour cells under non-neoplastic epithelium; the so called "cambium layer".

Rhabdomyosarcoma

Definition
A malignant tumour showing skeletal muscle differentiation.

ICD-O code   8910/3

Synonym
Sarcoma botryoides

Epidemiology
Rhabdomyosarcomas of the female genital tract are rare tumours, especially in adults. The cervix is the most common site in female reproductive organs in adults, and the vagina in children {543}. In both groups, embryonal rhabdomyosarcoma is the most common histological type. The peak incidence in the cervix is in the second and third decade, as opposed to a peak during infancy and childhood when it occurs in the vagina {420,435}.

Clinical features
Patients commonly present with a cervical polyp or vaginal bleeding {420,435,1087}.

Macroscopy
These are typically fleshy polyps that may show areas of haemorrhage.

Histopathology
Embryonal rhabdomyosarcoma is a polypoid tumour composed of small, round or spindle cells with hyperchromatic nuclei with subepithelial condensation of tumour cells (cambium layer). A variable degree of skeletal muscle differentiation can be appreciated. Nodules of cartilage are seen in up to 50% of tumours.

Tumour cells are positive for desmin (cytoplasmic) and myogenin (nuclear).

Genetic profile
Alveolar rhabdomyosarcomas have two characteristic translocations, t(2;13) and t(1:13) involving *FOXO1A*, *PAX7* and *PAX3* genes {1433,1899}.

Genetic susceptibility
A familial case involving siblings has been reported {1308}.

Prognosis and predictive factors
Patients with cervical, in comparison with vaginal embryonal rhabdomyosarcoma, have a more favourable outcome {420,435}; patients have been reported to remain disease free following conservative surgery and chemotherapy {435}.

Alveolar soft-part sarcoma

Definition
A sarcoma of unknown histogenesis composed of large, polygonal cells with granular, eosinophilic cytoplasm, growing in a solid or alveolar pattern.

ICD-O code   9581/3

Epidemiology
This is a very rare primary tumour of the cervix {682,1350}.

Clinical features
Patients typically present with abnormal uterine bleeding or a cervical nodule {714}.

Macroscopy
This tumour may have a yellow or greyish cut surface, often with areas of hemorrhage and necrosis. It can be polypoid or intramural.

Histopathology
Most tumours have a characteristic alveolar growth pattern with nests of tumour cells with loss of cellular cohesion centrally; sometimes the tumours can have a more solid growth pattern. A prominent, sinusoidal, vascular network separates the nests. PAS-D can demonstrate intracytoplasmic Shipkey crystals that can also be seen ultrastructurally. There is no specific immunohistochemical profile, except that there is frequently positive nuclear staining for TFE3 {1615}.

Genetic profile
This tumour shows t(X;17), resulting in *ASPL/TFE3* gene fusion {1022}.

Prognosis and predictive factors
Alveolar soft part sarcomas of the uterine cervix appear to have a better prognosis than their soft-tissue counterparts. Only rare cases metastasize {1350}.

Angiosarcoma

Definition
A malignant, mesenchymal tumour showing endothelial cell differentiation.

ICD-O code   9120/3

Macroscopy
The tumour grows as a flat or slightly raised violaceous plaque, oozing blood from the ulcerated areas {329}.

Histopathology

Angiosarcomas are characterized by the formation of infiltrative anastomosing vascular channels often combined with solid, poorly differentiated areas. The tumour cells are flat or cuboidal with atypical nuclei and inconspicuous cytoplasm. Mitoses are common. Haemorrhage and necrosis are usually present. A distinct morphological variant of angiosarcoma, known as the epithelioid variant, is composed of plump epithelioid endothelial cells with abundant acidophilic cytoplasm, large nuclei and very prominent nucleoli, the latter representing an important diagnostic clue. Immunohistochemically, there is positivity for endothelial markers, including CD31, CD34, Fli-1, ERG, and FVIII-related antigen. Ultrastructurally, some of the tumour cells contain a characteristic organelle known as Weibel-Palade body.

Histogenesis

The tumour is derived from endothelial cells.

Prognosis and predictive factors

Angiosarcoma is a highly aggressive neoplasm, prone to invade locally and metastasize distally. As a result, mortality is very high.

Malignant peripheral nerve sheath tumour

Definition

A malignant tumour showing nerve-sheath differentiation.

ICD-O code   9540/3

Epidemiology

Only few cases of cervical malignant peripheral nerve sheath tumour (MPNST) have been reported {144,898,1026,1272}.

Clinical features

Patients may present with irregular bleeding.

Macroscopy

They typically form a mass lesion or polyp.

Histopathology

Classic MPNST is composed of mitotically active spindle cells, growing in a fascicular pattern, often with alternating hypercellular and hypocellular areas.

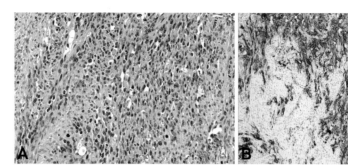

Fig. 7.34 Angiosarcoma. **A** This poorly differentiated tumour is composed of a solid proliferation of spindle cells that is focally vasoformative. **B** Positivity for CD31 is characteristic of angiosarcoma.

Immunohistochemically, approximately 50% show S100 expression. The recently described endocervical fibroblastic MPNST shows diffuse S100 expression in addition to CD34 expression {1272}.

Histogenesis

The tumours are of nerve sheath derivation.

Genetic susceptibility

Up to 50% of MPNSTs arise in patients with neurofibromatosis type 1 (NF1). No patient with cervical MPNST has been reported to have NF1.

Prognosis and predictive factors

Cervical tumours appear to behave better than soft-tissue MPNSTs. Only rare cases have been reported to metastasize {1272}.

Other sarcomas

Definition

Rare malignant sarcomas of the cervix include liposarcoma, undifferentiated endocervical sarcoma, and Ewing sarcoma {514}.

ICD-O codes

Liposarcoma	8850/3
Undifferentiated endocervical sarcoma	8805/3
Ewing sarcoma	9364/3

Tumour-like lesions

Postoperative spindle-cell nodule

Definition

A benign, non-neoplastic, reactive lesion that can mimic a sarcoma.

Synonym

Postoperative pseudosarcoma

Epidemiology

Only rare cases have been reported to arise in the cervix {893}.

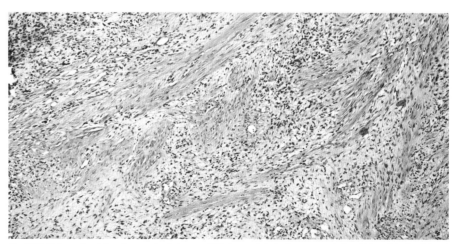

Fig. 7.35 Malignant peripheral nerve sheath tumour. This tumour is typically composed of variably cellular fascicles of spindle-shaped cells that infiltrate the cervical wall.

Clinical features
The lesion develops at the site of a prior operative procedure, usually several weeks after the surgery {1355,1530}. Clinically and pathologically it can mimic a sarcoma and is often diagnosed as such. A history of a previous procedure, such as curettage, is helpful when making the diagnosis.

Histopathology
The lesion is composed of intersecting fascicles of uniform, plump, spindle-shaped cells with a delicate network of small blood vessels and chronic inflammatory cells. The cells have abundant eosinophilic to amphophilic cytoplasm. Mitotic figures may be numerous (See vagina chapter, p. 221).

Histogenesis
This is a reactive myofibroblastic proliferation.

Prognosis and predictive factors
It is a benign lesion that can locally recur.

Lymphoma-like lesion

Definition
A florid, lymphoid, inflammatory infiltrate composed of large cells raising concern for lymphoma {2112}.

Epidemiology
This is a very rare lesion.

Etiology
Some patients may have Epstein Barr virus or other infections {2112}.

Clinical features
It affects patients with a wide age range, but patients are often premenopausal and present with vaginal bleeding or discharge, abnormal cytological smear or abdominal pain {1136,2112}.

Macroscopy
The cervix may be enlarged, erythematous, friable and/or eroded. It may rarely form a mass {2112}.

Histopathology
There is a subepithelial band-like infiltrate of large lymphoid cells forming sheets (more commonly) or vague nodules (rarely) extending below the level of endocervical glands. The infiltrate consists of a variable admixture of centrocytes, centroblasts, immunoblasts and tingible body macrophages. Mature lymphocytes, plasma cells and polymorphonuclear cells are also seen (polymorphic infiltrate). Adjacent acute and chronic or follicular cervicitis may be noted {2112}. By immunohistochemistry there is an admixture of B and T-cells and polyclonal plasma cells {629}.

Genetic profile
The lesion may harbour clonal immunoglobulin heavy-chain gene rearrangements {629}.

Prognosis and predictive factors
It is a self-limited process {629,1136}.

Mixed epithelial and mesenchymal tumours

M.R. Nucci   E. Oliva
M.L. Carcangiu   B. Quade

Adenomyoma

Definition
A benign, mixed, epithelial and mesenchymal tumour composed of endocervical-type glands and myomatous stroma.

ICD-O code   8932/0

Clinical features
Patients may be asymptomatic or present with symptoms related to a mass. The age at the time of pathological diagnosis ranges from 21–55 years old, with a mean age of 40 years {638,1267}.

Macroscopy
Adenomyomas in the cervix form well circumscribed masses ranging from 1–10 cm, and have grey-white or yellow-brown, trabecular cut surfaces, similar to those seen in the uterine corpus {638}. Mucin-filled cysts up to several centimetres in size may be visible. Some tumours grow as polypoid masses protruding into the endocervical canal.

Histopathology
The histopathology of adenomyoma in the cervix is similar to that in the corpus, with the notable exception that the epithelial component more frequently displays endocervical differentiation. In addition, the irregularly shaped glands often show papillary infoldings and a leaf-like architecture surrounded by smaller glands imparting a lobular appearance. Endometrioid and tubal differentiation in the glandular component is present in a minority of cases {638}. The combination of endocervical glands surrounded by smooth muscle cells may raise concern for minimal deviation endocervical adenocarcinoma (adenoma malignum). Gross circumscription, polypoid appearance, frequent lobular arrangement of glands, absence of invasive glands with a desmoplastic stromal reaction and lack of even focal atypia distinguish adenomyoma from endocervical adenocarcinoma {638,1267}. Unlike in the corpus, histological variants in the leiomyomatous component of cervical adenomyomas have not been reported.

Histogenesis
The precise nature of the neoplastic component (stromal versus epithelial) and the relationship between the two components have not been confirmed by molecular genetic methods.

Prognosis and predictive factors
This is a benign lesion.

Adenosarcoma

Definition
A biphasic tumour with an admixture of benign or, at most, mildly atypical Müllerian glands and low-grade malignant stroma {598}.

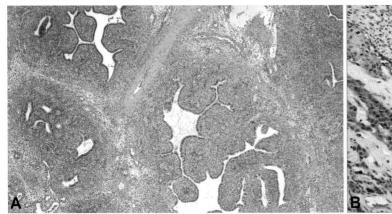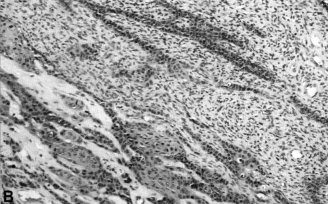

Fig. 7.36 A Adenosarcoma. This tumour is characterized by its leaf-like architecture (phyllodes-like growth), intraglandular polypoid projections and periglandular cuffing by cellular stroma. **B** Carcinosarcoma. Cervical carcinosarcomas often have a malignant component that resembles the most common primary cervical carcinomas, specifically squamous cell carcinoma.

ICD-O code   8933/3

Epidemiology
It is a rare tumour accounting for approximately 2% of adenosarcomas of the female reproductive organs {1983}.

Etiology
No relation to human papilloma virus has been reported, in contrast to most malignant tumours of the cervix {1315}.

Clinical features
Patients range widely in age but are often younger than those with uterine corpus tumours. They present with vaginal bleeding, abdominal or pelvic pain or a mass/polyp detected on routine gynaecological exam {598}. Patients may have a history of recurrent polyps {847}.

Macroscopy
It is frequently nodular, polypoid, or papillary.

Histopathology
Benign or atypical but not frankly malignant Müllerian glands are often uniformly distributed within the tumour, some of them showing a phyllodes or cystic appearance. The glands are most frequently lined by endocervical-type epithelium that may be associated with squamous metaplasia. They are surrounded by a cellular stroma that forms periglandular cuffs as well as intraluminal polypoid projections. The stroma is usually low-grade, resembling endometrial stromal sarcoma, with variable mitotic activity {598}. Sex cord-like areas and smooth muscle differentiation as well as heterologous el-

ements including fetal-type cartilage and rhabdomyoblasts (more common) or lipoblasts can be seen {598,847,1162,1558}. Sarcomatous overgrowth, defined as pure high-grade sarcoma comprising at least 25% of the tumour, has been reported {598,1315}. Rarely, tumours may be multifocal within the cervix or involve the cervix and endometrium simultaneously {338}.

Histogenesis
These tumours may arise from pre-existing endometriosis.

Prognosis and predictive factors
Outcome is related to invasion of the cervical wall and sarcomatous overgrowth {598,847}. If underdiagnosed as adenofibroma due to minimal mitotic activity, the tumour may recur and be associated with an unfavourable outcome. Thus, tumours with a typical low-power architecture should be diagnosed as adenosarcomas despite low mitotic activity {598}.

Carcinosarcoma

Definition
A malignant tumour of Müllerian derivation with an admixture of epithelial and mesenchymal elements.

ICD-O code   8980/3

Synonyms
Malignant mesodermal mixed tumour; malignant mixed Müllerian tumour; metaplastic carcinoma

Epidemiology
These tumours are considerably less frequent than those arising in the corpus or ovary.

Clinical features
They typically occur in postmenopausal women. Patients usually present with a large polypoid mass protruding into the cervical canal {350,668,1883}.

Macroscopy
These are large, fleshy masses often with haemorrhage and necrosis.

Histopathology
The carcinomatous component more commonly resembles a primary cervical epithelial tumour (basaloid squamous cell carcinoma, adenoid cystic carcinoma, adenoid basal carcinoma) and the mesenchymal component more commonly shows homologous differentiation (fibrosarcoma, endometrioid stromal sarcoma).

Histogenesis
Unlike uterine corpus carcinosarcoma, cervical tumours are associated with HPV infection, particularly type 16 {668,1883}.

Prognosis and predictive factors
Cervical carcinosarcomas are more commonly confined to the uterus than their corpus counterparts and thus may have a better prognosis {350}.

Melanocytic tumours

M.R. Nucci   J.A. Ferry
M.L. Carcangiu   E. Oliva
B. Quade

Blue naevus

Definition
A benign, melanocytic lesion composed of elongated, heavily pigmented cells with dendritic projections.

ICD-O code   8780/0

Clinical features
Blue naevi can occur anywhere in the lower genital tract, but most occur in the endocervical canal where they are found as incidental lesions in hysterectomy specimens from middle-aged women. In one series, only three cases were found in 2500 hysterectomy specimens {1469}. Rare cases coexisting with malignant melanoma have been described {1453}.

Macroscopy
Grossly, they appear as blue or black flat lesions, 2 or 3 mm in greatest dimension, with ill-defined borders centred in the stroma beneath an uninvolved mucosa.

Histopathology
The tumour cells are markedly elongated and contain a variable amount of melanin granules, many of which are located in dendritic projections of the tumour cells. The nuclei are bland and mitoses are absent. There is a tendency for the lesional cells to arrange themselves parallel to the skin surface. Melanin stains are strongly positive. Immunohistochemically, the tumour cells are positive for S100 protein but usually negative for HMB-45, Mart-1 (melan-A) and MiTF. Ultrastructurally, they are recognizable as melanocytes because of the presence

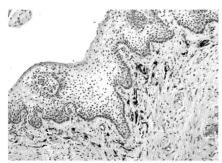

Fig. 7.37 Blue naevus. Heavily pigmented dendritic melanocytes are present in the cervical stroma.

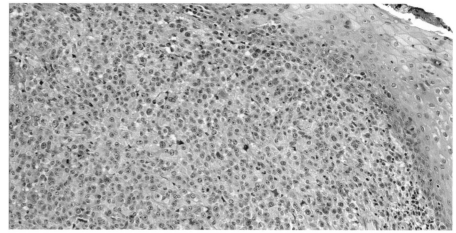

Fig. 7.38 Malignant melanoma. The tumour is composed of epithelioid cells with granular amphopilic cytoplasm, round nuclei and prominent nucleoli. Note the junctional component which helps identify the tumour as primary at this site.

of melanosomes (the melanin-producing organelles) in various stages of development {1469}.

Histogenesis
The lesion has a melanocytic derivation.

Prognosis and predictive factors
These are benign lesions.

Malignant melanoma

Definition
A malignant tumour composed of melanocytes.

ICD-O code   8720/3

Epidemiology
Malignant melanoma of the cervix is considerably less common than vulvar or vaginal melanoma.

Clinical features
All reported cases have been in adults, and approximately one-half had spread beyond the cervix at the time of presentation {1539}. Patients commonly present with abnormal vaginal bleeding.

Macroscopy
They are typically described as polypoid or fungating, pigmented masses. However, they may be amelanotic and nonspecific in appearance.

Histopathology
The cells of malignant melanoma vary in shape from epithelioid to spindled. Melanin production can be abundant, scanty, or altogether absent. Involvement of the basal layer of the overlying epithelium (so-called junctional activity) is present in about 50% of the cases, and it may be accompanied by transepithelial migration. In the absence of junctional activity, the possibility of the tumour being metastatic should be considered. A clear cell variant and a variant resembling a malignant peripheral nerve sheath tumour (MPNST) have been described in the uterine cervix {588,1538}. Immunohistochemically, there is usually reactivity for S100 protein, HMB-45, Mart 1 (melan-A) and MiTF. Ultrastructurally, the better-differentiated cells contain melanosomes and mature melanin granules.

Histogenesis
The tumour has a melanocytic derivation.

Prognosis and predictive factors
The prognosis of patients with cervical melanoma is extremely poor, and similar to that of melanomas of other sites such as vagina, vulva, anal canal, oral and nasal cavities and oesophagus {1539}.

Germer cell tumours

C.B. Gilks
S. Carinelli

Yolk sac tumour

Definition
A primitive malignant germ cell tumour characterized by a variety of distinctive histological patterns, some of which recapitulate phases in the development of the normal yolk sac.

Synonym
Endodermal sinus tumour.

Epidemiology
The tumour typically manifests in young children {2121}. Occurance in adults is exceptional {1165A}. The cervix is the second most common site in the lower female genital tract for yolk sac tumour after the vagina. It may be difficult or impossible to determine the primary site (vagina vs. cervix) in some cases {371}.

Clinical features
These tumours commonly present with abnormal vaginal bleeding. Yolk sac tumours are polypoid, friable masses, protruding into the vagina {284A,371}.

Histopathology
The histological features are the same as for vaginal yolk sac tumours {371,2121}.

Prognosis and predictive factors
The prognosis for patients with cervico-vaginal yolk sac tumours is good with modern chemotherapy {1189A}.

Lymphoid and myeloid tumours

M.R. Nucci   J.A. Ferry
M.L. Carcangiu   E. Oliva
                     B. Quade

Lymphomas

Definition
Malignant neoplasms composed of lymphoid cells.

Epidemiology
Primary cervical lymphoma is rare. Involvement of the cervix by a lymphoproliferative disorder is more commonly seen in the setting of systemic disease.

Clinical features
Primary cervical lymphoma affects adults, over a broad age range. They present most often with vaginal bleeding, but sometimes report local pain or dyspareunia. The lesions may invade surrounding tissues including vagina, bladder and parametria, and may extend to the pelvic sidewalls and compress the ureters and cause hydronephrosis {265,360,710,890}.

Macroscopy
Lymphomas are often bulky tumours, sometimes with circumferential enlargement of the cervix ("barrel-shaped" cervix). The lymphoma may form a discrete submucosal lesion {262,710}, a polypoid or multinodular lesion {265,604,710} or an exophytic mass. Surface epithelium usually remains intact {710}. The tumours are fleshy, rubbery, or firm and are usually white-tan to yellow in colour {710}.

Histopathology
Cervical diffuse large B-cell lymphomas are often associated with prominent sclerosis {604,1023,1970}, which may be associated with a cord-like arrangement or spindle-shaped tumour cells {710}. The spindle cell pattern may mimic a sarcoma; the terms "spindle cell variant" {231} and "sarcomatoid variant" {862} are suggested for such cases. Follicular lymphoma is the second most common type and all three grades have been reported {972,1970}. Like diffuse large B-cell lymphoma, cervical follicular lymphoma is also often associated with sclerosis. Neoplastic follicles are often found in a perivascular location.
Rare cervical marginal zone lymphomas (MALT lymphomas), Burkitt lymphomas {972,1970,1971} and extranodal NK/T-cell lymphomas, nasal-type {1970}, have been described. A variety of lymphomas can involve the cervix secondarily, in the setting of widespread disease {1970} (see Table 1.3, p. 80).

Histogenesis
The tumours have a haematopoietic origin.

Prognosis and predictive factors
Primary cervical lymphomas are usually localized and have a favourable prognosis. Outcome is less favourable with secondary involvement in the setting of widespread disease.

Myeloid neoplasms

Definition
Malignant neoplasms of haematopoietic origin, including myeloid leukaemias and myeloid sarcoma, a mass-forming lesion composed of primitive myeloid cells.

Synonyms
Myeloid sarcoma is also known as chloroma, granulocytic sarcoma or extramedullary myeloid tumour.

Epidemiology
Cervical involvement by myeloid neoplasia is rare but myeloid sarcoma involving the cervix has been described. Cervical involvement is more common than involvement of the uterine corpus {605}.

Clinical features
Cervical myeloid sarcoma may present as an isolated finding or with concurrent involvement of other extramedullary sites {605,1443}. Symptoms include vaginal

bleeding and dyspareunia {605,1443}.

Macroscopy
The cervix may appear diffusely enlarged or nodular.

Histopathology
Neoplasms are composed of a diffuse proliferation of primitive myeloid cells with oval, irregular, reniform or folded nuclei, fine chromatin, distinct to promi- nent nucleoli and scant to moderate cytoplasm. Maturing cells with recogniz- able myeloid differentiation may be seen. {605,1419,1443}.

Histogenesis
The tumours have a myeloid origin.

Genetic profile
Limited information is available, but one case of myeloid sarcoma confined to the cervix with a t(11;19)(q23;p13.3) involv- ing the *MLL* and *ELL* genes has been de- scribed {1443}.

Prognosis and predictive factors
Limited data on outcome are available, but prognosis is likely dependent on ex- tent of disease and on underlying genetic abnormalities.

Secondary tumours

M.R. Nucci
M.L. Carcangiu
J.A. Ferry
E. Oliva
B. Quade

Definition
Involvement by tumour that originates outside of the cervix.

Epidemiology
Secondary tumours of the cervix are un- common, representing less than 2% of metastases to the female reproductive organs {1072,1194}.

Clinical features
Secondary involvement of the cer- vix may cause abnormal bleeding or result in abnormal cervical cytology {1072,1151,1172}. The cervix may ap- pear enlarged, or have no recognizable clinical abnormality.

Macroscopy
Involvement may mimic a primary cervical malignancy appearing ei- ther as diffuse enlargement or a mass {1072,1151,1172}, or the cervix may be unremarkable {1892}.

Site of origin
Most commonly, secondary neoplasms represent contiguous spread from an endometrial primary {329,1892}. Ovary, gastrointestinal tract, breast and kidney are other common sites of origin in de- creasing order of frequency {1072}.

Histopathology
The neoplastic epithelium may involve any aspect of the cervix, including either su- perficial or deep cervical stroma. Features suggesting metastatic involvement include signet ring cells, lack of an in situ compo- nent, and extensive lymphovascular inva- sion. Secondary involvement by endome- trial adenocarcinoma can be deceptively bland and may be misinterpreted as be- nign {1892}.

WHO Classification of tumours of the vagina[a,b]

Epithelial tumours
Squamous cell tumours and precursors
  Squamous intraepithelial lesions
    Low-grade squamous intraepithelial lesion   8077/0
    High-grade squamous intraepithelial lesion 8077/2
  Squamous cell carcinoma, NOS   8070/3
    Keratinizing   8071/3
    Non-keratinizing   8072/3
    Papillary   8052/3
    Basaloid   8083/3
    Warty   8051/3
    Verrucous   8051/3
  Benign squamous lesions
    Condyloma acuminatum
    Squamous papilloma   8052/0
    Fibroepithelial polyp
    Tubulosquamous polyp   8560/0
    Transitional cell metaplasia
Glandular tumours
  Adenocarcinomas
    Endometrioid carcinoma   8380/3
    Clear cell carcinoma   8310/3
    Mucinous carcinoma   8480/3
    Mesonephric carcinoma   9110/3
  Benign glandular lesions
    Tubovillous adenoma   8263/0
    Villous adenoma   8261/0
    Müllerian papilloma
    Adenosis
    Endometriosis
    Endocervicosis
    Cysts
Other epithelial tumours
  Mixed tumour   8940/0
  Adenosquamous carcinoma   8560/3
  Adenoid basal carcinoma   8098/3
High-grade neuroendocrine carcinoma
  Small cell neuroendocrine carcinoma   8041/3
  Large cell neuroendocrine carcinoma   8013/3

Mesenchymal tumours
Leiomyoma   8890/0
Rhabdomyoma   8905/0
Leiomyosarcoma   8890/3
Rhabdomyosarcoma, NOS   8900/3
  Embryonal rhabdomyosarcoma   8910/3
Undifferentiated sarcoma   8805/3
Angiomyofibroblastoma   8826/0
Aggressive angiomyxoma   8841/0
Myofibroblastoma   8825/0

Tumour-like lesions
  Postoperative spindle cell nodule

Mixed epithelial and mesenchymal tumours
Adenosarcoma   8933/3
Carcinosarcoma   8980/3

Lymphoid and myeloid tumours
Lymphomas
Myeloid neoplasms

Melanocytic tumours
Naevi
  Melanocytic naevus   8720/0
  Blue naevus   8780/0
Malignant melanoma   8720/3

Miscellaneous tumours
Germ cell tumours
  Mature teratoma   9084/0
  Yolk sac tumour   9071/3
Others
  Ewing sarcoma   9364/3
  Paraganglioma   8693/1

Secondary tumours

---

[a] The morphology codes are from the International Classification of Diseases for Oncology (ICD-O) {575A}. Behaviour is coded /0 for benign tumours, /1 for unspecified, borderline or uncertain behaviour, /2 for carcinoma in situ and grade III intraepithelial neoplasia and /3 for malignant tumours; [b] The classification is modified from the previous WHO classification of tumours {1906A}, taking into account changes in our understanding of these lesions; *These new codes were approved by the IARC/WHO Committee for ICD-O in 2013.

TNM and FIGO classification of carcinomas of the vagina

T – Primary tumour

TNM	FIGO	
TX		Primary tumour cannot be assessed
T0		No evidence of primary tumour
Tis	a	Carcinoma in situ (preinvasive carcinoma)
T1	I	Tumour confined to vagina
T2	II	Tumour invades paravaginal tissues (paracolpium)
T3	III	Tumour extends to pelvic wall
T4	IVA	Tumour invades mucosa of bladder or rectum, or extends beyond the true pelvis[b]
M1	IVB	Distant metastasis

Note: [a]FIGO no longer includes stage 0 (Tis). [b]The presence of bullous oedema is not sufficient evidence to classify a tumour as T4

N – Regional Lymph Nodes

NX	Regional lymph nodes cannot be assessed
N0	No regional lymph node metastasis
N1	Regional lymph node metastasis

M – Distant Metastasis

M0	No distant metastasis
M1	Distant metastasis

Stage grouping[b]

Stage 0	Tis	N0	M0
Stage I	T1	N0	M0
Stage II	T2	N0	M0
Stage III	T3	N0	M0
	T1, T2, T3	N1	M0
Stage IVA	T4	Any N	M0
Stage IVB	Any T	Any N	M1

References

American Joint Committee on Cancer (AJCC) Cancer Staging Manual, 7th ed. (2011) Edge SB, Byrd DR, Compton CC, Fritz AG, Greene FL, Trotti III eds. Springer: New York

International Union against Cancer (UICC): TNM Classification of Malignant Tumours, 7th ed. (2009) Sobin LH, Gospodarowicz MK, Wittekind Ch eds. Wiley-Blackwell: Oxford

A help-desk for specific questions about the TNM classification is available at http://www.uicc.org.

Epithelial tumours

A.S. Ferenczy
T.J. Colgan
C.S. Herrington
L. Hirschowitz
T. Loening

K.J. Park
M. Stoler
M. Wells
D.C. Wilbur
T. Wright

Squamous cell tumours and precursors

Low-grade squamous intraepithelial lesion

Definition
An intraepithelial lesion of squamous epithelium that is the morphological manifestation of productive HPV infection. Low-grade refers to the low risk of concurrent or future cancer. See cervical low-grade squamous intraepithelial lesion (LSIL), p. 172, for further discussion.

ICD-O code   8077/0

Synonyms
Vaginal intraepithelial neoplasia grade 1 (VaIN-1); mild squamous dysplasia; flat condyloma; koilocytotic atypia; koilocytosis

Epidemiology
The exact prevalence of vaginal squamous intraepithelial lesion (SIL) is not known. The mean age of LSIL is similar to that observed for cervical LSIL {132,940}.

Etiology
LSIL is associated with both low and high-risk HPV types {1818}. It is the morphological manifestation of a productive, transient HPV infection and therefore tends to regress {1818}. The vaginal squamous epithelium is identical to the mature squamous ectocervical epithelium but may have fewer micro-openings. These are necessary for access to the basement membrane where the preferential binding of HPV takes place, before infecting the basal cells of vaginal (or cervical) epithelium {932}. This may explain why vaginal SIL is less common than cervical SIL.
Women exposed to diethylstilbestrol (DES) in-utero may have extensive vaginal transformation zones which provide access for HPV infection, although the majority of vaginal SIL is low-grade {1598} in these women.

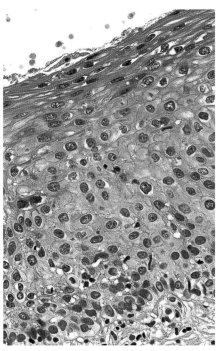

Fig. 8.01 Low-grade squamous intraepithelial lesion (VaIN-1). Flat-surfaced lesion in which the lower third of the epithelium contains a distinct basal cell layer, whereas the upper third is occupied by occasional cells with double nucleation, koilocytes and surface parakeratosis.

Clinical features
LSIL is usually asymptomatic and not detectable with the naked eye.

Macroscopy
Most vaginal SILs, including low-grade lesions, tend to be located in the upper third of the vagina and are only visible at colposcopy after the application of 3–5% acetic acid or half-strength Lugol's iodine solution. Unlike cervical SIL, vaginal SIL is often multifocal and multicentric, i.e. associated with cervical SIL and, less often, with high-grade vulvar SIL (VIN 2/3).

Histopathology
The use of a two-tier grading system is similar to that of the cervix, namely low-grade and high-grade SIL with corresponding modifiers; VaIN-1 for low-grade {1771} and VaIN-2/3 for high-grade lesions. The criteria are identical to the cervix (see cervical LSIL, p. 172).

Prognosis and predictive factors
LSIL typically regresses although it may progress to HSIL (VaIN-2/3), particularly if associated with high-risk HPV infection.

High-grade squamous intraepithelial lesion

Definition
A squamous intraepithelial lesion that carries a significant clinical risk of invasive cancer development if not treated {412,1586}. See cervical high-grade squamous intraepithelial lesion (HSIL), p. 174, for further discussion of HSIL.

ICD-O code   8077/2

Synonyms
Vaginal intraepithelial neoplasia grade 2 (VaIN-2); VaIN-3; moderate squamous dysplasia; severe squamous dysplasia; squamous carcinoma in situ

Epidemiology
About one-third of women with HSIL (VaIN-2/3) have a history of previous cervical HSIL (CIN-2/3) {1073}.

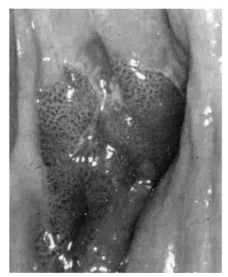

Fig. 8.02 Colposcopy of HSIL (VaIN-3). Sharply demarcated, slightly elevated, single, reddish lesion with prominent vascular punctation.

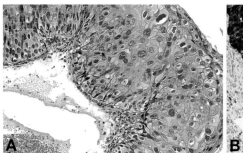
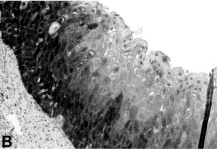
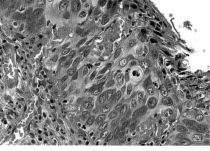

Fig. 8.03 High-grade squamous intraepithelial lesion (VaIN-2). **A** Atypical cells with pleomorphic nuclei and abnormal mitotic figures involve the lower half of the epithelium. The upper half contains koilocytes with perinuclear halos. **B** Strong and diffuse, block-type positivity for p16 is consistent with an HSIL.

Fig. 8.04 High-grade squamous intraepithelial lesion (VaIN-3). Transepithelial involvement by neoplastic, basaloid cells with several mitotic figures in the upper epithelium.

Etiology

HSIL (VaIN-3) is associated with high-risk HPV types {1818}. It is the morphological manifestation of a transforming type infection and therefore has greater potential to progress to invasive carcinoma than LSIL (VaIN-1) {1818}. HSIL (VaIN-2) is a heterogeneous lesion, similar to HSIL (CIN 2) (see cervical HSIL, p. 174).

Clinical features

HSIL (VaIN-2/3) is usually asymptomatic and not detectable with the naked eye.

Macroscopy

Most vaginal squamous intraepithelial lesions, including HSIL (VaIN-2/3), tend to be located in the upper third of the vagina and are only visible at colposcopy after the application of 3–5% acetic acid or half-strength Lugol's iodine solution. Unlike cervical SIL, vaginal SIL is often multifocal and multicentric, i.e. associated with cervical SIL and, less often, with high-grade vulvar SIL (VIN 2/3).

Histopathology

HSIL (VaIN-2) and HSIL (VaIN-3) show the same cellular alterations and p16 immunoprofile as their cervical counterparts (see cervical HSIL, p. 174).

Prognosis and predictive factors

Localized HSIL (VaIN-3) responds well to ablative or excisional procedures {1851}. Extensive, multifocal disease needs multiple ablational treatments with or without intravaginal 5-Fluorouracil chemotherapy or 5% imiquimod cream {2047}. Vaginectomy is reserved as a last treatment resort. The risk of progression of vaginal HSIL (VaIN-3) to invasion in immunocompetent patients is about 5%, significantly lower than that of cervical HSIL (CIN-3) {1775}.

Squamous cell carcinoma

Definition

An invasive epithelial tumour composed of squamous cells of varying degrees of differentiation without pre-existent cervical and/or vulvar carcinoma and no history of invasive squamous cell carcinomas of the cervix and/or vulva diagnosed for 10 years or more preceding the diagnosis of vaginal squamous cell carcinoma {2056}. See cervical squamous cell carcinoma (p. 176) for further discussion of HPV-associated squamous cell carcinoma.

ICD-O codes

Squamous cell carcinoma, NOS	8070/3
Keratinizing	8071/3
Non-keratinizing	8072/3
Papillary	8052/3
Basaloid	8083/3
Warty	8051/3
Verrucous	8051/3

Synonym

Epidermoid carcinoma

Epidemiology

Vaginal squamous cell carcinoma is rare {2056}. The age-adjusted incidence rate between 1998 and 2003 was 0.69/100 000 women (a figure so low that screening is impractical) and over 70% were diagnosed in women over 50 years of age with a median age of 68 years versus 58 years for high-grade intraepithelial lesion (VaIN-3). Squamous cell carcinoma (SCC) is the most common invasive malignancy of the vagina and the age-adjusted incidence is 72% higher in black than in white women {2056}.

Etiology

The majority of vaginal SCCs of all histological types are associated with high risk HPV {547,2056}. Similar to the vulva, an alternative HPV-negative pathway may exist especially in the lower vagina {36}. HPV-positive SCCs may have non-keratinizing, basaloid, squamotransitional or warty histology, are associated with HSIL (VaIN 2/3) and are p16 immunopositive. See p. 176 and p. 234.

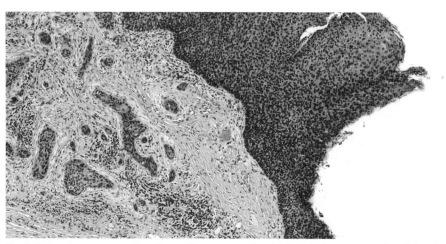

Fig. 8.05 Invasive squamous cell carcinoma. There are several nests of neoplastic squamous cells with irregular contours in the stroma beneath HSIL (VaIN-3).

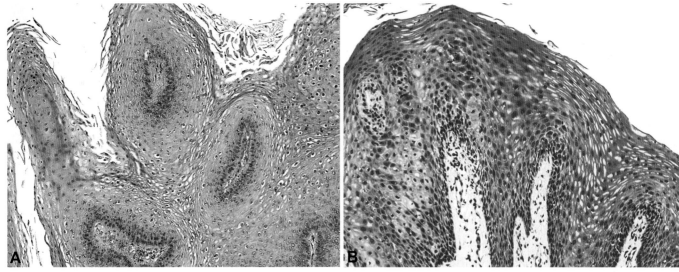

Fig. 8.06 A Condyloma acuminatum. Squamous papillary structures composed of stratified epithelium with surface parakeratosis and occasional koilocytes, supported by central fibrovascular stroma. B Squamous papilloma. Acanthotic epithelium with parakeratosis and elongated, non-anastomosing rete pegs without koilocytosis.

Clinical features

Most patients report painless vaginal bleeding (70%), dyspareunia or unusual vaginal discharge. Most vaginal SCCs are located in the posterior wall and upper third of the vagina. Tumours in the upper half of the vagina may give rise to pelvic node metastases as do cervical cancers whereas those arising in the lower half spread to the inguinofemoral nodes as do vulvar SCCs.

Macroscopy

Vaginal SCCs often display an ulcerated surface, exophytic growth and, less frequently, a constrictive, endophytic growth pattern.

Histopathology

The most frequent histological type is moderately differentiated, non-keratinizing, usual type squamous cell carcinoma. Rarely, it may be discovered at a superficially invasive stage, and lymph node metastasis is unlikely if no lymphovascular invasion is seen {1494}. Other variants include papillary (squamotransitional), basaloid, verrucous and warty (condylomatous) squamous cell carcinomas {1472}.

Prognosis and predictive factors

These depend on the FIGO/TNM stage, size, age and histotype of the tumour. In 314 patients, the overall 5-year survival rate was 45% with a 6-year follow-up whereas patients with stage I disease

had a 75% 5-year survival {735}. The three independent prognostic factors in the multivariate analysis in this study that predicted poor survival were old-age, tumour size (> 4 cm) and advanced stage (rectovaginal and inguinal node metastases) {735}. Several studies showed statistically better disease-free and overall survival rates in women with HPV-positive compared to HPV-negative SCCs that were independent of age and clinical stage {36}. Patients with verrucous carcinoma have excellent survival rates; lymph node metastasis after complete excision is rarely seen. The survival rates for the other variants of squamous cell carcinoma are not well known due to their rare occurrence, but are better than the usual type according to the limited experience available {36}. It is anticipated that with increasing use of prophylactic HPV vaccines, the incidence of HPV-related vaginal cancers will be greatly reduced {855}.

Benign squamous lesions

Condyloma acuminatum

Definition

A papillary, squamoproliferative lesion with HPV-associated koilocytosis supported by a fibrovascular stroma.

Synonyms

Vaginal wart; acuminate condyloma

Epidemiology

Vaginal condylomata are common, particularly in young women {1499}. Immunosuppressed patients are at high risk for developing anogenital/vaginal warts.

Etiology

Condyloma acuminatum is caused by HPV types 6/11. Infections with other HPV types may occur, particularly in immunosuppressed patients {148, 541}.

Macroscopy

Cauliflower-like lesions with verrucous surfaces are usually seen.

Histopathology

Papillary projections with club-shaped rete pegs merge towards "feeding" blood vessels. The epithelium displays features of productive HPV infection, in contrast to vestibular papillomatosis {564}. Condylomata are considered a variant of low-grade squamous intraepithelial lesion (see cervix chapter, p. 172).

Prognosis and predictive factors

Most resolve spontaneously or respond to topical chemotherapy or ablation {482}. Vaginal condylomata may be the source of juvenile recurrent respiratory papillomatosis in infants and young children delivered vaginally, yet molecular data are controversial for vertical HPV transmission {1036,1800}.

Squamous papilloma

Definition
Papillary lesion covered by normal to acanthotic squamous epithelium.

ICD-O code   8052/0

Synonyms
Squamous papillomatosis; micropapillomatosis vaginalis; vestibular papillomatosis

Clinical features
It may be associated with pruritus, burning and vaginal discharge.

Macroscopy
There are two variants. The most frequent form consists of multiple epithelial projections (micropapillomatosis). The other is a single papilloma, bearing multiple, grossly visible papillae on a single fibrovascular base. Lesions are localized or diffusely extend to the inner aspect of labia minora.

Histopathology
Epithelial papillae with parakeratosis and without koilocytosis are seen.

Histogenesis
This is a variant of physiological epithelium of the vagina and labia minora, not due to HPV infection. However, it may carry latent HPV detectable by molecular testing {137}.

Fibroepithelial polyp

Definition
Prominent central, fibrovascular tissue core covered by stratified squamous epithelium.

Synonyms
Mesodermal stromal polyp; pseudosarcoma botryoides (not recommended)

Epidemiology
These rare tumours are most frequent in women with a median age of 35 years {1396}. One-third are found during pregnancy.

Macroscopy
The tumours are single, pedunculated, smooth-surfaced, polypoid lesions often located on the lateral wall in the lower one-third of the vagina.

Histopathology
Fibrovascular tissue cores are covered by benign squamous epithelium. A variant has a hypercellular stroma with > 10 mitoses per 10 HPF with occasional abnormal forms and scattered with bizarre, stellate fibroblastic and multinucleated stromal ("fleurette") cells. This lesion may be confused with sarcoma botryoides (see vulva chapter, p. 248) {1396}.

Histogenesis
The polyp arises from focal polypoid hyperplasia of the so-called subepithelial stromal stellate cell layer that extends from the cervix to the vulva in adult women {495}.

Prognosis and predictive factors
The lesion has a benign clinical outcome including the hypercellular stromal variant with high mitotic activity.

Tubulosquamous polyp

Definition
Benign lesion composed of squamous epithelial and tubular structures set in a fibrovascular stroma.

ICD-O code   8560/0

Synonyms
Ectopic prostatic tissue; Skene duct cyst

Epidemiology
This is a rare entity. The polypoid variant occurs in postmenopausal women, whereas the cystic type is seen in premenopausal women {900}.

Clinical features
The polypoid type arises in the upper vagina. The cystic, single variant involves the lower vagina around the urethral ostium {900,1834}.

Macroscopy
In 50% of cases the polyps are solid or cystic, respectively.

Histopathology
Upper vaginal lesions contain solid squamous nests with central, microcystic areas and anastomosing cores of basaloid cells {1834}. Those in the lower vagina are cystic, lined by mucin-secreting glandular cells with central islands of squamous metaplasia. The glandular epithe-

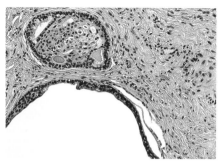

Fig. 8.07 Tubulosquamous polyp. These lesions contain cysts lined by mucinous epithelium and frequently exhibit central islands of squamous cells.

lium expresses prostate-specific antigen (PSA) and sometimes prostatic acid phosphatase (PrAP) {900,1834}.

Histogenesis
The lesion may arise from embryologically misplaced (upper vagina) or eutopic (lower vagina) Skene glands, the female counterpart of the prostate gland in males.

Prognosis and predictive factors
The clinical course after local excision is benign. Prostatic-type adenocarcinomas or Skene gland adenocarcinomas have rarely been reported {2150}.

Transitional cell metaplasia

Definition
Vaginal surface epithelium resembling transitional urothelium.

Epidemiology
The lesion is mainly seen in the elderly.

Histopathology
This entity should be distinguished from HSIL (VaIN-3) using p16 immunostaining (positive in HSIL) in equivocal cases {2016}.

Glandular tumours

Endometrioid carcinoma

Definition
An adenocarcinoma with the same histological features as those seen in the endometrium.

ICD-O code   8380/3

Epidemiology
Rare, anecdotal cases have been associated with adenosis of tubulo-endometrial type in women with history of in-utero diethylstilbestrol (DES) exposure while others were associated with vaginal endometriosis {718}.

Clear cell carcinoma

Definition
Malignant, glandular tumour composed of cells with clear cytoplasm with or without hobnail cells, growing in tubulocystic, papillary or solid patterns.

ICD-O code   8310/3

Synonym
Mesonephroma (not recommended)

Epidemiology
An increased risk of clear cell carcinoma has been observed in diethylstilbestrol (DES)-exposed offspring with a maternal history of spontaneous abortion {1991}. Prior to the use of DES, clear cell carcinoma of the vagina was almost never reported. Endogenous estrogens are also suspected to be a risk factor as most clear cell carcinomas are detected between puberty and 10 years thereafter. By 1999, 700 cases were recorded in the Registry for Research on Hormonal Transplacental Carcinogenesis {744}. These tumours had a bimodal age distribution, the first peak occurring at a mean age of 26 years. Two-thirds of these cases were vaginal whereas the second peak occurred at a mean age of 31 years and two-thirds of these women had cervical involvement {744}. The cancer risk in women < 24 years ranged between 0.014–0.14% as per the registry data {743}. The absolute risk was estimated to be 1:1000. Since the discontinuation of using DES to prevent abortions (particularly in the second trimester), the incidence of both cervical and vaginal clear cell carcinomas has markedly declined.

Etiology
About two-thirds of clear cell carcinomas occur before age 40 years and have been associated with transplacental DES exposure {745}. The relatively low frequency of clear cell carcinoma in female DES-exposed offspring suggests that DES is an incomplete carcinogen {745}.

Clinical features
The age distribution ranged from 6–42 years with a peak between 19 and 26 years. The majority were younger than 30 years old as per the registry data. Symptomatic patients had abnormal vaginal bleeding with or without excessive vaginal discharge; others were asymptomatic and were detected at pelvic examination or occasionally with screening cytology {745}. About two-thirds of clear cell carcinomas were confined to the vagina and most were located on the anterior wall of the upper third of the vagina.

Macroscopy
Most are exophytic, polypoid, nodular or papillary; some may be ulcerated or plaque-like lesions.

Histopathology
The growth and cytological patterns are similar to tumours in the cervix, endometrium and ovary. Vaginal clear cell carcinomas however, tend to be of the tubulocystic type and many of the lining cells are hobnail cells. Typically, mitotic activity is low and intracytoplasmic, hyaline bodies as well as psammoma bodies are often encountered.

Prognosis and predictive factors
Recurrence occurs in about 25% of cases of which one-third of cases occurs in the lungs and scalene lymph nodes following surgery and/or radiotherapy {1991}. Metastasis to pelvic lymph nodes occurs in 5% of patients with FIGO stage I disease and less than 3 mm stromal invasion. The rate is 16% overall with FIGO stage I lesions and the risk increases significantly if stromal invasion is greater than 3 mm. Positive nodes are reported in 50% of patients with stage II disease. Nevertheless, the overall survival rate of all stages is 80%, and 87% at 10 years with stage I lesions. Favourable prognosis is seen in women aged > 19 years, small-size lesions, minimal stromal invasion, a tubulocystic pattern, and asymptomatic at diagnosis.

Mucinous carcinoma

Definition
Malignant invasive glandular tumour of either endocervical or intestinal type, similar to those found in the cervix.

ICD-O code   8480/3

Synonym
Adenocarcinoma, NOS

Epidemiology
The incidence of non-clear cell adenocarcinoma is less than 10% of all vaginal cancers and this tumour is therefore extremely rare (incidence < 1/1'000'000) {1957}.

Clinical features
May present with vaginal discharge, bleeding, or be asymptomatic and discovered by screening cervical cytology.

Macroscopy
Tumours show exophytic, ulcerated growth, most commonly located on the anterior wall of the upper vagina.

Histopathology
A glandular tumour with either endocervical mucinous or intestinal type cells including goblet cells. It must be distinguished from metastatic adenocarcinoma of endocervical or gastrointestinal tract origin by clinical, pathological and immunohistochemical correlations.

Histogenesis
The histogenesis is not known; however, the intestinal variant may arise from cloacal remnants {1859}. Its relationship to HPV infection is unknown.

Prognosis and predictive factors
Because of the rarity of this tumour, prognosis is difficult to assess.

Mesonephric carcinoma

Definition
Tumours formed of tubules, lined by malignant cuboidal to columnar cells resembling those seen in mesonephric duct remnants.

ICD-O code   9110/3

Synonym
Mesonephroma (not recommended)

Epidemiology
Only rare examples have been reported {757}.

Clinical features
Vaginal bleeding and palpable lesions have been reported in the lateral wall of vagina.

Macroscopy
The tumours are mostly solid, nodular lesions.

Histopathology
The tumours show a mainly well differentiated tubular growth pattern. The neoplastic cells, resembling those of mesonephric remnants, are mitotically active and, unlike clear cell carcinoma, lack intracytoplasmic glycogen, clear cytoplasm and hobnail type cells. The tubules have a sharply defined PAS-positive basement membrane. Mesonephric adenocarcinomas are uniformly reactive for cytokeratin and epithelial membrane antigen, and often express calretinin, vimentin and CD10 (apical and luminal). They are typically negative for estrogen and progesterone receptors and CEA. They may express PAX8, TTF1 and p16 focally (see cervix chapter).

Histogenesis
They are thought to develop from mesonephric duct remnants via mesonephric hyperplasia, although their precise histogenesis is uncertain.

Prognosis and predictive factors
The rarity of mesonephric carcinoma precludes assessment of its clinical outcome.

Benign glandular lesions

Tubovillous and villous adenomas

Definition
Polyps that resemble colorectal adenomas.

ICD-O codes
Tubovillous adenoma   8263/0
Villous adenoma   8261/0

Synonyms
Adenomatous polyp; villous polyp

Epidemiology
Eight cases have been reported, most in women older than 40 years {1486}. They are not related to HPV {1486}.

Macroscopy
A polypoid growth near the introitus. Most measure less than 5 cm in diameter.

Histopathology
The lesions are identical to colonic adenomas with tubular, tubulovillous or villous growth patterns {1486}.

Histogenesis
The polyps may develop from misplaced intestinal, cloacal, urothelial or Müllerian (adenosis) epithelium.

Genetic profile
One case of congenital renal agenesis (Arnold-Chiari type II malformation) and another case without mutation in the KRAS, BRAF or LKB1/STK11 genes have been reported {1486}.

Prognosis and predictive factors
Two of eight cases were associated with invasive intestinal type adenocarcinoma and one with intraepithelial "dysplasia" {473,1486}.

Müllerian papilloma

Definition
Papilloma lined by Müllerian-type cuboidal or mucinous epithelium.

Epidemiology
The lesions are rare. Most occur in infants and young girls {1222}.

Clinical features
They may be associated with mucoid discharge or bleeding.

Macroscopy
The papillomas are of variable size.

Histopathology
Fibrovascular papillae covered by cuboidal, mucin-secreting cells and rarely, hobnail cells are seen (see cervix chapter, p. 189).

Histogenesis
The lesions have a Müllerian origin {1222}.

Prognosis and predictive factors
Two reported cases recurred; one was incompletely excised and the other had features resembling a low-grade ovarian tumour {464}.

Adenosis

Definition
This is defined as the presence of glandular structure(s) in the vagina.

Synonym
Adenomatosis vaginae

Epidemiology
After 1971, vaginal adenosis (VA) was found in 30% of offspring exposed to diethylstilbestrol (DES) in-utero {746} as opposed to 8% in the non-exposed population {1006}.

Macroscopy
Vaginal adenosis may or may not be visible to the naked eye. It can be accompanied by a transverse vaginal septum and obliterated vaginal fornices in the upper third of vagina in DES-exposed women {1399}.

Histopathology
Glands are of endocervical (upper vagina) or tubo-endometrial type (lower half). Rarely, these are cuboidal embryonic type cells (at the squamous epithelial-stromal interface) with little cytoplasm.

Histogenesis
DES administered before the 21st week of gestation inhibits normal upward migration of squamous epithelium and the pre-existing Müllerian epithelium develops into adenosis. Rarely, vaginal

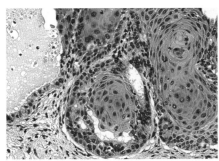
Fig. 8.08 Vaginal adenosis. Endocervical-type glands partially obliterated by immature squamous metaplastic epithelium.

adenosis occurs as a congenital anomaly due to endogenous estrogenic influence on normal epithelial development {1597}. It can also follow extensive epithelial denudation by intravaginal 5-FU cream therapy or CO_2 laser vapourization for condylomatosis {1721}.

Prognosis and predictive factors
Vaginal adenosis is obliterated by squamous metaplasia and needs no special treatment(s). Atypical tubo-endometrial vaginal adenosis is the precursor of clear cell carcinoma and needs long-term follow-up {1605}.

Endometriosis

Definition
The presence of endometrial stroma with or without endometrial type glands.

Clinical features
Occasionally, patients have vaginal spotting.

Macroscopy
Red or blue spots or cysts are seen, most frequently in the upper half of the vagina.

Histopathology
The lesion appears as endometrial tissue in the vaginal wall. During pregnancy, the glands may display an Arias-Stella reaction and simulate clear cell adenocarcinoma {1005}.

Histogenesis
The lesion results from endometrial tissue "implanted" in a previously denuded vagina or from Müllerian vestiges in the rectovaginal septum.

Prognosis and predictive factors
Local excision provides cure in most cases. It rarely gives rise to endometrioid adenocarcinoma {718}.

Endocervicosis

Definition
Endocervical glands in the vaginal wall.

Epidemiology
This is a rare lesion in the vagina {1226}.

Clinical features
These include pain and palpable vaginal nodules following hysterectomy.

Macroscopy
Tumour-like nodules can be seen on macroscopy.

Histopathology
Deeply located, cytologically benign endocervical-type glands are seen.

Histogenesis
The lesion results from displaced endocervical tissue during hysterectomy or from Müllerian vestiges.

Prognosis and predictive factors
A case of mucinous adenocarcinoma arising from endocervicosis has been reported {1226}.

Cysts

Definition
Subepithelial cystic structures lined by squamous, endocervical, mesonephric or transitional epithelium.

Synonyms
Inclusion cysts; Müllerian cysts; Gartner duct cysts; urothelial cysts {446}

Epidemiology
The most common variant is the squamous epithelial inclusion cyst.

Macroscopy
Single, simple cysts distended by serous or mucinous fluid are seen.

Histopathology
Squamous inclusion cysts are lined by stratified squamous epithelium, and the Müllerian variant by endocervical and tubo-endometrial type cells. Mesonephric cysts are lined by cuboidal cells which express calretinin. Urothelial cysts are lined by transitional epithelium.

Histogenesis
Squamous epithelial inclusion cysts, Müllerian and suburothelial cysts develop by invagination of surface epithelium after trauma. Mesonephric cysts derive from dilatation of the mesonephric (Gartner's) duct.

Prognosis and predictive factors
Simple excision of symptomatic cysts is curative.

Other epithelial tumours

Mixed tumour

Definition
A tumour composed of an admixture of benign epithelial and stromal cells.

ICD-O code   8940/0

Synonyms
Spindle cell epithelioma; benign mixed Müllerian tumour

Epidemiology
Up to 2003, only 50 cases had been reported in the English literature {1318, 1421}.

Clinical features
Most cases are asymptomatic and located near the hymenal ring.

Macroscopy
The tumours are circumscribed and measure 1.5–5.0 cm.

Histopathology
Vaginal mixed tumours should be distinguished from carcinosarcoma and the malignant tumour resembling synovial sarcoma, possibly using molecular studies. Both occur in the upper part of the vagina, contain cytonuclear atypia, mitotic figures and lack squamous metaplasia {1421}.

Histogenesis
A urogenital sinus-derived epithelial origin has been suggested {1421}. Using immunohistochemistry, tumours co-express epithelial and mesenchymal cell markers indicating a totipotential cell origin {1421}. The strong co-expression by the spindle cell component of CK-7 as well as CD10, Bcl-2, and ER/PR may favour a Müllerian derivation {1318}.

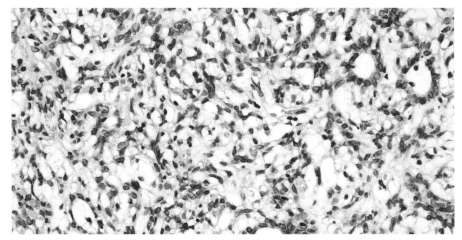

Fig. 8.09 Vaginal mixed tumour, which arose at the introitus. Both epithelial and stromal elements are present.

Prognosis and predictive factors
The tumours have a benign clinical course after complete local surgical excision {1318}.

Adenosquamous carcinoma

Definition
A malignant, epithelial tumour comprising both adenocarcinoma and squamous cell carcinoma.

ICD-O code   8560/3

Synonyms
Mixed adeno- and squamous cell carcinoma; adenocarcinoma with squamous differentiation

Epidemiology
Among 244 primary vaginal carcinomas, six (2.4%) were adenosquamous {1859}.

Clinical features
They are most commonly located on the anterior part of the vagina.

Histopathology
The histopathology is similar to cervical adenosquamous carcinoma. Some lesions may represent mucoepidermoid carcinomas and these harbour the *CRTC1-MAML2* fusion gene typical for these tumours {1074} (see cervix, p. 194).

Histogenesis
They may develop from pre-existing tuboendometrial adenosis or endometriosis or from minor vestibular glands or misplaced Bartholin glands. A cloacogenic origin has also been suggested {1859}.

Prognosis and predictive factors
The tumours are mainly locally aggressive with occasional pulmonary metastasis {1859}.

Adenoid basal carcinoma

Definition
A tumour composed of nests of peripherally located, basaloid cells with central glandular and squamous cell differentiation.

ICD-O code   8098/3

Synonyms
Adenoid basal cell tumour; adenoid basal epithelioma

Epidemiology
Rare case reports have been published {1336}.

High-grade neuroendocrine carcinoma

Definition
A high-grade, malignant, neuroendocrine tumour similar to those seen in lung or cervix.

ICD-O codes
Small cell neuroendocrine carcinoma
                                8041/3
Large cell neuroendocrine carcinoma
                                8013/3

Synonyms
For small cell neuroendocrine carcinoma: small cell carcinoma; oat cell carcinoma; neuroendocrine carcinoma, small cell type, grade 3;
For large cell neuroendocrine carcinoma: neuroendocrine carcinoma, large cell type, grade 3

Epidemiology
Up to 2004, 25 cases had appeared in the English literature {153}.

Clinical features
Most patients present with advanced FIGO stage disease, with bleeding, pelvic/back pain and dysuria.

Macroscopy
The tumours are usually ulcerated, 0.5–10 cm, exophytic or endophytic and found along the vaginal cavity.

Histopathology
The tumour has the same morphology and immunohistochemical profile as its cervical counterpart {153} (see cervix chapter, p. 197). Although other grades and types of neuroendocrine neoplasia in the vagina are theoretically possible, their occurrence is exceedingly rare.

Prognosis and predictive factors
Most patients die of disease (81%) within two years of diagnosis {153}.

Mesenchymal tumours

M.R. Nucci   G.P. Nielsen
W.G. McCluggage   E. Oliva

Leiomyoma

Definition
A benign mesenchymal neoplasm showing smooth muscle differentiation.

ICD-O code   8890/0

Epidemiology
It is the most common mesenchymal tumour of the vagina, although fewer than 300 cases have been reported.

Clinical features
Leiomyomas usually arise between the ages of 38–48 years {807} but can affect a wide age group. Depending on the size of the tumour, they may cause pain, bleeding, dyspareunia, urinary or rectal symptoms {807}. They may be hormonally dependent and recur during pregnancy {1659}.

Macroscopy
Most tumours are 3–4 cm in diameter and have a firm, solid or cystic cut surface.

Histopathology
Most have the typical features of a leiomyoma as seen elsewhere in the female reproductive organs, being composed of spindle-shaped cells demonstrating smooth muscle differentiation histologically or immunohistochemically. Variants of leiomyoma can also occur such as epithelioid leiomyoma and leiomyoma with bizarre nuclei {150,1907} and the possibility of a smooth muscle tumour should always be considered when dealing with an unusual mesenchymal tumour of the vagina.

Histogenesis
The tumours are derived from smooth muscle.

Prognosis and predictive factors
A benign tumour treated by local excision. Large tumours can recur.

Rhabdomyoma

Definition
Rhabdomyoma is a benign tumour exhibiting well-developed, skeletal muscle differentiation.

ICD-O code   8905/0

Synonym
Genital rhabdomyoma

Epidemiology
This is a rare tumour that most commonly occurs in the vagina, but may involve the cervix or vulva.

Clinical features
This tumour typically occurs in middle aged women with a median age of 42 years {257,705,822}. Symptoms can include dyspareunia and bleeding.

Macroscopy
This is typically a solitary polypoid or nodular lesion, usually less than 3 cm. It can be rubbery, with a grey, glistening cut surface.

Histopathology
It is characterized by a submucosal proliferation of spindle or strap-shaped cells arranged in a somewhat fascicular, but often haphazard, pattern. The tumour cells have abundant eosinophilic cytoplasm with distinct cross striations. Mitoses and nuclear pleomorphism are absent. The cells are positive for desmin and markers of skeletal muscle differentiation, such as myogenin and myoD1.

Prognosis and predictive factors
This tumour is benign and has an excellent prognosis. No recurrences have been reported.

Leiomyosarcoma

Definition
Malignant mesenchymal neoplasm showing smooth muscle differentiation.

ICD-O code   8890/3

Epidemiology
Leiomyosarcoma is the most common sarcoma of the vagina in adults although < 200 cases have been reported, comprising less than 2% of all malignant tumours of the vagina.

Clinical features
The age range is 22–86 years; most women are between the ages of 40–49 years {19,1343,1858}. Patients typically present with an enlarging mass, vaginal or rectal bleeding, dyspareunia, or urinary tract symptoms. The tumour most commonly arises in the posterior wall,

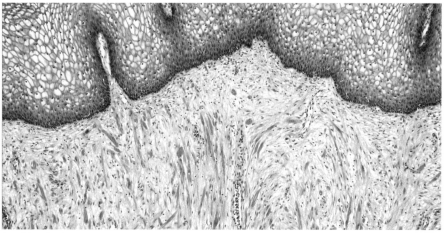

Fig. 8.10 Rhabdomyoma. Vaguely fascicular, haphazardly arranged, rhabdomyoblasts with abundant eosinophilic cytoplasmic processes are present within the submucosa.

followed by the anterior and lateral walls {19}. The overlying vaginal squamous mucosa may be intact or ulcerated.

Macroscopy
There are no specific gross features. The cut surface has a pink-grey, fleshy appearance often with areas of haemorrhage and necrosis.

Histopathology
Most are of the usual spindle cell type, similar in appearance to their uterine counterpart, although they can also be myxoid or epithelioid. Tumours that are greater than 3 cm, with significant cytological atypia and > 5 mitoses per 10 HPF, should be regarded as malignant; infiltrative margins are also associated with malignant behaviour {1907}.

Histogenesis
These tumours are derived from smooth muscle.

Prognosis and predictive factors
These are aggressive neoplasms that frequently recur locally and metastasize {396,1343}.

Rhabdomyosarcoma

Definition
A malignant tumour exhibiting skeletal (striated) muscle differentiation. This may be of embryonal, alveolar or pleomorphic subtype.

ICD-O code
Rhabdomyosarcoma, NOS 8900/3
Embryonal rhabdomyosarcoma 8910/3

Synonym
Sarcoma botryoides (embryonal subtype)

Epidemiology
Embryonal rhabdomyosarcoma is the most common vaginal sarcoma, the other subtypes being extremely rare.

Clinical features
Approximately 90% of embryonal rhabdomyosarcomas occur in infants and children < 5 years of age (mean 1.8 years) {50,51,727}. Rare examples occur in young adults. Presentation is usually with a vaginal mass which may protrude through the introitus. Symptoms related to this, such as vaginal bleeding, may occur.

Macroscopy
These are polypoid lesions, which often form multiple polypoid projections, sometimes with a "grape-like" appearance. They may be covered by intact vaginal mucosa or the surface may be ulcerated. Some contain obvious areas of haemorrhage, necrosis, oedema or gelatinous change.

Histopathology
Embryonal rhabdomyosarcomas are usually polypoid lesions that are partially covered by squamous epithelium, which may be ulcerated. At low power, there may be areas of alternating cellularity. The neoplasm is composed of cells with round, ovoid or spindle-shaped nuclei and generally scanty cytoplasm. Some tumour cells may have abundant eosinophilic cytoplasm. Rhabdomyoblasts with a round or strap-like appearance and cytoplasmic cross striations may be found in small numbers but these are not identified in all cases. Often there is a cellular cambium layer composed of closely packed cells with small, hyperchromatic nuclei just beneath the surface squamous epithelium. Occasionally a few multinucleate giant cells are present. Especially towards the centre of the neoplasm, hypocellular myxoid or oedematous areas may be present. The mitotic index is often high and there may be extravasation of erythrocytes. Islands of hyaline cartilage are sometimes present but are seen less commonly than in cervical embryonal rhabdomyosarcomas (see p. 200).

The neoplastic cells are usually positive with desmin and exhibit nuclear staining with the skeletal muscle markers myogenin and myoD1.

Genetic susceptibility
A case has been reported in a child with multiple congenital abnormalities and bilateral renal nephroblastomas, suggesting a possible genetic defect {936}.

Prognosis and predictive factors
The prognosis of vaginal embryonal rhabdomyosarcoma in the past was poor but combination chemotherapy, radiation and/or surgery have resulted in cure rates of 90–95% {50,51,727}.

Undifferentiated sarcoma

Definition
A malignant mesenchymal tumour, usually high-grade, lacking specific differentiation.

ICD-O code
8805/3

Epidemiology
Sarcomas of the vagina represent approximately 2% of all soft-tissue sarcomas and undifferentiated sarcoma is extremely rare.

Etiology
Patients may have a prior history of radiation {1861}.

Clinical features
The tumour affects patients in a wide age range, but most often adults. Symptoms and signs are non-specific, but are typically related to a rapidly growing mass.

Macroscopy
The tumour is large and fleshy with areas of haemorrhage and necrosis.

Histopathology
The tumour cells have a storiform, fascicular or diffuse growth and are typically associated with infiltrative borders. The cells are spindle to stellate and show variable degrees of pleomorphism and brisk mitotic activity. This should be a diagnosis of exclusion after eliminating the also rare, but more often reported, carcinosarcoma, adenosarcoma with sarcomatous overgrowth, specific sarcomas, gastrointestinal stromal tumour, melanoma, or even a mixed tumour of the vagina if the cytological features of the tumour are low-grade {1493}.

Prognosis and predictive factors
Patients have a poor prognosis.

Angiomyofibroblastoma

Definition
This is a benign tumour composed of myofibroblasts and blood vessels.

ICD-O code
8826/0

Epidemiology
This is a relatively uncommon, soft-tissue tumour of the vagina {1353}.

Clinical features

This is a tumour of adult women occurring in the vulvovaginal region (see also vulva chapter, p. 245).

Macroscopy

Most are small, usually < 5 cm, and limited by a pseudocapsule. They typically have a rubbery, solid and tan cut surface.

Histopathology

They are well circumscribed lesions with alternating hyper- and hypocellular areas composed of polygonal epithelioid and small spindle cells that tend to be clustered around numerous thin-walled small to medium-sized capillary-like vessels. Cytological atypia is rare and mitoses are infrequent. The stroma has a loose texture and contains mast cells. The cells are positive for vimentin, desmin, estrogen and progesterone receptors. CD34 is negative. Aggressive angiomyxomas can rarely show areas with angiomyofibroblastoma-like features {663}.

Histogenesis

Angiomyofibroblastoma is believed to originate from mesenchymal cells that are capable of myofibroblastic differentiation {585,762}.

Prognosis and predictive factors

These are usually benign, non-recurrent tumours.

Aggressive angiomyxoma

Definition

A non-metastasizing, locally infiltrative, hypocellular, myxoid neoplasm with potential for destructive, local recurrence.

ICD-O code   8841/0

Synonym

Deep angiomyxoma

Epidemiology

This is a rare soft-tissue tumour of the pelvicoperineal region {118,553,1824}.

Clinical features

This tumour most commonly occurs in patients in their fourth decade. They typically present with a soft-tissue swelling that may be mistaken for a cyst on clinical examination.

Macroscopy

It typically has a glistening and gelatinous cut surface. Recurrent tumours may be more fibrous in appearance as they infiltrate through scar tissue.

Histopathology

Characteristically, this is a hypocellular, myxoid neoplasm with interspersed, and often evenly spaced, small to medium-sized vessels, which may be thick-walled and hyalinised. The myxoid matrix also contains wispy collagen and small collections of smooth muscle, which are more commonly located near the vasculature. The stromal cells are typically bland spindle-shaped cells with ovoid nuclei and delicate uni- to bipolar cytoplasmic processes. These tumours typically have deceptively infiltrative borders (See vulva chapter, p. 246).

The stromal cells are positive for actin and desmin, particularly in the myxoid bundles. There can be nuclear positivity for HMGA2.

Genetic profile

Rearrangement of 12q15 has been shown by cytogenetic analysis and FISH {1257,1394,1549,1564}.

Prognosis and predictive factors

These tumours have a propensity to recur, particularly if incompletely excised.

Myofibroblastoma

Definition

This is a benign, mesenchymal neoplasm which is most common in the vagina but also occurs in the cervix and vulva.

ICD-O code   8825/0

Synonyms

Superficial myofibroblastoma of the lower female genital tract; superficial cervicovaginal myofibroblastoma {602,1038,1835}

Epidemiology

This is an uncommon, benign soft-tissue lesion. Occasional cases have been associated with tamoxifen, raising the possibility of a hormonal association {602,1038,1835}.

Clinical features

These occur in premenopausal or postmenopausal women {602,1038,1835}. Presentation is usually with a polypoid or "cystic" lesion in the vagina or vulva. The lesion may be an incidental finding on gynaecological examination.

Macroscopy

These are usually < 5 cm in maximum dimension. They are solid lesions but there are no distinctive gross features.

Histopathology

These are well-circumscribed but unencapsulated lesions growing beneath unremarkable squamous epithelium. Deep to the surface epithelium, there is usually a Grenz zone. There are typically areas of alternating cellularity with cells containing bland ovoid, spindle or stellate-shaped nuclei, often with a somewhat wavy appearance, embedded in a finely collagenous stroma, sometimes with thicker collagen bundles. Multiple patterns, including lace-like, sieve-like and fascicular are frequently present, resulting in a heterogeneous appearance. There is often stromal oedema or myxoid change. Few or no mitoses are present.

Immunohistochemistry

The cells are usually positive with vimentin, desmin (highlights ramifying dendritic cell processes), ER and PR and sometimes CD34 and smooth muscle actin {602,1038,1835}. HMGA2 is negative {1212}. This is a non-specific immunophenotype which is identical to many other vulvovaginal mesenchymal lesions.

Histogenesis

These are thought to arise from the subepithelial hormone receptor-positive mesenchymal region which extends from the endocervix to the vagina.

Prognosis and predictive factors

These are benign lesions which are treated by local excision. Although they may occasionally recur locally, there have been no reports of metastasis or malignant transformation.

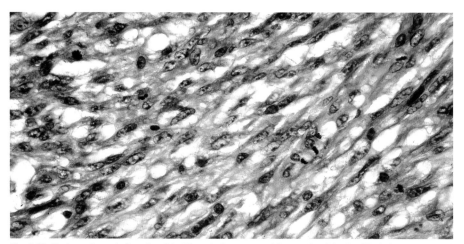

Fig. 8.11 Postoperative spindle cell nodule. These lesions are reminiscent of nodular fasciitis, being composed of spindled and stellate-shaped cells within an oedematous and inflamed stroma.

Tumour-like lesions

Postoperative spindle cell nodule

Definition
A benign non-neoplastic reactive lesion that resembles a sarcoma.

Synonym
Postoperative pseudosarcoma

Epidemiology
This is an uncommon lesion.

Clinical features
This lesion arises in young to middle-aged women {680,1530}. In the largest series, the patients ranged from 29–49 years of age. Three had a history of hysterectomy and one developed a postoperative spindle cell lesion eight weeks after an episiotomy {1530}.

It develops at the site of a prior operative procedure, usually within 3 months {1530}. Clinically and pathologically it can mimic a sarcoma. A history of a previous surgical procedure is helpful in making the correct diagnosis.

Macroscopy
The lesions can either be well- or poorly defined, measuring up to several centimetres in greatest diameter.

Histopathology
This lesion can be well- or poorly defined and is composed of intersecting fascicles of uniform, plump, spindle-shaped cells, a delicate network of small blood vessels and chronic inflammatory cells. The cells have abundant eosinophilic or amphophilic cytoplasm. Overlying ulceration is frequently present, associated with acute inflammation. Mitotic figures may be numerous. Oedema, haemorrhage and hemosiderin deposition may be present.

Histogenesis
The lesions presumably arise from myofibroblasts.

Prognosis and predictive factors
This is a benign lesion that can recur locally.

Mixed epithelial and mesenchymal tumours

M.R. Nucci   W.G. McCluggage
L. Hirschowitz   E. Oliva

Adenosarcoma

Definition
A biphasic tumour composed of benign or atypical epithelial cells of Müllerian type and a malignant, low-grade, mesenchymal component.

ICD-O code   8933/3

Epidemiology
This is an extremely rare tumour at this site {49,1109}.

Clinical features
Presentation is usually with a polypoid lesion in the vagina or symptoms such as vaginal bleeding. A history of endometriosis is common.

Macroscopy
These are polypoid tumours. Some examples contain cyst-like spaces or have a sponge-like cut surface.

Histopathology
Morphologically these are identical to their uterine counterparts {1207}. Occasional examples have arisen in endometriosis {49,1109}.

Prognosis and predictive factors
These are extremely rare and the behaviour is not well established.

Carcinosarcoma

Definition
Malignant biphasic tumour with a mixture of malignant epithelial and mesenchymal elements.

ICD-O code   8980/3

Synonyms
Malignant mixed mesodermal or Müllerian tumour; metaplastic carcinoma

Epidemiology
Fewer than 20 cases have been reported, most in post-menopausal patients (age range 48–75 years) {20,1757}. Because of the rarity of these tumours, no comprehensive epidemiological data are available.

Clinical features
Patients have a vaginal polyp/mass and may present with vaginal bleeding or discharge {20}. Prior pelvic irradiation has been reported in a few cases {1493}. Carcinosarcoma is not associated with tamoxifen or hormone replacement therapy {1338,1713,1757,1816}.

Macroscopy
The tumour is typically an ulcerated, polypoid mass 3–15 cm in diameter {1713}. Cut section reveals soft, fleshy tissue which may be partly necrotic.

Histopathology
The epithelial component (most often squamous carcinoma, followed by adenocarcinoma and anaplastic carcinoma) may arise from vaginal high-grade SIL (VaIN-3). Sarcomatous elements may be homologous (undifferentiated sarcoma) or heterologous (leiomyosarcoma, rhabdomyosarcoma, chondrosarcoma or osteosarcoma). Vaginal metastasis from another site in the female reproductive organs should always be excluded. *In situ* hybridization identified integrated high-risk HPV types 31/33/51 in both tumour components in one case {1713}.

Histogenesis
Carcinosarcomas are metaplastic carcinomas; the carcinomatous element drives the biphasic tumour growth {1202}.

Genetic profile
Unlike uterine carcinosarcomas, no *PIK-3CA, KRAS, CTNNB1* or *NRAS* mutations were identified in a single vaginal carcinosarcoma {673}.

Prognosis and predictive factors
Most patients present with stage I/II disease. The prognosis is poor with early, widespread metastasis and a 5-year survival of only 17% despite radical surgery and radiotherapy {1493}.

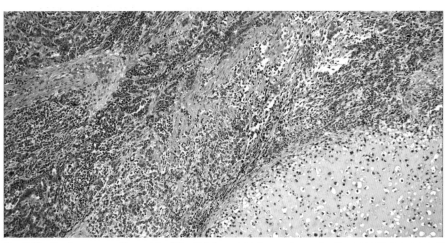

Fig. 8.12 Carcinosarcoma. The poorly differentiated carcinomatous component and sarcomatous component (chondrosarcoma) are intimately admixed but do not merge.

Lymphoid and myeloid tumours

J.A. Ferry

D. Cao
L. Hirschowitz

Lymphomas

Definition
Malignant neoplasms composed of lymphoid cells.

Epidemiology
Primary vaginal lymphoma is rare; secondary involvement of the vagina by lymphoma arising elsewhere is uncommon. Nearly all patients are adults, with a mean age in the fifth decade.

Clinical features
Patients present with vaginal bleeding, discharge, pain or a palpable mass {22, 1972}.

Macroscopy
Vaginal lymphomas typically take the form of induration of the vaginal wall, often with invasion of adjacent structures {1972}; extension to the pelvic side walls may occur {22,360}.

Histopathology
Nearly all primary lymphomas are diffuse large B-cell lymphomas. They are often associated with prominent sclerosis. The overlying epithelium is typically intact. Neoplastic cells sometimes have spindle cell morphology. Rare cases of follicular lymphoma {360,972}, Burkitt lymphoma, lymphoplasmacytic lymphoma {972}, marginal-zone lymphoma {2099} and B lymphoblastic lymphoma {549} have been reported. The majority of lymphomas secondarily involving the vagina are diffuse large B-cell lymphomas {1970} (see Table 1.3, p. 80).

Prognosis and predictive factors
Primary vaginal lymphoma usually presents with localized, although sometimes bulky, disease, and has a favourable prognosis. Secondary vaginal involvement in the setting of widespread lymphoma has a poor prognosis {22,360,972,1972}.

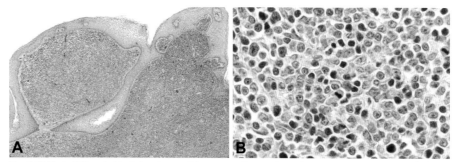

Fig. 8.13 Vaginal B lymphoblastic lymphoma. **A** Low-power shows a dense, lymphoid infiltrate filling the stroma, with intact surface epithelium. The surface has a vaguely papillary configuration; the lesion was thought to be a condyloma on physical examination. **B** High-power image shows medium-sized cells with irregular nuclei, fine chromatin, small nucleoli, scant cytoplasm and frequent mitoses.

Myeloid neoplasms

Definition
Myeloid neoplasms are defined as malignant neoplasms of haematopoietic origin, including myeloid leukaemias and myeloid sarcoma.

Synonyms
Myeloid sarcoma is also known as chloroma, granulocytic sarcoma or extramedullary myeloid tumour.

Epidemiology
Patients with acute myeloid leukaemia occasionally have vaginal involvement, but vaginal involvement by a discrete mass (myeloid sarcoma) is very uncommon. Vaginal myeloid sarcoma rarely occurs as an isolated finding or as the presenting sign of acute myeloid leukaemia. The vagina can be involved by myeloid sarcoma in women with a history of acute myeloid leukaemia {806,1419,1513,1794}.

Clinical features
Patients usually present with a mass.

Macroscopy
Myeloid sarcoma can form one or more lesions involving the vaginal wall or the recto-vaginal septum, impinging on the urethra, protruding into the lumen of the vagina or extending to adjacent structures {806,1419,1794}.

Histopathology
Similar to other sites (see ovary chapter for histopathology images, p. 79).

Genetic profile
Myeloid sarcoma with acute myeloid leukaemia with t(8;21)(q22;q22)(AML1-ETO) has been reported {806}.

Prognosis and predictive factors
Prognosis appears poor, with occasional long-term survival {806,1419,1794}.

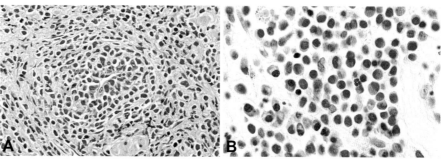

Fig. 8.14 Vaginal myeloid sarcoma. **A** Primitive cells with oval or irregular nuclei, fine chromatin and scant cytoplasm diffusely infiltrate the stroma and invade the wall of a small blood vessel. **B** The lesion contains blasts with scant cytoplasm and scattered cells with abundant bright red cytoplasm, indicating myeloid maturation.

Melanocytic tumours

D. Cao
L. Hirschowitz

Naevi

Definition
Melanocytic naevi result from the proliferation of nests of naevus cells. Blue naevus is a benign pigmented lesion derived from dermal melanocytes.

ICD-O codes
Melanocytic naevus	8720/0
Blue naevus	8780/0

Epidemiology
No well documented case of vaginal melanocytic naevus has been reported. Vaginal blue naevus is extremely rare with only six cases reported including one giant angiomatoid cellular blue naevus in the English literature {27,559}. The mean age of patients is 43 years (range 19–73 years).

Clinical features
Blue naevus is typically found during physical examination and does not present with specific symptoms. The lesion in one patient with angiomatoid giant cellular blue naevus was initially a pigmented lesion which grew to a soft vaginal mass during pregnancy {27}.

Macroscopy
Vaginal blue naevi are typically single or multiple, pigmented, blue to black macular lesions {559,732,1611}. The flat lesions may measure up to 20 mm. The angiomatoid giant cellular blue naevus was a 6 cm cystic mass {27}.

Histopathology
Vaginal blue naevi consist of bundles of heavily pigmented dendritic melanocytes in the dermis with no junctional activity. The cystic spaces in the angiomatoid cellular blue naevus were also lined by lesional cells {27}. No mitotic activity or necrosis is seen.

Histogenesis
Blue naevi are derived from either aberrantly migrated melanocytes or melanocytes transformed from stromal nerve cells {380}.

Prognosis and predictive factors
All reported vaginal blue naevi have been benign.

Malignant melanoma

Definition
A malignant neoplasm composed of malignant melanocytes.

ICD-O code
8720/3

Epidemiology
Vaginal melanomas account for less than 0.3% of melanomas and approximately 4% of vaginal malignancies {2015}. Most patients are postmenopausal with mean age around 60 years {576,685,1553,2015}.

Clinical features
The most common presenting symptom is vaginal bleeding, followed by a vaginal mass and discharge {576,685}. The tumour is typically located in the distal third of the vaginal wall (anterior and lateral) and uncommonly in the vaginal apex {685}.

Macroscopy
The majority of cases are polypoid and nodular and typically 2–3 cm in size {685}. Most vaginal melanomas are pigmented but a small percentage of tumours are amelanotic {685,1510}.

Histopathology
The majority of vaginal melanomas are of nodular type but lentiginous and unclassified types may be also seen {685}. The overlying mucosa is ulcerated in most cases and the tumours are usually deeply invasive {685,1274}. The vertical growth phase tumour cells of nodular melanoma are most commonly epithelioid but they may be purely spindled or mixed epithelioid and spindled {685}. There is marked nuclear pleomorphism in some cases. In most cases there is brisk mitotic activity. A small percentage of tumours may show a prominent lymphocytic response. Lymphovascular and perineural invasion are present in some tumours. In about 10% of cases, no melanin pigment is seen either grossly or microscopically {685}. Nodular melanoma does not have an associated in situ component, but the

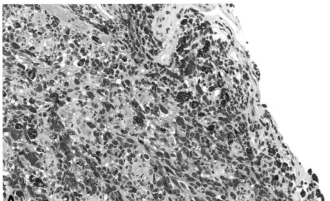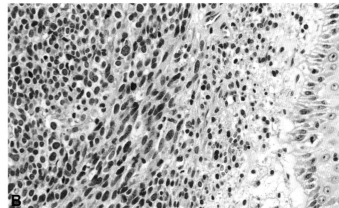

Fig. 8.15 Vaginal malignant melanoma. **A** The tumour cells are pigmented and pleomorphic with brisk mitotic activity. **B** The amelanotic tumour cells are mixed epithelioid and spindled with abundant mitotic figures.

lentiginous variant typically shows an associated lentiginous in situ component, which can be multifocal. Nearly all primary vaginal melanomas are positive for S100. Melan-A, HMB45, tyrosinase, and MITF1 are each positive in approximately 80% of cases {685}.

Histogenesis
The tumour is derived from aberrantly migrated melanocytes.

Genetic profile
Limited data have shown that, compared to sun-exposed skin melanomas, vaginal melanomas lack *BRAF* mutation and *c-KIT* mutation; however, approximately one-third of vaginal melanomas show *NRAS* mutation {1425,2045}.

Prognosis and predictive factors
The prognosis is poor regardless of treatment. The median survival is approximately 19–20 months and 5-year survival rate ranges from 0–21% {353,576,1264,1274}. Tumour size is the best predictive factor whereas tumour thickness does not significantly affect survival {205}. Lymph node metastasis is associated with a worse prognosis {576}. Surgical removal of gross disease is associated with improved clinical outcome {1274}.

Miscellaneous tumours

D. Cao
L. Hirschowitz

Germ cell tumours

Mature Teratoma

Definition
A tumour composed of tissue derived from more than one germ layer.

ICD-O code   9084/0

Synonyms
Dermoid cyst; mature cystic teratoma

Epidemiology
Primary vaginal teratoma is exceedingly rare. Only five cases of mature cystic teratoma (dermoid cyst) have been reported in the literature {760,1793}. Immature teratoma has not been reported.

Clinical features
The tumour typically presents with a slowly growing cyst in the vaginal wall.

Macroscopy
The cyst contains sebaceous material and hair.

Histopathology
The cyst is lined by squamous epithelium with underlying skin adnexal structures. Smooth and skeletal muscle may be also present {1793}.

Prognosis and predictive factors
Teratomas are benign but may recur if incompletely excised {760}.

Yolk sac tumour

Definition
A primitive, malignant, germ cell tumour with histological features recapitulating various development phases of the normal yolk sac.

ICD-O code   9071/3

Synonym
Endodermal sinus tumour

Epidemiology
Primary vaginal yolk sac tumour is very rare. Patients are almost exclusively under 4 years old {371,413,1903,2121}.

Clinical features
Most patients present with abnormal vaginal bleeding or bloody vaginal discharge {371,1903}. The serum α-fetoprotein level is almost always elevated {413,1903}.

Macroscopy
Primary yolk sac tumours typically present as a polypoid or sessile soft vaginal mass of 1–10 cm {371,1578,1903}. The tumours are variegated with tan-white to yellow appearance on cut surface {371}.

Histopathology
Primary vaginal yolk sac tumour shows identical histology to that of its ovarian counterpart. There are often various histological patterns in the same tumour with microcystic pattern being most common. The characteristic finding is the Schiller–Duval body which typically shows a papillary arrangement of columnar cells separated from central vascular channels by an acellular zone of connective tissue. The tumour cells are immunohistochemically positive for AFP, glypican-3, SALL4, and LIN28 {371,1999}.

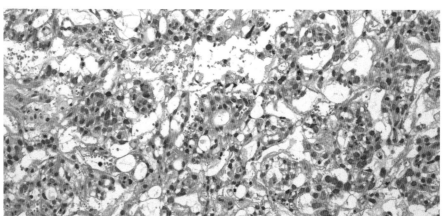

Fig. 8.16 Vaginal yolk sac tumour. The tumour displays a microcystic pattern.

Histogenesis

The histogenesis of primary vaginal yolk sac tumour is still uncertain. One plausible explanation is that primary vaginal yolk sac tumours arise from aberrantly migrated germ cells during early embryonic development {2141}.

Prognosis and predictive factors

The prognosis of primary vaginal yolk sac tumour has been markedly improved with the introduction of platinum-based chemotherapy {1578,1903}. Using the BEP protocol (bleomycin, etoposide, cisplastin) with or without conservative surgery, many patients achieve long-term disease-free survival {1578,1903}. Serum α-fetoprotein level can be used for monitoring therapy and follow-up. Recurrence is generally within 2 years after first-line treatment and is associated with a poor prognosis {413,1578}.

Others

Ewing sarcoma

Definition

Ewing sarcomas are composed of small round blue cells and are probably of mesenchymal stem cell origin {1866,1926}.

ICD-O code

Ewing tumour   9364/3

Synonym

Peripheral primitive neuroectodermal tumour (PNET)

Epidemiology

Primary vaginal Ewing sarcomas are rare.

Clinical features

Most vaginal Ewing sarcomas occur in the fourth decade {530,603,1093,1228}.

Histopathology

Like Ewing sarcomas at other sites, these tumours have a lobulated architecture and consist of sheets of uniform, small cells with round, hyperchromatic nuclei.

Nuclear chromatin is evenly dispersed, the nuclear to cytoplasmic ratio is high and mitotic activity is brisk. Occasional rosettes are present. Diffuse membranous expression of CD99 is demonstrable in almost all cases, and FLI-1 and cytokeratin AE1/AE3 in some. Desmin is not usually detectable. Rhabdomyosarcoma, non-Hodgkin lymphoma, undifferentiated, small cell squamous or neuroendocrine carcinoma (primary or metastatic), malignant melanoma, Merkel cell carcinoma and metastatic endometrial stromal sarcoma should be excluded by judicious use of immunohistochemistry and molecular studies if necessary.

Histogenesis

The tumour is of probable mesenchymal stem cell origin.

Genetic profile

The fused *EWS/FLI* transcript that results from t(11;22)(q24;q12) translocation is usually present in these tumours and can be demonstrated by fluorescence in situ hybridization (FISH) or quantitative real-time PCR.

Prognosis and predictive factors

Treatment involves a combination of surgery, chemotherapy and irradiation. Although Ewing sarcomas are aggressive tumours with a poor prognosis {1742}, limited outcome data suggest that tumours in the vagina may have a better outcome than Ewing sarcomas at other sites {1228}.

Paraganglioma

Definition

A tumour of neuroendocrine origin that originates from neural crest cells in autonomic paraganglia.

ICD-O code   8693/1

Epidemiology

Primary vaginal paraganglioma is exceedingly rare; fewer than ten cases have been reported {203, 720}.

Clinical features

Paraganglioma typically occurs in adults {24,720,1748} but one case has also been reported in a child {1466}. Tumours usually present as a vaginal mass and rarely as a pelvic mass {24}. Examples of functional paraganglioma associated with the development of hypertension and hypertensive crises have been reported {720,1748}.

Macroscopy

Excised tumours take the form of a soft, circumscribed mass with a pink-tan cut surface.

Histopathology

They have similar histological appearance and immunoprofile to paragangliomas occurring at other anatomical sites. The prominent vascularity and immunostaining for CD31 and CD34 may suggest a vasoformative tumour but non-reactive tumour cells between the vessels, some of which exhibit a typical "zellballen" growth pattern, express neuroendocrine markers and confirm the diagnosis.

Histogenesis

They are derived from neural crest cells in autonomic paraganglia.

Prognosis and predictive factors

Surgery is the main form of treatment. Most reported tumours have behaved in a benign fashion. Follow-up is recommended.

Other rare tumours

Other rare primary tumours in the vagina include alveolar soft-part sarcoma {1350}, angiosarcoma {1197,1528}, Brenner tumour {1347}, mixed adenocarcinoma-neuroendocrine tumour, carcinoid tumour {587}, malignant peripheral nerve sheath tumour {2157}, neurofibroma {115}, PEComa {563,2082}, schwannoma {410}, and synovial sarcoma.

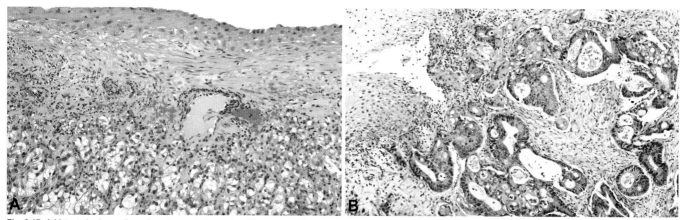

Fig. 8.17 A Metastatic clear cell renal carcinoma to the vagina. The tumour cells with clear cytoplasm form alveolar-like structures in the stroma beneath the squamous epithelium. **B** Metastatic colonic adenocarcinoma. In the stroma immediately beneath the squamous epithelium, the metastatic adenocarcinoma forms haphazardly distributed glands.

Secondary tumours

D. Cao
L. Hirschowitz

Definition
Tumours spreading to the vagina from other anatomical sites by direct extension, implantation from primary pelvic tumours or lymphovascular dissemination.

Epidemiology
Secondary involvement of the vagina as a result of spread of tumours from other sites is much more common than are primary vaginal tumours.

Clinical features
The most common symptom is vaginal bleeding. The primary tumour may be obvious clinically or patients may have a history of another pelvic or distant primary tumour.

Site of origin
Spread from primary cervical carcinomas is most common, but adenocarcinomas of the endometrium, colon, rectum and ovary may also spread to the vagina. Vulvar and urinary tract tumours (including rare cases of renal cell carcinoma {1091}) have been reported to spread to the vagina. Melanoma {686}, breast carcinoma {130}, uterine leiomyosarcoma {227} and gestational trophoblastic disease (mainly choriocarcinoma) {146,2089} may also spread to the vagina.

Histopathology
Histopathology varies with the type of secondary tumours. Vaginal cytology is sometimes useful to identify secondary tumours. In difficult cases, immunohistochemistry is helpful to confirm the diagnosis.

Prognosis and predictive factors
The prognosis is poor.

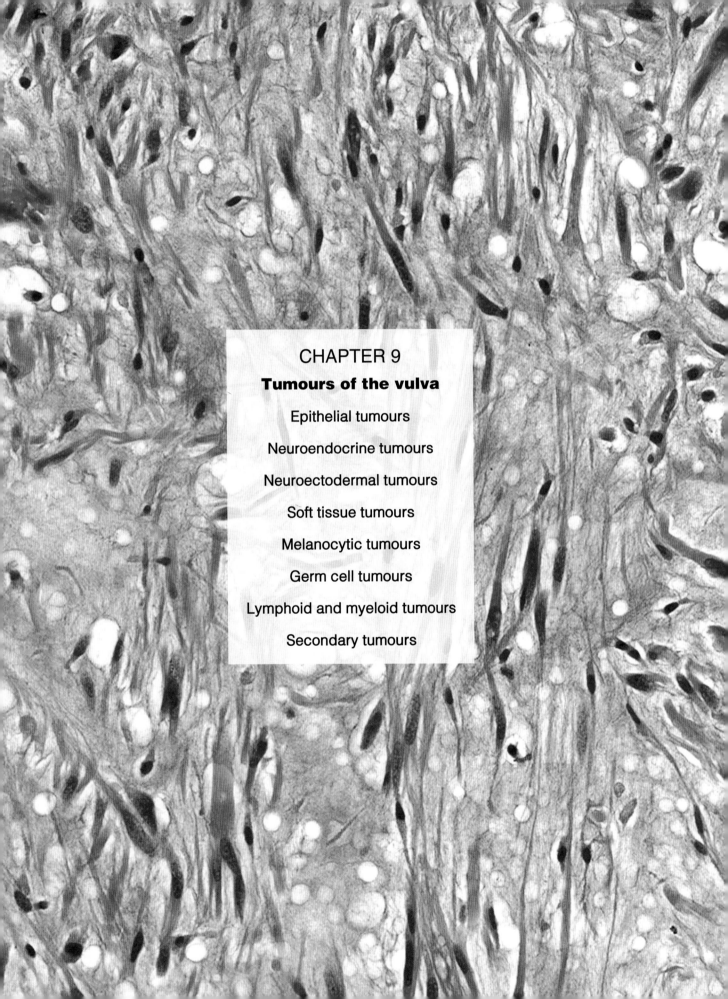

CHAPTER 9

Tumours of the vulva

Epithelial tumours

Neuroendocrine tumours

Neuroectodermal tumours

Soft tissue tumours

Melanocytic tumours

Germ cell tumours

Lymphoid and myeloid tumours

Secondary tumours

WHO Classification of tumours of the vulva[a,b]

Epithelial tumours
Squamous cell tumours and precursors
  Squamous intraepithelial lesions
    Low-grade squamous intraepithelial lesion 8077/0
    High-grade squamous intraepithelial lesion 8077/2
    Differentiated-type vulvar intraepithelial
      neoplasia 8071/2*
  Squamous cell carcinoma 8070/3
    Keratinizing 8071/3
    Non-keratinizing 8072/3
    Basaloid 8083/3
    Warty 8051/3
    Verrucous 8051/3
  Basal cell carcinoma 8090/3
  Benign squamous lesions
    Condyloma acuminatum
    Vestibular papilloma 8052/0
    Seborrheic keratosis
    Keratoacanthoma
Glandular tumours
  Paget disease 8542/3
  Tumours arising from Bartholin and
    other specialized anogenital glands
    Bartholin gland carcinomas
      Adenocarcinoma 8140/3
      Squamous cell carcinoma 8070/3
      Adenosquamous carcinoma 8560/3
      Adenoid cystic carcinoma 8200/3
      Transitional cell carcinoma 8120/3
    Adenocarcinoma of mammary gland type 8500/3
    Adenocarcinoma of Skene gland origin 8140/3
    Phyllodes tumour, malignant 9020/3
  Adenocarcinomas of other types
    Adenocarcinoma of sweat gland type 8140/3
    Adenocarcinoma of intestinal type 8140/3
  Benign tumours and cysts
    Papillary hidradenoma 8405/0
    Mixed tumour 8940/0
    Fibroadenoma 9010/0
    Adenoma 8140/0
    Adenomyoma 8932/0
    Bartholin gland cyst
    Nodular Bartholin gland hyperplasia
    Other vestibular gland cysts
    Other cysts
Neuroendocrine tumours
  High-grade neuroendocrine carcinoma
    Small cell neuroendocrine carcinoma 8041/3
    Large cell neuroendocrine carcinoma 8013/3
  Merkel cell tumour 8247/3

Neuroectodermal tumours
Ewing sarcoma 9364/3

Soft tissue tumours
Benign tumours
  Lipoma 8850/0
  Fibroepithelial stromal polyp
  Superficial angiomyxoma 8841/0*
  Superficial myofibroblastoma 8825/0
  Cellular angiofibroma 9160/0
  Angiomyofibroblastoma 8826/0
  Aggressive angiomyxoma 8841/0*
  Leiomyoma 8890/0
  Granular cell tumour 9580/0
  Other benign tumours
Malignant tumours
  Rhabdomyosarcoma
    Embryonal 8910/3
    Alveolar 8920/3
  Leiomyosarcoma 8890/3
  Epithelioid sarcoma 8804/3
  Alveolar soft part sarcoma 9581/3
  Other sarcomas
    Liposarcoma 8850/3
    Malignant peripheral nerve sheath tumour 9540/3
    Kaposi sarcoma 9140/3
    Fibrosarcoma 8810/3
    Dermatofibrosarcoma protuberans 8832/1*

Melanocytic tumours
Melanocytic naevi
  Congenital melanocytic naevus 8761/0
  Acquired melanocytic naevus 8720/0
  Blue naevus 8780/0
  Atypical melanocytic naevus of genital type 8720/0
  Dysplastic melanocytic naevus 8727/0
Malignant melanoma 8720/3

Germ cell tumours
Yolk sac tumour 9071/3

Lymphoid and myeloid tumours
Lymphomas
Myeloid neoplasms

Secondary tumours

---

[a] The morphology codes are from the International Classification of Diseases for Oncology (ICD-O) {575A}. Behaviour ¡s coded /0 for benign tumours, /1 for unspecified, borderline or uncertain behaviour, /2 for carcinoma in situ and grade III intraepithelial neoplasia and /3 for malignant tumours; [b] The classification is modified from the previous WHO classification of tumours {1906A}, taking into account changes in our understanding of these lesions; *These new codes were approved by the IARC/WHO Committee for ICD-O in 2013.

TNM and FIGO classification of carcinomas of the vulva

T – Primary tumour

TX	Primary tumour cannot be assessed
T0	No evidence of primary tumour
Tis	Carcinoma in situ (preinvasive carcinoma) intraepithelial neoplasia Grade III (VIN III)
T1	Tumour confined to vulva or vulva and perineum
T1a	Tumour 2 cm or less in greatest dimension and with stromal invasion no greater than 1.0 mm[1]
T1b	Tumour greater than 2 cm or with stromal invasion greater than 1.0 mm
T2	Tumour of any size with extension to adjacent perineal structures: lower third urethra, lower third vagina, anus
T3[2]	Tumour of any size with extension to the following structures: upper 2/3 urethra, upper 2/3 vagina, bladder mucosa, rectal mucosa, or fixed to the pelvic bone

Note: [1] The depth of invasion is defined as the measurement of the tumour from the epithelial-stromal junction of the adjacent most superficial dermal papilla to the deepest point of invasion. [2] T3 is not used by FIGO. They label it T4.

N – Regional Lymph Nodes

NX	Regional lymph nodes cannot be assessed
N0	No regional lymph node metastasis
N1	Regional lymph node metastasis with the following features:
N1a	1–2 lymph node metastasis each less than 5 mm
N1b	1 lymph node metastasis 5 mm or greater
N2	Regional lymph node metastasis with the following features:
N2a	3 or more lymph node metastases each less than 5 mm
N2b	2 or more lymph node metastases 5 mm or greater
N2c	Lymph node metastasis with extracapsular spread
N3	Fixed or ulcerated regional lymph node metastasis

M – Distant Metastasis

M0	No distant metastasis
M1	Distant metastasis (including pelvic lymph node metastasis)

Stage grouping

Stage 0[a]	Tis	N0	M0
Stage I	T1	N0	M0
Stage IA	T1a	N0	M0
Stage IB	T1b	N0	M0
Stage II	T2	N0	M0
Stage IIIA	T1, T2	N1a, N1b	M0
Stage IIIB	T1, T2	N2a, N2b	M0
Stage IIIC	T1, T2	N2c	M0
Stage IVA	T1, T2	N3	M0
	T3	Any N	M0
Stage IVB	Any T	Any N	M1

Note: [a] FIGO no longer includes stage 0 (Tis).

References

American Joint Committee on Cancer (AJCC) Cancer Staging Manual, 7th ed. (2011) Edge SB, Byrd DR, Compton CC, Fritz AG, Greene FL, Trotti III eds. Springer: New York

International Union against Cancer (UICC): TNM Classification of Malignant Tumours, 7th ed. (2009) Sobin LH, Gospodarowicz MK, Wittekind Ch eds. Wiley-Blackwell: Oxford

A help-desk for specific questions about the TNM classification is available at http://www.uicc.org.

Epithelial tumours

C.P. Crum
C.S. Herrington
W.G. McCluggage
S. Regauer
E.J. Wilkinson

Squamous cell tumours and precursors

Low-grade squamous intraepithelial lesion

Definition
Low-grade squamous intraepithelial lesion (LSIL) is an intraepithelial lesion of squamous epithelium that represents the clinical and morphological manifestation of a productive HPV infection. Low-grade refers to the associated low risk of concurrent or future cancer. See cervical LSIL (p. 172) for further discussion.

ICD-O code   8077/0

Synonyms
Vulvar intraepithelial neoplasia grade 1 (VIN 1); VIN 1 of usual type; mild squamous dysplasia; flat condyloma; koilocytotic atypia; koilocytosis

Epidemiology
This lesion is associated with a wide range of both low and high risk HPV types {1818}. It is most common during reproductive age.

Macroscopy
The lesion can appear macular, papular or hyperkeratotic.

Histopathology
Hyperplasia, anisonucleosis, parakeratosis, hyperkeratosis and variable koilocytotic atypia may be seen. Some lesions resemble seborrheic keratosis {1246}. Others exhibit apoptosis {1388}. Some are p16 positive. Only continuous linear horizontal (rather than vertical) staining involving the basal cell layer (also referred to as 'block-type' staining) is considered positive. Weak single cell or patchy staining should be interpreted as negative (see cervical LSIL for illustration and further dicussion, p. 172).

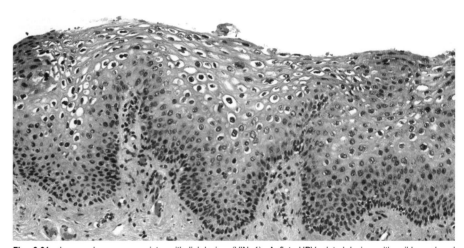

Fig. 9.01 Low-grade squamous intraepithelial lesion (VIN 1). A flat, HPV-related lesion with mild parabasal hypercellularity and koilocytotic atypia.

Prognosis and predictive factors
The lesions usually regress and have a very low risk of progression to cancer.

High-grade squamous intraepithelial lesion

Definition
High-grade squamous intraepithelial lesion (HSIL) is an intraepithelial lesion of squamous epithelium that carries a significant clinical risk of invasive cancer development if not treated {412,1586}.See cervical HSIL (p. 174) for further discussion.

ICD-O code   8077/2

Synonyms
Vulvar intraepithelial neoplasia grade 2 (VIN 2); vulvar intraepithelial neoplasia grade 3 (VIN 3); VIN 2 of usual type; VIN 3 of usual type; moderate squamous dysplasia; severe squamous dysplasia; carcinoma *in situ*; Bowen disease; Bowenoid dysplasia

Epidemiology
The incidence of the lesion increases in premenopausal women {85,459}. It is associated with an increased risk of cervical {829} and anal neoplasia {1681}. HIV infection confers a threefold higher frequency {657,1178}. Almost all these lesions contain HPV-16 {1047}.

Macroscopy
The lesions may be macular, papular or condylomatous. They may be acetowhite or pigmented and two-thirds are multifocal {258}. Multiple small pigmented lesions in young women correlate with the clinical syndrome of Bowenoid papulosis.

Histopathology
Epithelial cell hyperchromasia, crowding, anisonucleosis, acanthosis, parakeratosis, hyperkeratosis and variable HPV cytopathic effect may be seen. One-third of lesions involve skin appendages and this may mimic invasion {1745}. Grading is based on maturation. Both the basaloid and warty types are considered high-grade. p16 is almost always diffusely expressed, with a 'block-type' pattern of staining {1589}.

Prognosis and predictive factors
Older patients and those with large, clinically apparent lesions are at risk for concurrent carcinoma (20%) or eventual progression to invasive cancer {258,800,1398}. Treatments include excision, laser ablation, or medical therapy (e.g. topical imiquimod) {1487,1997}; 15% recur after complete excision, 50%

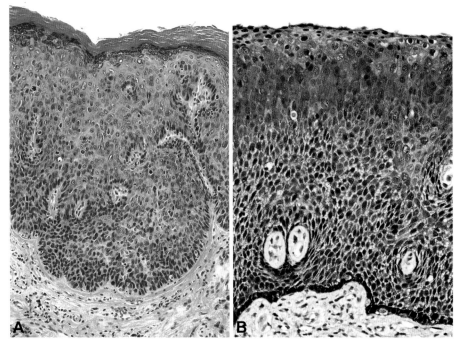

Fig. 9.02 High-grade squamous intraepithelial lesion (VIN 2/3). **A** Near full-thickness atypia with hypercellularity, and nuclear hyperchromasia with anisokaryosis and abnormal mitotic figures. **B** This lesion demonstrates diffuse nuclear and cytoplasmic p16 positivity.

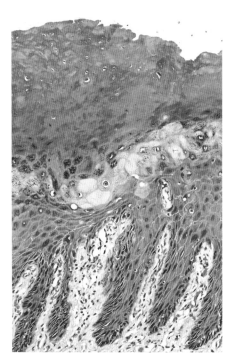

Fig. 9.03 Differentiated-type vulvar intraepithelial neoplasia. Elongation of rete ridges with overlying hyperkeratosis, basal keratinocyte atypia and abnormal keratinisation.

if margins are involved {850,1582}. Multifocal pigmented lesions (so-called Bowenoid papulosis) may spontaneously regress in young women {1828}. Recurrences are associated with cigarette smoking, large lesions and positive margins {1997}.

Differentiated-type vulvar intraepithelial neoplasia

Definition
HPV-negative squamous intraepithelial proliferation with abnormal keratinocyte differentiation and basal cell atypia.

ICD-O code   8071/2

Synonyms
Vulvar intraepithelial neoplasia (VIN) of differentiated-type; carcinoma in situ of simplex type

Epidemiology
This lesion is HPV negative, predominates in elderly women, is associated with lichen sclerosus and lichen planus, and is often associated with keratinizing carcinoma {302,1069,1678,1786}. The risk of cancer increases with age and duration of chronic anogenital inflammatory skin disease.

Etiology
Gene mutations (possibly *TP53*) may contribute in the setting of chronic vulvar disease. The contributing role of inflammation and clonal T-lymphocytes is unknown {1569,1570}.

Clinical features
Pruritis, irritation and pain commensurate with the associated vulvar inflammatory disorder or lichen sclerosus have been reported.

Macroscopy
The lesions can be hyperkeratotic, white or erythematous and are mostly solitary {1914}. Multicentricity is seen in the residual chronic inflammatory anogenital skin disease of women with a prior vulvar carcinoma {1569}.

Histopathology
Basal cell atypia with nuclear hyperchromasia, karyomegaly, prominent nucleoli, atypical mitosis in the basal layer, dyskeratosis and elongation and anastomosis of rete ridges may be found. Terminal differentiation (cornification) is often normal, but with dyskeratosis and individual cell keratosis {6,1956}. Hyperkeratosis is almost always present. p16 staining is negative (weak or patchy staining only). Although p53 immunohistochemistry may

be positive, it is highly variable and generally not useful in diagnosis {1430,1507}. Ki-67 staining is pronounced in the basal and parabasal layers but does not extend throughout the epithelium as in HSIL (VIN 2/3) {1961}. Differentiated VIN can be a difficult interpretation because of the morphological overlap with benign hyperplasia and hypertrophic variants of the dermatoses lichen sclerosus and lichen planus.

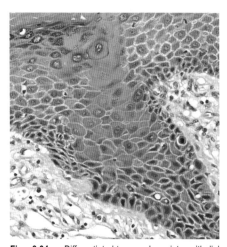

Fig. 9.04 Differentiated-type vulvar intraepithelial neoplasia. There is basal keratinocyte atypia with abnormal keratinisation. Reprinted from {1428A}.

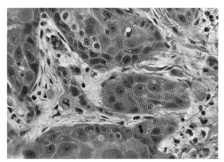

Fig. 9.05 Squamous cell carcinoma of the vulva. The tumour shows individual cell keratinization. Mitotic activity is generally most evident at the periphery of the nests of squamous epithelium.

Genetic profile
Mutations in *TP53* have been reported {1507,1589,2076} and linked to strong or absent immunohistochemical staining and aneuploidy {309,1960}.

Prognosis and predictive factors
These lesions are most strongly linked to cancer by association rather than outcome. Risk of progression to invasion is unclear but can be rapid, often < 6 months. Management is predicated on complete removal.

Squamous cell carcinoma

Definition
An invasive epithelial tumour composed of squamous cells of varying degrees of differentiation. Vulvar tumours may or may not be associated with HPV infection (see cervical squamous cell carcinoma (p. 176) for further discussion of HPV-associated tumours).

ICD-O codes
Squamous cell carcinoma	8070/3
Keratinizing	8071/3
Non-keratinizing	8072/3
Basaloid	8083/3
Warty	8051/3
Verrucous	8051/3

Epidemiology
Squamous cell carcinoma is the most common vulvar malignancy with incidence increasing with age {459,1853}.

Etiology
One group is linked to high risk HPV, cigarette smoking and HSIL (VIN 2/3) {615}, the second to chronic vulvar inflammatory disorders (lichen sclerosus (15–40%), lichen planus) and differentiated VIN {437,1069}. Up to 6% of patients with clinical lichen sclerosus develop carcinoma, and this risk is higher in symptomatic postmenopausal women {235,1568}. The presence of hyperplasia in association with lichen sclerosus may increase the risk of progression {1609,2022}. A third group, verrucous carcinoma, is occasionally linked to low-risk HPV types 6 and 11, but most are HPV negative {674,1246,1589}. Some are associated with squamous hyperplasias with altered differentiation {1333}.

Clinical features
Squamous cell carcinoma may present as an ulcer, nodule, macule or pedunculated mass. Symptoms in more advanced cases include discharge, bleeding and pain. Odour or self-palpation of a mass may bring the patient to the physician.

Macroscopy
Most vulvar squamous carcinomas are solitary. The tumours may be nodular, verruciform or ulcerated with raised firm edges.

Histopathology
As at other sites, squamous cell carcinoma is composed of infiltrating islands of malignant squamous cells. HPV positive tumours are often basaloid, composed of cohesive nests of immature basal-type squamous cells that may resemble HSIL (VIN 2/3). Warty (condylomatous) tumours have conspicuous superficial cell atypia, similar to that seen in HPV infected epithelium {1010}. Patterns may be mixed and include keratinizing histology. Tumours are usually HPV-16 and p16 positive {1589}.
Keratinizing carcinomas are variably mature with keratin pearls and the immature keratinocytes are strongly p53 positive {309,2078}. Most of these neoplasms tend to be well differentiated and the surface often shows minimal cytological atypia even when deeply invasive. As a result superficial biopsies may not be diagnostic of invasive carcinoma. Although these tumours may be associated with HPV, they are more often HPV and p16 negative and differentiated-type VIN may be present in the adjacent surface epithelium. Lichen sclerosus and lichen planus may also be present.
Verrucous carcinoma is warty-appearing, highly differentiated, variably keratinized and invades in the form of bulbous pegs with a pushing border. There is minimal atypia, abundant eosinophilic cytoplasm, normal mitotic figures and no increased p53 or p16 staining. Using these criteria, lesions with prominent koilocytotic atypia and HPV positivity are better classified as giant condyloma.
Rare variants of carcinoma include those with prominent spindle cells {1823} or prominent tumour giant cells, either of which can be confused with malignant melanoma {2031}.

Genetic profile
The principal molecular events are high-risk HPV infection or aberrant p53 function. Karyotypic abnormalities have been reported {991,2049} as well as altered promoter methylation with loss of gene expression {1827}. Poorer prognosis has been linked to expression of p14arf {1045} and cytoplasmic estrogen recep-

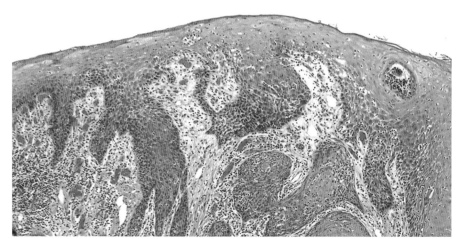

Fig. 9.06 Invasive squamous cell carcinoma. Infiltrative nests with an irregular growth pattern.

tor {2149}. Microsatellite instability is uncommon {209}.

Prognosis and predictive factors
Recurrence rates for FIGO stage IA tumours are low, with 5 and 10-year recurrence-free tumour specific survivals of 100% and 94.7%, respectively {1142}. Tumour diameter > 2.5 cm, multifocality, capillary-like space involvement, coexisting HSIL (VIN 2/3) and positive margins influence recurrence rate {671,770}. The most important factor predicting lymph node metastases is tumour depth and the strongest correlate of outcome is lymph node status {2040,2090}. The role of HPV status is unclear {437}. Carcinomas associated with differentiated VIN may be more likely to recur {510}.

Basal cell carcinoma

Definition
An infiltrating tumour composed predominantly of cells resembling the basal cells of the epidermis.

ICD-O code   8090/3

Clinical features
A slow growing ulcer or nodule. The most common symptom is pruritus {1313}. Lesions occasionally can be extensively pigmented {871}.

Histopathology
This tumour is composed of aggregates of uniform basal cells with peripheral palisading. Squamous cell differentiation may occur at the centre of the tumour nests. Half are infiltrative and a minority contains gland-like structures (adenoid basal cell carcinoma). Those containing infiltrating malignant-appearing squamous cells may be diagnosed as metatypical basal cell carcinoma or basosquamous carcinoma and should be managed similarly to squamous cell carcinoma {930}. This lesion must be distinguished from squamous cell carcinoma, basaloid type. The differential diagnosis of basal cell carcinoma also includes benign trichogenic tumours (trichoepithelioma).

Histogenesis
This tumour is derived from the basal cells of the epidermis or hair follicles.

Prognosis and predictive factors
Basal cell carcinoma of the vulva is usually

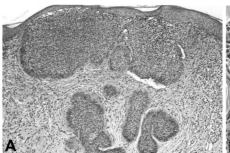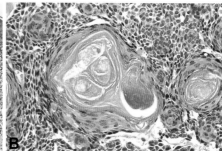

Fig. 9.07 A Basal cell carcinoma of the vulva. This tumour contains demarcated nests of palisaded basal cells originating at the epidermal–dermal junction. **B** Baso-squamous carcinoma. A basal cell carcinoma with prominent keratinization.

treated by local excision; however, groin metastases have been reported {534}.

Benign squamous lesions

Condyloma acuminatum

Definition
A benign verrucous papillary lesion associated with HPV infection.

Synonyms
Viral wart; genital wart; viral papilloma; low-grade squamous intraepithelial lesions (LSIL) with condylomatous features

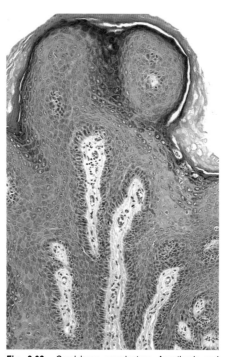

Fig. 9.08 Condyloma acuminatum. Acanthosis and papillomatosis with only focal viral cytopathic effect (centre right near the surface).

Epidemiology
This is a sexually transmitted disease of mostly young women affecting 0.1 – 0.2% yearly {567}. Ninety to 95% contain HPV-6 or 11 with a minority containing high-risk HPVs. Over 90% are theoretically preventable by the quadrivalent HPV vaccine {32,1852}.

Macroscopy
Papular or warty lesion may be seen on the introital, labial, perineal, and perianal mucosa. Lesions may be pruritic.

Histopathology
Acanthosis, papillomatosis, hyperkeratosis, parakaratosis, parabasal hyperplasia, delayed maturation and variable superficial (koilocytotic) atypia may be seen. In keratinized epithelium, koilocytotic atypia is not required for this diagnosis if the other criteria are present. Aetiologically-related lesions in young women associated with HPV-6 include seborrheic keratosis-like lesions and lesions resembling fibroepithelial papillomas {1246}.

Prognosis and predictive factors
The disease is managed by observation, local excision, topical imiquimod or trichoroacetic acid, and electro-cautery or superficial cryotherapy when larger. The majority resolve spontaneously or do not recur following removal. Recurrences are higher in immunosuppressed individuals in whom condylomata may co-exist with HSIL (VIN 2/3) {1159}.

Vestibular papilloma

Definition
A benign epithelial excrescence with a squamous epithelial mucosal surface that overlies a delicate fibrovascular stalk.

ICD-O code   8052/0

Synonyms

Micropapillomatosis labialis; vestibular micropapillomatosis; hirsuties papillaris genitalis (these terms are applicable when numerous frond-like excrescences are present)

Clinical features

The lesions may be solitary but frequently are multiple, often occurring in clusters near the hymenal ring and within the vulvar vestibule: this is termed vestibular papillomatosis or micropapillomatosis labialis. They do not display acanthosis or atypia and should not be treated as or mistaken for condyloma {137}.

Histopathology

These lesions have a papillary architecture and a smooth surface without acanthosis or koilocytotic atypia. They lack the complex arborizing architecture of condylomata.

Histogenesis

There is no relationship to HPV. The most plausible explanation is a simple variant of mucosal anatomy in the vulvar vestibule {1262}.

Seborrheic keratosis

Definition

A benign tumour characterized by proliferation of the parabasal cells of the squamous epithelium.

Histopathology

Acanthosis, hyperkeratosis and the formation of keratin-filled pseudohorn cysts may be seen. A variant, termed inverted follicular keratosis, contains prominent squamous eddies {1639}. Lesions with the morphology of seborrheic keratosis and that contain HPV (typically type 6) should be designated as condyloma acuminatum {1085} (see Condyloma acuminatum p. 235).

Keratoacanthoma

Definition

A neoplasm of keratinocytes thought to arise from follicular epithelium {632}.

Clinical features

Keratoacanthomas have been reported to arise rapidly, in some instances associated with prior trauma {1473}.

Macroscopy

Keratoacanthomas present as non-ulcerated lumps or nodules, typically 1–2 cm in diameter.

Histopathology

Keratoacanthomas are discrete, inverted, and form a crater of well differentiated keratinocytes with a resemblance to pseudoepitheliomatous hyperplasia.

Prognosis and predictive factors

Some regress spontaneously and most vulvar lesions have an uneventful outcome. However, many lesions classified as keratoacanthomas demonstrate some atypia and metastases have been reported. In this situation, the tumour is referred to as squamous cell carcinoma, keratoacanthoma type {765}.

Glandular tumours

Paget disease

Definition

An intraepithelial neoplasm of epithelial origin expressing apocrine or eccrine glandular-like features and characterized by distinctive large cells with prominent cytoplasm, referred to as Paget cells.

ICD-O code   8542/3

Synonym

Extramammary Paget disease

Epidemiology

Primary cutaneous Paget disease is an uncommon neoplasm, usually of postmenopausal Caucasian women. In a small proportion of women with vulvar Paget disease there is an invasive component or an underlying skin appendage adenocarcinoma {713}. A greater proportion of perianal Paget cases are associated with invasion {1198}.

Clinical features

The lesion is usually red, eczematoid, pruritic and may clinically resemble a dermatosis {529}. Paget disease of anorectal origin involves the perianal mucosa and skin as well as the adjacent vulva. Vulvar Paget disease typically presents on the labia majora and minora. Advanced cases extend onto extragenital skin or into the vagina. Most are non-invasive. Recurrence rates are high, even after complete initial resection. Metastasis to regional lymph nodes occurs in invasive disease.

Histopathology

Large round "Paget cells" with prominent pale cytoplasm and a prominent central nucleolus are distributed throughout the epithelium, either as single cells or clusters with variable extent. Extension into adnexal structures is common. The cytoplasm contains diastase resistant PAS-positive material.

Immunohistochemistry

Primary vulvar Paget cells consistently express CK7, CAM 5.2, carcinoembryonic antigen, GCDFP-15 (a marker of apocrine cells), HER2/neu, CA125 and androgen receptors. Estrogen and progesterone receptors are not expressed {80,1424}. Uroplakin-III, CK7 and CK20 are expressed in Paget disease secondary to urothelial carcinoma (Pagetoid urothelial intraepithelial neoplasia or PUIN) {2030}; and CK20, CDX2 and MUC-2 (but not CK7) in Paget disease associated with anorectal carcinoma {201,2152}. p53 protein overexpression in the intraepidermal component of primary vulvar Paget disease is associated with invasion {2153}. Lymphangiogenesis is a predictor of nodal metastases {1943}. An important morphological differential diagnosis is with malignant melanoma in situ. S-100 immunohistochemistry may be positive in the Paget cells, hence other melanoma markers (HMB45, melan A, etc.) should be used to resolve this differential diagnosis.

Histogenesis

Paget disease is an epithelial neoplasm arising from pluripotent epidermal stem cells, residing in interfollicular epidermis and in the folliculo-apocrine-sebaceous units. It may also be derived from an underlying skin appendage adenocarcinoma or anorectal or urothelial carcinoma {2030}.

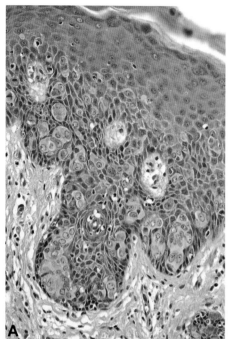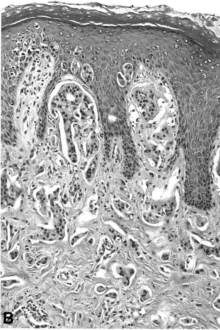

Fig. 9.09 A Paget Disease. Clusters of Paget cells with enlarged nuclei and abundant amphophilic cytoplasm are scattered through the epidermis. **B** Paget disease with an underlying invasive carcinoma.

Genetic profile

There are few data on the genetic profile of extramammary Paget disease. *Her-2/neu* gene amplification is more common in invasive and metastasized vulvar Paget disease (but is still rare). A single nucleotide polymorphism in the X-ray repair cross complementing group 1 (*XRCC1*) gene (Arg194Trp), aberrant *DLC1* methylation, *PIK3CA* mutations {303, 870}, gains of chromosome 7 and loss of the X chromosome are among other aberrations in case reports {1258}. Another study revealed recurrent amplification at chromosomes Xcent-q21 and 19, and loss at 10q24-qter {1062}.

Prognosis and predictive factors

At least one-third of cases will recur, particularly if resection margins are involved and recurrence can occur in transplanted skin {458,621}. Concomitant or subsequent invasion is reported in from 1–20% of cases but progression to invasion over time is uncommon {529,713,1286}. Overall, disease related mortality is well under 10% {842}. Dermal invasion and depth of dermal invasion are predictors for regional lymph nodes metastasis {381}. Significantly shorter disease-specific survival is associated with older age and advanced stage {876}. Approximately 40% of perianal Paget cases are associated with an underlying anorectal malignancy {1276}.

Tumours arising from Bartholin and other specialized anogenital glands

Bartholin gland carcinomas

Definition

An invasive epithelial tumour arising from the Bartholin gland.

ICD-O codes

Adenocarcinoma	8140/3
Squamous cell carcinoma	8070/3
Adenosquamous carcinoma	8560/3
Adenoid cystic carcinoma	8200/3
Transitional cell carcinoma	8120/3

Epidemiology and clinical features

These are rare neoplasms that occur in middle-aged to elderly women. They present as a painless swelling in the Bartholin gland area {103,234,1078,2025} and may be confused with Bartholin gland cyst or abscess. Adenocarcinomas and squamous cell carcinomas each account for approximately 40% and adenosquamous carcinomas for approximately 5%, of Bartholin gland carcinomas {103, 234, 1078, 2025}. Approximately 15% of Bartholin gland carcinomas are adenoid cystic carcinomas. Transitional cell carcinomas are rare.

Histopathology

Adenocarcinoma

These may be mucinous in type or have a papillary architecture. Clear cell adenocarcinoma has also been reported {103}. Occasional cases of Bartholin gland adenocarcinoma associated with vulvar extramammary Paget disease have been reported {721,1097}.

Squamous cell carcinoma

The histopathological features are similar to those of squamous cell carcinomas at other sites.

Adenosquamous carcinoma

Similar to adenosquamous carcinomas at other sites, these tumours are composed of malignant glandular and squamous elements.

Adenoid cystic carcinoma

The histopathological features are similar to those of adenoid cystic carcinomas at other sites {370,1913}. Rounded and cribriform islands of uniform epithelial cells are present within a hyaline stroma composed of basement membrane material. Cytogenetic analysis of an adenoid cystic carcinoma of Bartholin gland revealed a complex karyotype involving chromosomes 1, 4, 6, 11, 14 and 22 {2078}.

Transitional cell carcinoma

An invasive carcinoma composed of neoplastic cells with a transitional appearance. There may be a minor component of squamous or glandular differentiation. Cases associated with human papillomavirus type 16 or 18 have been reported {715,1706}.

Other carcinomas

Other types of carcinoma that have rarely been reported to arise in the Bartholin gland include small cell neuroendocrine carcinoma and Merkel cell carcinoma, as well as myoepithelial carcinoma, epithelial-myoepithelial carcinoma, salivary type basal cell adenocarcinoma, lymphoepithelioma-like carcinoma and undifferentiated carcinoma {538,808,843,861,912, 1015,1210,1477}.

Prognosis and predictive factors

Treatment may be surgery, radiotherapy, chemotherapy or chemoradiation alone or in combination depending on the tumour stage. Ipsilateral inguinofemoral lymph node metastasis is identified at presentation in approximately 20% of cases. In one series, the 5-year survival was 67% with 54.5% of patients suffering recurrence during a mean follow-up time of 73.5 months {234}. One study concluded that wide local excision followed by radiotherapy is the best treatment for advanced primary carcinoma of the Bartholin gland {103}.

Adenocarcinoma of mammary gland type

Definition
A primary invasive epithelial tumour showing morphological features of recognized breast adenocarcinomas.

ICD-O code
8500/3

Synonym
Adenocarcinoma of the vulva with breast carcinoma features

Epidemiology
Most patients reported are older than 60 years of age, with an age range from the mid-40s to more than 80 years {895}.

Macroscopy
The tumour typically presents as a single subcutaneous nodule most commonly involving the labium majus. Associated overlying extramammary Paget disease may be present.

Histopathology
Although such primary carcinomas are rare, several types of primary vulvar mammary-like carcinoma have been reported. Using terminology also applicable to primary breast adenocarcinomas, histopathological types include mammary-like ductal carcinoma, lobular carcinoma, tumours with mixed ductal and lobular features, tubulolobular carcinoma, mucinous carcinoma, and adenoid cystic-like adenocarcinoma. These tumours have morphological features similar to corresponding breast carcinomas {895}.

Histogenesis
These tumours are considered to arise from specialized anogenital mammary-like glands within the vulva, and are not considered to arise from ectopic breast tissue, or to represent metastatic breast adenocarcinoma. However, metastatic carcinoma should always be a differential diagnostic consideration {1958}.

Prognosis and predictive factors
Deep invasion with regional lymph node metastasis is reported in approximately 60% of cases. Common primary treatment is total, or partial, deep vulvectomy with or without chemotherapy and/or radiation therapy. Tumours may be positive for oestrogen and progesterone receptors and aromatase inhibitors or related anti-oestrogen therapies may have some role in management {1359}.

Adenocarcinoma of Skene gland origin

Definition
An invasive glandular epithelial tumour arising from Skene gland.

ICD-O code
8140/3

Synonym
Skene gland adenocarcinoma resembling prostate adenocarcinoma

Epidemiology
This is a rare tumour with few reported cases {1515}.

Clinical features
The tumour may present as a periurethral or anterior vaginal submucosal mass. Metastases to inguinal-femoral nodes may be present on initial presentation.

Macroscopy
A predominately solid tumour typically contiguous with and attached to, the urethra.

Histopathology
Skene gland adenocarcinoma has morphological features similar to prostate adenocarcinoma and usually expresses prostate specific antigen (PSA) that may be detected by immunohistochemistry, and in some cases within the serum {971}.

Histogenesis
The origin is from periurethral glands of Skene. These glands are the female homologue of the male prostate gland and express prostate specific antigen related products.

Prognosis and predictive factors
There is limited experience with these tumours, but regional lymph node involvement reflects more advanced stage and poorer prognosis.

Phyllodes tumour

Definition
Phyllodes tumour is a malignant tumour of either low or high-grade with mammary-like epithelium and predominant leaf-like stromal growth with periductal areas of hypercellularity with mitotic activity. The mass has a pushing interface with adjacent normal tissue.

ICD-O code
Phyllodes tumour, malignant 9020/3

Macroscopy
Phyllodes tumour may be very similar to fibroadenoma on gross examination, but the leaf-like pattern of growth is often evident grossly.

Histopathology
Phyllodes tumours have glandular elements lined by mammary-like epithelium that may have leaf-like stromal growth protruding into the glandular lumina. Tumour grade is based on the degree of stromal cellularity and atypical features. Both low- and high-grade neoplasms have stromal regional variability, typically with band-like areas of hypercellularity with increased mitotic activity around the epithelial components {896}.

Histogenesis
Phyllodes tumours arise from specialized anogenital glands that have features of mammary glandular tissue, but are not thought to represent ectopic breast tissue.

Prognosis and predictive factors
Phyllodes tumour of the vulva has a propensity for local recurrence but the overall prognosis is excellent with local complete excision {242,896}.

Adenocarcinomas of other types

Adenocarcinoma of sweat gland type

Definition
A primary, invasive, epithelial tumour of sweat gland type.

ICD-O code   8140/3

Epidemiology
These tumours are rare and their cause is unknown. The primary tumours in this group arise from vulvar skin sweat glands.

Clinical features
These tumours typically present as a painless cutaneous mass. In some cases, cutaneous Paget disease may be a manifestation of the underlying sweat gland tumour.

Macroscopy
The tumour primarily involves the skin and may be elevated or polypoid. The skin surface may be eroded or ulcerated.

Histopathology
Sweat gland adenocarcinomas may be ductal eccrine carcinoma, eccrine hidradenocarcinoma, eccrine porocarcinoma, apocrine carcinoma or other types {777,2026}. Primary sebaceous carcinoma, which may occur with vulvar intraepithelial neoplasia, is recognized {1540}.

Histogenesis
Skin appendages, primarily sweat glands, are the origin of the majority of these tumours.

Prognosis and predictive factors
Prognosis is primarily related to tumour stage.

Adenocarcinoma of intestinal type

Definition
A primary invasive glandular epithelial tumour of intestinal type.

ICD-O code   8140/3

Synonyms
Primary villoglandular mucinous adenocarcinoma arising in the surface epithelium of the vulva; cloacogenic carcinoma; cloacogenic adenocarcinoma

Epidemiology
These tumours are rare and their cause is unknown.

Clinical features
These tumours are typically solitary, but may be multiple at presentation. They form a superficial cutaneous mass that may be papular or polypoid {474A}.

Macroscopy
The tumour primarily involves the skin and may be elevated or polypoid. The skin surface may be eroded or ulcerated.

Histopathology
The microscopic features are typically those of a mucinous adenocarcinoma.

Histogenesis
Primary villoglandular mucinous adenocarcinoma arises in the surface epithelium of the vulva.

Prognosis and predictive factors
Prognosis is primarily related to tumour stage.

Benign tumours and cysts

Papillary hidradenoma

Definition
A benign tumour lined by epithelial secretory cells with subepithelial myoepithelial cells lining delicate fibrovascular, complex, branching papillae.

ICD-O code   8405/0

Synonyms
Hidradenoma papilliferum; mammary-like glandular adenoma

Epidemiology
This is the most common benign glandular neoplasm of the vulva.

Clinical features
The tumour presents as a mass or cyst, in or adjacent to the interlabial sulcus. There may be overlying epithelial ulceration or prolapse of the mass onto the surface, where it typically bleeds and may resemble an exophytic malignancy.

Macroscopy
With an intact epithelial surface the tumour is within the superficial dermis and well circumscribed. When prolapsed, it has a red, friable verrucoid-appearing surface, but is well circumscribed from the deeper tissue.

Histopathology
The tumour is composed of complex branching papillae with delicate fibrovascular stalks and associated glandular elements. The lining epithelial cells are uniform, columnar-epithelial secretory cells with underlying myoepithelial cells. Mitotic activity is often present and is occasionally prominent {1712,1958}. This lesion must be distinguished from adenocarcinoma.

Histogenesis
The origin within the vulva is from specialized anogenital glands that are located primarily in the interlabial sulcus, although they may be found anywhere

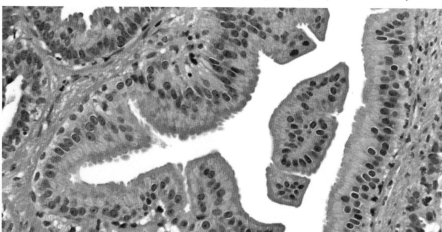

Fig. 9.10 Papillary hidradenoma. Papillae and gland-like spaces lined by uniform columnar epithelial secretory cells that have underlying myoepithelial cells in most areas. Mitotic activity is occasionally prominent.

from the lateral labium majus to the lateral labium minus {1958}.

Prognosis and predictive factors
This is a benign tumour, but may recur locally if incompletely excised. Ductal carcinoma in situ (DCIS) arising in papillary hidradenoma and resembling DCIS of the breast, as well as low-grade phyllodes tumour, have been reported in a few cases. Papillary hidradenoma as a source of invasive adenocarcinomas, although reported, has been challenged as an entity {895}.

Mixed tumour

Definition
A benign, mixed epithelial and stromal tumour.

ICD-O Code   8940/0

Synonyms
Pleomorphic adenoma; chondroid syringoma

Histopathology
A benign tumour of epithelial cells in tubules, associated with stroma that can contain chondroid, osseous and myxoid features.

Prognosis and predictive factors
The tumour may recur if not completely excised.

Fibroadenoma

Definition
Fibroadenoma is a benign, biphasic, circumscribed, epithelial-stromal neoplasm resembling the tumour of the same name in the breast.

ICD-O code   9010/0

Synonyms
Adenoma of anogenital mammary-like glands; ectopic breast fibroadenoma

Epidemiology
Occurrence is predominately in women of reproductive age, but they may be found in postmenopausal women and rarely in prepubertal girls {2156}.

Clinical features
Typically the lesion is a solitary, firm, subcutaneous nodule that is not fixed to deeper underlying tissues. The most common location is in the interlabial sulcus, but they also are found from the lateral labium majus or lateral labium minus, as well as in the perineum and perianal regions. Enlargement may occur during pregnancy. Rare cases have been reported with concurrent mammary and vulvar fibroadenomas {73,895}.

Macroscopy
Fibroadenomas of the vulva range in size from < 1 cm to 6 cm or larger, although most reported cases are < 4 cm in greatest dimension {896}. On cut section they are fibrous and may have cystic spaces.

Histopathology
Fibroadenomas have glandular elements lined by mammary-like epithelium within a relatively uniform, hypocellular stroma composed of spindled or stellate cells without nuclear atypia. There is rare or absent mitotic activity in the epithelial or stromal cellular elements. They express estrogen and progestogen receptors in both elements {73}.

Histogenesis
Fibroadenomas arise from specialized anogenital glands that have features of mammary glandular tissue, but are not considered to represent ectopic breast tissue.

Prognosis and predictive factors
Fibroadenomas are benign tumours, but may recur if not completely excised {242,896}.

Adenoma and adenomyoma

Definition
Bartholin gland adenoma and Bartholin gland adenomyoma are rare benign tumours of the Bartholin gland.

ICD-O codes
Adenoma   8140/0
Adenomyoma   8932/0

Histopathology
Bartholin gland adenoma consists of small, clustered, closely packed glands and tubules lined by columnar to cuboidal epithelium with colloid-like secretion, arranged in a lobular pattern and contiguous with identifiable Bartholin gland elements; it has been associated rarely with adenoid cystic carcinoma. Bartholin gland adenomyoma has a fibromuscular stromal element that is immunoreactive for smooth muscle actin and desmin as well as a lobular glandular architecture with glands lined by columnar mucin-secreting epithelial cells adjacent to tubules {956}. Adenomyomas are exceedingly rare.

Bartholin gland cyst

Definition
A cyst of the Bartholin duct.

Synonym
Bartholin duct cyst

Clinical features
Bartholin gland cysts are located in the postero-lateral introitus.

Histopathology
Bartholin gland cysts are lined by transitional or squamous epithelium. Inflammation is common, as is ulceration, and abscesses may form. A portion of Bartholin gland may also be present.

Histogenesis
Cysts are formed when the duct becomes obstructed, with secondary inflammation or infection.

Prognosis and predictive factors
Marsupialization and antibiotic therapy, when needed, are the standard management {1174}.

Nodular Bartholin gland hyperplasia

Definition
A benign expansion of normal Bartholin gland tissue and ducts.

Histopathology
There is a nodular proliferation of normal acini with preservation of the normal duct structures. Inflammation and squamous metaplasia may be present {956,1680}.

Other vestibular gland cysts

Definition
Cysts of vestibular ducts.

Synonym
Vestibular duct cysts

Clinical features
Vestibular gland cysts are located in the vestibule. Bartholin gland cysts are identified specifically from their anatomical location.

Histopathology
See Bartholin gland cyst.

Histogenesis
See Bartholin gland cyst.

Prognosis and predictive factors
See Bartholin gland cyst.

Other cysts

Definition
Mucinous and ciliated cysts are occasionally seen in the vulvar vestibule and have been proposed to be of urogenital sinus origin. Additional entities manifesting as cysts include epidermal inclusion cysts, urethral prolapse and hydrocele of the Canal of Nuck {158,881,1600,2094}. Phatidylinositol 4,5-bisphosphate 3-kinase, catalytic subunit, α isoform, have been found in subsets of Merkel cell carcinomas {177,1331}.

Prognosis and predictive factors
Prognosis is related to tumour size and stage, with better survival reported in individuals with tumours < 2 cm in greatest dimension {256}. Better survival is associated with fewer genetic aberrations but tumour-related mortality occurs in approximately one-third of patients {358,1607}. Regional lymph node and distant metastasis may be present at diagnosis or occur later. Primary treatment for localized tumour is wide local excision. Regional lymphadenectomy may be included. Adjuvant radiation therapy may be given. Chemotherapy is often employed for more extensive disease or recurrence.

Neuroendocrine tumours

C.P. Crum
C.S. Herrington
W.G. McCluggage
S. Regauer
E.J. Wilkinson

High-grade neuroendocrine carcinoma

Definition
A high-grade carcinoma exhibiting neuroendocrine differentiation.

ICD-O codes
Small cell neuroendocrine
   carcinoma   8041/3
Large cell neuroendocrine
   carcinoma   8013/3
Merkel cell tumour   8247/3

Synonyms
For small cell neuroendocrine carcinoma: small cell carcinoma; oat cell carcinoma; neuroendocrine carcinoma, small cell type, grade 3;
For large cell neuroendocrine carcinoma: neuroendocrine carcinoma, large cell type, grade 3

Epidemiology
In the vulva, as in the cervix, the term "small cell carcinoma" should be reserved for high-grade neuroendocrine carcinoma of small cell type (small cell neuroendocrine carcinoma, SCNEC). Most SCNECs of the vulva are examples of Merkel cell tumour and the existence of non-Merkel cell vulvar SCNEC, as seen in the vagina, cervix and lung, has been questioned, although there have been a few case reports {609}. Merkel cell tumour of the vulva is rare and the incidence increases with age. The incidence is significantly higher in HIV-positive individuals and those who have had organ transplantation {1607}.

Clinical features
Merkel cell tumour of the vulva typically presents as a cutaneous nodule, or nodules. The overlying skin may be erythematous or ulcerated. Regional lymph nodes may be involved. This tumour has been observed concurrently in women with SIL (VIN) or squamous cell carcinoma {1607}.

Macroscopy
The tumour is usually predominately intradermal and may have areas of haemorrhage and necrosis. Associated ulceration and induration of the immediately adjacent epithelium may be present {1746}.

Histopathology
Merkel cell tumours may show diverse differentiation patterns, but can be separated into two major types: those with morphological features of small cell carcinoma as seen within the lung; and those of non-pulmonary type ("classic type"). The latter display small, round to polygonal cells with scant cytoplasm and nuclei with pale and finely granular chromatin and small nucleoli, resembling lower grade neuroendocrine tumours (see also neuroendocrine tumours of the uterine cervix, p. 196) {256}. Distribution of the two types has not been studied. Glandular or squamous differentiation may be observed with Merkel cell tumour in the vulva {1711}. Pagetoid spread of the tumour cells may be observed within the adjacent squamous epithelium.

Immunohistochemistry
Immunohistochemical studies for cytokeratins, such as CAM 5.2, cytokeratin 20 and AE1/AE3, highlight a paranuclear cytoplasmic dot in many tumour cells. Reactivity for neuron-specific enolase (NSE) and NCAM/CD56 is usually present. Chromogranin and synaptopyhsin are positive in some, but not all cases. Tyrosine kinase receptor c-kit has been detected in the majority of Merkel cell tumours. HMB-45, S100, TTF1 and desmin are negative {630,1607}. Electron microscopy can be used to identify membrane-bound neurosecretory granules in the cells. Ectopic ACTH production by Merkel cell tumour may occur {256}.

Histogenesis

The origin of Merkel cell carcinoma is not well understood. Due to the heterogeneous histological differentiation of Merkel cell carcinoma and the post-mitotic character of Merkel cells, it is not very likely that Merkel cell carcinoma develops from differentiated Merkel cells. Stem cells of epidermal lineage or dermal stem cells derived from the neural crest lineage are more likely the cells of origin in Merkel cell carcinoma {1923}. Merkel cell polyomavirus (MCPyV) DNA has been reported in approximately two-thirds of cases studied {477,1283}.

Genetic profile

Numerous genetic abnormalities have been detected, including lost regions in chromosomes 3p, 4, 5q, 7, 10 and 13, but none specifically identify Merkel cell tumour {1607}. Additionally, mutations in several genes, including the tumour suppressor *ATOH1*, encoding a transcription factor involved in Merkel cell differentiation, and *PIK3CA*, which codes for phosphatidylinositol 4,5-bisphosphate 3-kinase, catalytic subunit, α isoform, have been found in subsets of Merkel cell carcinomas {177,1331}

Prognosis and predictive factors

Prognosis is related to tumour size and stage, with better survival reported in individuals with tumours > 2 cm in greatest dimension {256}. Better survival is associated with fewer genetic aberrations but tumour-related mortality occurs in approximately one-third of patients {358,1607}. Regional lymph node and distant metastasis may be present at diagnosis or occur later. Primary treatment for localized tumour is wide local excision. Regional lymphadenectomy may be included. Adjuvant radiation therapy may be given. Chemotherapy is often employed for more extensive disease or recurrence.

Neuroectodermal tumours

E.J. Wilkinson
C.P. Crum

C.S. Herrington
W.G. McCluggage
S. Regauer

Ewing sarcoma

Definition

A malignant soft-tissue tumour usually composed of small round cells and exhibiting variable neuroectodermal differentiation and demonstrating a chromosomal translocation, t(11;22)(q24;q12), in most cases.

ICD-O code   9364/3

Synonym

Peripheral primitive neuroectodermal tumour (PNET)

Epidemiology

Extraosseous Ewing sarcoma is a rare tumour of the vulva that has been observed predominantly in women of reproductive age but has been documented in children {256,406,1228}.

Clinical features

When involving the vulva, the tumour typically presents as a subcutaneous or polypoid mass that may resemble a Bartholin cyst. The overlying epithelium may be ulcerated {256,565}. The tumour on presentation is usually reported as localized to the labia minora or majora. The clinical presentation may vary from a small subcutanous nodule to a mass exceeding 20 cm in greatest dimension {406}.

Macroscopy

Ewing sarcoma is typically a soft, subcutaneous or polypoid mass that, on cut section, has a relatively nodular, uniform, lobulated appearance and appears circumscribed. There may be areas of necrosis. No capsule is present and gross margins with the adjacent tissues may not be well defined.

Histopathology

These tumours are composed of a well demarcated, but unencapsulated proliferation of small round blue cells often with a lobulated growth. The cells grow in sheets or solid aggregates and occasional rosettes may be seen. The tumour cells have minimal cytoplasm with round nuclei showing dispersed, finely granular chromatin {1228}.

Immunohistochemistry

The tumour cells are typically strongly and diffusely positive for CD99 (membranous pattern) {256,1228}. Nuclear FLI1 positivity and focal positivity for AE1/AE3 is common. Tumour cells are typically diffusely positive for vimentin, but negative for desmin {1228}.

Histogenesis

These tumours are thought to arise from cells deriving from the post-ganglionic cholinerigic neurons of the neural crest, although their precise origin is uncertain.

Genetic profile

Chromosome translocation t(11;22)(q24; q12) is identified in approximately 90% of cases. *EWS-FLI1* fusion product may be detected in some cases {256,1228}.

Prognosis and predictive factors

Patients typically have a poor prognosis, many developing pulmonary metastasis. Long-term survival (> 3 years) has been described in patients with complete surgical excision followed by adjuvant therapy {256,1228}.

Other tumours that may rarely occur on the vulva include paraganglioma and other neuroendocrine carcinomas, including one reported case with paraganglioma-like features {363,754,1397}. The morphological features are similar to those of the hononymous tumours when occuring in their respective sites.

Soft tissue tumours

M.R. Nucci   W.G. McCluggage
R. Ganesan   G.P. Nielsen

Benign tumours

Lipoma

Definition
This is a benign tumour composed of lobules of mature adipocytes.

ICD-O code   8850/0

Synonym
Fibrolipoma (a variant if predominantly fibrous)

Epidemiology
It is the most common soft-tissue tumour and can occur in visceral and non-visceral locations {1324,1657}; however, it is relatively uncommon in the vulva.

Clinical features
Lipomas generally occur in reproductive-aged women but can also occur in children {1409}. They typically present as slow-growing, soft, mobile, painless masses. In children, they most commonly occur in the right anterolateral aspect of the vulva {1409}.

Macroscopy
They are well demarcated, encapsulated tumours with a soft, yellow, homogeneous cut-surface.

Histopathology
Lipomas are typically composed of lobules of mature, uni-vacuolated adipocytes of uniform size. Fibrous septae and focal, myxoid change may be seen, and can sometimes be extensive. Cellular atypia and mitoses are not present. Variants of lipoma that may occur in the vulva include spindle cell lipoma {1575}; further, there is a case report on a benign lipoblastoma-like tumour {67}.

Histogenesis
They presumably arise from fat cells in the subcutaneous tissue.

Genetic profile
The most common cytogenetic aberration in lipomas involves chromosomal region 12q14.3. Deletion of a limited region of 13q14 has also been noted in lipomas {407}. Spindle cell lipomas show consistent rearrangements of chromosomes 13q and 16q {273}. Lipoblastomas show rearrangements of 8q11–13 {113}.

Genetic susceptibility
Familial multiple lipomatosis is a rare condition with proposed autosomal dominant inheritance {1978}.

Prognosis and predictive factors
Lipomas and spindle cell lipomas rarely recur after excision. An infiltrative margin in lipoblastomas is predictive for recurrence.

Fibroepithelial stromal polyp

Definition
A benign, polypoid growth of the distinctive subepithelial stroma of the distal female genital tract that is covered by stratified squamous epithelium.

Synonym
Fibroepithelial polyp

Clinical features
These polyps most commonly occur in the vagina, but they also occur in the vulva and, less commonly, the cervix {1387}. Stromal polyps typically occur in reproductive age women, most commonly during pregnancy but may also occur in postmenopausal women on hormone replacement therapy. Symptoms may include bleeding, discharge and sensation of a mass {1387}.

Macroscopy
These are typically solitary, polypoid or pedunculated lesions, and usually measure < 5 cm. On cut section, they are tan-white, soft and oedematous {1387}.

Histopathology
They are characteristically ill-defined, polypoid proliferations of variably cellular stroma with a central fibrovascular core and overlying variably hyperplastic squamous epithelium. The stroma is typically composed of bland, spindle-shaped cells with delicate uni- or bipolar cytoplasmic processes. Stellate or multinucleate stromal cells, which are often present near the epithelial-stromal interface or around the central vasculature, are characteristic. The stromal cells can exhibit a significant degree of nuclear pleomorphism, hyperchromasia and mitotic activity particularly, but not invariably, during pregnancy {1387,1396,1439}.

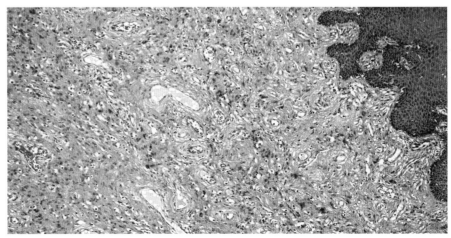

Fig. 9.11 Fibroepithelial stromal polyp. Stellate and multinucleate stromal cells extend up to the epithelial stromal interface.

Histogenesis

This lesion is thought to arise from the hormonally responsive subepithelial stromal cells of the distal female genital tract.

Prognosis and predictive factors

The lesions are benign. They may recur, particularly if incompletely excised, or with continued hormonal stimulation such as occurs with pregnancy.

Superficial angiomyxoma

Definition

A multilobulated, myxoid neoplasm of superficial skin and subcutaneous tissue with a propensity for local, non-destructive recurrence.

ICD-O code   8841/0

Clinical features

Superficial angiomyxoma occurs in young women, most commonly in the fourth decade as a slowly growing, painless polypoid mass {35,224,554}.

Macroscopy

It is an exophytic, polypoid mass, which typically measures < 5 cm and, on cut section, consists of one or more lobulated foci of relatively well circumscribed gelatinous tissue.

Histopathology

Superficial angiomyxoma is well demarcated but unencapsulated and consists of hypocellular myxoid nodules located in the dermis and superficial subcutaneous tissue. The tumour is composed of slender spindle or stellate cells, inflammatory cells (particularly and character-istically polymorphonuclear leukocytes) and numerous delicate, thin-walled and elongated vessels. Mitoses are uncommon. In about one-third of cases squamous epithelial-lined cysts or basaloid squamous buds or strands are noted adjacent to the myxoid nodules {554}.

Prognosis and predictive factors

These tumours have a propensity for local non-destructive recurrence (30%) if incompletely excised.

Superficial myofibroblastoma

Definition

A benign mesenchymal lesion composed of myofibroblasts {602,1038}.

ICD-O code   8825/0

Synonym

Vulvovaginal myofibroblastoma

Epidemiology

This lesion is uncommon.

Clinical features

This is a tumour of adult females and presents in the vulvovaginal region {602,1038,1143}. In most cases, the patients present with a unilateral painless swelling. There is reported to be an association with the use of tamoxifen and hormone replacement therapy.

Macroscopy

They are typically polypoid or nodular with a firm, white cut surface.

Histopathology

They are discrete, unencapsulated tumours that are separated from the overlying epidermis by a variably thick Grenz zone. The cells are oval or spindle-shaped with wavy nuclei and scant cytoplasm. The stroma is finely collagenous with variable amount of dense collagen. The vessels are centrally concentrated, thin-walled, dilated and often have a stag-horn pattern. Mitoses, necrosis, cytological atypia and entrapment of normal structures are not seen.
Immunohistochemically, the cells are positive for vimentin, desmin and CD99, variably positive for CD34 and oestrogen receptors and negative for α-smooth muscle actin.

Histogenesis

These tumours are believed to arise from a distinctive layer of stromal cells that extend from the endocervix to the vagina and vulva.

Genetic profile

13q14 chromosomal loss has been noted, similar to that seen in mammary myofibroblastoma, cellular angiofibroma and spindle cell lipoma {1144}, and there is a loss of nuclear staining for RB protein.

Prognosis and predictive factors

No recurrences have been reported.

Cellular angiofibroma

Definition

A benign mesenchymal neoplasm of fibroblastic lineage, which most commonly occurs on the vulva.

ICD-O code   9160/0

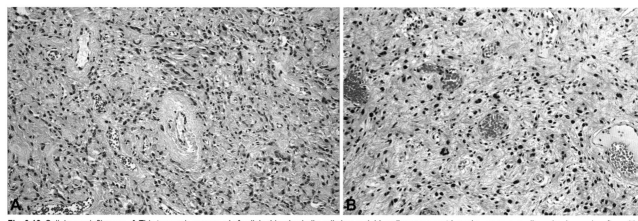

Fig. 9.12 Cellular angiofibroma. **A** This tumour is composed of cellular bland spindle cells in a variably collagenous matrix and numerous medium sized vessels, often with hyalinized walls. **B** Occasionally, this tumour can contain atypical stromal cells.

Clinical features

This tumour occurs at any age {823,1389}. Presentation is usually as a painless superficial mass or polypoid lesion.

Macroscopy

These are well circumscribed tumours that are usually < 5 cm in maximum dimension, but are occasionally larger {1389}. They are solid, usually with a firm grey-white cut surface, but there are no distinctive gross features.

Histopathology

These are well circumscribed but unencapsulated tumours covered by unremarkable squamous epithelium. Deep to the surface epithelium, there is usually a Grenz zone. There is often entrapped adipose tissue around the periphery of the tumours, which is usually moderately cellular and composed of a uniform population of bland spindle-shaped cells within a fibrous stroma. Occasionally, in the superficial portion, there are atypical stromal cells. Mitotic figures, although usually sparse, are easily identified in some cases. Numerous small to medium-sized blood vessels, often with thick hyalinised walls, are usually but not always present {823,1389}. Stromal mast cells may be present. In some cases, there are hypocellular, hyalinised areas, a haemangiopericytomatous-like vascular pattern, lymphoid aggregates, myxoid areas and focal marked nuclear atypia; the latter is often seen in association with adipocytes {1216}. In rare cases, there is sarcomatous transformation {274}.

Immunohistochemistry
The cells are usually positive with vimentin, ER and PR and often positive for CD34 (~50%). Desmin and smooth muscle actin are usually negative but sometimes focally positive {823,1216}. HMGA2 is negative {1212}. Overexpression of p16 may occur in areas of sarcomatous transformation {274}.

Histogenesis

These are thought to arise from the subepithelial, hormone receptor-positive mesenchymal region which exists in the lower female genital tract. Based on the morphological, immunohistochemical and electron microscopy findings, they are considered to exhibit a fibroblastic lineage.

Genetic profile

Abnormalities of chromosome 13q14, including deletions and allelic loss, have been demonstrated in these lesions {1140}, along with loss of immunohistochemical reactivity for RB protein. This is a similar genetic abnormality to that found in spindle cell lipoma, mammary myofibroblastoma and myofibroblastomas arising in the lower female genital tract, raising the possibility that these lesions represent a spectrum of a single entity.

Prognosis and predictive factors

These are usually benign lesions and are treated by local excision. They may occasionally recur locally. There have been occasional reports of overt sarcomatous transformation but this has not, as yet, been shown to be associated with malignant clinical behaviour {274}.

Angiomyofibroblastoma

Definition

This is a benign tumour composed of myofibroblasts and blood vessels.

ICD-O code   8826/0

Epidemiology

This is a relatively uncommon, soft-tissue tumour of the vulva {561,1037,1353}.

Clinical features

This is a tumour of adult women occurring in the vulvovaginal region. Patients present with painless swelling of the vulva that is often mistaken for a Bartholin cyst {1387}. They rarely present as a pedunculated mass {1787}.

Macroscopy

Most are small, usually < 5 cm, and limited by a pseudocapsule. They typically have a rubbery, solid and tan cut surface.

Histopathology

They are well circumscribed lesions with alternating hyper- and hypocellular areas composed of polygonal epithelioid and small spindle cells that tend to be clustered around numerous thin-walled small to medium-sized capillary-like vessels. Cytological atypia is rare and mitoses are infrequent. The stroma has a loose texture and contains mast cells. Intralesional adipose tissue is seen and, when dominant, the tumour is termed a lipomatous variant {230}. The cells are positive for vimentin, desmin, estrogen and progesterone receptors. CD34 is negative. Aggressive angiomyxomas can rarely show areas with angiomyofibroblastoma-like features {663}.

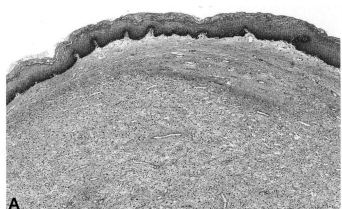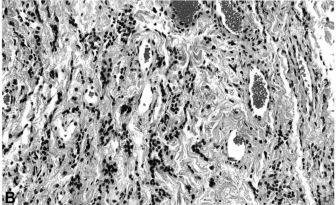

Fig. 9.13 Angiomyofibroblastoma. **A** The tumour is composed of epithelial stromal cells below the squamous epithelium. **B** This tumour characteristically contains numerous small capillaries around which the epithelioid-appearing stromal cells are clustered. Note the sharp border of this lesion.

Histogenesis

Angiomyofibroblastoma is believed to originate from mesenchymal cells that are capable of myofibroblastic differentiation {585,762}.

Genetic profile

Transcripts of *HMGI-C (HMGA-2)* were shown to be present by RT–PCR in one case {773}.

Prognosis and predictive factors

These are benign, non-recurrent tumours. There is one reported recurrence where typical angiomyofibroblastoma merged with high-grade sarcoma {1356}.

Aggressive angiomyxoma

Definition

A low-grade, hypocellular, infiltrative neoplasm of the deep soft-tissues of the vulvovaginal region, perineum and pelvis with a tendency to local recurrence following incomplete excision {118,553,1824}.

ICD-O code   8841/0

Synonyms

Deep angiomyxoma; aggressive (deep) angiomyxoma of the female pelvis and perineum

Clinical features

Aggressive angiomyxoma is most common in the reproductive years {118,553,1824}. Presentation is usually with a vulvar "cyst" or mass but because of their invasive growth these lesions can-not be easily "shelled out" and are therefore often incompletely excised; clinically they are frequently thought to represent a Bartholin gland cyst. The mass is usually large and painless and may cause pressure symptoms. Rapid growth may occur during pregnancy. Imaging often reveals the mass to be much larger than is apparent on clinical examination.

Macroscopy

These are usually large, poorly circumscribed lesions with irregular extension into surrounding tissues. They have a gelatinous, rubbery or myxoid consistency but some cases have a more fibrous appearance.

Histopathology

Aggressive angiomyxoma is paucicellular and is composed of cells with small bland ovoid to short spindle-shaped nuclei and inconspicuous cytoplasm. Occasional stellate nuclei may be present and the cells are embedded in an abundant myxoid stroma. Mitotic activity and nuclear atypia are virtually absent. Extravasated erythrocytes are common. Numerous blood vessels of varying calibre, ranging from thin-walled, capillary-like vessels of medium calibre, to large vessels with thick muscular walls are present. Perivascular smooth muscle fibres radiating from thick-walled blood vessels are present in some cases. The edge is infiltrative, with entrapment of adipose tissue and skeletal muscle at the periphery.

Immunohistochemistry

The cells are usually positive with vimentin, ER, PR and desmin and sometimes CD34 and smooth muscle actin {1225}. HMGA2 nuclear immunoreactivity is present in most cases {1212}. S100 is negative.

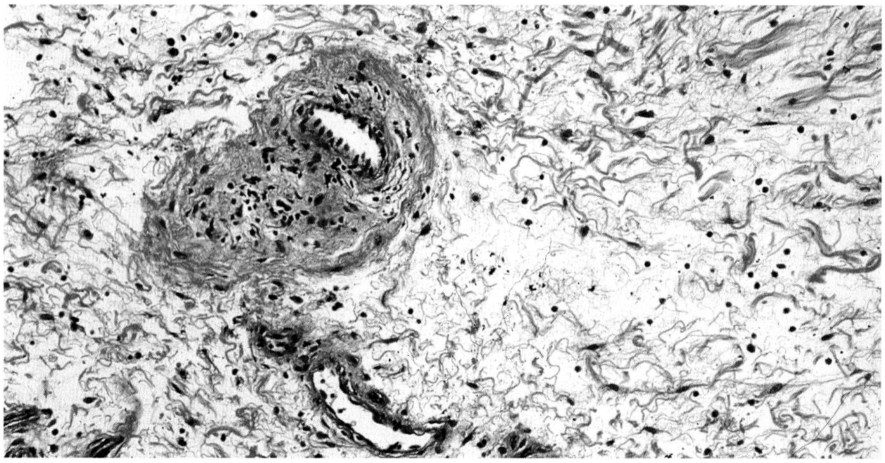

Histogenesis

These are thought to arise from the subepithelial, hormone receptor-positive mesenchymal region which exists in the lower female genital tract. They are considered to exhibit a myofibroblastic lineage.

Genetic profile

The architectural transcription factor HMGA2, located on chromosome 12q15, is rearranged in some cases of aggressive angiomyxoma {1244,1394}.

Prognosis and predictive factors

Treatment is predominantly surgical, by complete local excision. These lesions have a marked tendency to local recurrence if initial excision is incomplete. Adequate local excision may be difficult since there is often greater extension than can be appreciated on clinical examination. Gonadotrophin releasing hormone agonist therapy may be an option in lesions that are not amenable to excision or to shrink the tumour and make excision easier {1218}.

Leiomyoma

Definition

A benign mesenchymal neoplasm showing smooth-muscle differentiation.

ICD-O code   8890/0

Epidemiology

Leiomyoma is one of the more common soft-tissue tumours of the vulva.

Clinical features

Patients are typically in their fourth or fifth decade and most commonly present with a painless mass for which the most common clinical diagnosis is Bartholin gland cyst. A minority of patients with vulvar smooth muscle tumours have synchronous or metachronous oesophageal leiomyomas {767,1352}.

Macroscopy

Tumours are typically well circumscribed, subcutaneous masses with a grey-white to tan bulging cut surface. Some have a more homogeneous appearance with

Fig. 9.14 Aggressive angiomyxoma. Large thick-walled vessels are widely separated by a highly myxoid hypocellular stroma.

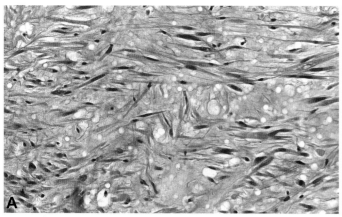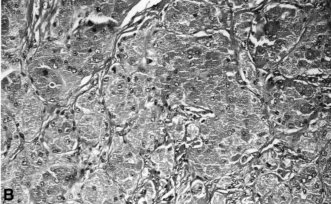

Fig. 9.15 A Myxoid leiomyoma. Smooth muscle tumours of the vagina and vulva often have a myxohyaline matrix. **B** Granular cell tumour. This tumour is composed of nests of polygonal cells with granular cytoplasm and small uniform hyperchromatic nuclei.

less prominent bulging surfaces. Most measure < 3 cm.

Histopathology
Most are of the usual spindle cell type as seen elsewhere in the female genital tract, with intersecting fascicles of morphologically bland spindle cells with abundant eosinophilic cytoplasm and blunt ended nuclei. Variable amounts of myxohyaline matrix may be present and is more common in smooth muscle tumours at this site.

Histogenesis
The tumour originates from smooth muscle.

Genetic susceptibility
Leiomyomatosis of the vulva, a condition in which patients have multiple ill-defined submucosal leiomyomas, has been associated with Alports syndrome {513,1387}. Patients may also have synchronous or metachronous oesophageal leiomyomas (oesophageal leiomyomatosis).

Prognosis and predictive factors
Leiomyomas can locally recur, sometimes after many years, particularly if incompletely excised.

Granular cell tumour

Definition
A benign tumour composed of round and polygonal cells with distinctive granular cytoplasm due to lysosome accumulation.

ICD-O code   9580/0

Synonyms
Granular cell myoblastoma; Abrikossoff tumour

Epidemiology
Vulvar granular tumours are uncommon {1080}. They occur mainly in middle-aged adults but can occur in children {1021,2154}. Multicentric tumours and familial tumours have also been reported {877,1146,1683}. They typically occur in the head and neck region but occasionally can occur in the vulva, most often the labium majus.

Clinical features
Patients typically present with a slowly enlarging mass in the vulva. They are usually asymptomatic but may present with pain or pruritus.

Macroscopy
They have a well circumscribed, firm, tan cut surface.

Histopathology
They are composed of nests of polygonal cells with granular cytoplasm and small, uniform, hyperchromatic nuclei. They typically have pushing borders but almost half show poorly defined or infiltrative margins. Tumour cell nests often are associated with small nerve twigs. The overlying squamous epithelium can show pseudoepitheliomatous hyperplasia {1021,2042}. Immunohistochemistry shows the tumour cells are positive for S100, CD68, NSE, Galectin-3 and HBME1 and negative for SMA and desmin {131}.

Histogenesis
Ultrastructural and immunohistochemical studies support a Schwann cell origin for most cases {1196}.

Prognosis and predictive factors
Granular cell tumours are generally benign and seldom recur although infiltrative margins, despite complete excision, are associated with recurrence {37}. Features indicating malignancy in granular cell tumours are necrosis, spindled tumour cells, increased nuclear to cytoplasmic ratio and vesicular nuclei with large nucleoli {526}.

Other benign tumours

The vulva can be the site of soft tissue tumours such as paraganglioma {363}, haemangioma, neurofibroma and rhabdomyoma. Recently described benign mesenchymal tumours and tumour-like conditions of the vulva include cyclist's nodule, myoepithelial neoplasm, prepubertal vulvar fibroma, solitary fibrous tumour, ischaemic fasciitis, massive vulvar oedema and childhood asymmetric labium majus enlargement {1221,1227, 1247,1690,1886,1976}.

Tumours that generally behave in a benign fashion but have low malignant potential include low-grade fibromyxoid sarcoma and angiomatoid fibrous histiocytoma {152,276}.

Malignant tumours

Embryonal rhabdomyosarcoma

Definition
A malignant embryonal tumour exhibiting skeletal (striated) muscle differentiation.

ICD-O code   8910/3

Synonym
Sarcoma botryoides

Epidemiology
Rhabdomyosarcomas are extremely rare as primary vulvar neoplasms and much less common than in the vagina {50,726}.

Clinical features
Embryonal rhabdomyosarcomas usually arise in children < 10 years of age. Presentation is usually with a vulvar mass, which may be polypoid and associated with bleeding or ulceration.

Macroscopy
These may be polypoid lesions, often in the form of multiple polyps and sometimes with a "grape-like" appearance. However, a polypoid appearance is less common than with vaginal primaries. Some contain obvious areas of haemorrhage, necrosis, oedema or myxoid change.

Histopathology
The morphological features of vulvar embryonal rhabdomyosarcomas are similar to those in the vagina. These are usually polypoid lesions which are partially covered by squamous epithelium which may be ulcerated. At low power, there may be areas of alternating cellularity. The neoplasm is composed of cells with round, ovoid or spindle-shaped nuclei and generally scanty cytoplasm. A proportion of the tumour cells may contain relatively abundant eosinophilic cytoplasm. Rhabdomyoblasts with a round or strap-like appearance and cytoplasmic cross striations may be found in small numbers but these are not identified in all cases. Often there is a cellular cambium layer composed of closely packed cells with small hyperchromatic nuclei just beneath the surface squamous epithelium. Occasionally a few multinucleated giant cells are present. Especially towards the centre

of the neoplasm, hypocellular myxoid or oedematous areas may be present. The mitotic rate is often high and there may be extravasation of erythrocytes.
The neoplastic cells usually stain positive for desmin and exhibit focal nuclear staining with the skeletal muscle markers myogenin and myoD1 (See rhabdomyosarcoma of vagina, p. 219).

Prognosis and predictive factors
The prognosis of embryonal rhabdomyosarcoma in the past was poor but combination chemotherapy, radiation and/or surgery have resulted in cure rates of 90–95% {50}.

Alveolar rhabdomyosarcoma

Definition
A malignant tumour exhibiting skeletal (striated) muscle differentiation with an alveolar pattern.

ICD-O code   8920/3

Epidemiology
Rhabdomyosarcomas are extremely rare as primary vulvar neoplasms and much less common than in the vagina {50,726}.

Clinical features
Alveolar rhabdomyosarcomas tend to occur at an older age than embryonal rhabdomyosarcoma. Presentation is usually with a vulvar mass, which may be associated with bleeding or ulceration.

Histopathology
The morphological features of alveolar rhabdomyosarcomas are identical to those that arise at more usual sites. Tumour cells grow in loosely cohesive nests separated by fibrous septae. The cells show loss of cohesion towards the centre of the nests and float freely while the cells at the periphery of the nests are adherent to the fibrous septae. Multinucleate cells may be present.
The neoplastic cells are usually positive for desmin and exhibit focal nuclear staining with the skeletal muscle markers myogenin and myoD1. Immunoreactivity with the latter two markers is typically more diffuse in alveolar than embryonal rhabdomyosarcomas.

Prognosis and predictive factors
The prognosis is poor.

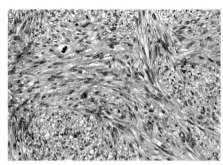
Fig. 9.16 Leiomyosarcoma. This tumour exhibits conventional spindle cell morphology, being composed of intersecting fascicles of atypical spindle cells with bright eosinophilic cytoplasm.

Leiomyosarcoma

Definition
A malignant mesenchymal neoplasm showing smooth muscle differentiation.

ICD-O code   8890/3

Epidemiology
Leiomyosarcoma of the vulva is rare, but does represent the most common soft-tissue sarcoma at this site.

Clinical features
Patients are usually in their fourth or fifth decade and present with an enlarging painless or painful mass.

Macroscopy
Tumours can be of varying size. They often have a tan or yellow cut surface with areas of necrosis.

Histopathology
Most vulvar leiomyosarcomas are of the conventional spindle cell type, although epithelioid and myxoid leiomyosarcoma can also occur {1927}. Criteria for malignancy are based on the presence of at least three of the following features: size > 5 cm, infiltrative growth pattern, moderate to severe cytological atypia and mitotic activity measuring > 5 per 10 HPF {1352,1908}.

Prognosis and predictive factors
Vulvar leiomyosarcoma can locally recur and metastasize.

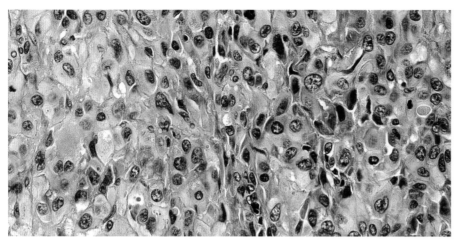

Fig. 9.17 Epithelioid sarcoma, proximal type. The neoplastic cells are large, with abundant eosinophilic cytoplasm, eccentric, vesicular nuclei and prominent nucleoli.

Epithelioid sarcoma

Definition
A malignant mesenchymal tumour of uncertain histogenesis composed of large epithelioid cells, often arranged in a granuloma-like fashion around areas of necrosis. The proximal (large cell) variant has a predilection for the genital areas and behaves more aggressively than the usual type.

ICD-O code   8804/3

Synonyms
Epithelioid sarcoma, proximal variant; proximal-type epithelioid sarcoma

Epidemiology
This is a rare primary malignant vulvar tumour.

Clinical features
Patients typically present in the fourth decade with symptoms related to a rapidly growing mass.

Macroscopy
Tumours usually measure < 6 cm and typically have a grey-white cut surface that may be multinodular.

Histopathology
This tumour may have a diffuse or multinodular growth pattern with common involvement of subcutaneous and deep soft tissue. The neoplastic cells are large, with abundant eosinophilic cytoplasm and eccentric nuclei with vesicular nuclei and prominent nucleoli. Rhabdoid inclusions are common. Immunohistochemically the tumour cells are positive for keratin, epithelial membrane antigen and vimentin and show loss of INI-1 expression {774,922}. Approximately half stain for CD34 and occasionally tumour cells are positive for actin and desmin.

Prognosis and predictive factors
Proximal type epithelioid sarcoma acts more aggressively than the usual (distal) type of epithelioid sarcoma, with more frequent recurrences and high incidence of metastasis {681,716,1428}.

Alveolar soft part sarcoma

Definition
Alveolar soft part sarcoma (ASPS) is a tumour of unknown histogenesis, composed of large, epithelioid cells with granular, eosinophilic cytoplasm, having a solid or alveolar growth pattern.

ICD-O code   9581/3

Epidemiology
ASPS is an exceedingly rare primary tumour of the vulva {1749}.

Clinical features
Patients typically present with a slowly growing tumour.

Macroscopy
Tumours typically have a yellow or grey cut surface often with areas of haemorrhage and necrosis.

Histopathology
Tumours typically have an alveolar growth pattern with tumour cell nests showing loss of cellular cohesion centrally; sometimes a solid growth pattern may be seen. A prominent sinusoidal vascular network separates the nests. PAS-D can demonstrate intracytoplasmic Shipkey crystals that can also be seen ultrastructurally. There is no specific immunohistochemical profile, except positive staining for TFE3.

Genetic profile
Alveolar soft part sarcoma has t(X;17), resulting in *ASPL/TFE3* fusion {1022}.

Prognosis and predictive factors
Generally, this is a slowly progressive disease in which metastases (usually to lungs, brain and bone) ultimately prove fatal.

Other sarcomas

Definition
A wide range of sarcomas, other than those specifically described, may occur on the vulva. All are rare at this location. Sarcomas specifically reported include malignant peripheral nerve sheath tumour (MPNST, malignant schwannoma, neurofibrosarcoma), liposarcoma, synovial sarcoma, angiosarcoma, Kaposi sarcoma, fibrosarcoma and dermatofibrosarcoma protuberans {481,1028,1141,1228,1247, 1386,1677,1861}. The morphological features are identical to those of the homonymous tumours occuring at more usual locations.

ICD-O codes
Liposarcoma	8850/3
Malignant peripheral nerve sheath tumour	9540/3
Kaposi sarcoma	9140/3
Fibrosarcoma	8810/3
Dermatofibrosarcoma protuberans	8832/1

Melanocytic tumours

M.R. Nucci   W.G. McCluggage
R. Ganesan

Melanocytic naevi

Definition
Benign melanocytic lesions occurring on the vulva.

ICD-O codes
Congenital melanocytic naevus	8761/0
Acquired melanocytic naevus	8720/0
Blue naevus	8780/0
Atypical melanocytic naevus of genital type	8720/0
Dysplastic melanocytic naevus	8727/0

Epidemiology
Melanocytic lesions of the genital area are common and include melanocytic naevi, lentigines, dysplastic naevi (naevi with architectural disorder and atypia of melanocytes) and atypical melanocytic naevi of the genital type, which are naevi that have overlapping histological features with melanoma.

Clinical features
The age range is wide. Presentation is with a pigmented lesion on the vulva, although naevi also occur less commonly on the perineum or mons pubis {1581}. In some cases, they may be an incidental finding during gynaecological examination. Atypical genital naevi most commonly arise on the labia minora of young women with a mean age of 26 years {321,646,1581}.

Macroscopy
These are similar to naevi arising at other cutaneous locations.

Histopathology
These are similar to naevi arising at other cutaneous locations. Variants that may occur include congenital naevi, acquired naevi (junctional, compound, intradermal), blue naevi, dysplastic naevi and atypical genital naevi. Vulvar naevi may grow or change during pregnancy and show occasional dermal mitoses.
Atypical genital naevus is regarded as a naevus of special sites. In one large series {646}, the dominant histological feature was a lentiginous and nested junctional component composed of prominent round or fusiform nests, which often showed retraction artefact and/or cellular dyscohesion. Cytological atypia was mild, moderate (most commonly) or severe. Pagetoid spread occurred in some cases. The atypical junctional melanocytic proliferation was often associated with a common dermal naevus component. Adnexal spread and nuclear atypia of melanocytes situated in the superficial dermis were relatively common but dermal mitoses were uncommon and maturation was present in all cases. A broad zone of dense eosinophilic fibrosis within the superficial dermis was a frequent finding.

Histogenesis
Naevi are of melanocytic origin.

Genetic susceptibility
Dysplastic naevi may occur in patients with the dysplastic naevus syndrome.

Prognosis and predictive factors
These are benign lesions, which are treated by local excision. Despite their worrisome histological appearance, atypical genital naevi exhibit a benign behaviour {646,1581}.

Malignant melanoma

Definition
A malignant tumour arising from melanocytes.

ICD-O code   8720/3

Synonym
Melanoma

Epidemiology
The vulva is the most common site of melanomas in the female genital tract and melanoma is the second most common malignant neoplasm of the vulva. Approximately 3% of all melanomas in women arise in the female genital tract and melanoma comprises approximately 5–10% of all vulvar cancers, occurring predominantly in Caucasians. The ratio of sun exposed skin melanoma to vulvar melanoma is 71:1 {1309,1553,1822,1857}.

Etiology
Most melanomas are caused by exposure to ultraviolet light {1071,1478} but melanomas of the vulva are likely to arise via an ultraviolet radiation-independent pathway {1279}.

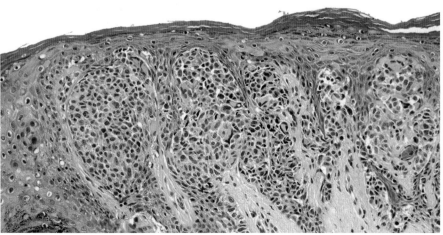

Fig. 9.18 Atypical genital naevus. This melanocytic lesion is characterized by a lentiginous and junctional component of round to fusiform nests which often show retraction artifact and/or cellular non-cohesion.

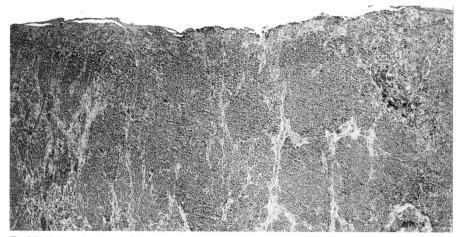

Fig. 9.19 Malignant melanoma. This melanoma shows expansile vertical growth. Note the melanin pigment which helps establish the diagnosis.

Clinical features

The median age for diagnosis of melanoma in sun exposed skin is 56 years and vulvar melanomas present a decade later. Most are pigmented; about 25% may be amelanotic. The most common symptoms at presentation are pruritus, bleeding or symptoms related to a mass. The glabrous skin, clitoris and labia majora are common sites {1554}.

Macroscopy

They are usually unevenly pigmented, asymmetric lesions with irregular borders that may be plaque like, nodular or polypoid. Tumours may show surface ulceration.

Histopathology

The melanoma cell can be spindled or epithelioid. The latter has abundant eosinophilic cytoplasm, large nuclei and multiple prominent nucleoli. Melanin can be seen as fine granular intracytoplasmic pigment. Radial growth-phase melanomas may show focal invasion by single cells and small nests of cells, which are smaller than the junctional nests. When there are invasive nests larger than the largest junctional nests or if there are dermal mitoses, the term vertical growth-phase may be applied. The common histological patterns are acral/mucosal lentiginous, nodular and superficial spreading. Mucosal lentiginous melanomas are characterized by a proliferation of atypical epithelioid melanocytes arranged in single cells and nests along the basal layer with pagetoid upward migration, which may be extensive. When they undergo vertical growth, they often elicit a pronounced desmoplastic response. Nodular melanomas show expansile vertical growth without a significant "shoulder" of intraepithelial spread beyond the confines of the tumour. Superficial spreading melanomas differ from nodular melanomas by the presence of a "shoulder" of melanoma in situ extending significantly beyond the confines of the nodular component. Melanoma cells are immunoreactive for S100, HMB-45 and Melan A. The main differential diagnoses include dysplastic naevi, which have pagetoid involvement confined to the central portion of the lesion; spindle cell squamous carcinoma, which lacks pigment, has intracellular bridges and is S100 negative; and extramammary Paget disease which has larger cells containing intracytoplasmic mucin and which are typically negative for S100. Important histological features include the growth phase, Breslow thickness, ulceration, mitotic index, lymphovascular invasion, microsatellite or in transit metastasis, perineural invasion, tumour infiltrating lymphocytes, regression, Clark level 4/5 and status of margins {669,1168}.

Histogenesis

The tumour arises from melanocytes in the surface epithelium.

Genetic profile

Genetic alterations in RAS-related pathways are present in most acral/mucosal lentiginous melanomas {1535}. c-KIT mutations may be seen in vulvar melanomas {1425}. Late stage melanomas overexpress epidermal growth factor receptor (EGFR) {970}.

Genetic susceptibility

Patients with familial atypical mole-melanoma (FAMM) syndrome have 9p21 deletions centered on CDKN2A, the familial melanoma gene {801}.

Prognosis and predictive factors

Five-year disease specific survival rates for patients with localized, regional and distant disease were 75.5%, 38.7% and 22.1% respectively in one large analysis {1857}. Advanced clinical stage of disease, Breslow thickness of greater than 1 mm, vertical growth phase, ulceration, and mitotic index > $1/mm^2$ are adverse prognostic factors. Presence of microsatellites and perineural invasion are associated with increased local recurrence. The prognostic value of tumour infiltrating lymphocytes and regression is unclear {841,1075,1135}.

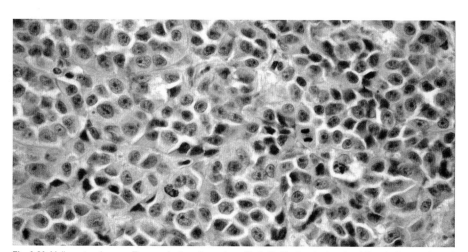

Fig. 9.20 Malignant melanoma. The neoplastic cells can be epithelioid with abundant eosinophilic cytoplasm and round nuclei with prominent nucleoli.

Germm cell tumours

M.R. Nucci   R. Ganesan
J.A. Ferry   W.G. McCluggage

Yolk sac tumour

Definition
Yolk sac tumour is a primitive germ cell tumour with a variety of distinctive patterns and which may also exhibit differentiation into endodermal structures, ranging from the primitive gut and mesenchyme to the derivatives of extraembryonal (secondary yolk sac and allantois) and embryonal somatic tissues (intestine, liver and mesenchyme). It is uncommon in the vulva {1949}.

ICD-O code   9071/3

Synonym
Endodermal sinus tumour

Epidemiology
This tumour is rarely primary in the vulva {560,1281,1949}.

Clinical features
Patients range in age from 1–52 years (mean 22 years) and either present with a rapidly or progressively growing mass or swelling of the labium majus (right side is more commonly affected than the left). On examination, the lesion is typically soft and freely mobile. Serum AFP levels are not consistently elevated at diagnosis.

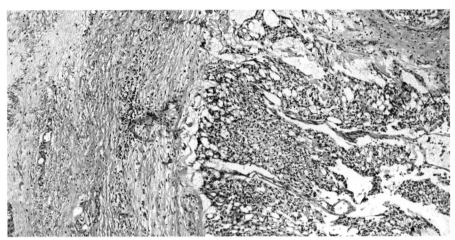

Fig. 9.21 Yolk sac tumour of vulva. This germ cell tumour, which rarely occurs in the vulva, has the typical appearance of its ovarian counterpart, with the reticular pattern being the most common.

Macroscopy
The tumours vary in size ranging from 4 – > 30 cm. Cut surface shows a solid, grey-white fleshy lesion with a variegated appearance. Haemorrhage and necrosis can be seen.

Histopathology
The tumour can show an admixture of architectural patterns with reticular being the most common. The tumour cells are large with hyperchromatic, irregular nuclei, prominent nucleoli and clear cytoplasm. PAS-positive, intracellular and extracellular hyaline globules are typically present. Schiller-Duval bodies, which resemble fetal glomeruli, can be seen {479}. The neoplastic cells are typically positive for α-fetoprotein, glypican-3 and SALL4.

Histogenesis
The tumour is believed to arise from germ cells in the vulva that persist following an error in migration {245}.

Prognosis and predictive factors
Tumour size of 5 cm or less may be a favourable prognostic feature {916}; outcome seems better than for ovarian tumours {1358}.

Lymphoid and myeloid tumours

Lymphomas

Definition
Malignant neoplasms composed of lymphoid cells.

Clinical features
Primary vulvar lymphoma is rare. Of the reported cases, many appear to be primary cutaneous lymphomas, but rare patients with Bartholin gland mass{1927A} or with a clitoral mass {972} are described. Patients are adults who present with a nodule, swelling, pruritis or induration of the vulva {552A,1970,1971A}. Patients are almost all middle-aged or older women {972}. Rare patients are HIV positive or iatrogenically immunosuppressed but most patients have no factor predisposing to the development of lymphoma.

Macroscopy
Most lesions are nodules beneath intact or ulcerated skin or mucosa.

Histopathology
Diffuse large B-cell lymphoma is by far the most common primary vulvar lymphoma {552A,1927A,1970,1971A}. A few cases of a variety of other types of lymphoma are reported {972}, and some of these, including at least some follicular lymphomas and extranodal marginal zone lymphomas {972}, are perhaps better considered primary cutaneous lymphomas rather than primary vulvar lymphomas. Lymphomas classified as primary cutaneous, but arising in the vulva, include primary cutaneous anaplastic large cell lymphoma {958A} and cutaneous diffuse large B-cell lymphoma (see Table 1.3, p. 80) {1510A}.

Lymphomas secondarily involving the vulva are also of a variety of types, with diffuse large B-cell lymphoma being the most common {972,1970}. Hodgkin lymphoma in the female reproductive organs is exceedingly rare but a case of classical Hodgkin lymphoma presenting with massive vulvar involvement in a patient with Crohn disease is reported; staging revealed widespread disease {2036A}.

Prognosis and predictive factors
Data are limited, and the lymphomas are heterogeneous, so it is difficult to draw firm conclusions, but lymphomas involving the vulva appear to be relatively aggressive {1971A}.

Myeloid neoplasms

Definition
Malignant neoplasms of haematopoietic origin, including myeloid leukaemias and myeloid sarcoma, a mass-forming lesion composed of primitive myeloid cells.

Synonyms
Myeloid sarcoma is also known as chloroma, granulocytic sarcoma or extramedullary myeloid tumour

Clinical features
In rare instances the vulva is involved by a myeloid sarcoma. This has been described as the first presentation of acute myeloid leukaemia {505A}, as an isolated relapse following therapy for acute myeloid leukaemia {1337A}, and in the setting of an established diagnosis of myelodysplastic syndrome/myeloproliferative neoplasm {605}. The lesions presented as a rash involving the clitoris or as a mass involving the labium majus or an unspecified portion of the vulva, with or without extension to involve the vagina and cervix.

Histopathology
The histological features are similar to those seen in other sites.

Prognosis and predictive factors
Outcome is variable, with prognosis likely due to underlying genetic abnormalities and extent of disease.

Secondary tumours

Definition
Secondary tumours of the vulva represent spread of neoplasms that originate outside of the vulva.

Epidemiology
Secondary involvement is rare and is estimated to constitute approximately 5–10% of all vulvar cancer {1340}.

Clinical features
In one large series, patients' age ranged from 18–84 (mean 55) years with most presenting with a mass in the labium majus, ulceration or pain {1340}. The metastases were detected on average 3 years after initial diagnosis; rarely, it is the first manifestation of disease {434,1340}.

Macroscopy
Tumours most commonly involve the dermis and subcutis and the size varies greatly, ranging from 0.5 to 11.9 cm in one series {1340}.

Site of origin
Vulvar metastases most often originate from primary gynaecological tumours, most commonly the cervix {1340}. Of non-gynaecological primaries, gastrointestinal tract and breast are the most common {660,858,1194,1340}.

Histopathology
The morphological features are similar to those of the primary tumour. Many tumours involve the epidermis.

Prognosis and predictive factors
Presence of metastases to the vulva is often associated with systemic metastasis and is a pre-terminal event. Isolated vulvar metastases may have a better prognosis.

Contributors

Dr Isabel ALVARADO-CABRERO
Guadalajara 94A-12 Col. Condesa
Delegacion Cuauhtemoc
Mexico DF
CP 06140
MEXICO
Tel. +52 555 574 23 22
keme2.tijax12@gmail.com

Dr Rebecca BAERGEN
NY-Presbyterian Hosp, Weill-Cornell Med Ctr
Surgical Pathology, Starr 1002
520 East 70th Street
New York, NY 10065
USA
Tel. +1 212 746 2768
Fax +1 212 746 0568
rbaergen@med.cornell.edu

Dr Debra A. BELL
Division of Anatomic Pathology-Hilton 11
Mayo Clinic - Rochester
200 First Street SW
Rochester, MN 55905
USA
Tel. +1 507 284 8746
Fax +1 507 284 1599
bell.debra@mayo.edu

Dr Christine BERGERON
Laboratoire CERBA
95066 Cergy Pontoise Cedex 9
FRANCE
Tel. +33 6 09 07 52 76
Fax +33 1 34 40 20 29
bergeron@lab-cerba.com

Dr Jonathan G. BIJRON
University Medical Center Utrecht
Department of Pathology H04.223
Heidelberglaan 100
3524 Utrecht TA
THE NETHERLANDS
Tel. + 31 88 751 693
Fax + 31 30 254 4990
j.g.bijron@umcutrecht.nl

Dr Dengfeng CAO*
Department of Pathology
Peking University Cancer Hospital
52 Fucheng Road, Haidian District
Beijing 100142
CHINA
Tel. +86 10 8819 6667, +86 10 0125 2716
Fax +86 10 8812 2437
dengfeng99@yahoo.com

Dr Maria Luisa CARCANGIU*
Department of Anatomical Pathology
Fondazione IRCCS
Istituto Nazionale dei Tumori
Via Venezian 1
20133, Milano
ITALY
Tel. +39 348 019 7903
Fax +39 022 390 2877
marialuisa.carcangiu@istitutotumori.mi.it

Dr Silvestro G. CARINELLI
Department of Pathology
Istituto Europeo di Oncologia
Via Ripamonti 435
20141 Milano
ITALY
Tel. +39 02 9437 2004
Fax +39 02 9437 9214
silvestro.carinelli@ieo.it

Dr Annie N.Y. CHEUNG
Department of Pathology
The University of Hong Kong
Room 322, University Pathology Building
Pokfulam Road
HONG KONG SAR CHINA
Tel. +852 2255 4876
Fax +852 2218 5202
anycheun@pathology.hku.hk

Dr Kathleen R. CHO
Department of Pathology
University of Michigan Medical School
1506 A. Alfred Taubman BSRB
109 Zina Pitcher
Ann Arbor, MI 48109
USA
Tel. +1 734 764 1549
Fax +1 734 647 7950
kathcho@umich.edu

Dr Terence J. COLGAN*
Room 6-502-3
Mount Sinai Hospital
600 University Avenue
Toronto, Ontario M5G 1X5
CANADA
Tel. +1 416 586 4522
Fax +1 416 586 8481
tcolgan@mtsinai.on.ca

Dr Christopher P. CRUM
Department of Pathology
Brigham and Women's Hospital
75 Francis Street
Boston, MA 02115
USA
Tel. +1 617 732 5481
Fax +1 617 264 5125
ccrum@partners.org

Dr Dean DAYA*
Department of Pathology
Jurawanski Hospital
Hamilton, Ontario
L9G 4S2
CANADA
Tel. +1 905 527 4322 ext 42036
Fax +1 905 389 1698
dayad@hhsc.ca

Dr Lora H. ELLENSON
Department of Pathology and Lab Medicine
Weill Cornell Medical College
1300 York Ave. Room F309D
New York, NY 10021
USA
Tel. +1 212 746 6447
Fax +1 212 746 8079
lora.ellenson@med.cornell.edu

Dr Charis ENG
Cleveland Clinic
Genomic Medicine Institute
9500 Euclid Ave., NE50
Cleveland, OH 44196
USA
Tel. +1 216 444 3440
Fax +1 216 636 0009
engc@ccf.org

---

* The asterix indicates participation in the Working Group Meeting on the Classification of Tumours of the Female Reproductive Organs that was held in Lyon, France, June 13–15, 2013.

Dr Alex S. FERENCZY
Department of Pathology
Jewish General Hospital
3755 Côte Ste-Catherine Road
Montreal, Quebec H3T 1E2
CANADA
Tel. +1 514 340 7526
Fax +1 514 340 8102
alex.ferenczy@mcgill.ca

Dr Judith A. FERRY
Department of Pathology
Massachusetts General Hospital
55 Fruit Street
Boston, MA 02114
USA
Tel. +1 617 726 4826
Fax +1 617 726 9312
jferry@partners.org

Dr Masaharu FUKUNAGA
Izumihoncho 4-11-1
Komaeski
Tokyo 201-8601
JAPAN
Tel. +81 3 3480 1151
Fax +81 3 3480 5700
maasafu@jikei.ac.jp

Dr Raji GANESAN
1st Floor Laboratories
Birmingham Womens' Hospital
Mindelsohn Way, Edgbaston
Birmingham B15 2TG
UK
Tel. +44 12 16 27 2724
Fax +44 12 16 07 4721
raji.ganesan@bwhct.nhs.uk

Dr Deborah GERSELL
St. John's Mercy Medical Center
615 S. New Ballas Rd
Department of Pathology
St. Louis, MO 63141
USA
Tel. +1 314 251 4715
Fax +1 314 251 4467
deborah.gersell@mercy.net

Dr C. Blake GILKS*
Department of Pathology and
Lab Medicine, Room 1503
Vancouver General Hospital
855 West 12th Ave
Vancouver BC V5Z1M9
CANADA
Tel. +1 604 875 4901
Fax +1 604 875 4797
blake.gilks@vch.ca

Dr C. Simon HERRINGTON*
Jaqui Wood Cancer Centre
James Arrott Drive
Ninewells Hospital and Medical School
Dundee DD1 9SY
UK
Tel. +44 13 82 38 3125
Fax +44 13 82 49 6361
s.herrington@dundee.ac.uk

Dr Lynn HIRSCHOWITZ
Department of Cellular Pathology, Level 1
Birmingham Women's NHS Foundation Trust
Mindelsohn Way, Edgbaston
Birmingham B15 2TG
UK
Tel. +44 79 73 31 0672
Fax +44 12 16 07 4721
lynn.hirschowitz@gmail.com

Dr Pei HUI*
Department of Pathology, BML 254B
Yale School of Medicine
310 Cedar St.
New Haven, CT 06520
USA
Tel. +1 203 785 6498
Fax +1 209 785 7146
pei.hui@yale.edu

Dr David HUNTSMAN
#3427 - 600 West 10th Ave
Vancouver, BC, V5Z 4E6
CANADA
Tel. +1 604 877 6000 ext 2148
Fax +1 604 877 6089
dhuntsma@bccancer.bc.ca

Dr Philip IP
Department of Pathology
The University of Hong Kong
Queen Mary Hospital
102 Pokfulam Road
HONG KONG SAR CHINA
Tel. +852 2255 4732
Fax +852 2872 8098
philipip@pathology.hku.hk

Dr Robert JAKOB*
Department of Classifications
Terminology and Standards
World Health Organization
Avenue Appia 20
1211 Geneva 27
SWITZERLAND
Tel. +41 22 79 15877
jakobr@who.int

Dr Hidetaka KATABUCHI
Department of Obstetrics and Gynecology
Faculty of Life Sciences
Kumamoto University
1-1-1 Honjo, Chuo-hu
Kumamoto, 860-8556
JAPAN
Tel. +81 96 373 5269
Fax +81 96 363 5164
buchi@kumamoto-u.ac.jp

Dr Surapan KHUNAMORNPONG
Department of Pathology
Faculty of Medicine
Chiang Mai University
Chiang Mai 50200
THAILAND
Tel. +66 89 854 8379
Fax +66 53 217 144
skhunamo@med.cmu.ac.th

Dr Insun KIM
125-1, 5 Ga
Anam Dong
Sungbuk Ku
Seoul
REPUBLIC OF KOREA
Tel. +82 2 920 6373
Fax +82 2 920 6576
iskim@korea.ac.kr

Dr Kyu-Rae KIM*
Department of Pathology, University of Ulsan
College of Medicine, Asan Medical Center
388-1 Pungnap-dong Songpa-gu
Seoul
REPUBLIC OF KOREA
Tel. +82 2 3010 4514
Fax +82 2 4727 898
krkim@amc.seoul.kr

Dr Takako KIYOKAWA
Department of Molecular Pathology
Chiba University School of Medicine
1-8-1 Inohana Chuo-ku
Chiba, 260-8670
JAPAN
Tel. +81 43 222 7171
Fax +81 43 226 2063
tkiyokawa@faculty.chiba-u.jp

Dr Martin KÖBEL*
Department of Pathology and Lab Medicine
Foothills Medical Centre
1403 29 ST NW
University of Calgary, CLS/AHS
Calgary, AB T2N 2T9
CANADA
Tel. +1 403 944 8504
Fax +1 403 944 4748
martin.koebel@cls.ab.ca

Dr Friedrich KOMMOSS
Institute of Pathology
Referral Centre for Gynecopathology
A2, 2
68159 Mannheim
GERMANY
Tel. +49 621 122 998 90
Fax +49 621 122 998 93 10
kommoss@gyn-patho.de

Dr Ikuo KONISHI
Department of Gynecology and Obstetrics
Kyoto University Graduate School of Medicine
54 Shogoin Kawahara-cho
Sakyo-ku, Kyoto 606-8507
JAPAN
Tel. +81 75 751 3267
Fax +81 75 761 3967
konishi@kuhp.kyoto-u.ac.jp

Dr Jolanta KUPRYJANCZYK
The Maria Sklodowska-Curie Memorial
Cancer Center and Institute of Oncology
Department of Pathology
Roentgena Street 5
02-781 Warsaw
POLAND
Tel. +48 22 546 21 22
Fax +48 22 546 29 84
jkupry@coi.waw.pl

Dr Robert J. KURMAN*
Departments of Pathology, Gyneology/
Obstetrics and Oncology
Division of Gynecologic Pathology
Johns Hopkins Hospital
401 N, Broadway
Baltimore, MD 21231
USA
Tel. +1 410 955 2804
Fax +1 410 614 1287
rkurman@jhmi.edu

Dr Janice M. LAGE
Department of Pathology
University of Mississippi Medical Center
2500 N State Street
Jackson, MS 39216
USA
Tel. +1 601 984 1540
Fax +1 601 984 1531
jlage@umc.edu

Dr Sunil R. LAKHANI*
Department of Molecular & Cellular Pathology
University of Queensland
The Royal Brisbane & Women's Hospital
Level 6, Building 71/918
Herston 4069 Brisbane, QLD
AUSTRALIA
Tel. +61 7 3346 6052
Fax +61 7 3346 5596
s.lakhani@uq.edu.au

Dr W. Dwayne LAWRENCE
Women & Infants Hospital of Rhode Island
Alpert Medical School of Brown University
101 Dudley Street
Providence, RI 02906
USA
Tel. +1 401 274 1122 ext. 1284
Fax +1 401 453 7681
dlawrence@wihri.org

Dr Sigurd LAX*
Department of Pathology
General Hospital Graz
Goestingerstrasse 22
8020 Graz
AUSTRIA
Tel. +43 316 5466 4650
Fax +43 316 5466 7465 2
sigurd.lax@medunigraz.at

Dr Douglas A. LEVINE*
Gynecology Service, Department of Surgery
Memorial Sloan-Kettering Cancer Center
1275 York Avenue
New York, NY 10065
USA
Tel. +1 212 639 7335
Fax +1 212 717 3789
levine2@mskcc.org

Dr Aijun LIU
Department of Pathology
Chinese PLA General Hospital
28# Fuxing Rd., Haidian District
Beijing 100853
CHINA
Tel. +86 10 6693 6253
Fax +86 10 6693 9820
aliu301@126.com

Dr Thomas LOENING*
Albertinen Pathologie
Fangdieckstr. 75a
22547 Hamburg
GERMANY
Tel. +40 70 708 51 20
Fax +40 70 708 51 10
loening@albertinenpathologie.de

Dr Teri A. LONGACRE*
Department of Pathology
Stanford University School of Medicine
300 Pasteur Drive, Room L-235
Stanford, CA 94305
USA
Tel. +1 650 498 6460
Fax +1 650 725 6902
longacre@stanford.edu

Dr Anais MALPICA
Department of Pathology
The University of Texas
MD Anderson Cancer Center
1515 Holcombe Blvd., Unit 85
Houston, TX 77030
USA
Tel. +1 713 792 4655
Fax +1 713 792 5529
amalpica@mdanderson.org

Dr Xavier MATIAS-GUIU
Hospital Universitari Arnau de Vilanova
Irblleida - University of Lleida
Alcalde rovira roure 80
25198 Lleida
SPAIN
Tel. +34 97 370 53 40 / +34 68 787 82 52
Fax +34 97 370 52 27
fjmatiasguiu.lleida.ics@gencat.cat

Dr W. Glenn McCLUGGAGE*
Department of Pathology
Royal Group of Hospitals
Grosvenor Road
Belfast BT12 6BA
UK
Tel. +44 28 90 632 563
Fax +44 28 90 233 643
glenn.mccluggage@belfasttrust.hscni.net

Dr Yoshiki MIKAMI*
Department of Diagnostic Pathology
Kyoto University Hospital
54 Shogoin Kawahara-cho, Sakyo-ku
Kyoto City, Kyoto 606-8507
JAPAN
Tel. +81 75 751 3488
Fax +81 75 751 3499
mika@kuhp.kyoto-u.ac.jp

Dr Eoghan E. MOONEY
Department of Pathology &
Laboratory Medicine
National Maternity Hospital
Holles St
Dublin 2
IRELAND
Tel. +353 1 637 3531
Fax +353 1 676 5048
emooney@nmh.ie

Dr George L. MUTTER
Department of Pathology
Brigham and Women's Hospital
75 Francis Street
Boston, MA 02115
USA
Tel. +1 617 732 6096
Fax +1 617 738 6996
gmutter@partners.org

Dr G. Petur NIELSEN
Department of Pathology
Massachusetts General Hospital
55 Fruit Street
Boston, MA 02478
USA
Tel. +1 617 724 1469
Fax +1 617 726 9312
gnielsen@mgh.harvard.edu

Dr Francisco F. NOGALES
Departamento de Anatomía Patológica
Facultad de Medicina
Av Madrid 11
18012 Granada
SPAIN
Tel. +34 95 824 35 08
Fax +34 95 824 35 10
fnogales@ugr.es

Dr Marisa R. NUCCI*
Division of Women's and Perinatal Pathology
Brigham and Women's Hospital
75 Francis Street
Boston, MA 02115
USA
Tel. +1 617 732 5054
Fax +1 617 277 9015
mnucci@partners.org

Dr Hiroko OHGAKI*
Section of Molecular Pathology
International Agency for Research on Cancer
150 Cours Albert Thomas
69372 Lyon
FRANCE
Tel. +33 4 72 73 85 34
Fax +33 4 72 73 86 98
ohgaki@iarc.fr

Dr Esther OLIVA*
Department of Pathology
Massachussetts General Hospital
55 Fruit Street
Boston, MA 02114
USA
Tel. +1 617 724 8272
Fax +1 617 724 6564
eoliva@partners.org

Dr José PALACIOS
Servicio de Anatomia Patologica
Hospital Universitario Ramon y Cajal
Carretera de Colmenar Viejo, Km 9,100
28034 Madrid
SPAIN
Tel. +34 65 178 82 87
Fax +34 91 336 87 94
jose.palacios@salud.madrid.org

Dr Kay J. PARK
Department of Pathology
Memorial Sloan-Kettering Cancer Center
1275 York Ave.
New York, NY 10065
USA
Tel. +1 212 639 5905
Fax +1 212 717 3203
parkk@mskcc.org

Dr Vinita PARKASH
Department of Pathology
Bridgeport Hospital
267 Grant Street
Bridgeport, CT 06610
USA
Tel. +1 203 384 4833
Fax +1 203 384 3237
vinita.parkash@yale.edu

Dr Barbara PASINI
Citta della Salute e della Scienza di Torino
SC Genetica Medica
Via Santena, 19
10126 Torino
ITALY
Tel. +39 01 16 33 44 79
Fax +39 01 16 33 51 81
barbara.pasini@unito.it

Dr William A. PETERS III
1101 Madison Street; Suite 1500
Seattle, WA 98104
USA
Tel. +1 206 965 1700
Fax +1 206 965 1735
wpeters@pacificgyn.com

Dr Jurgen M.J. PIEK
Comprehensive Cancer Center
South Location
TweeSteden Hospital
Doctor Deelenlaan 5
5042AD Tilburg
THE NETHERLANDS
Tel. +31 13 465 5655
jurgen.piek@gmail.com

Dr Jaime PRAT*
Department of Pathology
Hospital de la Santa Creu i Sant Pau
Autonomous University of Barcelona
Sant Quinti, 87-89
08041 Barcelona
SPAIN
Tel. +34 93 553 73 45
Fax +34 93 553 73 48
jprat@santpau.cat

Dr Bradley QUADE
Department of Pathology
Brigham and Women's Hospital
75 Francis Street
Boston, MA 02062
USA
Tel. +1 617 732 7980
Fax +1 617 738 6996
bquade@partners.org

Dr Sigrid REGAUER
Institute of Pathology
Medical University Graz
Auenbruggerplatz 25
8026 Graz
AUSTRIA
Tel. +43 316 380 4452 or +43 316 3858 3689
Fax +43 316 384 329
sigrid.regauer@medunigraz.at

Dr Cristina RIVA
Anatomia Patologica-Ospedale Di Circolo
University of Insubria
Viale Borri 57
21100 Varese
ITALY
Tel. +39 332 270 601
Fax +39 332 270 600
cristina.riva@uninsubria.it

Dr Brigitte M. RONNETT
The Johns Hopkins Hospital
Department of Pathology, Weinberg 2242
401 N. Broadway
Baltimore, MD 21231
USA
Tel. +1 410 614 2971
Fax +1 410 614 1287
bronnett@jhmi.edu

Dr Brian ROUS*
National Cancer Registration Service
Eastern Cancer Registration &
Information Centre, Unit C - Magog Court
Shelford Bottom
Cambridge CB22 3AD
UK
Tel. +44 1223 213 625
Fax +44 1223 213 571
brian.rous@ecric.nhs.uk

Dr Achim SCHNEIDER
Department of Gynecology
Charité University Hospital Campus Mitte
Charitéplatz 1
10117 Berlin
GERMANY
Tel. +49 30 450 564 172
Fax +49 30 450 564 931
achim.schneider@charite.de

Dr Neil J. SEBIRE
Trophoblastic Disease Unit
Department of Cancer Medicine
Charing Cross Hospital
Fulham Place Road, Hammersmith
London W6 8RF
UK
Tel. +44 207 829 863
Fax +44 207 829 787
neil.sebire@gosh.nhs.uk

Dr Jeffrey D. SEIDMAN*
Division of Immunology and Hematology
Office of In Vitro Diagnostics and
Radiological Health
Center for Devices and Radiological Health
Food and Drug Administration
10903 New Hampshire Ave.
Silver Spring, MD 20997
USA
Tel. +1 240 402 0349
jeffrey.seidman@fda.hhs.gov

Dr Patricia SHAW
University Health Network
Department of Pathology
TGH Eaton 11-444
200 Elizabeth St
Toronto, Ontario M5G 2C4
CANADA
Tel. +1 416 340 4673
Fax +1 416 340 5517
patricia.shaw@uhn.ca

Dr Mark E. SHERMAN
National Cancer Institute
Division of Cancer Epidemiology & Genetics
9609 Medical Center Drive
Bethesda, MD 20892
USA
Tel. +1 240 276 7051
shermanm@mail.nih.gov

Dr Ie-Ming SHIH
Departments of Pathology, Gynecology
and Obstetrics and Oncology
Johns Hopkins Medical Institutions, CRB2-305
1550 Orleans Street
Baltimore, MD 21029
USA
Tel. +1 410 502 7774
Fax +1 410 502 7943
ishih@jhmi.edu

Dr Gad SINGER
Institut für Pathologie
Kantonsspital Baden
5404 Baden
SWITZERLAND
Tel. +41 56 486 39 01
Fax +41 56 486 39 19
gad.singer@ksb.ch

Dr Robert SOSLOW
Memorial Sloan-Kettering Cancer Center
Department of Pathology
1275 York Avenue
New York, NY 10065
USA
Tel. +1 212 639 5905
Fax +1 646 422 2070
soslowr@mskcc.org

Dr Paul N. STAATS
Department of Pathology
University of Maryland School of Medicine
22 S. Greene Street, NBW43
Baltimore, MD 21201
USA
Tel. +1 410 328 5555
Fax +1 410 328 5508
pstaats@umm.edu

Dr Colin J.R. STEWART
Department of Histopathology
King Edward Memorial Hospital
374 Bagot Road
Subiaco WA 6008, Perth
AUSTRALIA
Tel. +61 608 9340 2715
Fax +61 608 9340 2636
colin.stewart@health.wa.gov.au

Dr Mark STOLER*
Department of Pathology, PO Box 800214
University of Virginia Health System
1215 Lee St. HEP Room 3032
Charlottesville, VA 22901
USA
Tel. +1 434 982 0284
Fax +1 434 924 9492
mhs2e@virginia.edu

Dr Hitoshi TSUDA
Department of Basic Pathology
National Defense Medical College
3-2 Namiki, Tokorozawa
Saitama 359-8513
JAPAN
Tel. +81 4 2995 1507
Fax +81 4 2996 5193
Email: htsuda@ndmc.ac.jp

Dr Paul J. van DIEST
University Medical Center Utrecht
Department of Pathology, H04.312
Heidelberglaan 100
3524 TA Utrecht
THE NETHERLANDS
Tel. +31 88 755 6565
Fax +31 30 254 4990
p.j.vandiest@umcutrecht.nl

Dr Russell VANG
The Johns Hopkins Hospital
Div. of Gynecologic Pathology
Weinberg Bldg., Rm. 2242
401 North Broadway
Baltimore, MD 21231
USA
Tel. +1 410 502 0532
Fax +1 410 614 1287
rvang1@jhmi.edu

Dr Michael WELLS*
Department of Oncology
Faculty of Medicine, Dentistry and Health
University of Sheffield
Beech Hill Road
Sheffield S10 2RX
UK
Tel. +44 114 271 2397
m.wells@sheffield.ac.uk

Dr David C. WILBUR*
55 Fruit Street
Warren 120
Massachusetts General Hospital
Boston, MA 02114
USA
Tel. +1 617 726 7943
Fax +1 617 724 6564
dwilbur@partners.org

Dr Edward J. WILKINSON
University of Florida
Department of Pathology
1600 SW Archer Road, Room 3113
Gainesville, FL 32610-0275
USA
Tel. +1 352 265 0238
Fax +1 352 265 0437
wilkinso@pathology.ufl.edu

Dr Thomas WRIGHT
84 Station Road
Irvington
New York, NY 10533
USA
Tel. +1 212 203 3961
Fax +1 212 648 4098
tcw1@columbia.edu

Dr Robert H. YOUNG*
James Homer Wright Pathology Laboratories
Massachusetts General Hospital
Harvard Medical School
55 Fruit Street
Boston, MA 02114
USA
Tel. +1 617 726 8892
Fax +1 617 726 9151
rhyoung@partners.org

Dr Richard ZAINO*
Penn State Milton S. Hershey Medical Center
Department of Pathology, MC H179
500 University Drive, PO Box 850
Hershey, PA 17033
USA
Tel. +1 717 531 1678
Fax +1 717 531 7741
rzaino@hmc.psu.edu

Dr Charles J. ZALOUDEK*
Department of Pathology
University of California, San Francisco
505 Parnassus Ave., M563
San Francisco, CA 94143
USA
Tel. +1 415 353 1734
Fax +1 415 353 1200
charles.zaloudek@ucsf.edu

Dr Gian Franco ZANNONI
Institute of Anatomical Pathology
Università Cattolica del Sacro Cuore
Largo F. Vito, 1
00186 Roma
ITALY
Tel. +39 63 015 4433
Fax +39 63 051 3433
gfzannoni@rm.unicatt.it

Dr Chengquan ZHAO
Department of Pathology
Magee-Womens Hospital, UPMC
300 Halket Street
Pittsburgh, PA 15213
USA
Tel. +1 412 641 6678
Fax +1 412 641 1675
czhao@mail.magee.edu

Dr Xianrong ZHOU
Department of Pathology
Obstetrics & Gynecology Hospital
Fudan University
419 Fangxie Road
Shanghai 200011
CHINA
Tel. +86 021 3318 9900
Fax +86 021 5512 2025
zhouxianrong@hotmail.com

IARC/WHO Committee for the International Classification of Diseases for Oncology (ICD-O)

Dr David FORMAN
Section of Cancer Information
International Agency for Research on Cancer
150 cours Albert Thomas
69372 Lyon cedex 08
FRANCE
Tel. +33 4 72 73 80 56
Fax +33 4 72 73 86 96
formand@iarc.fr

Mrs April FRITZ
A. Fritz and Associates, LLC
21361 Crestview Road
Reno, NV 89521
USA
Tel. +1 775 636 7243
Fax +1 888 891 3012
april@afritz.org

Dr Robert JAKOB
Classifications and Terminologies
Evidence and Information for Policy
World Health Organization (WHO)
20 Avenue Appia
1211 Geneva 27
SWITZERLAND
Tel. +41 22 791 58 77
Fax +41 22 791 48 94
jakobr@who.int

Dr Paul KLEIHUES
Medical Faculty
University of Zurich
Pestalozzistrasse 5
8032 Zurich
SWITZERLAND
Tel. +41 44 362 21 10
Fax +41 44 251 06 65
kleihues@pathol.uzh.ch

Dr Robert J. KURMAN
Department of Pathology
Gynecologic Pathology
Johns Hopkins Hospital
401 N, Broadway
Baltimore, MD 21231
USA
Tel. +1 410 955 2804
Fax +1 410 614 1287
rkurman@jhmi.edu

Dr Hiroko OHGAKI
Section of Molecular Pathology
International Agency for Research on Cancer
150 cours Albert Thomas
69372 Lyon cedex 08
FRANCE
Tel. +33 4 72 73 85 34
Fax +33 4 72 73 86 98
ohgaki@iarc.fr

Dr Brian ROUS
Eastern Cancer Registry and
Information Centre
Unit C - Magog Court
Shelford Bottom, Hinton Way
Cambridge CB22 3AD
UK
Tel. +1 223 213 625
Fax +1 223 213 571
brian.rous@ecric.nhs.uk

Dr Leslie H. SOBIN
The Cancer Human Biobank
National Cancer Institute
6110 Executive Blvd, Suite 250
Rockville, MD 20852
USA
Tel. +1 301 443 7947
Fax +1 301 402 9325
leslie.sobin@nih.gov

Dr Robert H. YOUNG
James Homer Wright Pathology Laboratories
Massachusetts General Hospital
Harvard Medical School
55 Fruit Street
Boston, MA 02114
USA
Tel. +1 617 726 8892
Fax +1 617 726 9151
rhyoung@partners.org

Sources of figures and tables

Sources of figures

1.01	Vang R.
1.02	Vang R.
1.03	Bell D.A.
1.04	Vang R.
1.05	Seidman J.D.
1.06	Bell D.A.
1.07 A	Bell D.A.
1.07 B	Vang R.
1.08	Vang R.
1.09 A,B	Vang R.
1.10 A,B	Vang R.
1.11 A	Singer G.
1.11 B	Gilks C.B.
1.12 A	Bell D.A.
1.12 B	Reprinted from: Yemelyanova A, Mao TL, Nakayama N, Shih I, Kurman RJ (2008). Low-grade serous carcinoma of the ovary displaying a macropapillary pattern of invasion. Am J Surg Pathol 32: 1800–1806.
1.13	Singer G.
1.14 A,B	Seidman J.D.
1.15	Reprinted from: Antoniou A, Pharoah PD, Narod S, Risch HA et al (2003). Average risks of breast and ovarian cancer associated with BRCA1 or BRCA2 mutations detected in case Series unselected for family history: a combined analysis of 22 Studies. Am J Hum Gen 72: 1117–1130. With permission from Elsevier
1.16	Seidman J.D.
1.17 A	Ronnett B.M.
1.17 B	Prat J.
1.18	Malpica A.
1.19 A,D	Bell D.A.
1.19 B	Longacre T.A.
1.19 C	Ronnett B.M.
1.20 A	Ronnett B.M.
1.20 B	Longacre T.A.
1.21 A	Prat J.
1.21 B	Longacre T.A.
1.22 A,B	Singer G.
1.23 A	Ronnett B.M.
1.23 B	Reprinted from: Seidman JD, Cho KR, Ronnett BM, Kurman RJ (2011). Surface epithelial tumours of the ovary. In: *Blaustein's Pathology of the Female Genital Tract*. Kurman RJ, Ellenson HK, Ronnett BM (Eds). Springer: New York 679–784. With permission from Springer Science and Business Media
1.24 A,B	Prat J.
1.25	Bell D.A.
1.26 A-C	Köbel M.
1.27 A,B	Gilks C.B.
1.28	Liu A.
1.29	Liu A.
1.30	Gilks C.B.
1.31	Prat J.
1.32	Vang R.
1.33 A,B	Köbel M.
1.33 C	Vang R.
1.33 D	Vang R.
1.34	Köbel M.
1.35	Köbel M.
1.36	Köbel M.
1.37 A,B	Kiyokawa T.
1.38	Kiyokawa T.
1.39 A,B	Staats P.N.
1.40 A,B	Staats P.N.
1.41	Young R.H.
1.42 A,B	Zaloudek C.J.
1.43	Staats P.N.
1.44 A,B	Zaloudek C.J.
1.45 A-C	Zaloudek C.J.
1.46 A,B	Zaloudek C.J.
1.47	Zaloudek C.J.
1.48	Young R.H.
1.49 A,B	Zaloudek C.J.
1.50	Zaloudek C.J.
1.51 A	Loening T.
1.51 B-D	Mooney E.E.
1.52	Mooney E.E.
1.53	Zaloudek C.J.
1.54 A-C	Zaloudek C.J.
1.55	Nogales F.F.
1.56 A	Zaloudek C.J.
1.56 B	Cao D..
1.57	Vang R.
1.58 A-D	Vang R.
1.59 A,B	Nogales F.F.
1.60	Vang R.
1.61 A	Young R.
1.61 B-D	Vang R.
1.62	Cao D..
1.63 A-C	Zaloudek C.J.
1.64 A-C	Prat J.
1.65	Nogales F.F.
1.66 A	Young R.H.
1.66 B	McCluggage W.G.
1.67 A	Oliva E.
1.67 B	Young R.H.
1.68	Sahin A., Department of Pathology, MD Anderson Cancer Center, Houston, TX, USA
1.69	Young R.H.
1.70	Oliva E.
1.71 A,B	McCluggage W.G.
1.72	Oliva E.
1.73 A	Lerwill M.F. Department of Pathology, Massachusetts General Hospital, Boston, MA, USA
1.73 B,C	Ip P.
1.74 A	Young R.H.
1.74 B	Zaloudek C.J.
1.75 A,B	Oliva E.
1.76 A,B	Oliva E.
1.77	Ferry J.A.
1.78	Ferry J.A.
1.79	Ferry J.A.
1.80	Ferry J.A.
1.81 A	Ronnett B.M.
1.81 B,C	Vang R.
1.82	Vang R.
1.83 A-C	Ronnett B.M.
1.84 A,B	Ronnett B.M.
1.85 A,B	Vang R.
1.86 A,B	Ronnett B.M.
2.01	Oliva E.
2.02	Daya D.
2.03	Daya D.
2.04	Daya D.
2.05	Prat J.
2.06 A	Carcangiu M.L.
2.06 B	Prat J.
2.07	Kim K.-R.
2.08	Kim K.-R.
2.09	Cao D..
2.10 A,B	Khunamornpong S.
2.11	Khunamornpong S.
2.12	Khunamornpong S.
2.13	Khunamornpong S.
2.14	Khunamornpong S.
2.15	Lerwill M.F. Department of Pathology, Massachusetts General Hospital, Boston, MA, USA
2.16	Cheung A.N.Y.
3.01 A	Cao D.
3.01 B	Crum C.P.
3.02 A-C	Lax S.
3.03 A	Alvarado-Cabrero I.
3.03 B	van Diest Paul J.
3.04 A	Crum C.P.
3.04 B	Reprinted from: Kurman R, Vang R, Junge J et al (2011). Papillary Tubal Hyperplasia: The Putative Precursor of Ovarian Atypical Proliferative (Borderline) Serous Tumors, Noninvasive Implants, and Endosalpingiosis. Am J Surg Pathol. 35(11):1605–1614. Copyright with permission from Wolters Kluwer Health.
3.05	Carcangiu M.L.
3.06	Crum C.P.
3.07	Crum C.P.
3.08	Crum C.P.
3.09 A,B	Ferry J.A.

Sources of tables

1.1	Köbel M.
1.2	Nogales F.F.
1.3	Ferry J.A.
1.4	Vang R.
5.1	Hui P.
6.1	Hui P.
6.2	Hui P.
6.3	Hui P.

Sources of figures for front cover

Top left	Singer G.
Top center	Mooney E.E.
Top right	Ip P.
Middle left	Oliva E.
Middle center	Reprinted from: Yemelyanova A, Mao TL, Nakayama N, Shih I, Kurman RJ (2008). Low-grade serous carcinoma of the ovary displaying a macropapillary pattern of invasion. Am J Surg Pathol 32: 1800–1806. With permission from Wolters Kluwer Health
Middle right	Zaloudek C.J.
Bottom left	Globocan, IARC
Bottom center	Stoler M.
Bottom right	Stoler M.

References

1. Abbott TM, Hermann WJ, Jr., Scully RE (1984). Ovarian fetiform teratoma (homunculus) in a 9-year-old girl. Int J Gynecol Pathol 2: 392-402.

2. Abeler VM, Holm R, Nesland JM, Kjorstad KE (1994). Small cell carcinoma of the cervix. A clinicopathologic study of 26 patients. Cancer 73: 672-677.

3. Abeler VM, Kjorstad KE (1991). Clear cell carcinoma of the endometrium: a histopathological and clinical study of 97 cases. Gynecol Oncol 40: 207-217.

4. Abeler VM, Royne O, Thoresen S, Danielsen HE, Nesland JM, Kristensen GB (2009). Uterine sarcomas in Norway. A histopathological and prognostic survey of a total population from 1970 to 2000 including 419 patients. Histopathology 54: 355-364.

5. Abeler VM, Vergote IB, Kjorstad KE, Trope CG (1996). Clear cell carcinoma of the endometrium. Prognosis and metastatic pattern. Cancer 78: 1740-1747.

6. Abell MR (1965). Intraepithelial carcinomas of epidermis and squamous mucosa of vulva and perineum. Surg Clin North Am 45: 1179-1198.

7. Abeln EC, Smit VT, Wessels JW, de Leeuw WJ, Cornelisse CJ, Fleuren GJ (1997). Molecular genetic evidence for the conversion hypothesis of the origin of malignant mixed mullerian tumours. J Pathol 183: 424-431.

7A. Abu-Rustum NR, Zhou Q, Gomez JD, Alektiar KM, Hensley ML, Soslow RA, Levine DA, Chi DS, Barakat RR, Iasonos A (2010). A nomogram for predicting overall survival of women with endometrial cancer following primary therapy: toward improving individualized cancer care. Gynecol Oncol 116: 399-403.

8. Acikalin MF, Tanir HM, Ozalp S, Dundar E, Ciftci E, Ozalp E (2009). Diffuse uterine adenomatoid tumor in a patient with chronic hepatitis C virus infection. Int J Gynecol Cancer 19: 242-244.

9. Adashi EY, Rosenshein NB, Parmley TH, Woodruff JD (1980). Histogenesis of the broad ligament adrenal rest. Int J Gynaecol Obstet 18: 102-104.

10. Adelman S, Benson CD, Hertzler JH (1975). Surgical lesions of the ovary in infancy and childhood. Surg Gynecol Obstet 141: 219-226.

11. Agaimy A, Wunsch PH, Schroeder J, Gaumann A, Dietmaier W, Hartmann A, Hofstaedter F, Mentzel T (2008). Low-grade abdominopelvic sarcoma with myofibroblastic features (low-grade myofibroblastic sarcoma): clinicopathological, immunohistochemical, molecular genetic and ultrastructural study of two cases with literature review. J Clin Pathol 61: 301-306.

12. Agarwal PK, Husain N, Chandrawati (1991). Adenofibroma of uterus and endocervix. Histopathology 18: 79-80.

13. Aggarwal N, Bhargava R, Elishaev E (2012). Uterine adenosarcomas: diagnostic use of the proliferation marker Ki-67 as an adjunct to morphologic diagnosis. Int J Gynecol Pathol 31: 447-452.

14. Agoff SN, Grieco VS, Garcia R, Gown AM (2001). Immunohistochemical distinction of endometrial stromal sarcoma and cellular leiomyoma. Appl Immunohistochem Mol Morphol 9: 164-169.

15. Agoff SN, Mendelin JE, Grieco VS, Garcia RL (2002). Unexpected gynecologic neoplasms in patients with proven or suspected BRCA-1 or -2 mutations: implications for gross examination, cytology, and clinical follow-up. Am J Surg Pathol 26: 171-178.

16. Aguirre P, Thor AD, Scully RE (1989). Ovarian small cell carcinoma. Histogenetic considerations based on immunohistochemical and other findings. Am J Clin Pathol 92: 140-149.

17. Ahmed MN, Kim K, Haddad B, Berchuck A, Qumsiyeh MB (2000). Comparative genomic hybridization studies in hydatidiform moles and choriocarcinoma: amplification of 7q21-q31 and loss of 8p12-p21 in choriocarcinoma. Cancer Genet Cytogenet 116: 10-15.

18. Ahn GH, Scully RE (1991). Clear cell carcinoma of the inguinal region arising from endometriosis. Cancer 67: 116-120.

19. Ahram J, Lemus R, Schiavello HJ (2006). Leiomyosarcoma of the vagina: case report and literature review. Int J Gynecol Cancer 16: 884-891.

20. Ahuja A, Safaya R, Prakash G, Kumar L, Shukla NK (2011). Primary mixed mullerian tumor of the vagina--a case report with review of the literature. Pathol Res Pract 207: 253-255.

21. Akahira J, Ito K, Kosuge S, Konno R, Sato S, Yajima A, Sasano H (1998). Ovarian mixed germ cell tumor composed of dysgerminoma, endodermal sinus tumor, choriocarcinoma and mature teratoma in a 44-year-old woman: case report and literature review. Pathol Int 48: 471-474.

22. Akbayir O, Gungorduk K, Gulkilik A, Yavuz E, Tekirdag AI, Odabas E (2008). Successful treatment of primary vaginal diffuse large B-cell lymphoma using chemotherapy. Taiwan J Obstet Gynecol 47: 334-337.

23. Akhan SE, Yavuz E, Tecer A, Iyibozkurt CA, Topuz S, Tuzlali S, Bengisu E, Berkman S (2005). The expression of Ki-67, p53, estrogen and progesterone receptors affecting survival in uterine leiomyosarcomas. A clinicopathologic study. Gynecol Oncol 99: 36-42.

24. Akl MN, Naidu SG, McCullough AE, Magtibay PM (2010). Vaginal paraganglioma presenting as a pelvic mass. Surgery 147: 169-171.

25. Al-Agha OM, Huwait HF, Chow C, Yang W, Senz J, Kalloger SE, Huntsman DG, Young RH, Gilks CB (2011). FOXL2 is a sensitive and specific marker for sex cord-stromal tumors of the ovary. Am J Surg Pathol 35: 484-494.

25A. Albores-Saavedra J, Gersell D, Gilks CB, Henson DE, Lindberg G, Santiago H, Scully RE, Silva E, Sobin LH, Tavassoli FJ, Travis WD, Woodruff JM (1997). Terminology of endocrine tumors of the uterine cervix: results of a workshop sponsored by the College of American Pathologists and the National Cancer Institute. Arch Pathol Lab Med 121: 34-39.

25B. Albores-Saavedra J, Martinez-Benitez B, Luevano E (2008). Small cell carcinomas and large cell neuroendocrine carcinomas of the endometrium and cervix: polypoid tumors and those arising in polyps may have a favorable prognosis. Int J Gynecol Pathol 27: 333-339.

25C. Albores-Saavedra J, Martinez-Benitez B, Luevano E (2008). Small cell carcinomas and large cell neuroendocrine carcinomas of the endometrium and cervix: polypoid tumors and those arising in polyps may have a favorable prognosis. Int J Gynecol Pathol 27: 333-339.

26. Al-Nafussi AI, Al-Yusif R (1998). Papillary squamotransitional cell carcinoma of the uterine cervix: an advanced stage disease despite superficial location: report of two cases and review of the literature. Eur J Gynaecol Oncol 19: 455-457.

27. Al-Shraim MM (2011). Angiomatoid giant cellular blue nevus of vaginal wall associated with pregnancy. Diagn Pathol 6: 32.

28. Al-Talib A, Tulandi T (2010). Pathophysiology and possible iatrogenic cause of leiomyomatosis peritonealis disseminata. Gynecol Obstet Invest 69: 239-244.

29. Alasiri SA, Ghahremani M, McComb PF (2012). Cornual polyps of the fallopian tube are associated with endometriosis and anovulation. Obstet Gynecol Int 2012: 561306.

30. Alenghat E, Okagaki T, Talerman A (1986). Primary mucinous carcinoid tumor of the ovary. Cancer 58: 777-783.

31. Alfsen GC, Kristensen GB, Skovlund E, Pettersen EO, Abeler VM (2001). Histologic subtype has minor importance for overall survival in patients with adenocarcinoma of the uterine cervix: a population-based study of prognostic factors in 505 patients with nonsquamous cell carcinomas of the cervix. Cancer 92: 2471-2483.

32. Ali H, Guy RJ, Wand H, Read TR, Regan DG, Grulich AE, Fairley CK, Donovan B (2013). Decline in in-patient treatments of genital warts among young Australians following the national HPV vaccination program. BMC Infect Dis 13: 140.

33. Ali RH, Seidman JD, Luk M, Kalloger S, Gilks CB (2012). Transitional cell carcinoma of the ovary is related to high-grade serous carcinoma and is distinct from malignant brenner tumor. Int J Gynecol Pathol 31: 499-506.

34. Alkushi A, Köbel M, Kalloger SE, Gilks CB (2010). High-grade endometrial carcinoma: serous and grade 3 endometrioid carcinomas have different immunophenotypes and outcomes. Int J Gynecol Pathol 29: 343-350.

35. Allen PW, Dymock RB, MacCormac LB (1988). Superficial angiomyxomas with and without epithelial components. Report of 30 tumors in 28 patients. Am J Surg Pathol 12: 519-530.

36. Alonso I, Felix A, Torne A, Fuste V, Del PM, Castillo P, Balasch J, Pahisa J, Rios J, Ordi J (2012). Human papillomavirus as a favorable prognostic biomarker in squamous cell carcinomas of the vagina. Gynecol Oncol 125: 194-199.

37. Althausen AM, Kowalski DP, Ludwig ME, Curry SL, Greene JF (2000). Granular cell tumors: a new clinically important histologic finding. Gynecol Oncol 77: 310-313.

38. Altman AD, Nelson GS, Ghatage P, McIntyre JB, Capper D, Chu P, Nation JG, Karnezis AN, Han G, Kalloger SE, Köbel M (2013). The diagnostic utility of TP53 and CDKN2A to distinguish ovarian high-grade serous carcinoma from low-grade serous ovarian tumors. Mod Pathol 26: 1255-1263.

39. Altrabulsi B, Malpica A, Deavers MT, Bodurka DC, Broaddus R, Silva EG (2005). Undifferentiated carcinoma of the endometrium. Am J Surg Pathol 29: 1316-1321.

39A. Alvarado-Cabrero I, Navani SS, Young RH, Scully RE (1997). Tumors of the fimbriated end of the fallopian tube: a clinicopathologic analysis of 20 cases, including nine carcinomas. Int J Gynecol Pathol 16: 189-196.

39B. Alvarado-Cabrero I, Stolnicu S, Kiyokawa T, Yamada K, Nikaido T, Santiago-Payán H (2013). Carcinoma of the fallopian tube: Results of a multi-institutional retrospective analysis of 127 patients with evaluation of staging and prognostic factors. Ann Diagn Pathol 17: 159-164.

39C. Alvarado-Cabrero I, Young RH, Vamvakas EC, Scully RE (1999). Carcinoma of the fallopian tube: a clinicopathological study of 105 cases with observations on staging and prognostic factors. Gynecol Oncol 72: 367-379.

40. Alvarez AA, Moore WF, Robboy SJ, Bentley RC, Gumbs C, Futreal PA, Berchuck A (2001). K-ras mutations in Mullerian inclusion cysts associated with serous borderline tumors of the ovary. Gynecol Oncol 80: 201-206.

40A. Amador-Ortiz C, Roma AA, Huettner PC, Becker N, Pfeifer JD (2011). JAZF1 and JJAZ1 gene fusion in primary extrauterine endometrial stromal sarcoma. Hum Pathol 42: 939-946.

41. Amant F, Moerman P, Vergote I (2005). Report of an unusual problematic uterine smooth muscle neoplasm, emphasizing the prognostic importance of coagulative tumor cell necrosis. Int J Gynecol Cancer 15: 1210-1212.

42. Amant F, Schurmans K, Steenkiste E, Verbist L, Abeler VM, Tulunay G, de Jonge E, Massuger L, Moerman P, Vergote I (2004). Immunohistochemical determination of estrogen and progesterone receptor positivity in uterine adenosarcoma. Gynecol Oncol 93: 680-685.

43. Amant F, Steenkiste E, Schurmans K, Verbist L, Abeler VM, Tulunay G, de Jonge E, Massuger L, Moerman P, Vergote I (2004). Immunohistochemical expression of CD10 antigen in uterine adenosarcoma. Int J Gynecol Cancer 14: 1118-1121.

44. Amant F, Tousseyn T, Coenegrachts L, Decloedt J, Moerman P, Debiec-Rychter M (2011). Case report of a poorly differentiated uterine tumour with t(10;17) translocation and neuroectodermal phenotype. Anticancer Res 31: 2367-2371.

45. Ambros RA, Sherman ME, Zahn CM, Bitterman P, Kurman RJ (1995). Endometrial intraepithelial carcinoma: a distinctive lesion specifically associated with tumors displaying serous differentiation. Hum Pathol 26: 1260-1267.

46. Amemiya S, Sekizawa A, Otsuka J, Tachikawa T, Saito H, Okai T (2004). Malignant transformation of endometriosis and genetic alterations of K-ras and microsatellite instability. Int J Gynaecol Obstet 86: 371-376.

47. An HJ, Kim KR, Kim IS, Kim DW, Park MH, Park IA, Suh KS, Seo EJ, Sung SH, Sohn JH, Yoon HK, Chang ED, Cho HI, Han JY, Hong SR, Ahn GH (2005). Prevalence of human papillomavirus DNA in various histological subtypes of cervical adenocarcinoma: a population-based study. Mod Pathol 18: 528-534.

48. An HJ, Logani S, Isacson C, Ellenson LH (2004). Molecular characterization of uterine clear cell carcinoma. Mod Pathol 17: 530-537.

49. Anderson J, Behbakht K, De GK, Bitterman P (2001). Adenosarcoma in a patient with vaginal endometriosis. Obstet Gynecol 98: 964-966.

50. Andrassy RJ, Hays DM, Raney RB, Wiener ES, Lawrence W, Lobe TE, Corpron CA, Smith M, Maurer HM (1995). Conservative surgical management of vaginal and vulvar pediatric rhabdomyosarcoma: a report from the Intergroup Rhabdomyosarcoma Study III. J Pediatr Surg 30: 1034-1036.

51. Andrassy RJ, Wiener ES, Raney RB, Hays DM, Arndt CA, Lobe TE, Lawrence W, Anderson JR, Qualman SJ, Crist WM (1999). Progress in the surgical management of vaginal rhabdomyosarcoma: a 25-year review from the Intergroup Rhabdomyosarcoma Study Group. J Pediatr Surg 34: 731-734.

51A. Angeles-Angeles A, Gutierrez-Villalobos LI, Lome-Maldonado C, Jimenez-Moreno A (2002). Polypoid Brenner tumor of the uterus. Int J Gynecol Pathol 21: 86-87.

52. Anglesio MS, Carey MS, Köbel M, Mackay H, Huntsman DG (2011). Clear cell carcinoma of the ovary: a report from the first Ovarian Clear Cell Symposium, June 24th, 2010. Gynecol Oncol 121: 407-415.

53. Anglesio MS, Kommoss S, Tolcher MC, Clarke B, Galletta L, Porter H, Damaraju S, Fereday S, Winterhoff BJ,Kalloger SE, Senz J, Yang W, Steed H, Allo G, Ferguson S, Shaw P, Teoman A, Garcia JJ, Schoolmeester JK, Bakkum-Gamez J, Tinker AV, Bowtell DD, Huntsman DG, Gilks CB, McAlpine JN (2013). Molecular characterization of mucinous ovarian tumours supports a stratified treatment approach with HER2 targeting in 19% of carcinomas. J Pathol 229: 111-120.

54. Anjarwalla S, Rollason TP, Rooney N, Hirschowitz L (2007). Atypical mucinous metaplasia and intraepithelial neoplasia of the female genital tract--a case report and review of the literature. Int J Gynecol Cancer 17: 1147-1150.

55. Anon (1971). Classification and staging of malignant tumours in the female pelvis. Acta Obstet Gynecol Scand 50: 1-7.

55A. Ansari-Lari MA, Staebler A, Zaino RJ, Shah KV, Ronnett BM (2004). Distinction of endocervical and endometrial adenocarcinomas: immunohistochemical p16 expression correlated with human papillomavirus (HPV) DNA detection. Am J Surg Pathol 28: 160-167.

55B. Antoniou A, Pharoah PD, Narod S, Risch HA et al (2003). Average risks of breast and ovarian cancer associated with BRCA 1or BRCA 2 mutations detected in case Series unselected for family history: a combined analysis of 22 Studies. Am J Hum Gen 72: 1117–1130.

56. Aoyama C, Peters J, Senadheera S, Liu P, Shimada H (1998). Uterine cervical dysplasia and cancer: identification of c-myc status by quantitative polymerase chain reaction. Diagn Mol Pathol 7: 324-330.

57. Arbyn M, Benoy I, Simoens C, Bogers J, Beutels P, Depuydt C (2009). Prevaccination distribution of human papillomavirus types in women attending at cervical cancer screening in Belgium. Cancer Epidemiol Biomarkers Prev 18: 321-330.

58. Arbyn M, Castellsague X, de Sanjose S., Bruni L, Saraiya M, Bray F, Ferlay J (2011). Worldwide burden of cervical cancer in 2008. Ann Oncol 22: 2675-2686.

59. Arbyn M, Martin-Hirsch P, Buntinx F, Van RM, Paraskevaidis E, Dillner J (2009). Triage of women with equivocal or low-grade cervical cytology results: a meta-analysis of the HPV test positivity rate. J Cell Mol Med 13: 648-659.

60. Arbyn M, Ronco G, Anttila A, Meijer CJ, Poljak M, Ogilvie G, Koliopoulos G, Naucler P, Sankaranarayanan R, Peto J (2012). Evidence regarding human papillomavirus testing in secondary prevention of cervical cancer. Vaccine 30 Suppl 5: F88-F99.

61. Arbyn M, Simoens C, Goffin F, Noehr B, Bruinsma F (2011). Treatment of cervical cancer precursors: influence of age, completeness of excision and cone depth on therapeutic failure, and on adverse obstetric outcomes. BJOG 118: 1274-1275.

62. Arend R, Bagaria M, Lewin SN, Sun X, Deutsch I, Burke WM, Herzog TJ, Wright JD (2010). Long-term outcome and natural history of uterine adenosarcomas. Gynecol Oncol 119: 305-308.

62A. Arias-Stella J (2002). The Arias-Stella reaction: facts and fancies four decades after. Adv Anat Pathol 9: 12-23.

63. Arici DS, Aker H, Yildiz E, Tasyurt A (2000). Mullerian adenosarcoma of the uterus associated with tamoxifen therapy. Arch Gynecol Obstet 264: 105-107.

64. Arif S, Ganesan R, Spooner D (2006). Intravascular leiomyomatosis and benign metastasizing leiomyoma: an unusual case. Int J Gynecol Cancer 16: 1448-1450.

65. Aslani M, Ahn GH, Scully RE (1988). Serous papillary cystadenoma of borderline malignancy of broad ligament. A report of 25 cases. Int J Gynecol Pathol 7: 131-138.

66. Aslani M, Scully RE (1989). Primary carcinoma of the broad ligament. Report of four cases and review of the literature. Cancer 64: 1540-1545.

67. Atallah D, Rouzier R, Chamoun ML, Mansour F, Nabaa T, Chababi M, Duvillard P, Chahine G (2007). Benign lipoblastomalike tumor of the vulva: report of a case affecting a young patient. J Reprod Med 52: 223-224.

68. Atkins KA, Arronte N, Darus CJ, Rice LW (2008). The Use of p16 in enhancing the histologic classification of uterine smooth muscle tumors. Am J Surg Pathol 32: 98-102.

69. Atlas I, Gajewski W, Falkenberry S, Granai CO, Steinhoff MM (1998). Absence of estrogen and progesterone receptors in glassy cell carcinoma of the cervix. Obstet Gynecol 91: 136-138.

70. Atrash HK, Hogue CJ, Grimes DA (1986). Epidemiology of hydatidiform mole during early gestation. Am J Obstet Gynecol 154: 906-909.

71. Attanoos RL, Webb R, Dojcinov SD, Gibbs AR (2002). Value of mesothelial and epithelial antibodies in distinguishing diffuse peritoneal mesothelioma in females from serous papillary carcinoma of the ovary and peritoneum. Histopathology 40: 237-244.

72. Attner B, Landin-Olsson M, Lithman T, Noreen D, Olsson H (2012). Cancer among patients with diabetes, obesity and abnormal blood lipids: a population-based register study in Sweden. Cancer Causes Control 23: 769-777.

73. Audisio T, Crespo-Roca F, Giraudo P, Ramallo R (2011). Fibroadenoma of the vulva-simultaneous with breast fibroadenomas and uterine myoma. J Low Genit Tract Dis 15: 75-79.

74. Auersperg N (2011). The origin of ovarian carcinomas: a unifying hypothesis. Int J Gynecol Pathol 30: 12-21.

75. Auersperg N, Wong AS, Choi KC, Kang SK, Leung PC (2001). Ovarian surface epithelium: biology, endocrinology, and pathology. Endocr Rev 22: 255-288.

76. Austin RM, Norris HJ (1987). Malignant Brenner tumor and transitional cell carcinoma of the ovary: a comparison. Int J Gynecol Pathol 6: 29-39.

77. Axiotis CA, Lippes HA, Merino MJ, deLanerolle NC, Stewart AF, Kinder B (1987). Corticotroph cell pituitary adenoma within an ovarian teratoma. A new cause of Cushing's syndrome. Am J Surg Pathol 11: 218-224.

78. Aydin H, Young RH, Ronnett BM, Epstein JI (2005). Clear cell papillary cystadenoma of the epididymis and mesosalpinx: immunohistochemical differentiation from metastatic clear cell renal cell carcinoma. Am J Surg Pathol 29: 520-523.

79. Ayhan A, Mao TL, Seckin T, Wu CH, Guan B, Ogawa H, Futagami M, Mizukami H, Yokoyama Y, Kurman RJ, Shih I (2012). Loss of ARID1A expression is an early molecular event in tumor progression from ovarian endometriotic cyst to clear cell and endometrioid carcinoma. Int J Gynecol Cancer 22: 1310-1315.

80. Diaz de Leon E, Carcangiu ML, Prieto VG, McCue PA, Burchette JL, To G, Norris BA, Kovatich AJ, Sanchez RL, Krigman HR, Gatalica Z (2000). Extramammary Paget disease is characterized by the consistent lack of estrogen and progesterone receptors but frequently expresses androgen receptor. Am J Clin Pathol 113: 572-575.

81. Baak JP, Mutter GL, Robboy S, van Diest PJ, Uyterlinde AM, Orbo A, Palazzo J, Fiane B, Lovslett K, Burger C, Voorhorst F, Verheijen RH (2005). The molecular genetics and morphometry-based endometrial intraepithelial neoplasia classification system predicts disease progression in endometrial hyperplasia more accurately than the 1994 World Health Organization classification system. Cancer 103: 2304-2312.

82. Baak JP, Nauta JJ, Wisse-Brekelmans EC, Bezemer PD (1988). Architectural and nuclear morphometrical features together are more important prognosticators in endometrial hyperplasias than nuclear morphometrical features alone. J Pathol 154: 335-341.

83. Baalbergen A, Ewing-Graham PC, Hop WC, Struijk P, Helmerhorst TJ (2004). Prognostic factors in adenocarcinoma of the uterine cervix. Gynecol Oncol 92: 262-267.

84. Baandrup L, Munk C, Andersen KK, Junge J, Iftner T, Kjaer SK (2012). HPV16 is associated with younger age in women with cervical intraepithelial neoplasia grade 2 and 3. Gynecol Oncol 124: 281-285.

85. Baandrup L, Varbo A, Munk C, Johansen C, Frisch M, Kjaer SK (2011). In situ and invasive squamous cell carcinoma of the vulva in Denmark 1978-2007-a nationwide population-based study. Gynecol Oncol 122: 45-49.

86. Baasanjav B, Usui H, Kihara M, Kaku H, Nakada E, Tate S, Mitsuhashi A, Matsui H, Shozu M (2010). The risk of post-molar gestational trophoblastic neoplasia is higher in heterozygous than in homozygous complete hydatidiform moles. Hum Reprod 25: 1183-1191.

87. Baergen RN, Kelly T, McGinniss MJ, Jones OW, Benirschke K (1996). Complete hydatidiform mole with a coexistent embryo. Hum Pathol 27: 731-734.

88. Baergen RN, Rutgers J, Young RH (2003). Extrauterine lesions of intermediate trophoblast. Int J Gynecol Pathol 22: 362-367.

89. Baergen RN, Rutgers JL, Young RH, Osann K, Scully RE (2006). Placental site trophoblastic tumor: A study of 55 cases and review of the literature emphasizing factors of prognostic significance. Gynecol Oncol 100: 511-520.

90. Bagshawe KD, Dent J, Webb J (1986). Hydatidiform mole in England and Wales 1973-83. Lancet 2: 673-677.

91. Bagshawe KD, Golding PR, Orr AH (1969). Choriocarcinoma after hydatidiform mole. Studies related to effectiveness of follow-up practice after hydatidiform mole. Br Med J 3: 733-737.

92. Bague S, Rodriguez IM, Prat J (2002). Sarcoma-like mural nodules in mucinous cystic tumors of the ovary revisited: a clinicopathologic analysis of 10 additional cases. Am J Surg Pathol 26: 1467-1476.

93. Bais AG, Kooi S, Teune TM, Ewing PC, Ansink AC (2005). Lymphoepithelioma-like carcinoma of the uterine cervix: absence of Epstein-Barr virus, but presence of a multiple human papillomavirus infection. Gynecol Oncol 97: 716-718.

94. Baker P, Oliva E (2007). Endometrial stromal tumours of the uterus: a practical approach using conventional morphology and ancillary techniques. J Clin Pathol 60: 235-243.

95. Baker PM, Clement PB, Young RH (2005). Malignant peritoneal mesothelioma in women: a study of 75 cases with emphasis on their morphologic spectrum and differential diagnosis. Am J Clin Pathol 123: 724-737.

96. Baker PM, Moch H, Oliva E (2005). Unusual morphologic features of endometrial stromal tumors: a report of 2 cases. Am J Surg Pathol 29: 1394-1398.

97. Baker PM, Oliva E, Young RH, Talerman A, Scully RE (2001). Ovarian mucinous carcinoids including some with a carcinomatous component: a report of 17 cases. Am J Surg Pathol 25: 557-568.

98. Baker PM, Rosai J, Young RH (2002). Ovarian teratomas with florid benign vascular proliferation: a distinctive finding associated with the neural component of teratomas that may be confused with a vascular neoplasm. Int J Gynecol Pathol 21: 16-21.

99. Baker PM, Young RH (2003). Brenner tumor of the ovary with striking microcystic change. Int J Gynecol Pathol 22: 185-188.

100. Baker RJ, Hildebrandt RH, Rouse RV, Hendrickson MR, Longacre TA (1999). Inhibin and CD99 (MIC2) expression in uterine stromal neoplasms with sex-cord-like elements. Hum Pathol 30: 671-679.

101. Baksu B, Akyol A, Davas I, Yazgan A, Ozgul J, Tanik C (2006). Recurrent mucinous cystadenoma in a 20-year-old woman: was hysterectomy inevitable? J Obstet Gynaecol Res 32: 615-618.

102. Balasa RW, Adcock LL, Prem KA, Dehner LP (1977). The Brenner tumor: a clinicopathologic review. Obstet Gynecol 50: 120-128.

103. Balat O, Edwards CL, Delclos L (2001). Advanced primary carcinoma of the Bartholin gland: report of 18 patients. Eur J Gynaecol Oncol 22: 46-49.

104. Balbi GC, Del PL, Labriola D, Visconti S, Monteverde A, Passaro M, Monaco R, Cardone A, Rossiello R, Panariello S, Montone L (2006). Female adnexal tumor of probable wolffian origin: clinicopathological, immunohistochemical and cytofluorimetric analyses of a 22-year-old virgin. case report. Eur J Gynaecol Oncol 27: 313-316.

105. Balci S, Saglam A, Usubutun A (2010). Primary signet-ring cell carcinoma of the cervix: case report and review of the literature. Int J Gynecol Pathol 29: 181-184.

106. Bandera CA, Muto MG, Schorge JO, Berkowitz RS, Rubin SC, Mok SC (1998). BRCA1 gene mutations in women with papillary serous carcinoma of the peritoneum. Obstet Gynecol 92: 596-600.

107. Bannatyne P, Russell P, Shearman RP (1990). Autoimmune oophoritis: a clinicopathologic assessment of 12 cases. Int J Gynecol Pathol 9: 191-207.

108. Barbieri RL, Hornstein MD (1988). Hyperinsulinemia and ovarian hyperandrogenism. Cause and effect. Endocrinol Metab Clin North Am 17: 685-703.

109. Barcena C, Oliva E (2011). WT1 expression in the female genital tract. Adv Anat Pathol 18: 454-465.

110. Barjot PJ, Refahi N, Berthet P, Delautre VD (1998). Intravenous leiomyomatosis of the uterus: a GnRH agonist utilisation before surgery. J Obstet Gynaecol 18: 492-493.

111. Barnetson RJ, Burnett RA, Downie I, Harper CM, Roberts F (2006). Immunohistochemical analysis of peritoneal mesothelioma and primary and secondary serous carcinoma of the peritoneum: antibodies to estrogen and progesterone receptors are useful. Am J Clin Pathol 125: 67-76.

112. Barrow E, Robinson L, Alduaij W, Shenton A, Clancy T, Lalloo F, Hill J, Evans DG (2009). Cumulative lifetime incidence of extracolonic cancers in Lynch syndrome: a report of 121 families with proven mutations. Clin Genet 75: 141-149.

113. Bartuma H, Domanski HA, Von Steyern FV, Kullendorff CM, Mandahl N, Mertens F (2008). Cytogenetic and molecular cytogenetic findings in lipoblastoma. Cancer Genet Cytogenet 183: 60-63.

114. Baschinsky DY, Isa A, Niemann TH, Prior TW, Lucas JG, Frankel WL (2000). Diffuse leiomyomatosis of the uterus: a case report with clonality analysis. Hum Pathol 31: 1429-1432.

115. Baulies S, Cusido MT, Grases PJ, Ubeda B, Pascual MA, Fabregas R (2008). Neurofibroma of the vaginal wall. Clin Exp Obstet Gynecol 35: 140-143.

116. Bazot M, Detchev R, Cortez A, Uzan S, Darai E (2003). Massive ovarian edema revealing gastric carcinoma: a case report. Gynecol Oncol 91: 648-650.

117. Beggs AD, Latchford AR, Vasen HF, Moslein G, Alonso A, Aretz S, Bertario L, Blanco I, Bulow S, Burn J, Capella G, Colas C, Friedl W, Moller P, Hes FJ, Jarvinen H, Mecklin JP, Nagengast FM, Parc Y, Phillips RK, Hyer W, Ponz de LM, Renkonen-Sinisalo L, Sampson JR, Stormorken A, Tejpar S, Thomas HJ, Wijnen JT, Clark SK, Hodgson SV (2010). Peutz-Jeghers syndrome: a systematic review and recommendations for management. Gut 59: 975-986.

118. Begin LR, Clement PB, Kirk ME, Jothy S, McCaughey WT, Ferenczy A (1985). Aggressive angiomyxoma of pelvic soft parts: a clinicopathologic study of nine cases. Hum Pathol 16: 621-628.

119. Bell DA (1991). Mucinous adenofibromas of the ovary. A report of 10 cases. Am J Surg Pathol 15: 227-232.

120. Bell DA, Longacre TA, Prat J, Kohn EC, Soslow RA, Ellenson LH, Malpica A, Stoler MH, Kurman RJ (2004). Serous borderline (low malignant potential, atypical proliferative) ovarian tumors: workshop perspectives. Hum Pathol 35: 934-948.

121. Bell DA, Scully RE (1985). Atypical and borderline endometrioid adenofibromas of the ovary. A report of 27 cases. Am J Surg Pathol 9: 205-214.

122. Bell DA, Scully RE (1985). Benign and borderline clear cell adenofibromas of the ovary. Cancer 56: 2922-2931.

123. Bell DA, Scully RE (1990). Ovarian serous borderline tumors with stromal microinvasion: a report of 21 cases. Hum Pathol 21: 397-403.

124. Bell DA, Scully RE (1990). Serous borderline tumors of the peritoneum. Am J Surg Pathol 14: 230-239.

125. Bell DA, Weinstock MA, Scully RE (1988). Peritoneal implants of ovarian serous borderline tumors. Histologic features and prognosis. Cancer 62: 2212-2222.

126. Bell DA, Woodruff JM, Scully RE (1984). Ependymoma of the broad ligament. A report of two cases. Am J Surg Pathol 8: 203-209.

127. Bell KA, Kurman RJ (2000). A clinicopathologic analysis of atypical proliferative (borderline) tumors and well-differentiated endometrioid adenocarcinomas of the ovary. Am J Surg Pathol 24: 1465-1479.

128. Bell KA, Smith Sehdev AE, Kurman RJ (2001). Refined diagnostic criteria for implants associated with ovarian atypical proliferative serous tumors (borderline) and micropapillary serous carcinomas. Am J Surg Pathol 25: 419-432.

129. Bell SW, Kempson RL, Hendrickson MR (1994). Problematic uterine smooth muscle neoplasms. A clinicopathologic study of 213 cases. Am J Surg Pathol 18: 535-558.

130. Bellati F, Palaia I, Gasparri ML, Musella A, Panici PB (2012). First case of isolated vaginal metastasis from breast cancer treated by surgery. BMC Cancer 12: 479.

131. Bellezza G, Colella R, Sidoni A, Del SR, Ferri I, Cioccoloni C, Cavaliere A (2008). Immunohistochemical expression of Galectin-3 and HBME-1 in granular cell tumors: a new finding. Histol Histopathol 23: 1127-1130.

132. Benedet JL, Sanders BH (1984). Carcinoma in situ of the vagina. Am J Obstet Gynecol 148: 695-700.

133. Benoit L, Arnould L, Cheynel N, Diane B, Causeret S, Machado A, Collin F, Fraisse J, Cuisenier J (2006). Malignant extraovarian endometriosis: a review. Eur J Surg Oncol 32: 6-11.

134. Beral V, Bull D, Reeves G (2005). Endometrial cancer and hormone-replacement therapy in the Million Women Study. Lancet 365: 1543-1551.

135. Beral V, Doll R, Hermon C, Peto R, Reeves G (2008). Ovarian cancer and oral contraceptives: collaborative reanalysis of data from 45 epidemiological studies including 23,257 women with ovarian cancer and 87,303 controls. Lancet 371: 303-314.

136. Berends MJ, Kleibeuker JH, de Vries EG, Mourits MJ, Hollema H, Pras E, van der Zee AG (1999). The importance of family history in young patients with endometrial cancer. Eur J Obstet Gynecol Reprod Biol 82: 139-141.

137. Bergeron C, Ferenczy A, Richart RM, Guralnick M (1990). Micropapillomatosis labialis appears unrelated to human papillomavirus. Obstet Gynecol 76: 281-286.

138. Bergeron C, Nogales FF, Masseroli M, Abeler V, Duvillard P, Muller-Holzner E, Pickartz H, Wells M (1999). A multicentric European study testing the reproducibility of the WHO classification of endometrial hyperplasia with a proposal of a simplified working classification for biopsy and curettage specimens. Am J Surg Pathol 23: 1102-1108.

139. Bergeron C, Ordi J, Schmidt D, Trunk MJ, Keller T, Ridder R (2010). Conjunctive p16INK4a testing significantly increases accuracy in diagnosing high-grade cervical intraepithelial neoplasia. Am J Clin Pathol 133: 395-406.

140. Berkowitz RS, Goldstein DP (1996). Chorionic tumors. N Engl J Med 335: 1740-1748.

141. Berkowitz RS, Goldstein DP (2009). Clinical practice. Molar pregnancy. N Engl J Med 360: 1639-1645.

142. Berkowitz RS, Goldstein DP, Bernstein MR (1984). Choriocarcinoma following term gestation. Gynecol Oncol 17: 52-57.

143. Bermudez A, Vighi S, Garcia A, Sardi J (2001). Neuroendocrine cervical carcinoma: a diagnostic and therapeutic challenge. Gynecol Oncol 82: 32-39.

144. Bernstein HB, Broman JH, Apicelli A, Kredentser DC (1999). Primary malignant schwannoma of the uterine cervix: a case report and literature review. Gynecol Oncol 74: 288-292.

145. Berretta R, Rolla M, Merisio C, Giordano G, Nardelli GB (2008). Uterine smooth muscle tumor of uncertain malignant potential: a three-case report. Int J Gynecol Cancer 18: 1121-1126.

146. Berry E, Hagopian GS, Lurain JR (2008). Vaginal metastases in gestational trophoblastic neoplasia. J Reprod Med 53: 487-492.

147. Bettaieb I, Mekni A, Bellil K, Haouet S, Bellil S, Kchir N, Chelly H, Zitouna M (2007). Endometrial adenofibroma: a rare entity. Arch Gynecol Obstet 275: 191-193.

148. Beutner KR, Ferenczy A (1997). Therapeutic approaches to genital warts. Am J Med 102: 28-37.

149. Bewtra C, Xie QM, Hunter WJ, Jurgensen W (2005). Ichthyosis uteri: a case report and review of the literature. Arch Pathol Lab Med 129: e124-e125.

150. Biankin SA, O'Toole VE, Fung C, Russell P (2000). Bizarre leiomyoma of the vagina: report of a case. Int J Gynecol Pathol 19: 186-187.

151. Bifulco C, Johnson C, Hao L, Kermalli H, Bell S, Hui P (2008). Genotypic analysis of hydatidiform mole: an accurate and practical method of diagnosis. Am J Surg Pathol 32: 445-451.

152. Billings SD, Giblen G, Fanburg-Smith JC (2005). Superficial low-grade fibromyxoid sarcoma (Evans tumor): a clinicopathologic analysis of 19 cases with a unique observation in the pediatric population. Am J Surg Pathol 29: 204-210.

153. Bing Z, Levine L, Lucci JA, Hatch SS, Eltorky MA (2004). Primary small cell neuroendocrine carcinoma of the vagina: a clinicopathologic study. Arch Pathol Lab Med 128: 857-862.

154. Biscuola M, Van de Vijver K, Castilla MA, Romero-Perez L, Lopez-Garcia MA, Diaz-Martin J, Matias-Guiu X, Oliva E, Palacios Calvo J. (2013). Oncogene alterations in endometrial carcinosarcomas. Hum Pathol 44: 852-859.

155. Bittinger SE, Nazaretian SP, Gook DA, Parmar C, Harrup RA, Stern CJ (2011). Detection of Hodgkin lymphoma within ovarian tissue. Fertil Steril 95: 803-806.

156. Bjorkholm E, Silfversward C (1980). Theca-cell tumors. Clinical features and prognosis. Acta Radiol Oncol 19: 241-244.

157. Blandamura S, Florea G, Chiarelli S, Rondinelli R, Ninfo V (2005). Myometrial leiomyoma with chondroid lipoma-like areas. Histopathology 46: 596-598.

158. Block RE (1975). Hydrocele of the canal of nuck. A report of five cases. Obstet Gynecol 45: 464-466.

159. Blom R, Guerrieri C, Stal O, Malmstrom H, Simonsen E (1998). Leiomyosarcoma of the uterus: A clinicopathologic, DNA flow cytometric, p53, and mdm-2 analysis of 49 cases. Gynecol Oncol 68: 54-61.

160. Blomberg M, Friis S, Munk C, Bautz A, Kjaer SK (2012). Genital warts and risk of cancer: a Danish study of nearly 50 000 patients with genital warts. J Infect Dis 205: 1544-1553.

161. Bocklage T, Lee KR, Belinson JL (1992). Uterine mullerian adenosarcoma following adenomyoma in a woman on tamoxifen therapy. Gynecol Oncol 44: 104-109.

162. Bodner-Adler B, Bartl M, Wagner G (2009). Intravenous leiomyomatosis of the uterus with pulmonary metastases or a case with benign metastasizing leiomyoma? Anticancer Res 29: 495-496.

163. Bodner-Adler B, Bodner K, Czerwenka K, Kimberger O, Leodolter S, Mayerhofer K (2005). Expression of p16 protein in patients with uterine smooth muscle tumors: an immunohistochemical analysis. Gynecol Oncol 96: 62-66.

164. Bokhman JV (1983). Two pathogenetic types of endometrial carcinoma. Gynecol Oncol 15: 10-17.

165. Bolton KL, Chenevix-Trench G, Goh C, Sadetzki S, Ramus SJ, Karlan BY, Lambrechts D, Despierre E, Barrowdale D, McGuffog L, Healey S, Easton DF, Sinilnikova O, Benitez J, Garcia MJ, Neuhausen S, Gail MH, Hartge P, Peock S, Frost D, Evans DG, Eeles R, Godwin AK, Daly MB, Kwong A, Ma ES, Lazaro C, Blanco I, Montagna M, D'Andrea E, Nicoletto MO, Johnatty SE, Kjaer SK, Jensen A, Hogdall E, Goode EL, Fridley BL, Loud JT, Greene MH, Mai PL, Chetrit A, Lubin F, Hirsh-Yechezkel G, Glendon G, Andrulis IL, Toland AE, Senter L, Gore ME, Gourley C, Michie CO, Song H, Tyrer J, Whittemore AS, McGuire V, Sieh W, Kristoffersson U, Olsson H, Borg A, Levine DA, Steele L, Beattie MS, Chan S, Nussbaum RL, Moysich KB, Gross J, Cass I, Walsh C, Li AJ, Leuchter R, Gordon O, Garcia-Closas M, Gayther SA, Chanock SJ, Antoniou AC, Pharoah PD (2012). Association between BRCA1 and BRCA2 mutations and survival in women with invasive epithelial ovarian cancer. JAMA 307: 382-390.

166. Bonadona V, Bonaiti B, Olschwang S, Grandjouan S, Huiart L, Longy M, Guimbaud R, Buecher B, Bignon YJ, Caron O, Colas C, Nogues C, Lejeune-Dumoulin S, Olivier-Faivre L, Polycarpe-Osaer F, Nguyen TD, Desseigne F, Saurin JC, Berthet P, Leroux D, Duffour J, Manouvrier S, Frebourg T, Sobol H, Lasset C, Bonaiti-Pellie C (2011). Cancer risks associated with germline mutations in MLH1, MSH2, and MSH6 genes in Lynch syndrome. JAMA 305: 2304-2310.

167. Bookman MA (2012). First-line chemotherapy in epithelial ovarian cancer. Clin Obstet Gynecol 55: 96-113.

168. Borah T, Mahanta RK, Bora BD, Saikia S (2011). Brenner tumor of ovary: An incidental finding. J Midlife Health 2: 40-41.

169. Albores-Saavedra J, Gersell D, Gilks CB, Henson DE, Lindberg G, Santiago H, Scully RE, Silva E, Sobin LH, Tavassoli FJ, Travis WD, Woodruff JM (1997). Terminology of endocrine tumors of the uterine cervix: results of a workshop sponsored by the College of American Pathologists and the National Cancer Institute. Arch Pathol Lab Med 121: 34-39.

170. Albores-Saavedra J, Martinez-Benitez B, Luevano E (2008). Small cell carcinomas and large cell neuroendocrine carcinomas of the endometrium and cervix: polypoid tumors and those arising in polyps may have a favorable prognosis. Int J Gynecol Pathol 27: 333-339.

171. Albores-Saavedra J, Young RH (1995). Transitional cell neoplasms (carcinomas and inverted papillomas) of the uterine cervix. A report of five cases. Am J Surg Pathol 19: 1138-1145.

172. Bosch FX, Lorincz A, Munoz N, Meijer CJ, Shah KV (2002). The causal relation between human papillomavirus and cervical cancer. J Clin Pathol 55: 244-265.

173. Bosincu L, Rocca PC, Martignoni G, Nogales FF, Longa L, Maccioni A, Massarelli G (2005). Perivascular epithelioid cell (PEC)

tumors of the uterus: a clinicopathologic study of two cases with aggressive features. Mod Pathol 18: 1336-1342.
174. Bosman FT, Carneiro F, Hruban RH, Theise ND (Eds) (2010). WHO Classification of Tumours of the Digestive System. IARC: Lyon.
175. Boss JH, Scully RE, Wegner KH, Cohen RB (1965). Structural variations in the adult ovary. Clinical significance. Obstet Gynecol 25: 747-764.
176. Bossuyt V, Medeiros F, Drapkin R, Folkins AK, Crum CP, Nucci MR (2008). Adenofibroma of the fimbria: a common entity that is indistinguishable from ovarian adenofibroma. Int J Gynecol Pathol 27: 390-397.
177. Bossuyt W, Kazanjian A, De GN, Van KS, De HG, Geboes K, Boivin GP, Luciani J, Fuks F, Chuah M, VandenDriessche T, Marynen P, Cools J, Shroyer NF, Hassan BA (2009). Atonal homolog 1 is a tumor suppressor gene. PLoS Biol 7: e39.
178. Bouraoui S, Mlika M, Blel A, Kamoun H, Mzabi-Regaya S (2008). Undifferentiated pleomorphic sarcoma of the broad ligament. Pathologica 100: 478-481.
179. Boutross-Tadross O, Saleh R, Asa SL (2007). Follicular variant papillary thyroid carcinoma arising in struma ovarii. Endocr Pathol 18: 182-186.
180. Bower M, Brock C, Fisher RA, Newlands ES, Rustin GJ (1995). Gestational choriocarcinoma. Ann Oncol 6: 503-508.
181. Boyd C, McCluggage WG (2011). Unusual morphological features of uterine leiomyomas treated with progestogens. J Clin Pathol 64: 485-489.
182. Boyd C, McCluggage WG (2012). Low-grade ovarian serous neoplasms (low-grade serous carcinoma and serous borderline tumor) associated with high-grade serous carcinoma or undifferentiated carcinoma: report of a series of cases of an unusual phenomenon. Am J Surg Pathol 36: 368-375.
183. Boyd C, Patel K, O'Sullivan B, Taniere P, McCluggage WG (2012). Pulmonary-type adenocarcinoma and signet ring mucinous adenocarcinoma arising in an ovarian dermoid cyst: report of a unique case. Hum Pathol 43: 2088-2092.
184. Boyle DP, McCluggage WG (2009). Peritoneal stromal endometriosis: a detailed morphological analysis of a large series of cases of a common and under-recognised form of endometriosis. J Clin Pathol 62: 530-533.
185. Bracken MB, Brinton LA, Hayashi K (1984). Epidemiology of hydatidiform mole and choriocarcinoma. Epidemiol Rev 6: 52-75.
186. Bradley RF, Stewart JH, Russell GB, Levine EA, Geisinger KR (2006). Pseudomyxoma peritonei of appendiceal origin: a clinicopathologic analysis of 101 patients uniformly treated at a single institution, with literature review. Am J Surg Pathol 30: 551-559.
187. Brady A, Nayar A, Cross P, Patel A, Naik R, Lee S, Kaushik S, Barton D, McCluggage WG (2012). A detailed immunohistochemical analysis of 2 cases of papillary cystadenoma of the broad ligament: an extremely rare neoplasm characteristic of patients with von Hippel-Lindau disease. Int J Gynecol Pathol 31: 133-140.
188. Brainard JA, Hart WR (1998). Adenoid basal epitheliomas of the uterine cervix: a reevaluation of distinctive cervical basaloid lesions currently classified as adenoid basal carcinoma and adenoid basal hyperplasia. Am J Surg Pathol 22: 965-975.
189. Bransilver BR, Ferenczy A, Richart RM (1974). Brenner tumors and Walthard cell nests. Arch Pathol 98: 76-86.
190. Brescia RJ, Dubin N, Demopoulos RI (1989). Endometrioid and clear cell carcinoma of the ovary. Factors affecting survival. Int J Gynecol Pathol 8: 132-138.
191. Brill LB, Kanner WA, Fehr A, Andren Y, Moskaluk CA, Loning T, Stenman G, Frierson HF Jr (2011). Analysis of MYB expression and MYB-NFIB gene fusions in adenoid cystic carcinoma and other salivary neoplasms. Mod Pathol 24: 1169-1176.
192. Brinck U, Jakob C, Bau O, Fuzesi L (2000). Papillary squamous cell carcinoma of the uterine cervix: report of three cases and a review of its classification. Int J Gynecol Pathol 19: 231-235.
193. Brinton LA, Bracken MB, Connelly RR (1986). Choriocarcinoma incidence in the United States. Am J Epidemiol 123: 1094-1100.
194. Brinton LA, Felix AS, McMeekin DS, Creasman WT, Sherman ME, Mutch D, Cohn DE, Walker JL, Moore RG, Downs LS, Soslow RA, Zaino R (2013). Etiologic heterogeneity in endometrial cancer: evidence from a Gynecologic Oncology Group trial. Gynecol Oncol 129: 277-284.
195. Bristow RE, Puri I, Chi DS (2009). Cytoreductive surgery for recurrent ovarian cancer: a meta-analysis. Gynecol Oncol 112: 265-274.
196. Broaddus RR, Lynch HT, Chen LM, Daniels MS, Conrad P, Munsell MF, White KG, Luthra R, Lu KH (2006). Pathologic features of endometrial carcinoma associated with HNPCC: a comparison with sporadic endometrial carcinoma. Cancer 106: 87-94.
197. Brooks JJ, Wells GB, Yeh IT, LiVolsi VA (1992). Bizarre epithelioid lipoleiomyoma of the uterus. Int J Gynecol Pathol 11: 144-149.
198. Brooks SE, Zhan M, Cote T, Baquet CR (2004). Surveillance, epidemiology, and end results analysis of 2677 cases of uterine sarcoma 1989-1999. Gynecol Oncol 93: 204-208.
199. Brotherton JM, Fridman M, May CL, Chappell G, Saville AM, Gertig DM (2011). Early effect of the HPV vaccination programme on cervical abnormalities in Victoria, Australia: an ecological study. Lancet 377: 2085-2092.
200. Brown E, Stewart M, Rye T, Al-Nafussi A, Williams AR, Bradburn M, Smyth J, Gabra H (2004). Carcinosarcoma of the ovary: 19 years of prospective data from a single center. Cancer 100: 2148-2153.
201. Brown HM, Wilkinson EJ (2002). Uroplakin-III to distinguish primary vulvar Paget disease from Paget disease secondary to urothelial carcinoma. Hum Pathol 33: 545-548.
202. Bruchim I, Amichay K, Kidron D, Attias Z, Biron-Shental T, Drucker L, Friedman E, Werner H, Fishman A (2010). BRCA1/2 germline mutations in Jewish patients with uterine serous carcinoma. Int J Gynecol Cancer 20: 1148-1153.
203. Brustmann H (2007). Paraganglioma of the vagina: report of a case. Pathol Res Pract 203: 189-192.
204. Abu-Rustum NR, Zhou Q, Gomez JD, Alektiar KM, Hensley ML, Soslow RA, Levine DA, Chi DS, Barakat RR, Iasonos A (2010). A nomogram for predicting overall survival of women with endometrial cancer following primary therapy: toward improving individualized cancer care. Gynecol Oncol 116: 399-403.
205. Buchanan DJ, Schlaerth J, Kurosaki T (1998). Primary vaginal melanoma: thirteen-year disease-free survival after wide local excision and review of recent literature. Am J Obstet Gynecol 178: 1177-1184.
206. Buchwalter CL, Jenison EL, Fromm M, Mehta VT, Hart WR (1997). Pure embryonal rhabdomyosarcoma of the fallopian tube. Gynecol Oncol 67: 95-101.
207. Buckley JD (1984). The epidemiology of molar pregnancy and choriocarcinoma. Clin Obstet Gynecol 27: 153-159.
208. Buell-Gutbrod R, Ivanovic M, Montag A, Lengyel E, Fadare O, Gwin K (2011). FOXL2 and SOX9 distinguish the lineage of the sex cord-stromal cells in gonadoblastomas. Pediatr Dev Pathol 14: 391-395.
209. Bujko M, Kowalewska M, Zub R, Radziszewski J, Bidzinski M, Siedlecki JA (2012). Lack of microsatellite instability in squamous cell vulvar carcinoma. Acta Obstet Gynecol Scand 91: 391-394.
210. Bullon A Jr., Arseneau J, Prat J, Young RH, Scully RE (1981). Tubular Krukenberg tumor. A problem in histopathologic diagnosis. Am J Surg Pathol 5: 225-232.
210A. Burandt E, Young RH (2014) Pregnancy luteoma. A study of 20 cases on occasion of the 50th anniversary of its description by Dr William Sternberg, with an emphasis on the common presence of follicle-like spaces and their diagnostic implications. Am J Surg Pathol 38: 239-244.
211. Burch DM, Tavassoli FA (2011). Myxoid leiomyosarcoma of the uterus. Histopathology 59: 1144-1155.
212. Burg J, Kommoss F, Bittinger F, Moll R, Kirkpatrick CJ (2002). Mature cystic teratoma of the ovary with struma and benign Brenner tumor: a case report with immunohistochemical characterization. Int J Gynecol Pathol 21: 74-77.
213. Burghardt E, Baltzer J, Tulusan AH, Haas J (1992). Results of surgical treatment of 1028 cervical cancers studied with volumetry. Cancer 70: 648-655.
214. Burghardt E, Pickel H, Girardi F (1998). Colposcopy, Cervical Pathology: Textbook and Atlas. 3rd Ed. Thieme: New York.
215. Burk RD, Terai M, Gravitt PE, Brinton LA, Kurman RJ, Barnes WA, Greenberg MD, Hadjimichael OC, Fu L, McGowan L, Mortel R, Schwartz PE, Hildesheim A (2003). Distribution of human papillomavirus types 16 and 18 variants in squamous cell carcinomas and adenocarcinomas of the cervix. Cancer Res 63: 7215-7220.
216. Burks RT, Kessis TD, Cho KR, Hedrick L (1994). Microsatellite instability in endometrial carcinoma. Oncogene 9: 1163-1166.
217. Burks RT, Sherman ME, Kurman RJ (1996). Micropapillary serous carcinoma of the ovary. A distinctive low-grade carcinoma related to serous borderline tumors. Am J Surg Pathol 20: 1319-1330.
218. Buza N, Hui P (2013). Partial hydatidiform mole: histologic parameters in correlation with DNA genotyping. Int J Gynecol Pathol 32: 307-315.
219. Caduff RF, Svoboda-Newman SM, Bartos RE, Ferguson AW, Frank TS (1998). Comparative analysis of histologic homologues of endometrial and ovarian carcinoma. Am J Surg Pathol 22: 319-326.
220. Cai B, Ronnett BM, Stoler M, Ferenczy A, Kurman RJ, Sadow D, Alvarez F, Pearson J, Sings HL, Barr E, Liaw KL (2007). Longitudinal evaluation of interobserver and intraobserver agreement of cervical intraepithelial neoplasia diagnosis among an experienced panel of gynecologic pathologists. Am J Surg Pathol 31: 1854-1860.
221. Cai KQ, Albarracin C, Rosen D, Zhong R, Zheng W, Luthra R, Broaddus R, Liu J (2004). Microsatellite instability and alteration of the expression of hMLH1 and hMSH2 in ovarian clear cell carcinoma. Hum Pathol 35: 552-559.
222. Callahan MJ, Crum CP, Medeiros F, Kindelberger DW, Elvin JA, Garber JE, Feltmate CM, Berkowitz RS, Muto MG (2007). Primary fallopian tube malignancies in BRCA-positive women undergoing surgery for ovarian cancer risk reduction. J Clin Oncol 25: 3985-3990.
223. Calle EE, Kaaks R (2004). Overweight, obesity and cancer: epidemiological evidence and proposed mechanisms. Nat Rev Cancer 4: 579-591.
224. Calonje E, Guerin D, McCormick D, Fletcher CD (1999). Superficial angiomyxoma: clinicopathologic analysis of a series of distinctive but poorly recognized cutaneous tumors with tendency for recurrence. Am J Surg Pathol 23: 910-917.
225. Campbell IG, Russell SE, Choong DY, Montgomery KG, Ciavarella ML, Hooi CS, Cristiano BE, Pearson RB, Phillips WA (2004). Mutation of the PIK3CA gene in ovarian and breast cancer. Cancer Res 64: 7678-7681.
226. Cancer Genome Atlas Research Network (2011). Integrated genomic analyses of ovarian carcinoma. Nature 474: 609-615.
227. Cantisani V, Mortele KJ, Kalantari BN, Glickman JN, Tempany C, Silverman SG (2003). Vaginal metastasis from uterine leiomyosarcoma. Magnetic resonance imaging features with pathological correlation. J Comput Assist Tomogr 27: 805-809.
228. Canzonieri V, D'Amore ES, Bartoloni G, Piazza M, Blandamura S, Carbone A (1994). Leiomyomatosis with vascular invasion. A unified pathogenesis regarding leiomyoma with vascular microinvasion, benign metastasizing leiomyoma and intravenous leiomyomatosis. Virchows Arch 425: 541-545.
229. Cao D, Guo S, Allan RW, Molberg KH, Peng Y (2009). SALL4 is a novel sensitive and specific marker of ovarian primitive germ cell tumors and is particularly useful in distinguishing yolk sac tumor from clear cell carcinoma. Am J Surg Pathol 33: 894-904.
230. Cao D, Srodon M, Montgomery EA, Kurman RJ (2005). Lipomatous variant of angiomyofibroblastoma: report of two cases and review of the literature. Int J Gynecol Pathol 24: 196-200.
231. Carbone A, Gloghini A, Libra M, Gasparotto D, Navolanic PM, Spina M, Tirelli U (2006). A spindle cell variant of diffuse large B-cell lymphoma possesses genotypic and phenotypic markers characteristic of a germinal center B-cell origin. Mod Pathol 19: 299-306.
232. Carcangiu ML, Peissel B, Pasini B, Spatti G, Radice P, Manoukian S (2006). Incidental carcinomas in prophylactic specimens in BRCA1 and BRCA2 germ-line mutation carriers, with emphasis on fallopian tube lesions: report of 6 cases and review of the literature. Am J Surg Pathol 30: 1222-1230.
233. Carcangiu ML, Radice P, Manoukian S, Spatti G, Gobbo M, Pensotti V, Crucianelli R, Pasini B (2004). Atypical epithelial proliferation in fallopian tubes in prophylactic salpingo-oophorectomy specimens from BRCA1 and BRCA2 germline mutation carriers. Int J Gynecol Pathol 23: 35-40.
234. Cardosi RJ, Speights A, Fiorica JV, Grendys EC Jr., Hakam A, Hoffman MS (2001). Bartholin's gland carcinoma: a 15-year experience. Gynecol Oncol 82: 247-251.
235. Carlson JA, Ambros R, Malfetano J, Ross J, Grabowski R, Lamb P, Figge H, Mihm MC Jr (1998). Vulvar lichen sclerosus and squamous cell carcinoma: a cohort, case control, and investigational study with historical perspective; implications for chronic inflammation and sclerosis in the development of neoplasia. Hum Pathol 29: 932-948.
236. Carlson JA Jr, Wheeler JE (1993). Primary ovarian melanoma arising in a dermoid stage IIIc: long-term disease-free survival with aggressive surgery and platinum therapy. Gynecol Oncol 48: 397-401.
237. Carlson JW, Mutter GL (2008). Endometrial intraepithelial neoplasia is

associated with polyps and frequently has metaplastic change. Histopathology 53: 325-332.
238. Carlson JW, Nucci MR, Brodsky J, Crum CP, Hirsch MS (2007). Biomarker-assisted diagnosis of ovarian, cervical and pulmonary small cell carcinomas: the role of TTF-1, WT-1 and HPV analysis. Histopathology 51: 305-312.
239. Carr KA, Roberts JA, Frank TS (1992). Progesterone receptors in bilateral ovarian ependymoma presenting in pregnancy. Hum Pathol 23: 962-965.
240. Carr NJ, Finch J, Ilesley IC, Chandrakumaran K, Mohamed F, Mirnezami A, Cecil T, Moran B (2012). Pathology and prognosis in pseudomyxoma peritonei: a review of 274 cases. J Clin Pathol 65: 919-923.
241. Carter J, Elliott P, Russell P (1992). Bilateral fibroepithelial polypi of labium minus with atypical stromal cells. Pathology 24: 37-39.
242. Carter JE, Mizell KN, Tucker JA (2008). Mammary-type fibroepithelial neoplasms of the vulva: a case report and review of the literature. J Cutan Pathol 35: 246-249.
243. Carvalho FM, Carvalho JP, Motta EV, Souen J (2000). Mullerian adenosarcoma of the uterus with sarcomatous overgrowth following tamoxifen treatment for breast cancer. Rev Hosp Clin Fac Med Sao Paulo 55: 17-20.
244. Carvalho JC, Thomas DG, Lucas DR (2009). Cluster analysis of immunohistochemical markers in leiomyosarcoma delineates specific anatomic and gender subgroups. Cancer 115: 4186-4195.
245. Castaldo TW, Petrilli ES, Ballon SC, Voet RL, Lagasse LD, Lubens R (1980). Endodermal sinus tumor of the clitoris. Gynecol Oncol 9: 376-380.
246. Castellsague X, Bosch FX, Munoz N, Meijer CJ, Shah KV, de Sanjose S, Eluf-Neto J, Ngelangel CA, Chichareon S, Smith JS, Herrero R, Moreno V, Franceschi S (2002). Male circumcision, penile human papillomavirus infection, and cervical cancer in female partners. N Engl J Med 346: 1105-1112.
247. Castellsague X, Munoz N (2003). Chapter 3: Cofactors in human papillomavirus carcinogenesis--role of parity, oral contraceptives, and tobacco smoking. J Natl Cancer Inst Monogr 20-28.
248. Castilla MA, Moreno-Bueno G, Romero-Perez L, Van de Vijver K, Biscuola M, Lopez-Garcia MA, Prat J, Matias-Guiu X, Cano A, Oliva E, Palacios J (2011). Micro-RNA signature of the epithelial-mesenchymal transition in endometrial carcinosarcoma. J Pathol 223: 72-80.
249. Castle PE, Gage JC, Wheeler CM, Schiffman M (2011). The clinical meaning of a cervical intraepithelial neoplasia grade 1 biopsy. Obstet Gynecol 118: 1222-1229.
250. Castle PE, Gravitt PE, Wentzensen N, Schiffman M (2012). A descriptive analysis of prevalent vs incident cervical intraepithelial neoplasia grade 3 following minor cytologic abnormalities. Am J Clin Pathol 138: 241-246.
251. Castle PE, Schiffman M, Wheeler CM, Wentzensen N, Gravitt PE (2010). Human papillomavirus genotypes in cervical intraepithelial neoplasia grade 3. Cancer Epidemiol Biomarkers Prev 19: 1675-1681.
252. Catasus L, Bussaglia E, Rodrguez I, Gallardo A, Pons C, Irving JA, Prat J (2004). Molecular genetic alterations in endometrioid carcinomas of the ovary: similar frequency of beta-catenin abnormalities but lower rate of microsatellite instability and PTEN alterations than in uterine endometrioid carcinomas. Hum Pathol 35: 1360-1368.
253. Cathro HP, Stoler MH (2005). The utility of calretinin, inhibin, and WT1 immunohistochemical staining in the differential diagnosis of ovarian tumors. Hum Pathol 36: 195-201.
254. Cenacchi G, Pasquinelli G, Montanaro L, Cerasoli S, Vici M, Bisceglia M, Giangaspero F, Martinelli GN, Derenzini M (1998). Primary endocervical extraosseous Ewing's sarcoma/PNET. Int J Gynecol Pathol 17: 83-88.
255. Cerruto CA, Brun EA, Chang D, Sugarbaker PH (2006). Prognostic significance of histomorphologic parameters in diffuse malignant peritoneal mesothelioma. Arch Pathol Lab Med 130: 1654-1661.
256. Cetiner H, Kir G, Gelmann EP, Ozdemirli M (2009). Primary vulvar Ewing sarcoma/primitive neuroectodermal tumor: a report of 2 cases and review of the literature. Int J Gynecol Cancer 19: 1131-1136.
257. Chabrel CM, Beilby JO (1980). Vaginal rhabdomyoma. Histopathology 4: 645-651.
258. Chafe W, Richards A, Morgan L, Wilkinson E (1988). Unrecognized invasive carcinoma in vulvar intraepithelial neoplasia (VIN). Gynecol Oncol 31: 154-165.
259. Chalvardjian A, Scully RE (1973). Sclerosing stromal tumors of the ovary. Cancer 31: 664-670.
260. Chan DP, Wong WP (1970). Extrauterine gestational choriocarcinoma. Report of two cases. Obstet Gynecol 35: 730-733.
261. Chan JK, Kawar NM, Shin JY, Osann K, Chen LM, Powell CB, Kapp DS (2008). Endometrial stromal sarcoma: a population-based analysis. Br J Cancer 99: 1210-1215.
262. Chan JK, Loizzi V, Magistris A, Hunter MI, Rutgers J, DiSaia PJ, Berman ML (2005). Clinicopathologic features of six cases of primary cervical lymphoma. Am J Obstet Gynecol 193: 866-872.
263. Chan JK, Loo KT, Yau BK, Lam SY (1997). Nodular histiocytic/mesothelial hyperplasia: a lesion potentially mistaken for a neoplasm in transbronchial biopsy. Am J Surg Pathol 21: 658-663.
264. Chan JK, Teoh D, Hu JM, Shin JY, Osann K, Kapp DS (2008). Do clear cell ovarian carcinomas have poorer prognosis compared to other epithelial cell types? A study of 1411 clear cell ovarian cancers. Gynecol Oncol 109: 370-376.
265. Chandy L, Kumar L, Dawar R (1998). Non-Hodgkin's lymphoma presenting as a primary lesion in uterine cervix: case report. J Obstet Gynaecol Res 24: 183-187.
266. Chang KL, Crabtree GS, Lim-Tan SK, Kempson RL, Hendrickson MR (1990). Primary uterine endometrial stromal neoplasms. A clinicopathologic study of 117 cases. Am J Surg Pathol 14: 415-438.
267. Chang KL, Crabtree GS, Lim-Tan SK, Kempson RL, Hendrickson MR (1993). Primary extrauterine endometrial stromal neoplasms: a clinicopathologic study of 20 cases and a review of the literature. Int J Gynecol Pathol 12: 282-296.
268. Chang MC, Vargas SO, Hornick JL, Hirsch MS, Crum CP, Nucci MR (2009). Embryonic stem cell transcription factors and D2-40 (podoplanin) as diagnostic immunohistochemical markers in ovarian germ cell tumors. Int J Gynecol Pathol 28: 347-355.
269. Chang SC, Lacey JV Jr, Brinton LA, Hartge P, Adams K, Mouw T, Carroll L, Hollenbeck A, Schatzkin A, Leitzmann MF (2007). Lifetime weight history and endometrial cancer risk by type of menopausal hormone use in the NIH-AARP diet and health study. Cancer Epidemiol Biomarkers Prev 16: 723-730.
270. Chang YL, Chang TC, Hsueh S, Huang KG, Wang PN, Liu HP, Soong YK (1999). Prognostic factors and treatment for placental site trophoblastic tumor-report of 3 cases and analysis of 88 cases. Gynecol Oncol 73: 216-222.
271. Chappell CA, Wiesenfeld HC (2012). Pathogenesis, diagnosis, and management of severe pelvic inflammatory disease and tuboovarian abscess. Clin Obstet Gynecol 55: 893-903.
272. Chelmow D, Waxman A, Cain JM, Lawrence HC, III (2012). The evolution of cervical screening and the specialty of obstetrics and gynecology. Obstet Gynecol 119: 695-699.
273. Chen BJ, Marino-Enriquez A, Fletcher CD, Hornick JL (2012). Loss of retinoblastoma protein expression in spindle cell/pleomorphic lipomas and cytogenetically related tumors: an immunohistochemical study with diagnostic implications. Am J Surg Pathol 36: 1119-1128.
274. Chen E, Fletcher CD (2010). Cellular angiofibroma with atypia or sarcomatous transformation: clinicopathologic analysis of 13 cases. Am J Surg Pathol 34: 707-714.
275. Chen EY, Mehra K, Mehrad M, Ning G, Miron A, Mutter GL, Monte N, Quade BJ, McKeon FD, Yassin Y, Xian W, Crum CP (2010). Secretory cell outgrowth, PAX2 and serous carcinogenesis in the Fallopian tube. J Pathol 222: 110-116.
276. Chen G, Folpe AL, Colby TV, Sittampalam K, Patey M, Chen MG, Chan JK (2011). Angiomatoid fibrous histiocytoma: unusual sites and unusual morphology. Mod Pathol 24: 1560-1570.
277. Chen KT (1985). Rhabdomyosarcomatous uterine adenosarcoma. Int J Gynecol Pathol 4: 146-152.
278. Chen KT (1999). Uterine leiomyohibernoma. Int J Gynecol Pathol 18: 96-97.
279. Chen KT (2003). Familial peritoneal multifocal calcifying fibrous tumor. Am J Clin Pathol 119: 811-815.
280. Chen KT, Kostich ND, Rosai J (1978). Peritoneal foreign body granulomas to keratin in uterine adenocanthoma. Arch Pathol Lab Med 102: 174-177.
281. Chen L, Yang B (2008). Immunohistochemical analysis of p16, p53, and Ki-67 expression in uterine smooth muscle tumors. Int J Gynecol Pathol 27: 326-332.
282. Chen RJ, Chen KY, Chang TC, Sheu BC, Chow SN, Huang SC (2008). Prognosis and treatment of squamous cell carcinoma from a mature cystic teratoma of the ovary. J Formos Med Assoc 107: 857-868.
283. Chen RJ, Lin YH, Chen CA, Huang SC, Chow SN, Hsieh CY (1999). Influence of histologic type and age on survival rates for invasive cervical carcinoma in Taiwan. Gynecol Oncol 73: 184-190.
284. Chen S, Leitao MM, Tornos C, Soslow RA (2005). Invasion patterns in stage I endometrioid and mucinous ovarian carcinomas: a clinicopathologic analysis emphasizing favorable outcomes in carcinomas without destructive stromal invasion and the occasional malignant course of carcinomas with limited destructive stromal invasion. Mod Pathol 18: 903-911.
284A. Chen SJ, Li YW, Tsai WY (1993). Endodermal sinus (yolk sac) tumor of vagina and cervix in an infant. Pediatr Radiol 23:57-58.
285. Chen TD, Chuang HC, Lee LY (2012). Adenoid basal carcinoma of the uterine cervix: clinicopathologic features of 12 cases with reference to CD117 expression. Int J Gynecol Pathol 31: 25-32.
286. Chen X, Sheng W, Wang J (2013). Well-differentiated papillary mesothelioma: a clinicopathological and immunohistochemical study of 18 cases with additional observation. Histopathology 62: 805-813.
287. Chen X, Zhang X, Zhang S, Lu B (2010). Angioleiomyomas in the bilateral broad ligaments. Int J Gynecol Pathol 29: 39-43.
288. Cheng EJ, Kurman RJ, Wang M, Oldt R, Wang BG, Berman DM, Shih I (2004). Molecular genetic analysis of ovarian serous cystadenomas. Lab Invest 84: 778-784.
289. Cheng L, Roth LM, Zhang S, Wang M, Morton MJ, Zheng W, Abdul Karim FW, Montironi R, Lopez-Beltran A (2011). KIT gene mutation and amplification in dysgerminoma of the ovary. Cancer 117: 2096-2103.
290. Cheng L, Thomas A, Roth LM, Zheng W, Michael H, Karim FW (2004). OCT4: a novel biomarker for dysgerminoma of the ovary. Am J Surg Pathol 28: 1341-1346.
291. Cheng L, Zhang S, Talerman A, Roth LM (2010). Morphologic, immunohistochemical, and fluorescence in situ hybridization study of ovarian embryonal carcinoma with comparison to solid variant of yolk sac tumor and immature teratoma. Hum Pathol 41: 716-723.
292. Chestnut DH, Szpak CA, Fortier KJ, Hammond CB (1988). Uterine hemangioma associated with infertility. South Med J 81: 926-928.
293. Chetty R, Clark SP, Bhathal PS (1993). Carcinoid tumour of the uterine corpus. Virchows Arch A Pathol Anat Histopathol 422: 93-95.
294. Cheuk W, Beavon I, Chui DT, Chan JK (2011). Extrapancreatic solid pseudopapillary neoplasm: report of a case of primary ovarian origin and review of the literature. Int J Gynecol Pathol 30: 539-543.
295. Cheung AN (2003). Pathology of gestational trophoblastic diseases. Best Pract Res Clin Obstet Gynaecol 17: 849-868.
296. Cheung LW, Hennessy BT, Li J, Yu S, Myers AP, Djordjevic B, Lu Y, Stemke-Hale K, Dyer MD, Zhang F, Ju Z, Cantley LC, Scherer SE, Liang H, Lu KH, Broaddus RR, Mills GB (2011). High frequency of PIK3R1 and PIK3R2 mutations in endometrial cancer elucidates a novel mechanism for regulation of PTEN protein stability. Cancer Discov 1: 170-185.
297. Chiang AJ, La V, Peng J, Yu KJ, Teng NN (2011). Squamous cell carcinoma arising from mature cystic teratoma of the ovary. Int J Gynecol Cancer 21: 466-474.
298. Chiang S, Ali R, Melnyk N, McAlpine JN, Huntsman DG, Gilks CB, Lee CH, Oliva E (2011). Frequency of known gene rearrangements in endometrial stromal tumors. Am J Surg Pathol 35: 1364-1372.
299. Chiesa AG, Deavers MT, Veras E, Silva EG, Gershenson D, Malpica A (2010). Ovarian intestinal type mucinous borderline tumors: are we ready for a nomenclature change? Int J Gynecol Pathol 29: 108-112.
300. Chikkamuniyappa S, Herrick J, Jagirdar JS (2004). Nodular histiocytic/mesothelial hyperplasia: a potential pitfall. Ann Diagn Pathol 8: 115-120.
301. Chittenden BG, Fullerton G, Maheshwari A, Bhattacharya S (2009). Polycystic ovary syndrome and the risk of gynaecological cancer: a systematic review. Reprod Biomed Online 19: 398-405.
302. Chiu TL, Jones RW (2011). Multifocal multicentric squamous cell carcinomas arising in vulvovaginal lichen planus. J Low Genit Tract Dis 15: 246-247.
303. Chiyomaru K, Nagano T, Nishigori C (2012). XRCC1 Arg194Trp polymorphism, risk of nonmelanoma skin cancer and extramammary Paget's disease in a Japanese population. Arch Dermatol Res 304: 363-370.
304. Cho KR (2009). Ovarian cancer update: lessons from morphology, molecules, and mice. Arch Pathol Lab Med 133: 1775-1781.
305. Cho KR, Shih I (2009). Ovarian cancer. Annu Rev Pathol 4: 287-313.
306. Cho KR, Woodruff JD, Epstein JI (1989). Leiomyoma of the uterus with multiple

extrauterine smooth muscle tumors: a case report suggesting multifocal origin. Hum Pathol 20: 80-83.

307. Chong AL, Ngan BY, Weitzman S, Abla O (2009). Anaplastic large cell lymphoma of the ovary in a pediatric patient. J Pediatr Hematol Oncol 31: 702-704.

308. Chopra R, Al-Mulhim AR, Hashish H (2003). Parametrial angiomyolipoma with multicystic change. Gynecol Oncol 90: 220-223.

309. Choschzick M, Hantaredja W, Tennstedt P, Gieseking F, Wolber L, Simon R (2011). Role of TP53 mutations in vulvar carcinomas. Int J Gynecol Pathol 30: 497-504.

310. Chou HH, Lai CH, Wang PN, Tsai KT, Liu HP, Hsueh S (1997). Combination of high-dose chemotherapy, autologous bone marrow/ peripheral blood stem cell transplantation, and thoracoscopic surgery in refractory nongestational choriocarcinoma of a 45XO/46XY female: a case report. Gynecol Oncol 64: 521-525.

311. Christman JE, Ballon SC (1990). Ovarian fibrosarcoma associated with Maffucci's syndrome. Gynecol Oncol 37: 290-291.

312. Christopherson WM, Alberhasky RC, Connelly PJ (1982). Carcinoma of the endometrium: I. A clinicopathologic study of clear-cell carcinoma and secretory carcinoma. Cancer 49: 1511-1523.

313. Chu DZ, Lang NP, Thompson C, Osteen PK, Westbrook KC (1989). Peritoneal carcinomatosis in nongynecologic malignancy. A prospective study of prognostic factors. Cancer 63: 364-367.

314. Chu PG, Arber DA, Weiss LM, Chang KL (2001). Utility of CD10 in distinguishing between endometrial stromal sarcoma and uterine smooth muscle tumors: an immunohistochemical comparison of 34 cases. Mod Pathol 14: 465-471.

315. Chu PG, Chung L, Weiss LM, Lau SK (2011). Determining the site of origin of mucinous adenocarcinoma: an immunohistochemical study of 175 cases. Am J Surg Pathol 35: 1830-1836.

316. Chuaqui R, Silva M, Emmert-Buck M (2001). Allelic deletion mapping on chromosome 6q and X chromosome inactivation clonality patterns in cervical intraepithelial neoplasia and invasive carcinoma. Gynecol Oncol 80: 364-371.

317. Chumas JC, Scully RE (1991). Sebaceous tumors arising in ovarian dermoid cysts. Int J Gynecol Pathol 10: 356-363.

318. Churg A, Galateau-Salle F (2012). The separation of benign and malignant mesothelial proliferations. Arch Pathol Lab Med 136: 1217-1226.

319. Cibula D, Widschwendter M, Majek O, Dusek L (2011). Tubal ligation and the risk of ovarian cancer: review and meta-analysis. Hum Reprod Update 17: 55-67.

320. Clark DH, Weed JC (1977). Metastasizing leiomyoma: a case report. Am J Obstet Gynecol 127: 672-673.

321. Clark WH, Jr., Hood AF, Tucker MA, Jampel RM (1998). Atypical melanocytic nevi of the genital type with a discussion of reciprocal parenchymal-stromal interactions in the biology of neoplasia. Hum Pathol 29: S1-24.

322. Clarke B, Tinker AV, Lee CH, Subramanian S, van de Rijn M, Turbin D, Kalloger S, Han G, Ceballos K, Cadungog MG, Huntsman DG, Coukos G, Gilks CB (2009). Intraepithelial T cells and prognosis in ovarian carcinoma: novel associations with stage, tumor type, and BRCA1 loss. Mod Pathol 22: 393-402.

323. Clarke BA, Mulligan AM, Irving JA, McCluggage WG, Oliva E (2011). Mullerian adenosarcomas with unusual growth patterns: staging issues. Int J Gynecol Pathol 30: 340-347.

324. Clarke BA, Rahimi K, Chetty R (2010). Leiomyosarcoma of the broad ligament with osteoclast-like giant cells and rhabdoid cells. Int J Gynecol Pathol 29: 432-437.

325. Clarke MA, Rodriguez AC, Gage JC, Herrero R, Hildesheim A, Wacholder S, Burk R, Schiffman M (2012). A large, population-based study of age-related associations between vaginal pH and human papillomavirus infection. BMC Infect Dis 12: 33.

326. Clavero PA, Nogales FF, Ruiz-Avila I, Linares J, Concha A (1992). Regression of peritoneal leiomyomatosis after treatment with gonadotropin releasing hormone analogue. Int J Gynecol Cancer 2: 52-54.

327. Clement PB (1988). Intravenous leiomyomatosis of the uterus. Pathol Annu 23 Pt 2: 153-183.

328. Clement PB (1989). Mullerian adenosarcomas of the uterus with sarcomatous overgrowth. A clinicopathological analysis of 10 cases. Am J Surg Pathol 13: 28-38.

329. Clement PB (1990). Miscellaneous primary tumors and metastatic tumors of the uterine cervix. Semin Diagn Pathol 7: 228-248.

330. Clement PB (2007). The pathology of endometriosis: a survey of the many faces of a common disease emphasizing diagnostic pitfalls and unusual and newly appreciated aspects. Adv Anat Pathol 14: 241-260.

331. Clement PB, Dimmick JE (1979). Endodermal variant of mature cystic teratoma of the ovary: report of a case. Cancer 43: 383-385.

332. Clement PB, Oliva E, Young RH (1996). Mullerian adenosarcoma of the uterine corpus associated with tamoxifen therapy: a report of six cases and a review of tamoxifen-associated endometrial lesions. Int J Gynecol Pathol 15: 222-229.

333. Clement PB, Scully RE (1974). Mullerian adenosarcoma of the uterus. A clinicopathologic analysis of ten cases of a distinctive type of mullerian mixed tumor. Cancer 34: 1138-1149.

334. Clement PB, Scully RE (1976). Uterine tumors resembling ovarian sex-cord tumors. A clinicopathologic analysis of fourteen cases. Am J Clin Pathol 66: 512-525.

335. Clement PB, Scully RE (1978). Extrauterine mesodermal (mullerian) adenosarcoma: a clinicopathologic analysis of five cases. Am J Clin Pathol 69: 276-283.

336. Clement PB, Scully RE (1980). Large solitary luteinized follicle cyst of pregnancy and puerperium: A clinicopathological analysis of eight cases. Am J Surg Pathol 4: 431-438.

337. Clement PB, Scully RE (1990). Mullerian adenofibroma of the uterus with invasion of myometrium and pelvic veins. Int J Gynecol Pathol 9: 363-371.

338. Clement PB, Scully RE (1990). Mullerian adenosarcoma of the uterus: a clinicopathologic analysis of 100 cases with a review of the literature. Hum Pathol 21: 363-381.

339. Clement PB, Scully RE (1992). Endometrial stromal sarcomas of the uterus with extensive endometrioid glandular differentiation: a report of three cases that caused problems in differential diagnosis. Int J Gynecol Pathol 11: 163-173.

340. Clement PB, Young RH (1987). Atypical polypoid adenomyoma of the uterus associated with Turner's syndrome. A report of three cases, including a review of "estrogen-associated" endometrial neoplasms and neoplasms associated with Turner's syndrome. Int J Gynecol Pathol 6: 104-113.

341. Clement PB, Young RH (1987). Diffuse leiomyomatosis of the uterus: a report of four cases. Int J Gynecol Pathol 6: 322-330.

342. Clement PB, Young RH (1993). Florid mesothelial hyperplasia associated with ovarian tumors: a potential source of error in tumor diagnosis and staging. Int J Gynecol Pathol 12: 51-58.

343. Clement PB, Young RH, Hanna W, Scully RE (1994). Sclerosing peritonitis associated with luteinized thecomas of the ovary. A clinicopathological analysis of six cases. Am J Surg Pathol 18: 1-13.

344. Clement PB, Young RH, Keh P, Ostor AG, Scully RE (1995). Malignant mesonephric neoplasms of the uterine cervix. A report of eight cases, including four with a malignant spindle cell component. Am J Surg Pathol 19: 1158-1171.

345. Clement PB, Young RH, Scully RE (1987). Endometrioid-like variant of ovarian yolk sac tumor. A clinicopathological analysis of eight cases. Am J Surg Pathol 11: 767-778.

346. Clement PB, Young RH, Scully RE (1988). Intravenous leiomyomatosis of the uterus. A clinicopathological analysis of 16 cases with unusual histologic features. Am J Surg Pathol 12: 932-945.

347. Clement PB, Young RH, Scully RE (1988). Ovarian granulosa cell proliferations of pregnancy: a report of nine cases. Hum Pathol 19: 657-662.

348. Clement PB, Young RH, Scully RE (1992). Diffuse, perinodular, and other patterns of hydropic degeneration within and adjacent to uterine leiomyomas. Problems in differential diagnosis. Am J Surg Pathol 16: 26-32.

349. Clement PB, Young RH, Scully RE (1996). Malignant mesotheliomas presenting as ovarian masses. A report of nine cases, including two primary ovarian mesotheliomas. Am J Surg Pathol 20: 1067-1080.

350. Clement PB, Zubovits JT, Young RH, Scully RE (1998). Malignant mullerian mixed tumors of the uterine cervix: a report of nine cases of a neoplasm with morphology often different from its counterpart in the corpus. Int J Gynecol Pathol 17: 211-222.

351. Clifford GM, Smith JS, Plummer M, Munoz N, Franceschi S (2003). Human papillomavirus types in invasive cervical cancer worldwide: a meta-analysis. Br J Cancer 88: 63-73.

352. Coakley FV, Choi PH, Gougoutas CA, Pothuri B, Venkatraman E, Chi D, Bergman A, Hricak H (2002). Peritoneal metastases: detection with spiral CT in patients with ovarian cancer. Radiology 223: 495-499.

353. Cobellis L, Calabrese E, Stefanon B, Raspagliesi F (2000). Malignant melanoma of the vagina. A report of 15 cases. Eur J Gynaecol Oncol 21: 295-297.

354. Cobellis L, Schurfeld K, Ignacchiti E, Santopietro R, Petraglia F (2004). An ovarian mucinous adenocarcinoma arising from mature cystic teratoma associated with respiratory type tissue: a case report. Tumori 90: 521-524.

355. Coffin CM, Patel A, Perkins S, Elenitoba-Johnson KS, Perlman E, Griffin CA (2001). ALK1 and p80 expression and chromosomal rearrangements involving 2p23 in inflammatory myofibroblastic tumor. Mod Pathol 14: 569-576.

356. Coffin CM, Watterson J, Priest JR, Dehner LP (1995). Extrapulmonary inflammatory myofibroblastic tumor (inflammatory pseudotumor). A clinicopathologic and immunohistochemical study of 84 cases. Am J Surg Pathol 19: 859-872.

357. Cohen D, Mazur MT, Jozefczyk MA, Badawy SZ (1994). Hyalinization and cellular changes in uterine leiomyomata after gonadotropin releasing hormone agonist therapy. J Reprod Med 39: 377-380.

358. Cohen JG, Chan JK, Kapp DS (2012). The management of small-cell carcinomas of the gynecologic tract. Curr Opin Oncol 24: 572-579.

359. Cohen MB, Mulchahey KM, Molnar JJ (1986). Ovarian endodermal sinus tumor with intestinal differentiation. Cancer 57: 1580-1583.

360. Cohn DE, Resnick KE, Eaton LA, deHart J, Zanagnolo V (2007). Non-Hodgkin's lymphoma mimicking gynecological malignancies of the vagina and cervix: a report of four cases. Int J Gynecol Cancer 17: 274-279.

361. Cole L, Stoler MH (2012). Issues and inconsistencies in the revised gynecologic staging systems. Semin Diagn Pathol 29: 167-173.

362. Colgan TJ (2003). Challenges in the early diagnosis and staging of Fallopian-tube carcinomas associated with BRCA mutations. Int J Gynecol Pathol 22: 109-120.

363. Colgan TJ, Dardick I, O'Connell G (1991). Paraganglioma of the vulva. Int J Gynecol Pathol 10: 203-208.

364. Colgan TJ, Murphy J, Cole DE, Narod S, Rosen B (2001). Occult carcinoma in prophylactic oophorectomy specimens: prevalence and association with BRCA germline mutation status. Am J Surg Pathol 25: 1283-1289.

365. Colgan TJ, Pendergast S, LeBlanc M (1993). The histopathology of uterine leiomyomas following treatment with gonadotropin-releasing hormone analogues. Hum Pathol 24: 1073-1077.

366. Colgan TJ, Pron G, Mocarski EJ, Bennett JD, Asch MR, Common A (2003). Pathologic features of uteri and leiomyomas following uterine artery embolization for leiomyomas. Am J Surg Pathol 27: 167-177.

367. Comin CE, Saieva C, Messerini L (2007). h-caldesmon, calretinin, estrogen receptor, and Ber-EP4: a useful combination of immunohistochemical markers for differentiating epithelioid peritoneal mesothelioma from serous papillary carcinoma of the ovary. Am J Surg Pathol 31: 1139-1148.

368. Connolly DC, Katabuchi H, Cliby WA, Cho KR (2000). Somatic mutations in the STK11/LKB1 gene are uncommon in rare gynecological tumor types associated with Peutz-Jegher's syndrome. Am J Pathol 156: 339-345.

369. Cook HT, Boylston AW (1988). Plasmacytoma of the ovary. Gynecol Oncol 29: 378-381.

370. Copeland LJ, Sneige N, Gershenson DM, Saul PB, Stringer CA, Seski JC (1986). Adenoid cystic carcinoma of Bartholin gland. Obstet Gynecol 67: 115-120.

371. Copeland LJ, Sneige N, Ordonez NG, Hancock KC, Gershenson DM, Saul PB, Kavanagh JJ (1985). Endodermal sinus tumor of the vagina and cervix. Cancer 55: 2558-2565.

372. Cossu-Rocca P, Zhang S, Roth LM, Eble JN, Zheng W, Karim FW, Michael H, Emerson RE, Jones TD, Hattab EM, Cheng L (2006). Chromosome 12p abnormalities in dysgerminoma of the ovary: a FISH analysis. Mod Pathol 19: 611-615.

373. Costa MJ, Ames PF, Walls J, Roth LM (1997). Inhibin immunohistochemistry applied to ovarian neoplasms: a novel, effective, diagnostic tool. Hum Pathol 28: 1247-1254.

374. Costa MJ, Guinee D, Jr. (2000). CD34 immunohistochemistry in female genital tract carcinosarcoma (malignant mixed mullerian tumors) supports a dominant role of the carcinomatous component. Appl Immunohistochem Mol Morphol 8: 293-299.

375. Costa MJ, McIlnay KR, Trelford J (1995). Cervical carcinoma with glandular differentiation: histological evaluation predicts disease recurrence in clinical stage I or II patients. Hum Pathol 26: 829-837.

376. Costa MJ, Morris R, DeRose PB, Cohen C (1993). Histologic and immunohistochemical evidence for considering ovarian myxoma as a variant of the thecoma-fibroma group of ovarian stromal tumors. Arch Pathol Lab Med 117: 802-808.
377. Costa MJ, Thomas W, Majmudar B, Hewan-Lowe K (1992). Ovarian myxoma: ultrastructural and immunohistochemical findings. Ultrastruct Pathol 16: 429-438.
378. Costa-Sison H (1958). The relative frequency of various anatomic sites as the point of first metastasis in 32 cases of chorionepithelioma. Am J Obstet Gynecol 75: 1149-1152.
379. Cox JT, Schiffman M, Solomon D (2003). Prospective follow-up suggests similar risk of subsequent cervical intraepithelial neoplasia grade 2 or 3 among women with cervical intraepithelial neoplasia grade 1 or negative colposcopy and directed biopsy. Am J Obstet Gynecol 188: 1406-1412.
380. Craddock KJ, Bandarchi B, Khalifa MA (2007). Blue nevi of the Mullerian tract: case series and review of the literature. J Low Genit Tract Dis 11: 284-289.
381. Crawford D, Nimmo M, Clement PB, Thomson T, Benedet JL, Miller D, Gilks CB (1999). Prognostic factors in Paget's disease of the vulva: a study of 21 cases. Int J Gynecol Pathol 18: 351-359.
382. Creasman W (2009). Revised FIGO staging for carcinoma of the endometrium. Int J Gynaecol Obstet 105: 109.
383. Creasman WT, Morrow CP, Bundy BN, Homesley HD, Graham JE, Heller PB (1987). Surgical pathologic spread patterns of endometrial cancer. A Gynecologic Oncology Group Study. Cancer 60: 2035-2041.
384. Creasman WT, Odicino F, Maisonneuve P, Quinn MA, Beller U, Benedet JL, Heintz AP, Ngan HY, Pecorelli S (2006). Carcinoma of the corpus uteri. FIGO 26th Annual Report on the Results of Treatment in Gynecological Cancer. Int J Gynaecol Obstet 95 Suppl 1: S105-S143.
385. Crispens MA, Bodurka D, Deavers M, Lu K, Silva EG, Gershenson DM (2002). Response and survival in patients with progressive or recurrent serous ovarian tumors of low malignant potential. Obstet Gynecol 99: 3-10.
386. Crosbie EJ, Zwahlen M, Kitchener HC, Egger M, Renehan AG (2010). Body mass index, hormone replacement therapy, and endometrial cancer risk: a meta-analysis. Cancer Epidemiol Biomarkers Prev 19: 3119-3130.
387. Crow J, Gardner RL, McSweeney G, Shaw RW (1995). Morphological changes in uterine leiomyomas treated by GnRH agonist goserelin. Int J Gynecol Pathol 14: 235-242.
388. Crum CP, Fu YS, Levine RU, Richart RM, Townsend DE, Fenoglio CM (1982). Intraepithelial squamous lesions of the vulva: biologic and histologic criteria for the distinction of condylomas from vulvar intraepithelial neoplasia. Am J Obstet Gynecol 144: 77-83.
388A. Crum CP, Herfs M, Ning G, Bijron JG, Howitt BE, Jimenez CA, Hanamornroongruang S, McKeon FD, Xian W (2013). Through the glass darkly: intraepithelial neoplasia, top-down differentiation and the road to ovarian cancer. J Pathol 231: 402-412.
389. Cuatrecasas M, Catasus L, Palacios J, Prat J (2009). Transitional cell tumors of the ovary: a comparative clinicopathologic, immunohistochemical, and molecular genetic analysis of Brenner tumors and transitional cell carcinomas. Am J Surg Pathol 33: 556-567.
390. Cuatrecasas M, Erill N, Musulen E, Costa I, Matias-Guiu X, Prat J (1998). K-ras mutations in nonmucinous ovarian epithelial tumors: a molecular analysis and clinicopathologic study of 144 patients. Cancer 82: 1088-1095.
391. Cuatrecasas M, Villanueva A, Matias-Guiu X, Prat J (1997). K-ras mutations in mucinous ovarian tumors: a clinicopathologic and molecular study of 95 cases. Cancer 79: 1581-1586.
392. Cubilla AL, Lloveras B, Alemany L, Alejo M, Vidal A, Kasamatsu E, Clavero O, Alvarado-Cabrero I, Lynch C, Velasco-Alonso J, Ferrera A, Chaux A, Klaustermeier J, Quint W, de Sanjose S, Munoz N, Bosch FX (2012). Basaloid squamous cell carcinoma of the penis with papillary features: a clinicopathologic study of 12 cases. Am J Surg Pathol 36: 869-875.
393. Cuff J, Longacre TA (2012). Endometriosis does not confer improved prognosis in ovarian carcinoma of uniform cell type. Am J Surg Pathol 36: 688-695.
394. Cui S, Lespinasse P, Cracchiolo B, Sama J, Kreitzer MS, Heller DS (2001). Large cell neuroendocrine carcinoma of the cervix associated with adenocarcinoma in situ: evidence of a common origin. Int J Gynecol Pathol 20: 311-312.
395. Culton LK, Deavers MT, Silva EG, Liu J, Malpica A (2006). Endometrioid carcinoma simultaneously involving the uterus and the fallopian tube: a clinicopathologic study of 13 cases. Am J Surg Pathol 30: 844-849.
396. Curtin JP, Saigo P, Slucher B, Venkatraman ES, Mychalczak B, Hoskins WJ (1995). Soft-tissue sarcoma of the vagina and vulva: a clinicopathologic study. Obstet Gynecol 86: 269-272.
397. Czernobilsky B (2008). Uterine tumors resembling ovarian sex cord tumors: an update. Int J Gynecol Pathol 27: 229-235.
398. Czernobilsky B, Hohlweg-Majert P, Dallenbach-Hellweg G (1983). Uterine adenosarcoma: a clinicopathologic study of 11 cases with a reevaluation of histologic criteria. Arch Gynecol 233: 281-294.
399. D'Angelo E, Ali RH, Espinosa I, Lee CH, Huntsman DG, Gilks B, Prat J (2013). Endometrial stromal sarcomas with sex cord differentiation are associated with PHF1 rearrangement. Am J Surg Pathol 37: 514-521.
400. D'Angelo E, Espinosa I, Ali R, Gilks CB, Rijn M, Lee CH, Prat J (2011). Uterine leiomyosarcomas: tumor size, mitotic index, and biomarkers Ki67, and Bcl-2 identify two groups with different prognosis. Gynecol Oncol 121: 328-333.
401. D'Angelo E, Mozos A, Nakayama D, Espinosa I, Catasus L, Munoz J, Prat J (2011). Prognostic significance of FOXL2 mutation and mRNA expression in adult and juvenile granulosa cell tumors of the ovary. Mod Pathol 24: 1360-1367.
402. D'Angelo E, Prat J (2011). Pathology of mixed Mullerian tumours. Best Pract Res Clin Obstet Gynaecol 25: 705-718.
403. D'Angelo E, Spagnoli LG, Prat J (2009). Comparative clinicopathologic and immunohistochemical analysis of uterine sarcomas diagnosed using the World Health Organization classification system. Hum Pathol 40: 1571-1585.
404. D'Ippolito G, Huizing MT, Tjalma WA (2012). Desmoplastic small round cell tumor (DSRCT) arising in the ovary: report of a case diagnosed at an early stage and review of the literature. Eur J Gynaecol Oncol 33: 96-100.
405. Dabbs DJ, Sturtz K, Zaino RJ (1996). The immunohistochemical discrimination of endometrioid adenocarcinomas. Hum Pathol 27: 172-177.
406. Dadhwal V, Bahadur A, Gupta R, Bansal S, Mittal S (2010). Peripheral neuroectodermal tumor of the vulva: a case report. J Low Genit Tract Dis 14: 59-62.
407. Dahlen A, Debiec-Rychter M, Pedeutour F, Domanski HA, Hoglund M, Bauer HC, Rydholm A, Sciot R, Mandahl N, Mertens F (2003). Clustering of deletions on chromosome 13 in benign and low-malignant lipomatous tumors. Int J Cancer 103: 616-623.
408. Daly MB (1992). The epidemiology of ovarian cancer. Hematol Oncol Clin North Am 6: 729-738.
409. Damjanov I, Amenta PS, Zarghami F (1984). Transformation of an AFP-positive yolk sac carcinoma into an AFP-negative neoplasm. Evidence for in vivo cloning of the human parietal yolk sac carcinoma. Cancer 53: 1902-1907.
410. Dane B, Dane C, Basaran S, Erginbas M, Cetin A (2010). Vaginal Schwannoma in a case with uterine myoma. Ann Diagn Pathol 14: 137-139.
411. Danon M, Robboy SJ, Kim S, Scully R, Crawford JD (1975). Cushing syndrome, sexual precocity, and polyostotic fibrous dysplasia (Albright syndrome) in infancy. J Pediatr 87: 917-921.
412. Darragh TM, Colgan TJ, Cox JT, Heller DS, Henry MR, Luff RD, McCalmont T, Nayar R, Palefsky JM, Stoler MH, Wilkinson EJ, Zaino RJ, Wilbur DC (2012). The Lower Anogenital Squamous Terminology Standardization Project for HPV-Associated Lesions: background and consensus recommendations from the College of American Pathologists and the American Society for Colposcopy and Cervical Pathology. J Low Genit Tract Dis 16: 205-242.
413. Davidoff AM, Hebra A, Bunin N, Shochat SJ, Schnaufer L (1996). Endodermal sinus tumor in children. J Pediatr Surg 31: 1075-1078.
414. Davis GL (1996). Malignant melanoma arising in mature ovarian cystic teratoma (dermoid cyst). Report of two cases and literature analysis. Int J Gynecol Pathol 15: 356-362.
415. Davis KP, Hartmann LK, Keeney GL, Shapiro H (1996). Primary ovarian carcinoid tumors. Gynecol Oncol 61: 259-265.
416. Daya D (1994). Malignant female adnexal tumor of probable wolffian origin with review of the literature. Arch Pathol Lab Med 118: 310-312.
417. Daya D, Lukka H, Clement PB (1992). Primitive neuroectodermal tumors of the uterus: a report of four cases. Hum Pathol 23: 1120-1129.
418. Daya D, McCaughey WT (1990). Well-differentiated papillary mesothelioma of the peritoneum. A clinicopathologic study of 22 cases. Cancer 65: 292-296.
418A. Daya D, Nazerali L, Frank GL (1992). Metastatic ovarian carcinoma of large intestinal origin simulating primary ovarian carcinoma. A clinicopathologic study of 25 cases. Am J Clin Pathol 97: 751-758.
419. Daya D, Young RH, Scully RE (1992). Endometrioid carcinoma of the fallopian tube resembling an adnexal tumor of probable wolffian origin: a report of six cases. Int J Gynecol Pathol 11: 122-130.
420. Daya DA, Scully RE (1988). Sarcoma botryoides of the uterine cervix in young women: a clinicopathological study of 13 cases. Gynecol Oncol 29: 290-304.
421. de Boer MA, Peters LA, Aziz MF, Siregar B, Cornain S, Vrede MA, Jordanova ES, Fleuren GJ (2005). Human papillomavirus type 18 variants: histopathology and E6/E7 polymorphisms in three countries. Int J Cancer 114: 422-425.
422. de Brito PA, Silverberg SG, Orenstein JM (1993). Carcinosarcoma (malignant mixed mullerian (mesodermal) tumor) of the female genital tract: immunohistochemical and ultrastructural analysis of 28 cases. Hum Pathol 24: 132-142.
423. de la Torre FJ, Rojo F, Garcia A (2002). Clear cells carcinoma of fallopian tubes associated with tubal endometriosis. Case report and review. Arch Gynecol Obstet 266: 172-174.
423A. de Leval L, Lim GS, Waltregny D, Oliva E (2010). Diverse phenotypic profile of uterine tumors resembling ovarian sex cord tumors: an immunohistochemical study of 12 cases. Am J Surg Pathol 34: 1749-1761.
423B. de Leval L, Waltregny D, Boniver J, Young RH, Castronovo V, Oliva E (2006). Use of histone deacetylase 8 (HDAC8), a new marker of smooth muscle differentiation, in the classification of mesenchymal tumors of the uterus. Am J Surg Pathol 30: 319-327.
424. de Lima GR, de Lima OA, Baracat EC, Vasserman J, Burnier M, Jr. (1989). Virilizing Brenner tumor of the ovary: case report. Obstet Gynecol 73: 895-898.
425. de Ruiter GC, Scheithauer BW, Amrami KK, Spinner RJ (2006). Benign metastasizing leiomyomatosis with massive brachial plexus involvement mimicking neurofibromatosis type 1. Clin Neuropathol 25: 282-287.
426. de Waal YR, Thomas CM, Oei AL, Sweep FC, Massuger LF (2009). Secondary ovarian malignancies: frequency, origin, and characteristics. Int J Gynecol Cancer 19: 1160-1165.
427. de Leval L, Lim GS, Waltregny D, Oliva E (2010). Diverse phenotypic profile of uterine tumors resembling ovarian sex cord tumors: an immunohistochemical study of 12 cases. Am J Surg Pathol 34: 1749-1761.
428. de Leval L, Waltregny D, Boniver J, Young RH, Castronovo V, Oliva E (2006). Use of histone deacetylase 8 (HDAC8), a new marker of smooth muscle differentiation, in the classification of mesenchymal tumors of the uterus. Am J Surg Pathol 30: 319-327.
429. de Sanjose S., Quint WG, Alemany L, Geraets DT, Klaustermeier JE, Lloveras B, Tous S, Felix A, Bravo LE, Shin HR, Vallejos CS, de Ruiz PA, Lima MA, Guimera N, Clavero O, Alejo M, Llombart-Bosch A, Cheng-Yang C, Tatti SA, Kasamatsu E, Iljazovic E, Odida M, Prado R, Seoud M, Grce M, Usubutun A, Jain A, Suarez GA, Lombardi LE, Banjo A, Menendez C, Domingo EJ, Velasco J, Nessa A, Chichareon SC, Qiao YL, Lerma E, Garland SM, Sasagawa T, Ferrera A, Hammouda D, Mariani L, Pelayo A, Steiner I, Oliva E, Meijer CJ, Al-Jassar WF, Cruz E, Wright TC, Puras A, Llave CL, Tzardi M, Agorastos T, Garcia-Barriola V, Clavel C, Ordi J, Andujar M, Castellsague X, Sanchez GI, Nowakowski AM, Bornstein J, Munoz N, Bosch FX (2010). Human papillomavirus genotype attribution in invasive cervical cancer: a retrospective cross-sectional worldwide study. Lancet Oncol 11: 1048-1056.
430. Deacon JM, Evans CD, Yule R, Desai M, Binns W, Taylor C, Peto J (2000). Sexual behaviour and smoking as determinants of cervical HPV infection and of CIN3 among those infected: a case-control study nested within the Manchester cohort. Br J Cancer 83: 1565-1572.
431. Deavers MT, Malpica A, Liu J, Broaddus R, Silva EG (2003). Ovarian sex cord-stromal tumors: an immunohistochemical study including a comparison of calretinin and inhibin. Mod Pathol 16: 584-590.
432. Deen S, Duncan TJ, Hammond RH (2007). Malignant female adnexal tumors of probable Wolffian origin. Int J Gynecol Pathol 26: 383-386.
433. Dehari R, Kurman RJ, Logani S, Shih I (2007). The development of high-grade serous carcinoma from atypical proliferative (borderline) serous tumors and low-grade micropapillary serous carcinoma: a morphologic and molecular genetic analysis. Am J Surg Pathol 31: 1007-1012.

434. Dehner LP (1973). Metastatic and secondary tumors of the vulva. Obstet Gynecol 42: 47-57.
435. Dehner LP, Jarzembowski JA, Hill DA (2012). Embryonal rhabdomyosarcoma of the uterine cervix: a report of 14 cases and a discussion of its unusual clinicopathological associations. Mod Pathol 25: 602-614.
436. Dei Tos AP, Maestro R, Doglioni C, Piccinin S, Libera DD, Boiocchi M, Fletcher CD (1996). Tumor suppressor genes and related molecules in leiomyosarcoma. Am J Pathol 148: 1037-1045.
437. Del PM, Rodriguez-Carunchio L, Ordi J (2013). Pathways of vulvar intraepithelial neoplasia and squamous cell carcinoma. Histopathology 62: 161-175.
438. DeLair D, Oliva E, Köbel M, Macias A, Gilks CB, Soslow RA (2011). Morphologic spectrum of immunohistochemically characterized clear cell carcinoma of the ovary: a study of 155 cases. Am J Surg Pathol 35: 36-44.
439. Delbaere A, Smits G, Olatunbosun O, Pierson R, Vassart G, Costagliola S (2004). New insights into the pathophysiology of ovarian hyperstimulation syndrome. What makes the difference between spontaneous and iatrogenic syndrome? Hum Reprod 19: 486-489.
440. Delgado G, Bundy B, Zaino R, Sevin BU, Creasman WT, Major F (1990). Prospective surgical-pathological study of disease-free interval in patients with stage IB squamous cell carcinoma of the cervix: a Gynecologic Oncology Group study. Gynecol Oncol 38: 352-357.
441. Dellas A, Schultheiss E, Holzgreve W, Oberholzer M, Torhorst J, Gudat F (1997). Investigation of the Bcl-2 and C-myc expression in relationship to the Ki-67 labelling index in cervical intraepithelial neoplasia. Int J Gynecol Pathol 16: 212-218.
442. DeMatteo RP, Lewis JJ, Leung D, Mudan SS, Woodruff JM, Brennan MF (2000). Two hundred gastrointestinal stromal tumors: recurrence patterns and prognostic factors for survival. Ann Surg 231: 51-58.
443. Demopoulos RI, Touger L, Dubin N (1987). Secondary ovarian carcinoma: a clinical and pathological evaluation. Int J Gynecol Pathol 6: 166-175.
444. Denton AS, Bond SJ, Matthews S, Bentzen SM, Maher EJ (2000). National audit of the management and outcome of carcinoma of the cervix treated with radiotherapy in 1993. Clin Oncol (R Coll Radiol) 12: 347-353.
445. Deodhar KK, Kerkar RA, Suryawanshi P, Menon H, Menon S (2011). Large cell neuroendocrine carcinoma of the endometrium: an extremely uncommon diagnosis, but worth the efforts. J Cancer Res Ther 7: 211-213.
446. Deppisch LM (1975). Cysts of the vagina: Classification and clinical correlations. Obstet Gynecol 45: 632-637.
447. DePriest PD, Banks ER, Powell DE, van Nagell JR Jr, Gallion HH, Puls LE, Hunter JE, Kryscio RJ, Royalty MB (1992). Endometrioid carcinoma of the ovary and endometriosis: the association in postmenopausal women. Gynecol Oncol 47: 71-75.
448. Deshpande V, Oliva E, Young RH (2010). Solid pseudopapillary neoplasm of the ovary: a report of 3 primary ovarian tumors resembling those of the pancreas. Am J Surg Pathol 34: 1514-1520.
449. Devor EJ, DE Mik JN, Ramachandran S, Goodheart MJ, Leslie KK (2012). Global dysregulation of the chromosome 14q32 imprinted region in uterine carcinosarcoma. Exp Ther Med 3: 677-682.
449A. Devouassoux-Shisheboran M, Silver SA, Tavassoli FA (1999). Wolffian adnexal tumor, so-called female adnexal tumor of probable Wolffian origin (FATWO): immunohistochemical evidence in support of a Wolffian origin. Hum Pathol 30: 856-863.
450. DeWaay DJ, Syrop CH, Nygaard IE, Davis WA, Van Voorhis BJ (2002). Natural history of uterine polyps and leiomyomata. Obstet Gynecol 100: 3-7.
451. Dharkar DD, Kraft JR, Gangadharam D (1981). Uterine lipomas. Arch Pathol Lab Med 105: 43-45.
451A. Diaz de Leon E, Carcangiu ML, Prieto VG, McCue PA, Burchette JL, To G, Norris BA, Kovatich AJ, Sanchez RL, Krigman HR, Gatalica Z (2000). Extramammary Paget disease is characterized by the consistent lack of estrogen and progesterone receptors but frequently expresses androgen receptor. Am J Clin Pathol 113: 572-575.
452. Dickersin GR, Kline IW, Scully RE (1982). Small cell carcinoma of the ovary with hypercalcemia: a report of eleven cases. Cancer 49: 188-197.
453. Dickersin GR, Young RH, Scully RE (1995). Signet-ring stromal and related tumors of the ovary. Ultrastruct Pathol 19: 401-419.
454. Dickson MA, Schwartz GK, Antonescu CR, Kwiatkowski DJ, Malinowska IA (2013). Extrarenal perivascular epithelioid cell tumors (PEComas) respond to mTOR inhibition: clinical and molecular correlates. Int J Cancer 132: 1711-1717.
455. Dietl J, Horny HP, Ruck P, Kaiserling E (1993). Dysgerminoma of the ovary. An immunohistochemical study of tumor-infiltrating lymphoreticular cells and tumor cells. Cancer 71: 2562-2568.
456. Dimopoulos MA, Daliani D, Pugh W, Gershenson D, Cabanillas F, Sarris AH (1997). Primary ovarian non-Hodgkin's lymphoma: outcome after treatment with combination chemotherapy. Gynecol Oncol 64: 446-450.
456A. Diniz da Costa AT, Coelho AM, Lourenco AV, Bernardino M, Ribeirinho AL, Jorge CC (2012). Primary breast cancer of the vulva: a case report. J Low Genit Tract Dis 16: 155-157.
457. Dionigi A, Oliva E, Clement PB, Young RH (2002). Endometrial stromal nodules and endometrial stromal tumors with limited infiltration: a clinicopathologic study of 50 cases. Am J Surg Pathol 26: 567-581.
458. DiSaia PJ, Dorion GE, Cappuccini F, Carpenter PM (1995). A report of two cases of recurrent Paget's disease of the vulva in a split-thickness graft and its possible pathogenesis-labeled "retrodissemination". Gynecol Oncol 57: 109-112.
459. Dittmer C, Katalinic A, Mundhenke C, Thill M, Fischer D (2011). Epidemiology of vulvar and vaginal cancer in Germany. Arch Gynecol Obstet 284: 169-174.
460. Djordjevic B, Clement-Kruzel S, Atkinson NE, Malpica A (2010). Nodal endosalpingiosis in ovarian serous tumors of low malignant potential with lymph node involvement: a case for a precursor lesion. Am J Surg Pathol 34: 1442-1448.
461. Djordjevic B, Gien LT, Covens A, Malpica A, Khalifa MA (2009). Polypoid or non-polypoid? A novel dichotomous approach to uterine carcinosarcoma. Gynecol Oncol 115: 32-36.
462. Djordjevic B, Hennessy BT, Li J, Barkoh BA, Luthra R, Mills GB, Broaddus RR (2012). Clinical assessment of PTEN loss in endometrial carcinoma: immunohistochemistry outperforms gene sequencing. Mod Pathol 25: 699-708.
463. Djordjevic B, Malpica A (2012). Ovarian serous tumors of low malignant potential with nodal low-grade serous carcinoma. Am J Surg Pathol 36: 955-963.
464. Dobbs SP, Shaw PA, Brown LJ, Ireland D (1998). Borderline malignant change in recurrent mullerian papilloma of the vagina. J Clin Pathol 51: 875-877.
465. Doorbar J, Quint W, Banks L, Bravo IG, Stoler M, Broker TR, Stanley MA (2012). The biology and life-cycle of human papillomaviruses. Vaccine 30 Suppl 5: F55-F70.
466. Dos Santos LA, Garg K, Diaz JP, Soslow RA, Hensley ML, Alektiar KM, Barakat RR, Leitao MM Jr (2011). Incidence of lymph node and adnexal metastasis in endometrial stromal sarcoma. Gynecol Oncol 121: 319-322.
467. Dos Santos L, Mok E, Iasonos A, Park K, Soslow RA, Aghajanian C, Alektiar K, Barakat RR, Abu-Rustum NR (2007). Squamous cell carcinoma arising in mature cystic teratoma of the ovary: a case series and review of the literature. Gynecol Oncol 105: 321-324.
468. Dossus L, Allen N, Kaaks R, Bakken K, Lund E, Tjonneland A, Olsen A, Overvad K, Clavel-Chapelon F, Fournier A, Chabbert-Buffet N, Boeing H, Schutze M, Trichopoulou A, Trichopoulos D, Lagiou P, Palli D, Krogh V, Tumino R, Vineis P, Mattiello A, Bueno-de-Mesquita HB, Onland-Moret NC, Peeters PH, Dumeaux V, Redondo ML, Duell E, Sanchez-Cantalejo E, Arriola L, Chirlaque MD, Ardanaz E, Manjer J, Borgquist S, Lukanova A, Lundin E, Khaw KT, Wareham N, Key T, Chajes V, Rinaldi S, Slimani N, Mouw T, Gallo V, Riboli E (2010). Reproductive risk factors and endometrial cancer: the European Prospective Investigation into Cancer and Nutrition. Int J Cancer 127: 442-451.
469. Downes KA, Hart WR (1997). Bizarre leiomyomas of the uterus: a comprehensive pathologic study of 24 cases with long-term follow-up. Am J Surg Pathol 21: 1261-1270.
470. Downey GO, Okagaki T, Ostrow RS, Clark BA, Twiggs LB, Faras AJ (1988). Condylomatous carcinoma of the vulva with special reference to human papillomavirus DNA. Obstet Gynecol 72: 68-73.
471. Drake A, Dhundee J, Buckley CH, Woolas R (2001). Disseminated leiomyomatosis peritonealis in association with oestrogen secreting ovarian fibrothecoma. BJOG 108: 661-664.
472. Dreisler E, Stampe SS, Ibsen PH, Lose G (2009). Prevalence of endometrial polyps and abnormal uterine bleeding in a Danish population aged 20-74 years. Ultrasound Obstet Gynecol 33: 102-108.
473. Dubé V, Lickrish GM, MacNeill KN, Colgan TJ (2006). Villoglandular adenocarcinoma in situ of intestinal type of the hymen: de novo origin from squamous mucosa? J Low Genit Tract Dis 10: 156-160.
474. Dubé V, Roy M, Plante M, Renaud MC, Têtu B (2005). Mucinous ovarian tumors of Mullerian-type: an analysis of 17 cases including borderline tumors and intraepithelial, microinvasive, and invasive carcinomas. Int J Gynecol Pathol 24: 138-146.
474A. Dubé V, Veilleux C, Plante M, Têtu B (2004). Primary villoglandular adenocarcinoma of cloacogenic origin of the vulva. Hum Pathol 35: 377-379.
475. Duggan BD, Felix JC, Muderspach LI, Tourgeman D, Zheng J, Shibata D (1994). Microsatellite instability in sporadic endometrial carcinoma. J Natl Cancer Inst 86: 1216-1221.
476. Dunaif A, Hoffman AR, Scully RE, Flier JS, Longcope C, Levy LJ, Crowley WF Jr (1985). Clinical, biochemical, and ovarian morphologic features in women with acanthosis nigricans and masculinization. Obstet Gynecol 66: 545-552.
477. Duncavage EJ, Le BM, Wang D, Pfeifer JD (2009). Merkel cell polyomavirus: a specific marker for Merkel cell carcinoma in histologically similar tumors. Am J Surg Pathol 33: 1771-1777.
478. Duska LR, Garrett L, Henretta M, Ferriss JS, Lee L, Horowitz N (2010). When 'never-events' occur despite adherence to clinical guidelines: the case of venous thromboembolism in clear cell cancer of the ovary compared with other epithelial histologic subtypes. Gynecol Oncol 116: 374-377.
479. Duval M (1891). Le placenta des rongeurs. Journal de l'anatomie et de la physiologie normales et pathologiques de l'homme et des animaux 24-73, 344-395, 513-612.
480. Easton DF, Matthews FE, Ford D, Swerdlow AJ, Peto J (1996). Cancer mortality in relatives of women with ovarian cancer: the OPCS Study. Office of Population Censuses and Surveys. Int J Cancer 65: 284-294.
481. Edelweiss M, Malpica A (2010). Dermatofibrosarcoma protuberans of the vulva: a clinicopathologic and immunohistochemical study of 13 cases. Am J Surg Pathol 34: 393-400.
481A. Edge S (ed.) (2002). AJCC Cancer Staging Manual. Springer Verlag: New York.
482. Edwards L, Ferenczy A, Eron L, Baker D, Owens ML, Fox TL, Hougham AJ, Schmitt KA (1998). Self-administered topical 5% imiquimod cream for external anogenital warts. HPV Study Group. Human PapillomaVirus. Arch Dermatol 134: 25-30.
483. Egger H, Weigmann P (1982). Clinical and surgical aspects of ovarian endometriotic cysts. Arch Gynecol 233: 37-45.
484. Ehrlich CE, Roth LM (1971). The Brenner tumor. A clinicopathologic study of 57 cases. Cancer 27: 332-342.
485. Eichhorn JH, Bell DA, Young RH, Scully RE (1999). Ovarian serous borderline tumors with micropapillary and cribriform patterns: a study of 40 cases and comparison with 44 cases without these patterns. Am J Surg Pathol 23: 397-409.
486. Eichhorn JH, Bell DA, Young RH, Swymer CM, Flotte TJ, Preffer RI, Scully RE (1992). DNA content and proliferative activity in ovarian small cell carcinomas of the hypercalcemic type. Implications for diagnosis, prognosis, and histogenesis. Am J Clin Pathol 98: 579-586.
487. Eichhorn JH, Scully RE (1991). Ovarian myxoma: clinicopathologic and immunocytologic analysis of five cases and a review of the literature. Int J Gynecol Pathol 10: 156-169.
488. Eichhorn JH, Scully RE (1996). Endometrioid ciliated-cell tumors of the ovary: a report of five cases. Int J Gynecol Pathol 15: 248-256.
489. Eichhorn JH, Young RH, Clement PB, Scully RE (2002). Mesodermal (mullerian) adenosarcoma of the ovary: a clinicopathologic analysis of 40 cases and a review of the literature. Am J Surg Pathol 26: 1243-1258.
490. Eichhorn JH, Young RH, Scully RE (1992). Primary ovarian small cell carcinoma of pulmonary type. A clinicopathologic, immunohistologic, and flow cytometric analysis of 11 cases. Am J Surg Pathol 16: 926-938.
491. Eisenkop SM, Spirtos NM, Lin WC (2006). "Optimal" cytoreduction for advanced epithelial ovarian cancer: a commentary. Gynecol Oncol 103: 329-335.
492. El-Ghobashy AA, Shaaban AM, Innes J, Prime W, Herrington CS (2007). Differential expression of cyclin-dependent kinase inhibitors and apoptosis-related proteins in endocervical lesions. Eur J Cancer 43: 2011-2018.
493. Elishaev E, Gilks CB, Miller D, Srodon M, Kurman RJ, Ronnett BM (2005). Synchronous and metachronous endocervical and ovarian neoplasms: evidence supporting interpretation

of the ovarian neoplasms as metastatic endocervical adenocarcinomas simulating primary ovarian surface epithelial neoplasms. Am J Surg Pathol 29: 281-294.

494. Elliot VJ, Shaw EC, Walker M, Jaynes E, Theaker JM (2012). Ovarian paraganglioma arising from mature cystic teratoma. Int J Gynecol Pathol 31: 545-546.

495. Elliott GB, Elliott JD (1973). Superficial stromal reactions of lower genital tract. Arch Pathol 95: 100-101.

496. Eltabbakh GH (2007). Broad ligament lipoma presenting as a pelvic mass: a case report. J Reprod Med 52: 543-544.

497. Emerson RE, Wang M, Roth LM, Zheng W, Abdul-Karim FW, Liu F, Ulbright TM, Eble JN, Cheng L (2007). Molecular genetic evidence supporting the neoplastic nature of the Leydig cell component of ovarian Sertoli-Leydig cell tumors. Int J Gynecol Pathol 26: 368-374.

498. Emery JD, Kennedy AW, Tubbs RR, Castellani WJ, Hussein MA (1999). Plasmacytoma of the ovary: a case report and literature review. Gynecol Oncol 73: 151-154.

499. Emoto M, Charnock-Jones DS, Licence DR, Ishiguro M, Kawai M, Yanaihara A, Saito T, Hachisuga T, Iwasaki H, Kawarabayashi T, Smith SK (2004). Localization of the VEGF and angiopoietin genes in uterine carcinosarcoma. Gynecol Oncol 95: 474-482.

500. Emoto M, Iwasaki H, Kawarabayashi T, Egami D, Yoshitake H, Kikuchi M, Shirakawa K (1994). Primary osteosarcoma of the uterus: report of a case with immunohistochemical analysis. Gynecol Oncol 54: 385-388.

501. Eng C (2003). PTEN: one gene, many syndromes. Hum Mutat 22: 183-198.

502. Enomoto T, Haba T, Fujita M, Hamada T, Yoshino K, Nakashima R, Wada H, Kurachi H, Wakasa K, Sakurai M, Murata Y, Shroyer KR (1997). Clonal analysis of high-grade squamous intra-epithelial lesions of the uterine cervix. Int J Cancer 73: 339-344.

503. Enomoto T, Weghorst CM, Inoue M, Tanizawa O, Rice JM (1991). K-ras activation occurs frequently in mucinous adenocarcinomas and rarely in other common epithelial tumors of the human ovary. Am J Pathol 139: 777-785.

504. Epplein M, Reed SD, Voigt LF, Newton KM, Holt VL, Weiss NS (2008). Risk of complex and atypical endometrial hyperplasia in relation to anthropometric measures and reproductive history. Am J Epidemiol 168: 563-570.

505. Epps CH, Hanan EB (1952). Metastasis of rectal carcinoid to the broad ligament. J Am Med Assoc 149: 1205-1209.

505A. Erşahin C, Omeroglu G, Potkul RK, Salhadar A (2007). Myeloid sarcoma of the vulva as the presenting symptom in a patient with acute myeloid leukemia. Gynecol Oncol 106: 259-261.

506. Escobar J, Klimowicz AC, Dean M, Chu P, Nation JG, Nelson GS, Ghatage P, Kalloger SE, Köbel M (2013). Quantification of ER/PR expression in ovarian low-grade serous carcinoma. Gynecol Oncol 128: 371-376.

507. Esheba GE, Longacre TA, Atkins KA, Higgins JP (2009). Expression of the urothelial differentiation markers GATA3 and placental S100 (S100P) in female genital tract transitional cell proliferations. Am J Surg Pathol 33: 347-353.

508. Esteller M, Levine R, Baylin SB, Ellenson LH, Herman JG (1998). MLH1 promoter hypermethylation is associated with the microsatellite instability phenotype in sporadic endometrial carcinomas. Oncogene 17: 2413-2417.

509. Euscher ED, Deavers MT, Lopez-Terrada D, Lazar AJ, Silva EG, Malpica A (2008). Uterine tumors with neuroectodermal

differentiation: a series of 17 cases and review of the literature. Am J Surg Pathol 32: 219-228.

510. Eva LJ, Ganesan R, Chan KK, Honest H, Malik S, Luesley DM (2008). Vulval squamous cell carcinoma occurring on a background of differentiated vulval intraepithelial neoplasia is more likely to recur: a review of 154 cases. J Reprod Med 53: 397-401.

511. Evans HL, Chawla SP, Simpson C, Finn KP (1988). Smooth muscle neoplasms of the uterus other than ordinary leiomyoma. A study of 46 cases, with emphasis on diagnostic criteria and prognostic factors. Cancer 62: 2239-2247.

512. Evans MJ, Langlois NE, Kitchener HC, Miller ID (1995). Is there an association between long-term tamoxifen treatment and the development of carcinosarcoma (malignant mixed Mullerian tumor) of the uterus? Int J Gynecol Cancer 5: 310-313.

513. Faber K, Jones MA, Spratt D, Tarraza HM Jr (1991). Vulvar leiomyomatosis in a patient with esophagogastric leiomyomatosis: review of the syndrome. Gynecol Oncol 41: 92-94.

514. Fadare O (2006). Uncommon sarcomas of the uterine cervix: a review of selected entities. Diagn Pathol 1: 30.

515. Fadare O (2011). Heterologous and rare homologous sarcomas of the uterine corpus: a clinicopathologic review. Adv Anat Pathol 18: 60-74.

516. Fadare O, Bonvicino A, Martel M, Renshaw IL, Azodi M, Parkash V (2010). Pleomorphic rhabdomyosarcoma of the uterine corpus: a clinicopathologic study of 4 cases and a review of the literature. Int J Gynecol Pathol 29: 122-134.

517. Fadare O, McCalip B, Mariappan MR, Hileeto D, Parkash V (2005). An endometrial stromal tumor with osteoclast-like giant cells. Ann Diagn Pathol 9: 160-165.

518. Fadare O, Parkash V, Carcangiu ML, Hui P (2006). Epithelioid trophoblastic tumor: clinicopathological features with an emphasis on uterine cervical involvement. Mod Pathol 19: 75-82.

519. Fadare O, Parkash V, Yilmaz Y, Mariappan MR, Ma L, Hileeto D, Qumsiyeh MB, Hui P (2004). Perivascular epithelioid cell tumor (PEComa) of the uterine cervix associated with intraabdominal "PEComatosis": A clinicopathological study with comparative genomic hybridization analysis. World J Surg Oncol 2: 35.

520. Fadare O, Zheng W (2005). Well-differentiated papillary villoglandular adenocarcinoma of the uterine cervix with a focal high-grade component: is there a need for reassessment? Virchows Arch 447: 883-887.

521. Fader AN, Arriba LN, Frasure HE, von Gruenigen V (2009). Endometrial cancer and obesity: epidemiology, biomarkers, prevention and survivorship. Gynecol Oncol 114: 121-127.

522. Fagundes H, Perez CA, Grigsby PW, Lockett MA (1992). Distant metastases after irradiation alone in carcinoma of the uterine cervix. Int J Radiat Oncol Biol Phys 24: 197-204.

523. Falkenberry SS, Steinhoff MM, Gordinier M, Rappoport S, Gajewski W, Granai CO (1996). Synchronous endometrioid tumors of the ovary and endometrium. A clinicopathologic study of 22 cases. J Reprod Med 41: 713-718.

524. Famoriyo A, Sawant S, Banfield PJ (2004). Abnormal uterine bleeding as a presentation of metastatic breast disease in a patient with advanced breast cancer on tamoxifen therapy. Arch Gynecol Obstet 270: 192-193.

525. Fan LD, Zang HY, Zhang XS (1996). Ovarian epidermoid cyst: report of eight cases. Int J Gynecol Pathol 15: 69-71.

526. Fanburg-Smith JC, Meis-Kindblom JM, Fante R, Kindblom LG (1998). Malignant granular cell tumor of soft tissue: diagnostic criteria and clinicopathologic correlation. Am J Surg Pathol 22: 779-794.

527. Fang YM, Gomes J, Lysikiewicz A, Maulik D (2005). Massive luteinized follicular cyst of pregnancy. Obstet Gynecol 105: 1218-1221.

528. Fanghong L, Szallasi A, Young RH (2008). Wolffian tumor of the ovary with a prominent spindle cell component: report of a case with brief discussion of unusual problems in differential diagnosis, and literature review. Int J Surg Pathol 16: 222-225.

529. Fanning J, Lambert HC, Hale TM, Morris PC, Schuerch C (1999). Paget's disease of the vulva: prevalence of associated vulvar adenocarcinoma, invasive Paget's disease, and recurrence after surgical excision. Am J Obstet Gynecol 180: 24-27.

530. Farley J, O'Boyle JD, Heaton J, Remmenga S (2000). Extraosseous Ewing sarcoma of the vagina. Obstet Gynecol 96: 832-834.

531. Farley JH, Hickey KW, Carlson JW, Rose GS, Kost ER, Harrison TA (2003). Adenosquamous histology predicts a poor outcome for patients with advanced-stage, but not early-stage, cervical carcinoma. Cancer 97: 2196-2202.

532. Faul C, Kounelis S, Karasek K, Papadaki H, Greenberger J, Jones MW (1996). Small cell carcinoma of the uterine cervix: overexpression of p53, BCL-2 and CD-44. International Journal of Gynecological Cancer 369-375.

533. Fawcett FJ, Kimbell NK (1971). Phaeochromocytoma of the ovary. J Obstet Gynaecol Br Commonw 78: 458-459.

534. Feakins RM, Lowe DG (1997). Basal cell carcinoma of the vulva: a clinicopathologic study of 45 cases. Int J Gynecol Pathol 16: 319-324.

535. Fearnley EJ, Marquart L, Spurdle AB, Weinstein P, Webb PM (2010). Polycystic ovary syndrome increases the risk of endometrial cancer in women aged less than 50 years: an Australian case-control study. Cancer Causes Control 21: 2303-2308.

536. Feeley KM, Wells M (2001). Precursor lesions of ovarian epithelial malignancy. Histopathology 38: 87-95.

537. Fehr A, Meyer A, Heidorn K, Roser K, Loning T, Bullerdiek J (2009). A link between the expression of the stem cell marker HMGA2, grading, and the fusion CRTC1-MAML2 in mucoepidermoid carcinoma. Genes Chromosomes Cancer 48: 777-785.

538. Felix A, Moura Nunes JF, Soares J (2002). Salivary gland-type basal cell adenocarcinoma of presumed bartholin's gland origin: a case report. Int J Gynecol Pathol 21: 194-197.

539. Feltmate CM, Genest DR, Wise L, Bernstein MR, Goldstein DP, Berkowitz RS (2001). Placental site trophoblastic tumor: a 17-year experience at the New England Trophoblastic Disease Center. Gynecol Oncol 82: 415-419.

540. Feltmate CM, Growdon WB, Wolfberg AJ, Goldstein DP, Genest DR, Chinchilla ME, Lieberman ES, Berkowitz RS (2006). Clinical characteristics of persistent gestational trophoblastic neoplasia after partial hydatidiform molar pregnancy. J Reprod Med 51: 902-906.

541. Ferenczy A (1995). Epidemiology and clinical pathophysiology of condylomata acuminata. Am J Obstet Gynecol 172: 1331-1339.

542. Ferguson AW, Katabuchi H, Ronnett BM, Cho KR (2001). Glial implants in gliomatosis peritonei arise from normal tissue, not from the associated teratoma. Am J Pathol 159: 51-55.

543. Ferguson SE, Gerald W, Barakat RR, Chi DS, Soslow RA (2007). Clinicopathologic features of rhabdomyosarcoma of gynecologic origin in adults. Am J Surg Pathol 31: 382-389.

544. Ferguson SE, Tornos C, Hummer A, Barakat RR, Soslow RA (2007). Prognostic features of surgical stage I uterine carcinosarcoma. Am J Surg Pathol 31: 1653-1661.

545. Ferlay J, Shin HR, Bray F, Forman D, Mathers C, Parkin DM (2008). Cancer incidence and mortality worldwide: IARC CancerBase. IARC.

546. Ferlay J, Shin HR, Bray F, Forman D, Mathers C, Parkin DM (2010). Estimates of worldwide burden of cancer in 2008: GLOBOCAN 2008. Int J Cancer 127: 2893-2917.

547. Ferreira M, Crespo M, Martins L, Felix A (2008). HPV DNA detection and genotyping in 21 cases of primary invasive squamous cell carcinoma of the vagina. Mod Pathol 21: 968-972.

548. Ferris DG, Litaker M (2005). Interobserver agreement for colposcopy quality control using digitized colposcopic images during the ALTS trial. J Low Genit Tract Dis 9: 29-35.

549. Ferry J (2011). Lymphomas of the Female Genital Tract. In: Extranodal Lymphomas. Ferry J, ed. Elsevier Saunders: Philadelphia PA, pp. 259-280.

550. Ferry JA (1997). Adenoid basal carcinoma of the uterine cervix: evolution of a distinctive clinicopathologic entity. Int J Gynecol Pathol 16: 299-300.

551. Ferry JA, Harris NL, Scully RE (1989). Uterine leiomyomas with lymphoid infiltration simulating lymphoma. A report of seven cases. Int J Gynecol Pathol 8: 263-270.

552. Ferry JA, Scully RE (1990). Mesonephric remnants, hyperplasia, and neoplasia in the uterine cervix. A study of 49 cases. Am J Surg Pathol 14: 1100-1111.

552A. Ferry JA, Young R (1997). Malignant lymphoma of the genitourinary tract. Curr Diagn Pathol 4: 145-169.

553. Fetsch JF, Laskin WB, Lefkowitz M, Kindblom LG, Meis-Kindblom JM (1996). Aggressive angiomyxoma: a clinicopathologic study of 29 female patients. Cancer 78: 79-90.

554. Fetsch JF, Laskin WB, Tavassoli FA (1997). Superficial angiomyxoma (cutaneous myxoma): a clinicopathologic study of 17 cases arising in the genital region. Int J Gynecol Pathol 16: 325-334.

555. Finch A, Shaw P, Rosen B, Murphy J, Narod SA, Colgan TJ (2006). Clinical and pathologic findings of prophylactic salpingo-oophorectomies in 159 BRCA1 and BRCA2 carriers. Gynecol Oncol 100: 58-64.

556. Fine C, Bundy AL, Berkowitz RS, Boswell SB, Berezin AF, Doubilet PM (1989). Sonographic diagnosis of partial hydatidiform mole. Obstet Gynecol 73: 414-418.

557. Finke NM, Lae ME, Lloyd RV, Gehani SK, Nascimento AG (2002). Sinonasal desmoplastic small round cell tumor: a case report. Am J Surg Pathol 26: 799-803.

558. Finkler NJ (1991). Placental site trophoblastic tumor. Diagnosis, clinical behavior and treatment. J Reprod Med 36: 27-30.

559. Fitzhugh VA, Houck K, Heller DS (2011). Vaginal blue nevus: report of a case and review of the literature. J Low Genit Tract Dis 15: 325-327.

560. Flanagan CW, Parker JR, Mannel RS, Min KW, Kida M (1997). Primary endodermal sinus tumor of the vulva: a case report and review of the literature. Gynecol Oncol 66: 515-518.

561. Fletcher CD, Tsang WY, Fisher C, Lee KC, Chan JK (1992). Angiomyofibroblastoma of the vulva. A benign neoplasm distinct from

aggressive angiomyxoma. Am J Surg Pathol 16: 373-382.
562. Fletcher JA, Morton CC, Pavelka K, Lage JM (1990). Chromosome aberrations in uterine smooth muscle tumors: potential diagnostic relevance of cytogenetic instability. Cancer Res 50: 4092-4097.
563. Folpe AL, Mentzel T, Lehr HA, Fisher C, Balzer BL, Weiss SW (2005). Perivascular epithelioid cell neoplasms of soft tissue and gynecologic origin: a clinicopathologic study of 26 cases and review of the literature. Am J Surg Pathol 29: 1558-1575.
564. Fonder MA, Hunter-Yates J, Lawrence WD, Telang GH (2012). Vestibular papillomatosis: a benign condition mimicking genital warts. Cutis 90: 300-301.
565. Fong YE, Lopez-Terrada D, Zhai QJ (2008). Primary Ewing sarcoma/peripheral primitive neuroectodermal tumor of the vulva. Hum Pathol 39: 1535-1539.
566. Forde GK, Harrison C, Doss BJ, Forde AE, Carlson JW (2010). Bilateral and multinodular signet-ring stromal tumor of the ovary. Obstet Gynecol 116 Suppl 2: 556-558.
567. Forman D, de MC, Lacey CJ, Soerjomataram I, Lortet-Tieulent J, Bruni L, Vignat J, Ferlay J, Bray F, Plummer M, Franceschi S (2012). Global burden of human papillomavirus and related diseases. Vaccine 30 Suppl 5: F12-F23.
568. Forouzanfar MH, Foreman KJ, Delossantos AM, Lozano R, Lopez AD, Murray CJ, Naghavi M (2011). Breast and cervical cancer in 187 countries between 1980 and 2010: a systematic analysis. Lancet 378: 1461-1484.
569. Foster R, Solano S, Mahoney J, Fuller A, Oliva E, Seiden MV (2006). Reclassification of a tubal leiomyosarcoma as an eGIST by molecular evaluation of c-KIT. Gynecol Oncol 101: 363-366.
570. Fowler DJ, Lindsay I, Seckl MJ, Sebire NJ (2007). Histomorphometric features of hydatidiform moles in early pregnancy: relationship to detectability by ultrasound examination. Ultrasound Obstet Gynecol 29: 76-80.
571. Fox H, Agrawal K, Langley FA (1972). The Brenner tumour of the ovary. A clinicopathological study of 54 cases. J Obstet Gynaecol Br Commonw 79: 661-665.
572. Franco EL, Villa LL, Sobrinho JP, Prado JM, Rousseau MC, Desy M, Rohan TE (1999). Epidemiology of acquisition and clearance of cervical human papillomavirus infection in women from a high-risk area for cervical cancer. J Infect Dis 180: 1415-1423.
573. Franquemont DW, Frierson HF Jr, Mills SE (1991). An immunohistochemical study of normal endometrial stroma and endometrial stromal neoplasms. Evidence for smooth muscle differentiation. Am J Surg Pathol 15: 861-870.
574. Freeman C, Berg JW, Cutler SJ (1972). Occurrence and prognosis of extranodal lymphomas. Cancer 29: 252-260.
575. Frisch M, Biggar RJ, Goedert JJ (2000). Human papillomavirus-associated cancers in patients with human immunodeficiency virus infection and acquired immunodeficiency syndrome. J Natl Cancer Inst 92: 1500-1510.
575A. Fritz A, Percy C, Jack A, Shanmugaratnam K, Sobin L, Parkin DM, Whelan S (2000). International Classification of Diseases for Oncology (ICD-O). Third edition. World Health Organization: Geneva.
576. Frumovitz M, Etchepareborda M, Sun CC, Soliman PT, Eifel PJ, Levenback CF, Ramirez PT (2010). Primary malignant melanoma of the vagina. Obstet Gynecol 116: 1358-1365.
577. Fujii H, Yoshida M, Gong ZX, Matsumoto T, Hamano Y, Fukunaga M, Hruban RH, Gabrielson E, Shirai T (2000). Frequent genetic heterogeneity in the clonal evolution of gynecological carcinosarcoma and its influence on phenotypic diversity. Cancer Res 60: 114-120.
578. Fujii S, Okamura H, Nakashima N, Bann C, Aso T, Nishimura T (1980). Leiomyomatosis peritonealis disseminata. Obstet Gynecol 55: 79S-83S.
579. Fukunaga M (2003). Benign "metastasizing" lipoleiomyoma of the uterus. Int J Gynecol Pathol 22: 202-204.
580. Fukunaga M (2011). Pure alveolar rhabdomyosarcoma of the uterine corpus. Pathol Int 61: 377-381.
581. Fukunaga M, Endo Y, Miyazawa Y, Ushigome S (1997). Small cell neuroendocrine carcinoma of the ovary. Virchows Arch 430: 343-348.
582. Fukunaga M, Endo Y, Ushigome S (1996). Clinicopathologic study of tetraploid hydropic villous tissues. Arch Pathol Lab Med 120: 569-572.
583. Fukunaga M, Endo Y, Ushigome S, Ishikawa E (1995). Atypical polypoid adenomyomas of the uterus. Histopathology 27: 35-42.
584. Fukunaga M, Nomura K, Ishikawa E, Ushigome S (1997). Ovarian atypical endometriosis: its close association with malignant epithelial tumours. Histopathology 30: 249-255.
585. Fukunaga M, Nomura K, Matsumoto K, Doi K, Endo Y, Ushigome S (1997). Vulval angiomyofibroblastoma. Clinicopathologic analysis of six cases. Am J Clin Pathol 107: 45-51.
586. Fukunishi H, Murata K, Takeuchi S, Kitazawa S (1996). Ovarian fibromatosis with minor sex cord elements. Arch Gynecol Obstet 258: 207-211.
587. Fukushima M, Twiggs LB, Okagaki T (1986). Mixed intestinal adenocarcinoma-argentaffin carcinoma of the vagina. Gynecol Oncol 23: 387-394.
588. Furuya M, Shimizu M, Nishihara H, Ito T, Sakuragi N, Ishikura H, Yoshiki T (2001). Clear cell variant of malignant melanoma of the uterine cervix: a case report and review of the literature. Gynecol Oncol 80: 409-412.
589. Gaber LW, Redline RW, Mostoufi-Zadeh M, Driscoll SG (1986). Invasive partial mole. Am J Clin Pathol 85: 722-724.
590. Gadducci A, Landoni F, Sartori E, Zola P, Maggino T, Lissoni A, Bazzurini L, Arisio R, Romagnolo C, Cristofani R (1996). Uterine leiomyosarcoma: analysis of treatment failures and survival. Gynecol Oncol 62: 25-32.
591. Gaffan J, Herbertson R, Davis P, Dogan A, Jones A (2004). Bilateral peripheral T-cell lymphoma of the fallopian tubes. Gynecol Oncol 95: 736-738.
592. Gaffey MJ, Mills SE, Boyd JC (1994). Aggressive papillary tumor of middle ear/temporal bone and adnexal papillary cystadenoma. Manifestations of von Hippel-Lindau disease. Am J Surg Pathol 18: 1254-1260.
593. Gage JC, Hanson VW, Abbey K, Dippery S, Gardner S, Kubota J, Schiffman M, Solomon D, Jeronimo J (2006). Number of cervical biopsies and sensitivity of colposcopy. Obstet Gynecol 108: 264-272.
594. Gagnon Y, Tetu B (1989). Ovarian metastases of breast carcinoma. A clinicopathologic study of 59 cases. Cancer 64: 892-898.
595. Galgano MT, Castle PE, Atkins KA, Brix WK, Nassau SR, Stoler MH (2010). Using biomarkers as objective standards in the diagnosis of cervical biopsies. Am J Surg Pathol 34: 1077-1087.
596. Galgano MT, Castle PE, Stoler MH, Solomon D, Schiffman M (2008). Can HPV-16 genotyping provide a benchmark for cervical biopsy specimen interpretation? Am J Clin Pathol 130: 65-70.
597. Gallardo A, Matias-Guiu X, Lagarda H, Catasus L, Bussaglia E, Gras E, Suarez D, Prat J (2002). Malignant mullerian mixed tumor arising from ovarian serous carcinoma: a clinicopathologic and molecular study of two cases. Int J Gynecol Pathol 21: 268-272.
598. Gallardo A, Prat J (2009). Mullerian adenosarcoma: a clinicopathologic and immunohistochemical study of 55 cases challenging the existence of adenofibroma. Am J Surg Pathol 33: 278-288.
599. Gamallo C, Palacios J, Moreno G, Calvo de MJ, Suarez A, Armas A (1999). beta-catenin expression pattern in stage I and II ovarian carcinomas : relationship with beta-catenin gene mutations, clinicopathological features, and clinical outcome. Am J Pathol 155: 527-536.
600. Gancberg D, Scourneau M, Verdebout JM, Larsimont D, Verhest A (2001). Detection of extra chromosomes 12 by fluorescent in situ hybridization (FISH) in ovarian stromal tumors. Study of 12 cases and review of the literature. Ann Pathol 21: 393-398.
601. Gandhi N, Soomro IN, O'Connor S, Sovani V (2012). Primary lymphoma arising in a mature cystic teratoma of the ovary. Histopathology 61: 1238-1240.
602. Ganesan R, McCluggage WG, Hirschowitz L, Rollason TP (2005). Superficial myofibroblastoma of the lower female genital tract: report of a series including tumours with a vulval location. Histopathology 46: 137-143.
603. Gaona-Luviano P, Unda-Franco E, Gonzalez-Jara L, Romero P, Medina-Franco H (2003). Primitive neuroectodermal tumor of the vagina. Gynecol Oncol 91: 456-458.
604. Garavaglia E, Taccagni G, Montoli S, Panacci N, Ponzoni M, Frigerio L, Mangili G (2005). Primary stage I-IIE non-Hodgkin's lymphoma of uterine cervix and upper vagina: evidence for a conservative approach in a study on three patients. Gynecol Oncol 97: 214-218.
605. Garcia MG, Deavers MT, Knoblock RJ, Chen W, Tsimberidou AM, Manning JT Jr, Medeiros LJ (2006). Myeloid sarcoma involving the gynecologic tract: a report of 11 cases and review of the literature. Am J Clin Pathol 125: 783-790.
606. Garcia-Bunuel R, Berek JS, Woodruff JD (1975). Luteomas of pregnancy. Obstet Gynecol 45: 407-414.
607. Garcia-Galvis OF, Stolnicu S, Munoz E, Aneiros-Fernandez J, Alaggio R, Nogales FF (2009). Adult extrarenal Wilms tumor of the uterus with teratoid features. Hum Pathol 40: 418-424.
608. Gardella C, Chumas JC, Pearl ML (1996). Ovarian lipoma of teratomatous origin. Obstet Gynecol 87: 874-875.
609. Gardner GJ, Reidy-Lagunes D, Gehrig PA (2011). Neuroendocrine tumors of the gynecologic tract: A Society of Gynecologic Oncology (SGO) clinical document. Gynecol Oncol 122: 190-198.
610. Garg K, Leitao MM Jr, Kauff ND, Hansen J, Kosarin K, Shia J, Soslow RA (2009). Selection of endometrial carcinomas for DNA mismatch repair protein immunohistochemistry using patient age and tumor morphology enhances detection of mismatch repair abnormalities. Am J Surg Pathol 33: 925-933.
611. Garg K, Leitao MM Jr, Wynveen CA, Sica GL, Shia J, Shi W, Soslow RA (2010). p53 overexpression in morphologically ambiguous endometrial carcinomas correlates with adverse clinical outcomes. Mod Pathol 23: 80-92.
612. Garg K, Soslow RA (2009). Lynch syndrome (hereditary non-polyposis colorectal cancer) and endometrial carcinoma. J Clin Pathol 62: 679-684.
613. Garg K, Soslow RA, Rivera M, Tuttle MR, Ghossein RA (2009). Histologically bland "extremely well differentiated" thyroid carcinomas arising in struma ovarii can recur and metastasize. Int J Gynecol Pathol 28: 222-230.
614. Garg MM, Arora VK (2012). Clear cell adenosquamous carcinoma of the cervix: a case report with discussion of the differential diagnosis. Int J Gynecol Pathol 31: 294-296.
615. Gargano JW, Wilkinson EJ, Unger ER, Steinau M, Watson M, Huang Y, Copeland G, Cozen W, Goodman MT, Hopenhayn C, Lynch CF, Hernandez BY, Peters ES, Saber MS, Lyu CW, Sands LA, Saraiya M (2012). Prevalence of human papillomavirus types in invasive vulvar cancers and vulvar intraepithelial neoplasia 3 in the United States before vaccine introduction. J Low Genit Tract Dis 16: 471-479.
616. Garrett AP, Lee KR, Colitti CR, Muto MG, Berkowitz RS, Mok SC (2001). k-ras mutation may be an early event in mucinous ovarian tumorigenesis. Int J Gynecol Pathol 20: 244-251.
617. Garrett LA, Garner EI, Feltmate CM, Goldstein DP, Berkowitz RS (2008). Subsequent pregnancy outcomes in patients with molar pregnancy and persistent gestational trophoblastic neoplasia. J Reprod Med 53: 481-486.
618. Gatta G, Lasota MB, Verdecchia A (1998). Survival of European women with gynaecological tumours, during the period 1978-1989. EUROCARE Working Group. Eur J Cancer 34: 2218-2225.
619. Geas FL, Tewari DS, Rutgers JK, Tewari KS, Berman ML (2004). Surgical cytoreduction and hormone therapy of an advanced endometrial stromal sarcoma of the ovary. Obstet Gynecol 103: 1051-1054.
620. Geiersbach KB, Jarboe EA, Jahromi MS, Baker CL, Paxton CN, Tripp SR, Schiffman JD (2011). FOXL2 mutation and large-scale genomic imbalances in adult granulosa cell tumors of the ovary. Cancer Genet 204: 596-602.
621. Geisler JP, Stowell MJ, Melton ME, Maloney CD, Geisler HE (1995). Extramammary Paget's disease of the vulva recurring in a skin graft. Gynecol Oncol 56: 446-447.
622. Genest DR (2001). Partial hydatidiform mole: clinicopathological features, differential diagnosis, ploidy and molecular studies, and gold standards for diagnosis. Int J Gynecol Pathol 20: 315-322.
623. Geng L, Connolly DC, Isacson C, Ronnett BM, Cho KR (1999). Atypical immature metaplasia (AIM) of the cervix: is it related to high-grade squamous intraepithelial lesion (HSIL)? Hum Pathol 30: 345-351.
624. Gentile G, Formelli G, Pelusi G, Flamigni C (1997). Is vestibular micropapillomatosis associated with human papillomavirus infection? Eur J Gynaecol Oncol 18: 523-525.
625. Gersell DJ, King TC (1988). Papillary cystadenoma of the mesosalpinx in von Hippel-Lindau disease. Am J Surg Pathol 12: 145-149.
626. Gershenson DM, Del JG, Copeland LJ, Rutledge FN (1984). Mixed germ cell tumors of the ovary. Obstet Gynecol 64: 200-206.
627. Gershenson DM, Sun CC, Bodurka D, Coleman RL, Lu KH, Sood AK, Deavers M, Malpica AL, Kavanagh JJ (2009). Recurrent low-grade serous ovarian carcinoma is relatively chemoresistant. Gynecol Oncol 114: 48-52.
628. Gershenson DM, Sun CC, Lu KH, Coleman RL, Sood AK, Malpica A, Deavers MT, Silva EG, Bodurka DC (2006). Clinical behavior of stage II-IV low-grade serous carcinoma of the ovary. Obstet Gynecol 108: 361-368.
629. Geyer JT, Ferry JA, Harris NL, Young RH, Longtine JA, Zukerberg LR (2010). Florid reactive lymphoid hyperplasia of the lower

female genital tract (lymphoma-like lesion): a benign condition that frequently harbors clonal immunoglobulin heavy chain gene rearrangements. Am J Surg Pathol 34: 161-168.
630. Gil-Moreno A, Garcia-Jimenez A, Gonzalez-Bosquet J, Esteller M, Castellvi-Vives J, Martinez Palones JM, Xercavins J (1997). Merkel cell carcinoma of the vulva. Gynecol Oncol 64: 526-532.
631. Gilbert L, Basso O, Sampalis J, Karp I, Martins C, Feng J, Piedimonte S, Quintal L, Ramanakumar AV, Takefman J, Grigorie MS, Artho G, Krishnamurthy S (2012). Assessment of symptomatic women for early diagnosis of ovarian cancer: results from the prospective DOvE pilot project. Lancet Oncol 13: 285-291.
632. Gilbey S, Moore DH, Look KY, Sutton GP (1997). Vulvar keratoacanthoma. Obstet Gynecol 89: 848-850.
633. Gilks CB, Alkushi A, Yue JJ, Lanvin D, Ehlen TG, Miller DM (2003). Advanced-stage serous borderline tumors of the ovary: a clinicopathological study of 49 cases. Int J Gynecol Pathol 22: 29-36.
634. Gilks CB, Bell DA, Scully RE (1990). Serous psammocarcinoma of the ovary and peritoneum. Int J Gynecol Pathol 9: 110-121.
635. Gilks CB, Clement PB, Hart WR, Young RH (2000). Uterine adenomyomas excluding atypical polypoid adenomyomas and adenomyomas of endocervical type: a clinicopathologic study of 30 cases of an underemphasized lesion that may cause diagnostic problems with brief consideration of adenomyomas of other female genital tract sites. Int J Gynecol Pathol 19: 195-205.
636. Gilks CB, Taylor GP, Clement PB (1987). Inflammatory pseudotumor of the uterus. Int J Gynecol Pathol 6: 275-286.
637. Gilks CB, Young RH, Aguirre P, DeLellis RA, Scully RE (1989). Adenoma malignum (minimal deviation adenocarcinoma) of the uterine cervix. A clinicopathological and immunohistochemical analysis of 26 cases. Am J Surg Pathol 13: 717-729.
638. Gilks CB, Young RH, Clement PB, Hart WR, Scully RE (1996). Adenomyomas of the uterine cervix of of endocervical type: a report of ten cases of a benign cervical tumor that may be confused with adenoma malignum [corrected]. Mod Pathol 9: 220-224.
639. Gilks CB, Young RH, Gersell DJ, Clement PB (1997). Large cell neuroendocrine [corrected] carcinoma of the uterine cervix: a clinicopathologic study of 12 cases. Am J Surg Pathol 21: 905-914.
640. Giordano G, Pizzi S, Berretta R, D'Adda T (2012). A new case of primary signet-ring cell carcinoma of the cervix with prominent endometrial and myometrial involvement: Immunohistochemical and molecular studies and review of the literature. World J Surg Oncol 10: 7.
641. Gisser SD (1986). Obstructing fallopian tube papilloma. Int J Gynecol Pathol 5: 179-182.
642. Giuliano AR, Sedjo RL, Roe DJ, Harri R, Baldwi S, Papenfuss MR, Abrahamsen M, Inserra P (2002). Clearance of oncogenic human papillomavirus (HPV) infection: effect of smoking (United States). Cancer Causes Control 13: 839-846.
643. Giuntoli RL, Gerardi MA, Yemelyanova AV, Ueda SM, Fleury AC, Diaz-Montes TP, Bristow RE (2012). Stage I noninvasive and minimally invasive uterine serous carcinoma: comprehensive staging associated with improved survival. Int J Gynecol Cancer 22: 273-279.
644. Giuntoli RL, Gostout BS, DiMarco CS, Metzinger DS, Keeney GL (2007). Diagnostic criteria for uterine smooth muscle tumors: leiomyoma variants associated with malignant behavior. J Reprod Med 52: 1001-1010.
645. Giuntoli RL, Metzinger DS, DiMarco CS, Cha SS, Sloan JA, Keeney GL, Gostout BS (2003). Retrospective review of 208 patients with leiomyosarcoma of the uterus: prognostic indicators, surgical management, and adjuvant therapy. Gynecol Oncol 89: 460-469.
646. Gleason BC, Hirsch MS, Nucci MR, Schmidt BA, Zembowicz A, Mihm MC Jr, McKee PH, Brenn T (2008). Atypical genital nevi. A clinicopathologic analysis of 56 cases. Am J Surg Pathol 32: 51-57.
647. Gleason BC, Hornick JL (2008). Inflammatory myofibroblastic tumours: where are we now? J Clin Pathol 61: 428-437.
648. Goff BA, Mandel LS, Melancon CH, Muntz HG (2004). Frequency of symptoms of ovarian cancer in women presenting to primary care clinics. JAMA 291: 2705-2712.
649. Goff BA, Sainz de la Cuesta R, Muntz HG, Fleischhacker D, Ek M, Rice LW, Nikrui N, Tamimi HK, Cain JM, Greer BE, Fuller AF Jr (1996). Clear cell carcinoma of the ovary: a distinct histologic type with poor prognosis and resistance to platinum-based chemotherapy in stage III disease. Gynecol Oncol 60: 412-417.
650. Goldblum J, Hart WR (1995). Localized and diffuse mesotheliomas of the genital tract and peritoneum in women. A clinicopathologic study of nineteen true mesothelial neoplasms, other than adenomatoid tumors, multicystic mesotheliomas, and localized fibrous tumors. Am J Surg Pathol 19: 1124-1137.
651. Gonzalez-Bosquet E, Gonzalez-Bosquet J, Garcia JA, Gil A, Xercavins J (1998). Carcinoid tumor of the uterine corpus. A case report. J Reprod Med 43: 844-846.
652. Gonzalez-Crussi F, deMello DE, Sotelo-Avila C (1983). Omental-mesenteric myxoid hamartomas. Infantile lesions simulating malignant tumors. Am J Surg Pathol 7: 567-578.
653. Gonzalez-Moreno S, Yan H, Alcorn KW, Sugarbaker PH (2002). Malignant transformation of "benign" cystic mesothelioma of the peritoneum. J Surg Oncol 79: 243-251.
654. Goodlad JR, MacPherson S, Jackson R, Batstone P, White J (2004). Extranodal follicular lymphoma: a clinicopathological and genetic analysis of 15 cases arising at non-cutaneous extranodal sites. Histopathology 44: 268-276.
655. Gopalan A, Dhall D, Olgac S, Fine SW, Korkola JE, Houldsworth J, Chaganti RS, Bosl GJ, Reuter VE, Tickoo SK (2009). Testicular mixed germ cell tumors: a morphological and immunohistochemical study using stem cell markers, OCT3/4, SOX2 and GDF3, with emphasis on morphologically difficult-to-classify areas. Mod Pathol 22: 1066-1074.
656. Gorlin RJ (1987). Nevoid basal-cell carcinoma syndrome. Medicine (Baltimore) 66: 98-113.
657. Gormley RH, Kovarik CL (2012). Human papillomavirus-related genital disease in the immunocompromised host: Part I. J Am Acad Dermatol 66: 867-14.
658. Goswami D, Sharma K, Zutshi V, Tempe A, Nigam S (2001). Nongestational pure ovarian choriocarcinoma with contralateral teratoma. Gynecol Oncol 80: 262-266.
659. Gotlieb WH, Chetrit A, Menczer J, Hirsh-Yechezkel G, Lubin F, Friedman E, Modan B, Ben-Baruch G (2005). Demographic and genetic characteristics of patients with borderline ovarian tumors as compared to early stage invasive ovarian cancer. Gynecol Oncol 97: 780-783.
660. Grabiec M, Walentowicz M, Marszalek A (2010). Multiple skin metastases to vulva from carcinoma of the cervical stump. Ginekol Pol 81: 140-143.
661. Grammatikakis I, Evangelinakis N, Salamalekis G, Tziortzioti V, Samaras C, Chrelias C, Kassanos D (2009). Prevalence of severe pelvic inflammatory disease and endometriotic ovarian cysts: a 7-year retrospective study. Clin Exp Obstet Gynecol 36: 235-236.
662. Grandjean M, Legrand L, Waterkeyn M, Baurain JF, Jadoul P, Donnez J, Marbaix E (2007). Small cell carcinoma of pulmonary type inside a microinvasive mucinous cystadenocarcinoma of the ovary: a case report. Int J Gynecol Pathol 26: 426-431.
663. Granter SR, Nucci MR, Fletcher CD (1997). Aggressive angiomyxoma: reappraisal of its relationship to angiomyofibroblastoma in a series of 16 cases. Histopathology 30: 3-10.
664. Gray HJ, Garcia R, Tamimi HK, Koh WJ, Goff BA, Greer BE, Paley PJ (2002). Glassy cell carcinoma of the cervix revisited. Gynecol Oncol 85: 274-277.
665. Grayson W, Cooper K (2002). A reappraisal of "basaloid carcinoma" of the cervix, and the differential diagnosis of basaloid cervical neoplasms. Adv Anat Pathol 9: 290-300.
666. Grayson W, Taylor LF, Cooper K (1997). Adenoid basal carcinoma of the uterine cervix: detection of integrated human papillomavirus in a rare tumor of putative "reserve cell" origin. Int J Gynecol Pathol 16: 307-312.
667. Grayson W, Taylor LF, Cooper K (1999). Adenoid cystic and adenoid basal carcinoma of the uterine cervix: comparative morphologic, mucin, and immunohistochemical profile of two rare neoplasms of putative 'reserve cell' origin. Am J Surg Pathol 23: 448-458.
668. Grayson W, Taylor LF, Cooper K (2001). Carcinosarcoma of the uterine cervix: a report of eight cases with immunohistochemical analysis and evaluation of human papillomavirus status. Am J Surg Pathol 25: 338-347.
669. Edge S (eds.) (2002). AJCC Cancer Staging Manual. Springer Verlag: New York.
670. Grigsby PW, Perez CA, Kuske RR, Camel HM, Kao MS, Galakatos AE, Hederman MA (1988). Adenocarcinoma of the uterine cervix: lack of evidence for a poor prognosis. Radiother Oncol 12: 289-296.
671. Groenen SM, Timmers PJ, Burger CW (2010). Recurrence rate in vulvar carcinoma in relation to pathological margin distance. Int J Gynecol Cancer 20: 869-873.
672. Groisman GM, Meir A, Sabo E (2004). The value of Cdx2 immunostaining in differentiating primary ovarian carcinomas from colonic carcinomas metastatic to the ovaries. Int J Gynecol Pathol 23: 52-57.
673. Growdon WB, Roussel BN, Scialabba VL, Foster R, Dias-Santagata D, Iafrate AJ, Ellisen LW, Tambouret RH, Rueda BR, Borger DR (2011). Tissue-specific signatures of activating PIK3CA and RAS mutations in carcinosarcomas of gynecologic origin. Gynecol Oncol 121: 212-217.
674. Gualco M, Bonin S, Foglia G, Fulcheri E, Odicino F, Prefumo F, Stanta G, Ragni N (2003). Morphologic and biologic studies on ten cases of verrucous carcinoma of the vulva supporting the theory of a discrete clinico-pathologic entity. Int J Gynecol Cancer 13: 317-324.
675. Guan B, Mao TL, Panuganti PK, Kuhn E, Kurman RJ, Maeda D, Chen E, Jeng YM, Wang TL, Shih I (2011). Mutation and loss of expression of ARID1A in uterine low-grade endometrioid carcinoma. Am J Surg Pathol 35: 625-632.
676. Guerrieri C, Hogberg T, Wingren S, Fristedt S, Simonsen E, Boeryd B (1994). Mucinous borderline and malignant tumors of the ovary. A clinicopathologic and DNA ploidy study of 92 cases. Cancer 74: 2329-2340.
677. Gui T, Cao D, Shen K, Yang J, Zhang Y, Yu Q, Wan X, Xiang Y, Xiao Y, Guo L (2012). A clinicopathological analysis of 40 cases of ovarian Sertoli-Leydig cell tumors. Gynecol Oncol 127: 384-389.
678. Guido R, Schiffman M, Solomon D, Burke L (2003). Postcolposcopy management strategies for women referred with low-grade squamous intraepithelial lesions or human papillomavirus DNA-positive atypical squamous cells of undetermined significance: a two-year prospective study. Am J Obstet Gynecol 188: 1401-1405.
679. Guido RS, Jeronimo J, Schiffman M, Solomon D (2005). The distribution of neoplasia arising on the cervix: results from the ALTS trial. Am J Obstet Gynecol 193: 1331-1337.
680. Guillou L, Gloor E, De Grandi P, Costa J (1989). Post-operative pseudosarcoma of the vagina. A case report. Pathol Res Pract 185: 245-248.
681. Guillou L, Wadden C, Coindre JM, Krausz T, Fletcher CD (1997). "Proximal-type" epithelioid sarcoma, a distinctive aggressive neoplasm showing rhabdoid features. Clinicopathologic, immunohistochemical, and ultrastructural study of a series. Am J Surg Pathol 21: 130-146.
682. Guntupalli S, Anderson ML, Bodurka DC (2009). Alveolar soft part sarcoma of the cervix: case report and literature review. Arch Gynecol Obstet 279: 263-265.
683. Guo Z, Thunberg U, Sallstrom J, Wilander E, Ponten J (1998). Clonality analysis of cervical cancer on microdissected archival materials by PCR-based X-chromosome inactivation approach. Int J Oncol 12: 1327-1332.
684. Gupta D, Deavers MT, Silva EG, Malpica A (2004). Malignant melanoma involving the ovary: a clinicopathologic and immunohistochemical study of 23 cases. Am J Surg Pathol 28: 771-780.
685. Gupta D, Malpica A, Deavers MT, Silva EG (2002). Vaginal melanoma: a clinicopathologic and immunohistochemical study of 26 cases. Am J Surg Pathol 26: 1450-1457.
686. Gupta D, Neto AG, Deavers MT, Silva EG, Malpica A (2003). Metastatic melanoma to the vagina: clinicopathologic and immunohistochemical study of three cases and literature review. Int J Gynecol Pathol 22: 136-140.
687. Hackethal A, Brueggmann D, Bohlmann MK, Franke FE, Tinneberg HR, Munstedt K (2008). Squamous-cell carcinoma in mature cystic teratoma of the ovary: systematic review and analysis of published data. Lancet Oncol 9: 1173-1180.
688. Hafezi-Bakhtiari S, Morava-Protzner I, Burnell MJ, Reardon E, Colgan TJ (2010). Choriocarcinoma arising in a serous carcinoma of ovary: an example of histopathology driving treatment. J Obstet Gynaecol Can 32: 698-702.
689. Halabi M, Oliva E, Mazal PR, Breitenecker G, Young RH (2002). Prostatic tissue in mature cystic teratomas of the ovary: a report of four cases, including one with features of prostatic adenocarcinoma, and cytogenetic studies. Int J Gynecol Pathol 21: 261-267.
690. Halbwedl I, Ullmann R, Kremser ML, Man YG, Isadi-Moud N, Lax S, Denk H, Popper HH, Tavassoli FA, Moinfar F (2005). Chromosomal alterations in low-grade endometrial stromal sarcoma and undifferentiated endometrial sarcoma as detected by comparative genomic hybridization. Gynecol Oncol 97: 582-587.
691. Hall KL, Teneriello MG, Taylor RR, Lemon S, Ebina M, Linnoila RI, Norris JH, Park RC, Birrer MJ (1997). Analysis of Ki-ras, p53, and MDM2 genes in uterine leiomyomas and leiomyosarcomas. Gynecol Oncol 65: 330-335.
692. Hallak M, Peipert JF, Heller PB, Sedlacek TV, Schauer GM (1992). Mullerian

adenosarcoma of the uterus with sarcomatous overgrowth. J Surg Oncol 51: 68-70.
693. Hallatt JG, Steele CH, Jr., Snyder M (1984). Ruptured corpus luteum with hemoperitoneum: a study of 173 surgical cases. Am J Obstet Gynecol 149: 5-9.
694. Hallgrimsson J, Scully RE (1972). Borderline and malignant Brenner tumours of the ovary. A report of 15 cases. Acta Pathol Microbiol Scand Suppl 233: 56-66.
695. Halperin D, Visscher DW, Wallis T, Lawrence WD (1995). Evaluation of chromosome 12 copy number in ovarian granulosa cell tumors using interphase cytogenetics. Int J Gynecol Pathol 14: 319-323.
696. Halperin R, Zehavi S, Habler L, Hadas E, Bukovsky I, Schneider D (2001). Comparative immunohistochemical study of endometrioid and serous papillary carcinoma of endometrium. Eur J Gynaecol Oncol 22: 122-126.
697. Hamazaki S, Nakamoto S, Okino T, Tsukayama C, Mori M, Taguchi K, Okada S (1999). Epithelioid trophoblastic tumor: morphological and immunohistochemical study of three lung lesions. Hum Pathol 30: 1321-1327.
698. Hameed K (1972). Brenner tumor of the ovary with Leydig cell hyperplasia. A histologic and ultrastructural study. Cancer 30: 945-952.
699. Hameed K, Burslem MR (1970). A melanotic ovarian neoplasm resembling the "retinal anlage" tumor. Cancer 25: 564-567.
700. Hampton GM, Penny LA, Baergen RN, Larson A, Brewer C, Liao S, Busby-Earle RM, Williams AW, Steel CM, Bird CC, and al. (1994). Loss of heterozygosity in cervical carcinoma: subchromosomal localization of a putative tumor-suppressor gene to chromosome 11q22-q24. Proc Natl Acad Sci U S A 91: 6953-6957.
701. Hampton HL, Huffman HT, Meeks GR (1992). Extraovarian Brenner tumor. Obstet Gynecol 79: 844-846.
702. Hanada S, Okumura Y, Kaida K (2003). Multicentric adenomatoid tumors involving uterus, ovary, and appendix. J Obstet Gynaecol Res 29: 234-238.
703. Haning RV Jr, Strawn EY, Nolten WE (1985). Pathophysiology of the ovarian hyperstimulation syndrome. Obstet Gynecol 66: 220-224.
704. Hannibal CG, Vang R, Jung J, Frederiksen K, Kjaerbye-Thygesern A, Andersen KK, Tabor A, Kurman RJ, Kjaer SK (2013). A Nationwide Study of Serous Borderline Ovarian Tumors in Denmark 1978–2002: Centralized Pathology Review, Long-Term Follow-up and Overall Survival. Gynecol Oncol. In Press.
705. Hanski W, Hagel-Lewicka E, Daniszewski K (1991). Rhabdomyomas of female genital tract. Report on two cases. Zentralbl Pathol 137: 439-442.
705A. Harada O, Ota H, Takagi K, Matsuura H, Hidaka E, Nakayama J (2006). Female adnexal tumor of probable wolffian origin: morphological, immunohistochemical, and ultrastructural study with c-kit gene analysis. Pathol Int 56: 95-100.
706. Hardisson D, Simon RS, Burgos E (2001). Primary osteosarcoma of the uterine corpus: report of a case with immunohistochemical and ultrastructural study. Gynecol Oncol 82: 181-186.
707. Hardman WJ, III, Majmudar B (1996). Leiomyomatosis peritonealis disseminata: clinicopathologic analysis of five cases. South Med J 89: 291-294.
708. Harlow BL, Weiss NS, Lofton S (1986). The epidemiology of sarcomas of the uterus. J Natl Cancer Inst 76: 399-402.
709. Harnden P, Kennedy W, Andrew AC, Southgate J (1999). Immunophenotype of transitional metaplasia of the uterine cervix. Int J Gynecol Pathol 18: 125-129.
710. Harris NL, Scully RE (1984). Malignant lymphoma and granulocytic sarcoma of the uterus and vagina. A clinicopathologic analysis of 27 cases. Cancer 53: 2530-2545.
711. Hart WR (2005). Mucinous tumors of the ovary: a review. Int J Gynecol Pathol 24: 4-25.
712. Hart WR, Billman JK Jr (1978). A reassessment of uterine neoplasms originally diagnosed as leiomyosarcomas. Cancer 41: 1902-1910.
713. Hart WR, Millman JB (1977). Progression of intraepithelial Paget's disease of the vulva to invasive carcinoma. Cancer 40: 2333-2337.
714. Hasegawa K, Ichikawa R, Ishii R, Oe S, Kato R, Kobayashi Y, Kuroda M, Udagawa Y (2011). A case of primary alveolar soft part sarcoma of the uterine cervix and a review of the literature. Int J Clin Oncol 16: 751-758.
715. Hasegawa K, Minegishi K, Sugihara K, Toyoshima K, Itoh K, Nishino R, Kitai H (1995). [A case of primary transitional cell carcinoma of the Bartholin gland with human papillomavirus type 18 infection]. Nihon Sanka Fujinka Gakkai Zasshi 47: 1385-1388.
716. Hasegawa T, Matsuno Y, Shimoda T, Umeda T, Yokoyama R, Hirohashi S (2001). Proximal-type epithelioid sarcoma: a clinicopathologic study of 20 cases. Mod Pathol 14: 655-663.
717. Hashimoto K, Azuma C, Kamiura S, Kimura T, Nobunaga T, Kanai T, Sawada M, Noguchi S, Saji F (1995). Clonal determination of uterine leiomyomas by analyzing differential inactivation of the X-chromosome-linked phosphoglycerokinase gene. Gynecol Obstet Invest 40: 204-208.
718. Haskel S, Chen SS, Spiegel G (1989). Vaginal endometrioid adenocarcinoma arising in vaginal endometriosis: a case report and literature review. Gynecol Oncol 34: 232-236.
719. Hassadia A, Gillespie A, Tidy J, Everard RGNJ, Wells M, Coleman R, Hancock B (2005). Placental site trophoblastic tumour: clinical features and management. Gynecol Oncol 99: 603-607.
720. Hassan A, Bennet A, Bhalla S, Ylagan LR, Mutch D, Dehner LP (2003). Paraganglioma of the vagina: report of a case, including immunohistochemical and ultrastructural findings. Int J Gynecol Pathol 22: 404-406.
721. Hastrup N, Andersen ES (1988). Adenocarcinoma of Bartholin's gland associated with extramammary Paget's disease of the vulva. Acta Obstet Gynecol Scand 67: 375-377.
722. Hayasaka K, Morita K, Saitoh T, Tanaka Y (2006). Uterine adenofibroma and endometrial stromal sarcoma associated with tamoxifen therapy: MR findings. Comput Med Imaging Graph 30: 315-318.
723. Hayashi K, Bracken MB, Freeman DH Jr, Hellenbrand K (1982). Hydatidiform mole in the United States (1970-1977): a statistical and theoretical analysis. Am J Epidemiol 115: 67-77.
724. Hayes MC, Scully RE (1987). Ovarian steroid cell tumors (not otherwise specified). A clinicopathological analysis of 63 cases. Am J Surg Pathol 11: 835-845.
725. Hayes MC, Scully RE (1987). Stromal luteoma of the ovary: a clinicopathological analysis of 25 cases. Int J Gynecol Pathol 6: 313-321.
726. Hays DM, Shimada H, Raney RB Jr, Tefft M, Newton W, Crist WM, Lawrence W Jr, Ragab A, Beltangady M, Maurer HM (1988). Clinical staging and treatment results in rhabdomyosarcoma of the female genital tract among children and adolescents. Cancer 61: 1893-1903.
727. Hays DM, Shimada H, Raney RB Jr, Tefft M, Newton W, Crist WM, Lawrence W Jr, Ragab A, Maurer HM (1985). Sarcomas of the vagina and uterus: the Intergroup Rhabdomyosarcoma Study. J Pediatr Surg 20: 718-724.
728. Heatley MK (2000). Adenomatous hyperplasia of the rete ovarii. Histopathology 36: 383-384.
729. Heatley MK (2006). Atypical polypoid adenomyoma: a systematic review of the English literature. Histopathology 48: 609-610.
730. Heatley MK (2009). Is female adnexal tumour of probable wolffian origin a benign lesion? A systematic review of the English literature. Pathology 41: 645-648.
731. Heeren JH, Croonen AM, Pijnenborg JM (2008). Primary extranodal marginal zone B-cell lymphoma of the female genital tract: a case report and literature review. Int J Gynecol Pathol 27: 243-246.
732. Heim K, Hopfl R, Muller-Holzner E, Bergant A, Dapunt O (2000). Multiple blue nevi of the vagina. A case report. J Reprod Med 45: 42-44.
733. Heintz AP, Odicino F, Maisonneuve P, Beller U, Benedet JL, Creasman WT, Ngan HY, Pecorelli S (2003). Carcinoma of the ovary. Int J Gynaecol Obstet 83 Suppl 1: 135-166.
734. Helland A, Karlsen F, Due EU, Holm R, Kristensen G, Borresen-Dale A (1998). Mutations in the TP53 gene and protein expression of p53, MDM 2 and p21/WAF-1 in primary cervical carcinomas with no or low human papillomavirus load. Br J Cancer 78: 69-72.
735. Hellman K, Lundell M, Silfversward C, Nilsson B, Hellstrom AC, Frankendal B (2006). Clinical and histopathologic factors related to prognosis in primary squamous cell carcinoma of the vagina. Int J Gynecol Cancer 16: 1201-1211.
736. Hemalatha AL, Rao SM, Kumar DB, Vani M (2007). Papillary serous carcinoma of the broad ligament: a rare case report. Indian J Pathol Microbiol 50: 555-557.
737. Hemminki K, Bermejo JL, Granstrom C (2005). Endometrial cancer: population attributable risks from reproductive, familial and socioeconomic factors. Eur J Cancer 41: 2155-2159.
738. Hemminki K, Dong C, Vaittinen P (1999). Familial risks in cervical cancer: is there a hereditary component? Int J Cancer 82: 775-781.
739. Hendrickson MR, Kempson RL (1983). Ciliated carcinoma--a variant of endometrial adenocarcinoma: a report of 10 cases. Int J Gynecol Pathol 2: 1-12.
740. Hensleigh PA, Woodruff JD (1978). Differential maternal-fetal response to androgenizing luteoma or hyperreactio luteinalis. Obstet Gynecol Surv 33: 262-271.
741. Heravi-Moussavi A, Anglesio MS, Cheng SW, Senz J, Yang W, Prentice L, Fejes AP, Chow C, Tone A, Kalloger SE, Hamel N, Roth A, Ha G, Wan AN, Maines-Bandiera S, Salamanca C, Pasini B, Clarke BA, Lee AF, Lee CH, Zhao C, Young RH, Aparicio SA, Sorensen PH, Woo MM, Boyd N, Jones SJ, Hirst M, Marra MA, Gilks B, Shah SP, Foulkes WD, Morin GB, Huntsman DG (2012). Recurrent somatic DICER1 mutations in nonepithelial ovarian cancers. N Engl J Med 366: 234-242.
742. Herbst AL (2000). Behavior of estrogen-associated female genital tract cancer and its relation to neoplasia following intrauterine exposure to diethylstilbestrol (DES). Gynecol Oncol 76: 147-156.
743. Herbst AL, Cole P, Colton T, Robboy SJ, Scully RE (1977). Age-incidence and risk of diethylstilbestrol-related clear cell adenocarcinoma of the vagina and cervix. Am J Obstet Gynecol 128: 43-50.
744. Herbst AL, Kurman RJ, Scully RE, Poskanzer DC (1972). Clear-cell adenocarcinoma of the genital tract in young females. Registry report. N Engl J Med 287: 1259-1264.
745. Herbst AL, Robboy SJ, Scully RE, Poskanzer DC (1974). Clear-cell adenocarcinoma of the vagina and cervix in girls: analysis of 170 registry cases. Am J Obstet Gynecol 119: 713-724.
746. Herbst AL, Ulfelder H, Poskanzer DC, Longo LD (1999). Adenocarcinoma of the vagina. Association of maternal stilbestrol therapy with tumor appearance in young women. 1971. Am J Obstet Gynecol 181: 1574-1575.
747. Herfs M, Yamamoto Y, Laury A, Wang X, Nucci MR, Laughlin-Drubin ME, Munger K, Feldman S, McKeon FD, Xian W, Crum CP (2012). A discrete population of squamocolumnar junction cells implicated in the pathogenesis of cervical cancer. Proc Natl Acad Sci USA 109: 10516-10521.
748. Herrington CS, Graham D, Southern SA, Bramdev A, Chetty R (1999). Loss of retinoblastoma protein expression is frequent in small cell neuroendocrine carcinoma of the cervix and is unrelated to HPV type. Hum Pathol 30: 906-910.
749. Hersmus R, Kalfa N, de Leeuw B, Stoop H, Oosterhuis JW, de Krijger R, Wolffenbuttel KP, Drop SL, Veitia RA, Fellous M, Jaubert F, Looijenga LH (2008). FOXL2 and SOX9 as parameters of female and male gonadal differentiation in patients with various forms of disorders of sex development (DSD). J Pathol 215: 31-38.
750. Hersmus R, Stoop H, van de Geijn GJ, Eini R, Biermann K, Oosterhuis JW, Dhooge C, Schneider DT, Meijssen IC, Dinjens WN, Dubbink HJ, Drop SL, Looijenga LH (2012). Prevalence of c-KIT mutations in gonadoblastoma and dysgerminomas of patients with disorders of sex development (DSD) and ovarian dysgerminomas. PLoS One 7: e43952.
751. Hersmus R, van der Zwan YG, Stoop H, Bernard P, Sreenivasan R, Oosterhuis JW, Bruggenwirth HT, De Boer S, White S, Wolffenbuttel KP, Alders M, McElreavy K, Drop SL, Harley VR, Looijenga LH (2012). A 46,XY female DSD patient with bilateral gonadoblastoma, a novel SRY missense mutation combined with a WT1 KTS splice-site mutation. PLoS One 7: e40858.
752. Hertel JD, Huettner PC, Dehner LP, Pfeifer JD (2010). The chromosome Y-linked testis-specific protein locus TSPY1 is characteristically present in gonadoblastoma. Hum Pathol 41: 1544-1549.
753. Hesseling MH, De Wilde RL (2000). Endosalpingiosis in laparoscopy. J Am Assoc Gynecol Laparosc 7: 215-219.
754. Hierro I, Blanes A, Matilla A, Munoz S, Vicioso L, Nogales FF (2000). Merkel cell (neuroendocrine) carcinoma of the vulva. A case report with immunohistochemical and ultrastructural findings and review of the literature. Pathol Res Pract 196: 503-509.
755. Hildesheim A, Hadjimichael O, Schwartz PE, Wheeler CM, Barnes W, Lowell DM, Willett J, Schiffman M (1999). Risk factors for rapid-onset cervical cancer. Am J Obstet Gynecol 180: 571-577.
756. Hillard JB, Malpica A, Ramirez PT (2004). Conservative management of a uterine tumor resembling an ovarian sex cord-stromal tumor. Gynecol Oncol 92: 347-352.
757. Hinchey WW, Silva EG, Guarda LA, Ordonez NG, Wharton JT (1983). Paravaginal wolffian duct (mesonephros) adenocarcinoma:

a light and electron microscopic study. Am J Clin Pathol 80: 539-544.
758. Hirai Y, Takeshima N, Haga A, Arai Y, Akiyama F, Hasumi K (1998). A clinicocytopathologic study of adenoma malignum of the uterine cervix. Gynecol Oncol 70: 219-223.
759. Hirakawa T, Tsuneyoshi M, Enjoji M (1989). Squamous cell carcinoma arising in mature cystic teratoma of the ovary. Clinicopathologic and topographic analysis. Am J Surg Pathol 13: 397-405.
760. Hirose R, Imai A, Kondo H, Itoh K, Tamaya T (1991). A dermoid cyst of the paravaginal space. Arch Gynecol Obstet 249: 39-41.
761. Hirst JE, Gard GB, McIllroy K, Nevell D, Field M (2009). High rates of occult fallopian tube cancer diagnosed at prophylactic bilateral salpingo-oophorectomy. Int J Gynecol Cancer 19: 826-829.
762. Hisaoka M, Kouho H, Aoki T, Daimaru Y, Hashimoto H (1995). Angiomyofibroblastoma of the vulva: a clinicopathologic study of seven cases. Pathol Int 45: 487-492.
763. Ho CL, Kurman RJ, Dehari R, Wang TL, Shih I (2004). Mutations of BRAF and KRAS precede the development of ovarian serous borderline tumors. Cancer Res 64: 6915-6918.
764. Ho GY, Bierman R, Beardsley L, Chang CJ, Burk RD (1998). Natural history of cervicovaginal papillomavirus infection in young women. N Engl J Med 338: 423-428.
765. Hodak E, Jones RE, Ackerman AB (1993). Solitary keratoacanthoma is a squamous-cell carcinoma: three examples with metastases. Am J Dermatopathol 15: 332-342.
766. Hoei-Hansen CE, Kraggerud SM, Abeler VM, Kaern J, Rajpert-De ME, Lothe RA (2007). Ovarian dysgerminomas are characterised by frequent KIT mutations and abundant expression of pluripotency markers. Mol Cancer 6: 12.
767. Hoelscher AC, Hoelscher AH, Drebber U, Bludau M, Schroeder W (2012). Hereditary esophageal-vulvar syndrome. Ann Thorac Surg 94: e65-e67.
768. Hoerl HD, Hart WR (1998). Primary ovarian mucinous cystadenocarcinomas: a clinicopathologic study of 49 cases with long-term follow-up. Am J Surg Pathol 22: 1449-1462.
769. Holtz F, Hart WR (1982). Krukenberg tumors of the ovary: a clinicopathologic analysis of 27 cases. Cancer 50: 2438-2447.
770. Homesley HD, Bundy BN, Sedlis A, Yordan E, Berek JS, Jahshan A, Mortel R (1993). Prognostic factors for groin node metastasis in squamous cell carcinoma of the vulva (a Gynecologic Oncology Group study). Gynecol Oncol 49: 279-283.
771. Honoré LH (2003). Pathology of the Fallopian Tube and broad ligament. In: Haines & Taylor Obstetrical and Gynaecological Pathology. Fox H, Wells M, eds. 585-634.
772. Hopkins MP, Morley GW (2004). Glassy cell adenocarcinoma of the uterine cervix. Am J Obstet Gynecol 190: 67-70.
773. Horiguchi H, Matsui-Horiguchi M, Fujiwara M, Kaketa M, Kawano M, Ohtsubo-Shimoyamada R, Ohse H (2003). Angiomyofibroblastoma of the vulva: report of a case with immunohistochemical and molecular analysis. Int J Gynecol Pathol 22: 277-284.
774. Hornick JL, Dal Cin P, Fletcher CD (2009). Loss of INI1 expression is characteristic of both conventional and proximal-type epithelioid sarcoma. Am J Surg Pathol 33: 542-550.
775. Hornick JL, Fletcher CD (2008). Sclerosing PEComa: clinicopathologic analysis of a distinctive variant with a predilection for the retroperitoneum. Am J Surg Pathol 32: 493-501.
776. Hoskins WJ, McGuire WP, Brady MF, Homesley HD, Creasman WT, Berman M, Ball H, Berek JS (1994). The effect of diameter of largest residual disease on survival after primary cytoreductive surgery in patients with suboptimal residual epithelial ovarian carcinoma. Am J Obstet Gynecol 170: 974-979.
777. Hou JL, Wu LY, Zhang HT, Lv NN, Huang Y, Yu GZ (2010). Clinicopathologic characteristics of 12 patients with vulvar sweat gland carcinoma. Int J Gynecol Cancer 20: 874-878.
778. Houghton O, Jamison J, Wilson R, Carson J, McCluggage WG (2010). p16 Immunoreactivity in unusual types of cervical adenocarcinoma does not reflect human papillomavirus infection. Histopathology 57: 342-350.
779. Hristov AC, Young RH, Vang R, Yemelyanova AV, Seidman JD, Ronnett BM (2007). Ovarian metastases of appendiceal tumors with goblet cell carcinoidlike and signet ring cell patterns: a report of 30 cases. Am J Surg Pathol 31: 1502-1511.
780. Hrzenjak A, Moinfar F, Tavassoli FA, Strohmeier B, Kremser ML, Zatloukal K, Denk H (2005). JAZF1/JJAZ1 gene fusion in endometrial stromal sarcomas: molecular analysis by reverse transcriptase-polymerase chain reaction optimized for paraffin-embedded tissue. J Mol Diagn 7: 388-395.
781. Hsueh S, Chang TC (1996). Malignant rhabdoid tumor of the uterine corpus. Gynecol Oncol 61: 142-146.
782. Hu J, Khanna V, Jones M, Surti U (2001). Genomic alterations in uterine leiomyosarcomas: potential markers for clinical diagnosis and prognosis. Genes Chromosomes Cancer 31: 117-124.
783. Huang HY, Ladanyi M, Soslow RA (2004). Molecular detection of JAZF1-JJAZ1 gene fusion in endometrial stromal neoplasms with classic and variant histology: evidence for genetic heterogeneity. Am J Surg Pathol 28: 224-232.
784. Huang YT, Wang CC, Tsai CS, Lai CH, Chang TC, Chou HH, Lee SP, Hong JH (2012). Clinical behaviors and outcomes for adenocarcinoma or adenosquamous carcinoma of cervix treated by radical hysterectomy and adjuvant radiotherapy or chemoradiotherapy. Int J Radiat Oncol Biol Phys 84: 420-427.
785. Hubalek M, Ramoni A, Mueller-Holzner E, Marth C (2004). Malignant mixed mesodermal tumor after tamoxifen therapy for breast cancer. Gynecol Oncol 95: 264-266.
786. Huettner PC, Gersell DJ (1994). Arias-Stella reaction in nonpregnant women: a clinicopathologic study of nine cases. Int J Gynecol Pathol 13: 241-247.
787. Huettner PC, Gersell DJ (1994). Placental site nodule: a clinicopathologic study of 38 cases. Int J Gynecol Pathol 13: 191-198.
788. Hui P (2010). Molecular diagnosis of gestational trophoblastic disease. Expert Rev Mol Diagn 10: 1023-1034.
789. Hui P, Parkash V, Perkins AS, Carcangiu ML (2000). Pathogenesis of placental site trophoblastic tumor may require the presence of a paternally derived X chromosome. Lab Invest 80: 965-972.
790. Hui P, Riba A, Pejovic T, Johnson T, Baergen RN, Ward D (2004). Comparative genomic hybridization study of placental site trophoblastic tumour: a report of four cases. Mod Pathol 17: 248-251.
791. Hui P, Wang HL, Chu P, Yang B, Huang J, Baergen RN, Sklar J, Yang XJ, Soslow RA (2007). Absence of Y chromosome in human placental site trophoblastic tumor. Mod Pathol 20: 1055-1060.
792. Hunn J, Rodriguez GC (2012). Ovarian cancer: etiology, risk factors, and epidemiology. Clin Obstet Gynecol 55: 3-23.
793. Hunt CR, Hale RJ, Armstrong C, Rajkumar T, Gullick WJ, Buckley CH (1995). c-erbB-3 proto-oncogene expression in uterine cervical carcinoma. Int J Gynecol Cancer 5: 282-285.
794. Hunter SM, Anglesio MS, Sharma R, Gilks CB, Melnyk N, Chiew YE, deFazio A, Longacre TA, Huntsman DG, Gorringe KL, Campbell IG (2011). Copy number aberrations in benign serous ovarian tumors: a case for reclassification? Clin Cancer Res 17: 7273-7282.
795. Huntsman DG, Clement PB, Gilks CB, Scully RE (1994). Small-cell carcinoma of the endometrium. A clinicopathological study of sixteen cases. Am J Surg Pathol 18: 364-375.
796. Hurrell DP, McCluggage WG (2007). Uterine tumour resembling ovarian sex cord tumour is an immunohistochemically polyphenotypic neoplasm which exhibits coexpression of epithelial, myoid and sex cord markers. J Clin Pathol 60: 1148-1154.
797. Hurwitz JL, Fenton A, McCluggage WG, McKenna S (2007). Squamous cell carcinoma arising in a dermoid cyst of the ovary: a case series. BJOG 114: 1283-1287.
798. Husaini AL, Soudy H, El Din DA, Ahmed M, Eltigani A, Mubarak AL, Sabaa AA, Edesa W, Tweigeri T, Al-Badawi IA (2012). Pure dysgerminoma of the ovary: a single institutional experience of 65 patients. Med Oncol 29: 2944-2948.
799. Huss S, Nehles J, Binot E, Wardelmann E, Mittler J, Kleine MA, Kunstlinger H, Hartmann W, Hohenberger P, Merkelbach-Bruse S, Buettner R, Schildhaus HU (2013). beta-catenin (CTNNB1) mutations and clinicopathological features of mesenteric desmoid-type fibromatosis. Histopathology 62: 294-304.
800. Husseinzadeh N, Recinto C (1999). Frequency of invasive cancer in surgically excised vulvar lesions with intraepithelial neoplasia (VIN 3). Gynecol Oncol 73: 119-120.
801. Hussussian CJ, Struewing JP, Goldstein AM, Higgins PA, Ally DS, Sheahan MD, Clark WH, Jr., Tucker MA, Dracopoli NC (1994). Germline p16 mutations in familial melanoma. Nat Genet 8: 15-21.
802. Huusom LD, Frederiksen K, Hogdall EV, Glud E, Christensen L, Hogdall CK, Blaakaer J, Kjaer SK (2006). Association of reproductive factors, oral contraceptive use and selected lifestyle factors with the risk of ovarian borderline tumors: a Danish case-control study. Cancer Causes Control 17: 821-829.
803. Ichikawa Y, Nishida M, Suzuki H, Yoshida S, Tsunoda H, Kubo T, Uchida K, Miwa M (1994). Mutation of K-ras protooncogene is associated with histological subtypes in human mucinous ovarian tumors. Cancer Res 54: 33-35.
804. Idowu MO, Rosenblum MK, Wei XJ, Edgar MA, Soslow RA (2008). Ependymomas of the central nervous system and adult extra-axial ependymomas are morphologically and immunohistochemically distinct--a comparative study with assessment of ovarian carcinomas for expression of glial fibrillary acidic protein. Am J Surg Pathol 32: 710-718.
805. Ikota H, Kaneko K, Takahashi S, Kawarai M, Tanaka Y, Yokoo H, Nakazato Y (2012). Malignant transformation of ovarian mature cystic teratoma with a predominant pulmonary type small cell carcinoma component. Pathol Int 62: 276-280.
806. Imagawa J, Harada Y, Yoshida T, Sakai A, Sasaki N, Kimura A, Harada H (2010). Giant granulocytic sarcoma of the vagina concurrent with acute myeloid leukemia with t(8;21)(q22;q22) translocation. Int J Hematol 92: 553-555.
807. Imai A, Furui T, Hatano Y, Suzuki M, Suzuki N, Goshima S (2008). Leiomyoma and rhabdomyoma of the vagina. Vaginal myoma. J Obstet Gynaecol 28: 563-566.
808. Imperiale A, Heymann S, Claria M, Cimarelli S, Sellem DB, Goetz C, Onea A, Blondet C, Constantinesco A (2007). F-18 FDG PET-CT in a rare case of Bartholin's gland undifferentiated carcinoma managed with chemoradiation and interstitial brachytherapy. Clin Nucl Med 32: 498-500.
809. Insinga RP, Perez G, Wheeler CM, Koutsky LA, Garland SM, Leodolter S, Joura EA, Ferris DG, Steben M, Brown DR, Elbasha EH, Paavonen J, Haupt RM (2010). Incidence, duration, and reappearance of type-specific cervical human papillomavirus infections in young women. Cancer Epidemiol Biomarkers Prev 19: 1585-1594.
810. Insinga RP, Perez G, Wheeler CM, Koutsky LA, Garland SM, Leodolter S, Joura EA, Ferris DG, Steben M, Hernandez-Avila M, Brown DR, Elbasha E, Munoz N, Paavonen J, Haupt RM (2011). Incident cervical HPV infections in young women: transition probabilities for CIN and infection clearance. Cancer Epidemiol Biomarkers Prev 20: 287-296.
811. Ip PP, Cheung AN, Clement PB (2009). Uterine smooth muscle tumors of uncertain malignant potential (STUMP): a clinicopathologic analysis of 16 cases. Am J Surg Pathol 33: 992-1005.
812. Ip PP, Irving JA, McCluggage WG, Clement PB, Young RH (2013). Papillary proliferation of the endometrium: a clinicopathologic study of 59 cases of simple and complex papillae without cytologic atypia. Am J Surg Pathol 37: 167-177.
813. Ip PP, Lam KW, Cheung CL, Yeung MC, Pun TC, Chan QK, Cheung AN (2007). Tranexamic acid-associated necrosis and intralesional thrombosis of uterine leiomyomas: a clinicopathologic study of 147 cases emphasizing the importance of drug-induced necrosis and early infarcts in leiomyomas. Am J Surg Pathol 31: 1215-1224.
814. Ip PP, Tse KY, Tam KF (2010). Uterine smooth muscle tumors other than the ordinary leiomyomas and leiomyosarcomas: a review of selected variants with emphasis on recent advances and unusual morphology that may cause concern for malignancy. Adv Anat Pathol 17: 91-112.
815. Irving JA, Alkushi A, Young RH, Clement PB (2006). Cellular fibromas of the ovary: a study of 75 cases including 40 mitotically active tumors emphasizing their distinction from fibrosarcoma. Am J Surg Pathol 30: 929-938.
816. Irving JA, Carinelli S, Prat J (2006). Uterine tumors resembling ovarian sex cord tumors are polyphenotypic neoplasms with true sex cord differentiation. Mod Pathol 19: 17-24.
817. Irving JA, Catasus L, Gallardo A, Bussaglia E, Romero M, Matias-Guiu X, Prat J (2005). Synchronous endometrioid carcinomas of the uterine corpus and ovary: alterations in the beta-catenin (CTNNB1) pathway are associated with independent primary tumors and favorable prognosis. Hum Pathol 36: 605-619.
818. Irving JA, Young RH (2008). Granulosa cell tumors of the ovary with a pseudopapillary pattern: a study of 14 cases of an unusual morphologic variant emphasizing their distinction from transitional cell neoplasms and other papillary ovarian tumors. Am J Surg Pathol 32: 581-586.
819. Irving JA, Young RH (2009). Microcystic stromal tumor of the ovary: report of 16 cases of a hitherto uncharacterized distinctive ovarian neoplasm. Am J Surg Pathol 33: 367-375.
820. Isaac MA, Vijayalakshmi S, Madhu CS, Bosincu L, Nogales FF (2000). Pure cystic nephroblastoma of the ovary with a review

of extrarenal Wilms' tumors. Hum Pathol 31: 761-764.
821. Itamochi H, Kigawa J, Terakawa N (2008). Mechanisms of chemoresistance and poor prognosis in ovarian clear cell carcinoma. Cancer Sci 99: 653-658.
822. Iversen UM (1996). Two cases of benign vaginal rhabdomyoma. Case reports. APMIS 104: 575-578.
823. Iwasa Y, Fletcher CD (2004). Cellular angiofibroma: clinicopathologic and immunohistochemical analysis of 51 cases. Am J Surg Pathol 28: 1426-1435.
824. Iyengar P, Deodhare S (2004). Primary extranodal marginal zone B-cell lymphoma of MALT type of the endometrium. Gynecol Oncol 93: 238-241.
825. Jackson-York GL, Ramzy I (1992). Synchronous papillary mucinous adenocarcinoma of the endocervix and fallopian tubes. Int J Gynecol Pathol 11: 63-67.
826. Jacobs PA, Szulman AE, Funkhouser J, Matsuura JS, Wilson CC (1982). Human triploidy: relationship between parental origin of the additional haploid complement and development of partial hydatidiform mole. Ann Hum Genet 46: 223-231.
827. Jacobs VR, Zemzoum I, Kremer M, Gottschalk N, Baumgartner AK, Krol J, Kiechle M (2010). Primary metastatic leiomyosarcoma of the fallopian tube: a rare case report. Onkologie 33: 49-52.
828. Jakate K, Azimi F, Ali RH, Lee CH, Clarke BA, Rasty G, Shaw PA, Melnyk N, Huntsman DG, Laframboise S, Rouzbahman M (2013). Endometrial sarcomas: an immunohistochemical and JAZF1 re-arrangement study in low-grade and undifferentiated tumors. Mod Pathol 26: 95-105.
829. Jakobsson M, Pukkala E, Paavonen J, Tapper AM, Gissler M (2011). Cancer incidence among Finnish women with surgical treatment for cervical intraepithelial neoplasia, 1987-2006. Int J Cancer 128: 1187-1191.
830. Jamieson S, Butzow R, Andersson N, Alexiadis M, Unkila-Kallio L, Heikinheimo M, Fuller PJ, Anttonen M (2010). The FOXL2 C134W mutation is characteristic of adult granulosa cell tumors of the ovary. Mod Pathol 23: 1477-1485.
831. Jarboe E, Folkins A, Nucci MR, Kindelberger D, Drapkin R, Miron A, Lee Y, Crum CP (2008). Serous carcinogenesis in the fallopian tube: a descriptive classification. Int J Gynecol Pathol 27: 1-9.
832. Jeffers MD, Farquharson MA, Richmond JA, McNicol AM (1995). p53 immunoreactivity and mutation of the p53 gene in smooth muscle tumours of the uterine corpus. J Pathol 177: 65-70.
833. Jeffers MD, Richmond JA, Macaulay EM (1995). Overexpression of the c-myc proto-oncogene occurs frequently in uterine sarcomas. Mod Pathol 8: 701-704.
834. Jenkins CS, Williams SR, Schmidt GE (1993). Salpingitis isthmica nodosa: a review of the literature, discussion of clinical significance, and consideration of patient management. Fertil Steril 60: 599-607.
835. Jensen KC, Mariappan MR, Putcha GV, Husain A, Chun N, Ford JM, Schrijver I, Longacre TA (2008). Microsatellite instability and mismatch repair protein defects in ovarian epithelial neoplasms in patients 50 years of age and younger. Am J Surg Pathol 32: 1029-1037.
836. Jeronimo J, Massad LS, Schiffman M (2007). Visual appearance of the uterine cervix: correlation with human papillomavirus detection and type. Am J Obstet Gynecol 197: 47-48.
837. Jessop FA, Roberts PF (2000). Mullerian adenosarcoma of the uterus in association with tamoxifen therapy. Histopathology 36: 91-92.
838. Ji H, Isacson C, Seidman JD, Kurman RJ, Ronnett BM (2002). Cytokeratins 7 and 20, Dpc4, and MUC5AC in the distinction of metastatic mucinous carcinomas in the ovary from primary ovarian mucinous tumors: Dpc4 assists in identifying metastatic pancreatic carcinomas. Int J Gynecol Pathol 21: 391-400.
839. Jiang L, Malpica A, Deavers MT, Guo M, Villa LL, Nuovo G, Merino MJ, Silva EG (2010). Endometrial endometrioid adenocarcinoma of the uterine corpus involving the cervix: some cases probably represent independent primaries. Int J Gynecol Pathol 29: 146-156.
840. Jin Z, Ogata S, Tamura G, Katayama Y, Fukase M, Yajima M, Motoyama T (2003). Carcinosarcomas (malignant mullerian mixed tumors) of the uterus and ovary: a genetic study with special reference to histogenesis. Int J Gynecol Pathol 22: 368-373.
841. Johnson TL, Kumar NB, White CD, Morley GW (1986). Prognostic features of vulvar melanoma: a clinicopathologic analysis. Int J Gynecol Pathol 5: 110-118.
842. Jones IS, Crandon A, Sanday K (2011). Paget's disease of the vulva: Diagnosis and follow-up key to management; a retrospective study of 50 cases from Queensland. Gynecol Oncol 122: 42-44.
843. Jones MA, Mann EW, Caldwell CL, Tarraza HM, Dickersin GR, Young RH (1990). Small cell neuroendocrine carcinoma of Bartholin's gland. Am J Clin Pathol 94: 439-442.
844. Jones MA, Young RH, Scully RE (1991). Diffuse laminar endocervical glandular hyperplasia. A benign lesion often confused with adenoma malignum (minimal deviation adenocarcinoma). Am J Surg Pathol 15: 1123-1129.
845. Jones MW, Harri R, Dabbs DJ, Carter GJ (2010). Immunohistochemical profile of steroid cell tumor of the ovary: a study of 14 cases and a review of the literature. Int J Gynecol Pathol 29: 315-320.
846. Jones MW, Kounelis S, Papadaki H, Bakker A, Swalsky PA, Finkelstein SD (1997). The origin and molecular characterization of adenoid basal carcinoma of the uterine cervix. Int J Gynecol Pathol 16: 301-306.
847. Jones MW, Lefkowitz M (1995). Adenosarcoma of the uterine cervix: a clinicopathological study of 12 cases. Int J Gynecol Pathol 14: 223-229.
848. Jones MW, Norris HJ (1995). Clinicopathologic study of 28 uterine leiomyosarcomas with metastasis. Int J Gynecol Pathol 14: 243-249.
849. Jones MW, Silverberg SG, Kurman RJ (1993). Well-differentiated villoglandular adenocarcinoma of the uterine cervix: a clinicopathological study of 24 cases. Int J Gynecol Pathol 12: 1-7.
850. Jones RW, Rowan DM, Stewart AW (2005). Vulvar intraepithelial neoplasia: aspects of the natural history and outcome in 405 women. Obstet Gynecol 106: 1319-1326.
851. Jones S, Wang TL, Kurman RJ, Nakayama K, Velculescu VE, Vogelstein B, Kinzler KW, Papadopoulos N, Shih I (2012). Low-grade serous carcinomas of the ovary contain very few point mutations. J Pathol 226: 413-420.
852. Jones S, Wang TL, Shih I, Mao TL, Nakayama K, Roden R, Glas R, Slamon D, Diaz LA Jr, Vogelstein B, Kinzler KW, Velculescu VE, Papadopoulos N (2010). Frequent mutations of chromatin remodeling gene ARID1A in ovarian clear cell carcinoma. Science 330: 228-231.
853. Jordan LB, Al-Nafussi A, Beattie G (2002). Cotyledonoid hydropic intravenous leiomyomatosis: a new variant leiomyoma. Histopathology 40: 245-252.
854. Jordan SJ, Green AC, Whiteman DC, Moore SP, Bain CJ, Gertig DM, Webb PM (2008). Serous ovarian, fallopian tube and primary peritoneal cancers: a comparative epidemiological analysis. Int J Cancer 122: 1598-1603.
855. Joura EA, Leodolter S, Hernandez-Avila M, Wheeler CM, Perez G, Koutsky LA, Garland SM, Harper DM, Tang GW, Ferris DG, Steben M, Jones RW, Bryan J, Taddeo FJ, Bautista OM, Esser MT, Sings HL, Nelson M, Boslego JW, Sattler C, Barr E, Paavonen J (2007). Efficacy of a quadrivalent prophylactic human papillomavirus (types 6, 11, 16, and 18) L1 virus-like-particle vaccine against high-grade vulval and vaginal lesions: a combined analysis of three randomised clinical trials. Lancet 369: 1693-1702.
856. Jovanovic AS, Boynton KA, Mutter GL (1996). Uteri of women with endometrial carcinoma contain a histopathological spectrum of monoclonal putative precancers, some with microsatellite instability. Cancer Res 56: 1917-1921.
857. Judd HL, Scully RE, Herbst AL, Yen SS, Ingersol FM, Kliman B (1973). Familial hyperthecosis: comparison of endocrinologic and histologic findings with polycystic ovarian disease. Am J Obstet Gynecol 117: 976-982.
857A. Judson K, McCormick C, Vang R, Yemelyanova AV, Wu LS, Bristow RE, Ronnett BM (2008). Women with undiagnosed colorectal adenocarcinomas presenting with ovarian metastases: clinicopathologic features and comparison with women having known colorectal adenocarcinomas and ovarian involvement. Int J Gynecol Pathol 27: 182-190.
858. Julien V, Labadie M, Gauthier G, Ronger-Savle S (2012). Clitoral metastasis from ductal breast cancer revealing metastases in multiple sites and review of the literature. J Low Genit Tract Dis 16: 66-69.
859. Jung WY, Shin BK, Kim I (2002). Uterine adenomyoma with uterus-like features: a report of two cases. Int J Surg Pathol 10: 163-166.
860. Kaaks R, Lukanova A, Kurzer MS (2002). Obesity, endogenous hormones, and endometrial cancer risk: a synthetic review. Cancer Epidemiol Biomarkers Prev 11: 1531-1543.
861. Kacerovska D, Nemcova J, Petrik R, Michal M, Kazakov DV (2008). Lymphoepithelioma-like carcinoma of the Bartholin gland. Am J Dermatopathol 30: 586-589.
862. Kahlifa M, Buckstein R, Perez-Ordonez B (2003). Sarcomatoid variant of B-cell lymphoma of the uterine cervix. Int J Gynecol Pathol 22: 289-293.
863. Kajii T, Ohama K (1977). Androgenetic origin of hydatidiform mole. Nature 268: 633-634.
864. Kaku T, Silverberg SG, Major FJ, Miller A, Fetter B, Brady MF (1992). Adenosarcoma of the uterus: a Gynecologic Oncology Group clinicopathologic study of 31 cases. Int J Gynecol Pathol 11: 75-88.
865. Kalir T, Goldstein M, Dottino P, Brodman M, Gordon R, Deligdisch L, Wu H, Gil J (1998). Morphometric and electron-microscopic analyses of the effects of gonadotropin-releasing hormone agonists on uterine leiomyomas. Arch Pathol Lab Med 122: 442-446.
866. Kallenberg GA, Pesce CM, Norman B, Ratner RE, Silvergerg SG (1990). Ectopic hyperprolactinemia resulting from an ovarian teratoma. JAMA 263: 2472-2474.
867. Kaminski PF, Maier RC (1983). Clear cell adenocarcinoma of the cervix unrelated to diethylstilbestrol exposure. Obstet Gynecol 62: 720-727.
868. Kandoth C, Schultz N, Cherniack AD, Akbani R, Liu Y, Shen H, Robertson AG, Pashtan I, Shen R, Benz CC, Yau C, Laird PW, Ding L, Zhang W, Mills GB, Kucherlapati R, Mardis ER, Levine DA (2013). Integrated genomic characterization of endometrial carcinoma. Nature 497: 67-73.
869. Kane S, Mehta J (2005). Primary epithelioid hemangioendothelioma of the peritoneum – a diagnostic dilemma. Virchows Arch 446: 93-94.
870. Kang Z, Xu F, Zhang QA, Lin J, Wu Z, Zhang X, Luo Y, Xu J, Guan M (2012). Correlation of DLC1 gene methylation with oncogenic PIK3CA mutations in extramammary Paget's disease. Mod Pathol 25: 1160-1168.
871. Kanitakis J, Arbona-Vidal E, Faure M (2011). Extensive pigmented vulvar basal-cell carcinoma presenting as pruritus in an elderly woman. Dermatol Online J 17: 8.
872. Kao CS, Idrees MT, Young RH, Ulbright TM (2012). Solid pattern yolk sac tumor: a morphologic and immunohistochemical study of 52 cases. Am J Surg Pathol 36: 360-367.
873. Kao GF, Norris HJ (1978). Benign and low grade variants of mixed mesodermal tumor (adenosarcoma) of the ovary and adnexal region. Cancer 42: 1314-1324.
874. Kao GF, Norris HJ (1979). Unusual cystadenofibromas: endometrioid, mucinous, and clear cell types. Obstet Gynecol 54: 729-736.
875. Karageorgi S, Hankinson SE, Kraft P, De Vivo I (2010). Reproductive factors and postmenopausal hormone use in relation to endometrial cancer risk in the Nurses' Health Study cohort 1976-2004. Int J Cancer 126: 208-216.
876. Karam A, Dorigo O (2012). Treatment outcomes in a large cohort of patients with invasive Extramammary Paget's disease. Gynecol Oncol 125: 346-351.
877. Kardhashi A, Assunta DM, Renna A, Trojano G, Zito FA, Trojano V (2012). Benign granular cell tumor of the vulva: first report of multiple cases in a family. Gynecol Obstet Invest 73: 341-348.
878. Karnezis AN, Aysal A, Zaloudek CJ, Rabban JT (2013). Transitional cell-like morphology in ovarian endometrioid carcinoma: morphologic, immunohistochemical, and behavioral features distinguishing it from high-grade serous carcinoma. Am J Surg Pathol 37: 24-37.
879. Karseladze AI, Kulinitch SI (1994). Peritoneal strumosis. Pathol Res Pract 190: 1082-1085.
880. Karvouni E, Papakonstantinou K, Dimopoulou C, Kairi-Vassilatou E, Hasiakos D, Gennatas CG, Kondi-Paphiti A (2009). Abnormal uterine bleeding as a presentation of metastatic breast disease in a patient with advanced breast cancer. Arch Gynecol Obstet 279: 199-201.
881. Kasby CB, Parsons KF (1980). Prolapsed ureterocele presenting as a vulval mass in a child. Case report. Br J Obstet Gynaecol 87: 1178-1180.
882. Kashima T, Matsushita H, Kuroda M, Takeuchi H, Udagawa H, Ishida T, Hara M, Machinami R (1997). Biphasic synovial sarcoma of the peritoneal cavity with t(X;18) demonstrated by reverse transcriptase polymerase chain reaction. Pathol Int 47: 637-641.
883. Kaspersen P, Buhl L, Moller BR (1988). Fallopian tube papilloma in a patient with primary sterility. Acta Obstet Gynecol Scand 67: 93-94.
884. Katagiri A, Nakayama K, Rahman MT, Rahman M, Katagiri H, Ishikawa M, Ishibashi T, Iida K, Otsuki Y, Nakayama S, Miyazaki K (2012). Frequent loss of tumor suppressor ARID1A protein expression in

adenocarcinomas/adenosquamous carcinomas of the uterine cervix. Int J Gynecol Cancer 22: 208-212.

885. Kato N, Katayama Y, Kaimori M, Motoyama T (2002). Glassy cell carcinoma of the uterine cervix: histochemical, immunohistochemical, and molecular genetic observations. Int J Gynecol Pathol 21: 134-140.

886. Kato N, Takeda J, Fukase M, Motoyama T (2010). Alternate mucoid and hyalinized stroma in clear cell carcinoma of the ovary: manifestation of serial stromal remodeling. Mod Pathol 23: 881-888.

887. Kaur H, Levinsky E, Colgan TJ (2013). Papillary syncytial metaplasia of fallopian tube endometriosis: a potential pitfall in the diagnosis of serous tubal intraepithelial carcinoma. Arch Pathol Lab Med 137: 126-129.

888. Kawaguchi K, Oda Y, Saito T, Yamamoto H, Tamiya S, Takahira T, Miyajima K, Iwamoto Y, Tsuneyoshi M (2003). Mechanisms of inactivation of the p16INK4a gene in leiomyosarcoma of soft tissue: decreased p16 expression correlates with promoter methylation and poor prognosis. J Pathol 201: 487-495.

889. Kawauchi S, Fukuda T, Miyamoto S, Yoshioka J, Shirahama S, Saito T, Tsukamoto N (1998). Peripheral primitive neuroectodermal tumor of the ovary confirmed by CD99 immunostaining, karyotypic analysis, and RT-PCR for EWS/FLI-1 chimeric mRNA. Am J Surg Pathol 22: 1417-1422.

890. Kawauchi S, Fukuma F, Morioka H, Okuda S, Sasaki K (2002). Malignant lymphoma arising as a primary tumor of the uterine corpus. Pathol Int 52: 423-424.

891. Kawauchi S, Okuda S, Morioka H, Iwasaki F, Fukuma F, Chochi Y, Furuya T, Oga A, Sasaki K (2005). Large cell neuroendocrine carcinoma of the uterine cervix with cytogenetic analysis by comparative genomic hybridization: a case study. Hum Pathol 36: 1096-1100.

892. Kawauchi S, Tsuji T, Kaku T, Kamura T, Nakano H, Tsuneyoshi M (1998). Sclerosing stromal tumor of the ovary: a clinicopathologic, immunohistochemical, ultrastructural, and cytogenetic analysis with special reference to its vasculature. Am J Surg Pathol 22: 83-92.

893. Kay S, Schneider V (1985). Reactive spindle cell nodule of the endocervix simulating uterine sarcoma. Int J Gynecol Pathol 4: 255-257.

894. Kayser K, Zink S, Schneider T, Dienemann H, Andre S, Kaltner H, Schuring MP, Zick Y, Gabius HJ (2000). Benign metastasizing leiomyoma of the uterus: documentation of clinical, immunohistochemical and lectin-histochemical data of ten cases. Virchows Arch 437: 284-292.

895. Kazakov DV, Spagnolo DV, Kacerovska D, Michal M (2011). Lesions of anogenital mammary-like glands: an update. Adv Anat Pathol 18: 1-28.

896. Kazakov DV, Spagnolo DV, Stewart CJ, Thompson J, Agaimy A, Magro G, Bisceglia M, Vazmitel M, Kacerovska D, Kutzner H, Mukensnabl P, Michal M (2010). Fibroadenoma and phyllodes tumors of anogenital mammary-like glands: a series of 13 neoplasms in 12 cases, including mammary-type juvenile fibroadenoma, fibroadenoma with lactation changes, and neurofibromatosis-associated pseudoangiomatous stromal hyperplasia with multinucleated giant cells. Am J Surg Pathol 34: 95-103.

897. Keating JT, Cviko A, Riethdorf S, Riethdorf L, Quade BJ, Sun D, Duensing S, Sheets EE, Munger K, Crum CP (2001). Ki-67, cyclin E, and p16INK4 are complimentary surrogate biomarkers for human papilloma virus-related cervical neoplasia. Am J Surg Pathol 25: 884-891.

898. Keel SB, Clement PB, Prat J, Young RH (1998). Malignant schwannoma of the uterine cervix: a study of three cases. Int J Gynecol Pathol 17: 223-230.

899. Keep D, Zaragoza MV, Hassold T, Redline RW (1996). Very early complete hydatidiform mole. Hum Pathol 27: 708-713.

900. Kelly P, McBride HA, Kennedy K, Connolly LE, McCluggage WG (2011). Misplaced Skene's glands: glandular elements in the lower female genital tract that are variably immunoreactive with prostate markers and that encompass vaginal tubulosquamous polyp and cervical ectopic prostatic tissue. Int J Gynecol Pathol 30: 605-612.

901. Kendall BS, Ronnett BM, Isacson C, Cho KR, Hedrick L, Diener-West M, Kurman RJ (1998). Reproducibility of the diagnosis of endometrial hyperplasia, atypical hyperplasia, and well-differentiated carcinoma. Am J Surg Pathol 22: 1012-1019.

902. Kennedy MM, Baigrie CF, Manek S (1999). Tamoxifen and the endometrium: review of 102 cases and comparison with HRT-related and non-HRT-related endometrial pathology. Int J Gynecol Pathol 18: 130-137.

903. Kenny SL, McBride HA, Jamison J, McCluggage WG (2012). Mesonephric adenocarcinomas of the uterine cervix and corpus: HPV-negative neoplasms that are commonly PAX8, CA125, and HMGA2 positive and that may be immunoreactive with TTF1 and hepatocyte nuclear factor 1-beta. Am J Surg Pathol 36: 799-807.

904. Kerdraon O, Cornelius A, Farine MO, Boulanger L, Wacrenier A (2012). Adenoid basal hyperplasia of the uterine cervix: a lesion of reserve cell type, distinct from adenoid basal carcinoma. Hum Pathol 43: 2255-2265.

905. Kerner H, Lichtig C (1993). Mullerian adenosarcoma presenting as cervical polyps: a report of seven cases and review of the literature. Obstet Gynecol 81: 655-659.

906. Kersemaekers AM, Hermans J, Fleuren GJ, Van de Vijver K (1998). Loss of heterozygosity for defined regions on chromosomes 3, 11 and 17 in carcinomas of the uterine cervix. Br J Cancer 77: 192-200.

907. Kersemaekers AM, Van de Vijver K, Kenter GG, Fleuren GJ (1999). Genetic alterations during the progression of squamous cell carcinomas of the uterine cervix. Genes Chromosomes Cancer 26: 346-354.

908. Ketabi Z, Bartuma K, Bernstein I, Malander S, Gronberg H, Bjorck E, Holck S, Nilbert M (2011). Ovarian cancer linked to Lynch syndrome typically presents as early-onset, non-serous epithelial tumors. Gynecol Oncol 121: 462-465.

909. Khalifa MA, Hansen CH, Moore JL Jr, Rusnock EJ, Lage JM (1996). Endometrial stromal sarcoma with focal smooth muscle differentiation: recurrence after 17 years: a follow-up report with discussion of the nomenclature. Int J Gynecol Pathol 15: 171-176.

910. Khosla D, Gupta R, Srinivasan R, Patel FD, Rajwanshi A (2012). Sarcomas of uterine cervix: clinicopathological features, treatment, and outcome. Int J Gynecol Cancer 22: 1026-1030.

911. Khosravi MR, Margulies DR, Alsabeh R, Nissen N, Phillips EH, Morgenstern L (2004). Consider the diagnosis of splenosis for soft tissue masses long after any splenic injury. Am Surg 70: 967-970.

912. Khoury-Collado F, Elliott KS, Lee YC, Chen PC, Abulafia O (2005). Merkel cell carcinoma of the Bartholin's gland. Gynecol Oncol 97: 928-931.

913. Khunamornpong S, Lerwill MF, Siriaunkgul S, Suprasert P, Pojchamarnwiputh S, Chiangmai WN, Young RH (2008). Carcinoma of extrahepatic bile ducts and gallbladder metastatic to the ovary: a report of 16 cases. Int J Gynecol Pathol 27: 366-379.

914. Khunamornpong S, Russell P, Dalrymple JC (1999). Proliferating (LMP) mucinous tumors of the ovaries with microinvasion: morphologic assessment of 13 cases. Int J Gynecol Pathol 18: 238-246.

915. Khunamornpong S, Settakorn J, Sukpan K, Suprasert P, Siriaunkgul S (2011). Mucinous tumor of low malignant potential ("borderline" or "atypical proliferative" tumor) of the ovary: a study of 171 cases with the assessment of intraepithelial carcinoma and microinvasion. Int J Gynecol Pathol 30: 218-230.

916. Khunamornpong S, Siriaunkgul S, Suprasert P, Chitapanarux I (2005). Yolk sac tumor of the vulva: a case report with long-term disease-free survival. Gynecol Oncol 97: 238-242.

917. Khunamornpong S, Siriaunkgul S, Suprasert P, Pojchamarnwiputh S, Na CW, Young RH (2007). Intrahepatic cholangiocarcinoma metastatic to the ovary: a report of 16 cases of an underemphasized form of secondary tumor in the ovary that may mimic primary neoplasia. Am J Surg Pathol 31: 1788-1799.

918. Khunamornpong S, Suprasert P, Chiangmai WN, Siriaunkgul S (2006). Metastatic tumors to the ovaries: a study of 170 cases in northern Thailand. Int J Gynecol Cancer 16 Suppl 1: 132-138.

919. Kido A, Togashi K, Konishi I, Kataoka ML, Koyama T, Ueda H, Fujii S, Konishi J (1999). Dermoid cysts of the ovary with malignant transformation: MR appearance. AJR Am J Roentgenol 172: 445-449.

920. Kilic G, Boruban MC, Bueco-Ramos C, Konoplev SN (2007). Granulocytic sarcoma involving the uterus and right fallopian tube with negative endometrial biopsy. Eur J Gynaecol Oncol 28: 270-272.

921. Killeen VB, Reich H, McGlynn F, Virgilio LA, Krawitz MA, Sekel L (1997). Pelvic gliomatosis within foci of endometriosis. JSLS 1: 267-268.

922. Kim HJ, Kim MH, Kwon J, Kim JY, Park K, Ro JY (2012). Proximal-type epithelioid sarcoma of the vulva with INI1 diagnostic utility. Ann Diagn Pathol 16: 411-415.

923. Kim KR, Lee HI, Lee SK, Ro JY, Robboy SJ (2007). Is stromal microinvasion in primary mucinous ovarian tumors with "mucin granuloma" true invasion? Am J Surg Pathol 31: 546-554.

924. Kim KR, Peng R, Ro JY, Robboy SJ (2004). A diagnostically useful histopathologic feature of endometrial polyp: the long axis of endometrial glands arranged parallel to surface epithelium. Am J Surg Pathol 28: 1057-1062.

925. Kim KR, Scully RE (1990). Peritoneal keratin granulomas with carcinomas of endometrium and ovary and atypical polypoid adenomyoma of endometrium. A clinicopathological analysis of 22 cases. Am J Surg Pathol 14: 925-932.

926. Kim MD, Lee M, Jung DC, Park SI, Lee MS, Won JY, Lee dY, Lee KH (2012). Limited efficacy of uterine artery embolization for cervical leiomyomas. J Vasc Interv Radiol 23: 236-240.

927. Kim MS, Hur SY, Yoo NJ, Lee SH (2010). Mutational analysis of FOXL2 codon 134 in granulosa cell tumour of ovary and other human cancers. J Pathol 221: 147-152.

928. Kim SA, Jung JS, Ju SJ, Kim YT, Kim KR (2011). Mullerian adenosarcoma with sarcomatous overgrowth in the pelvic cavity extending into the inferior vena cava and the right atrium. Pathol Int 61: 445-448.

929. Kim YH, Kim MA, Park IA, Park WY, Kim JW, Kim SC, Park NH, Song YS, Kang SB (2010). VEGF polymorphisms in early cervical cancer susceptibility, angiogenesis, and survival. Gynecol Oncol 119: 232-236.

930. Kimball KJ, Straughn JM, Conner MG, Kirby TO (2006). Recurrent basosquamous cell carcinoma of the vulva. Gynecol Oncol 102: 400-402.

931. Kindelberger DW, Lee Y, Miron A, Hirsch MS, Feltmate C, Medeiros F, Callahan MJ, Garner EO, Gordon RW, Birch C, Berkowitz RS, Muto MG, Crum CP (2007). Intraepithelial carcinoma of the fimbria and pelvic serous carcinoma: Evidence for a causal relationship. Am J Surg Pathol 31: 161-169.

932. Kines RC, Thompson CD, Lowy DR, Schiller JT, Day PM (2009). The initial steps leading to papillomavirus infection occur on the basement membrane prior to cell surface binding. Proc Natl Acad Sci U S A 106: 20458-20463.

933. King ME, Dickersin GR, Scully RE (1982). Myxoid leiomyosarcoma of the uterus. A report of six cases. Am J Surg Pathol 6: 589-598.

934. King ME, Micha JP, Allen SL, Mouradian JA, Chaganti RS (1985). Immature teratoma of the ovary with predominant malignant retinal anlage component. A parthenogenically derived tumor. Am J Surg Pathol 9: 221-231.

935. Kinney W, Fetterman B, Cox JT, Lorey T, Flanagan T, Castle PE (2011). Characteristics of 44 cervical cancers diagnosed following Pap-negative, high risk HPV-positive screening in routine clinical practice. Gynecol Oncol 121: 309-313.

936. Kinoshita T, Nakamura Y, Kinoshita M, Fukuda S, Nakashima H, Hashimoto T (1986). Bilateral cystic nephroblastomas and botryoid sarcoma in a child with Dandy-Walker syndrome. Arch Pathol Lab Med 110: 150-152.

937. Kir G, Eren S, Akoz I, Kir M (2003). Leiomyosarcoma of the broad ligament arising in a pre-existing pure neurilemmoma-like leiomyoma. Eur J Gynaecol Oncol 24: 505-506.

938. Kirchhoff M, Rose H, Petersen BL, Maahr J, Gerdes T, Lundsteen C, Bryndorf T, Kryger-Baggesen N, Christensen L, Engelholm SA, Philip J (1999). Comparative genomic hybridization reveals a recurrent pattern of chromosomal aberrations in severe dysplasia/carcinoma in situ of the cervix and in advanced-stage cervical carcinoma. Genes Chromosomes Cancer 24: 144-150.

939. Kirk CM, Naumann RW, Hartmann CJ, Brown CA, Banks PM (2001). Primary endometrial T-cell lymphoma. A case report. Am J Clin Pathol 115: 561-566.

940. Kirkbride P, Fyles A, Rawlings GA, Manchul L, Levin W, Murphy KJ, Simm J (1995). Carcinoma of the vagina--experience at the Princess Margaret Hospital (1974-1989). Gynecol Oncol 56: 435-443.

941. Kirkham JC, Nero CJ, Tambouret RH, Yoon SS (2008). Leiomyoma and leiomyosarcoma arising from the round ligament of the uterus. J Am Coll Surg 207: 452.

942. Kiyokawa T, Young RH, Scully RE (2006). Krukenberg tumors of the ovary: a clinicopathologic analysis of 120 cases with emphasis on their variable pathologic manifestations. Am J Surg Pathol 30: 277-299.

943. Kjaer SK, Svare EI, Worm AM, Walboomers JM, Meijer CJ, van den Brule AJ (2000). Human papillomavirus infection in Danish female sex workers. Decreasing prevalence with age despite continuously high sexual activity. Sex Transm Dis 27: 438-445.

944. Kleinman GM, Young RH, Scully RE (1993). Primary neuroectodermal tumors of the ovary. A report of 25 cases. Am J Surg Pathol 17: 764-778.

945. Klemi PJ, Gronroos M (1979). Endometrioid carcinoma of the ovary. A clinicopathologic, histochemical, and electron microscopic study. Obstet Gynecol 53: 572-579.

946. Kline RC, Wharton JT, Atkinson EN, Burke TW, Gershenson DM, Edwards CL (1990). Endometrioid carcinoma of the ovary: retrospective review of 145 cases. Gynecol Oncol 39: 337-346.

947. Kloos I, Delaloge S, Pautier P, Di PM, Goupil A, Duvillard P, Cailleux PE, Lhomme C (2002). Tamoxifen-related uterine carcinosarcomas occur under/after prolonged treatment: report of five cases and review of the literature. Int J Gynecol Cancer 12: 496-500.

948. Kloppel G (2011). Classification and pathology of gastroenteropancreatic neuroendocrine neoplasms. Endocr Relat Cancer 18 Suppl 1: S1-S16.

949. Klug SJ, Ressing M, Koenig J, Abba MC, Agorastos T, Brenna SM, Ciotti M, Das BR, Del Mistro A, Dybikowska A, Giuliano AR, Gudleviciene Z, Gyllensten U, Haws AL, Helland A, Herrington CS, Hildesheim A, Humbey O, Jee SH, Kim JW, Madeleine MM, Menczer J, Ngan HY, Nishikawa A, Niwa Y, Pegoraro R, Pillai MR, Ranzani G, Rezza G, Rosenthal AN, Roychoudhury S, Saranath D, Schmitt VM, Sengupta S, Settheetham-Ishida W, Shirasawa H, Snijders PJ, Stoler MH, Suárez-Rincón AE, Szarka K, Tachezy R, Ueda M, van der Zee AG, von Knebel Doeberitz M, Wu MT, Yamashita T, Zehbe I, Blettner M (2009). TP53 codon 72 polymorphism and cervical cancer: a pooled analysis of individual data from 49 studies. Lancet Oncol 10: 772-784.

950. Köbel M, Kalloger SE, Baker PM, Ewanowich CA, Arseneau J, Zherebitskiy V, Abdulkarim S, Leung S, Duggan MA, Fontaine D, Parker R, Huntsman DG, Gilks CB (2010). Diagnosis of ovarian carcinoma cell type is highly reproducible: a transcanadian study. Am J Surg Pathol 34: 984-993.

951. Köbel M, Kalloger SE, Huntsman DG, Santos JL, Swenerton KD, Seidman JD, Gilks CB (2010). Differences in tumor type in low-stage versus high-stage ovarian carcinomas. Int J Gynecol Pathol 29: 203-211.

951A. Köbel M, Kalloger SE, Lee S, Duggan MA, Kelemen LE, Prentice L, Kalli KR, Fridley BL, Visscher DW, Keeney GL, Vierkant RA, Cunningham JM, Chow C, Ness RB, Moysich K, Edwards R, Modugno F, Bunker C, Wozniak EL, Benjamin E, Gayther SA, Gentry-Maharaj A, Menon U, Gilks CB, Huntsman DG, Ramus SJ, Goode EL; Ovarian Tumor Tissue Analysis consortium (2013). Biomarker-based ovarian carcinoma typing: a histologic investigation in the ovarian tumor tissue analysis consortium. Cancer Epidemiol Biomarkers Prev 22: 1677-1686.

952. Köbel M, Kalloger SE, Santos JL, Huntsman DG, Gilks CB, Swenerton KD (2010). Tumor type and substage predict survival in stage I and II ovarian carcinoma: insights and implications. Gynecol Oncol 116: 50-56.

953. Köbel M, Reuss A, Bois Ad, Kommoss S, Kommoss F, Gao D, Kalloger SE, Huntsman DG, Gilks CB (2010). The biological and clinical value of p53 expression in pelvic high-grade serous carcinomas. J Pathol 222: 191-198.

954. Koch CA, Azumi N, Furlong MA, Jha RC, Kehoe TE, Trowbridge CH, O'Dorisio TM, Chrousos GP, Clement SC (1999). Carcinoid syndrome caused by an atypical carcinoid of the uterine cervix. J Clin Endocrinol Metab 84: 4209-4213.

955. Kocova L, Michal M, Sulc M, Zamecnik M (1997). Calcifying fibrous pseudotumour of visceral peritoneum. Histopathology 31: 182-184.

956. Koenig C, Tavassoli FA (1998). Nodular hyperplasia, adenoma, and adenomyoma of Bartholin's gland. Int J Gynecol Pathol 17: 289-294.

957. Koenig C, Turnicky RP, Kankam CF, Tavassoli FA (1997). Papillary squamotransitional cell carcinoma of the cervix: a report of 32 cases. Am J Surg Pathol 21: 915-921.

958. Kofinas AD, Suarez J, Calame RJ, Chipeco Z (1984). Chondrosarcoma of the uterus. Gynecol Oncol 19: 231-237.

958A. Koh LP, Wong LC, Ng SB, Poon ML, Low JJ (2009). Primary cutaneous anaplastic large cell lymphoma of the vulva: a typical cutaneous lesion with an 'atypical' presenting site. Int J Hematol 90: 388-391.

959. Kohorn EI (2001). The new FIGO 2000 staging and risk factor scoring system for gestational trophoblastic disease: description and critical assessment. Int J Gynecol Cancer 11: 73-77.

960. Kohrenhagen N, Eck M, Holler S, Dietl J (2008). Lymphoepithelioma-like carcinoma of the uterine cervix: absence of Epstein-Barr virus and high-risk human papilloma virus infection. Arch Gynecol Obstet 277: 175-178.

961. Kojima A, Mikami Y, Sudo T, Yamaguchi S, Kusanagi Y, Ito M, Nishimura R (2007). Gastric morphology and immunophenotype predict poor outcome in mucinous adenocarcinoma of the uterine cervix. Am J Surg Pathol 31: 664-672.

962. Kolusari A, Ugurluer G, Kosem M, Kurdoglu M, Yildizhan R, Adali E (2009). Leiomyosarcoma of the broad ligament: a case report and review of the literature. Eur J Gynaecol Oncol 30: 332-334.

963. Kommoss F, Oliva E, Bhan AK, Young RH, Scully RE (1998). Inhibin expression in ovarian tumors and tumor-like lesions: an immunohistochemical study. Mod Pathol 11: 656-664.

964. Kondi-Pafiti A, Grapsa D, Kontogianni-Katsarou K, Papadias K, Kairi-Vassilatou E (2005). Ectopic decidua mimicking metastatic lesions--report of three cases and review of the literature. Eur J Gynaecol Oncol 26: 459-461.

965. Kondi-Pafiti A, Kairi-Vasilatou E, Iavazzo C, Dastamani C, Bakalianou K, Liapis A, Hassiakos D, Fotiou S (2011). Metastatic neoplasms of the ovaries: a clinicopathological study of 97 cases. Arch Gynecol Obstet 284: 1283-1288.

966. Kondo T, Hashi A, Murata SI, Fischer SE, Nara M, Nakazawa T, Yuminamochi T, Hoshi K, Katoh R (2007). Gastric mucin is expressed in a subset of endocervical tunnel clusters: type A tunnel clusters of gastric phenotype. Histopathology 50: 843-850.

967. Konis EE, Belsky RD (1966). Metastasizing leiomyoma of the uterus. Report of a case. Obstet Gynecol 27: 442-446.

968. Koonings PP, Campbell K, Mishell DR Jr, Grimes DA (1989). Relative frequency of primary ovarian neoplasms: a 10-year review. Obstet Gynecol 74: 921-926.

969. Koontz JI, Soreng AL, Nucci M, Kuo FC, Pauwels P, van den Berghe H, Dal Cin P, Fletcher JA, Sklar J (2001). Frequent fusion of the JAZF1 and JJAZ1 genes in endometrial stromal tumors. Proc Natl Acad Sci U S A 98: 6348-6353.

970. Koprowski H, Herlyn M, Balaban G, Parmiter A, Ross A, Nowell P (1985). Expression of the receptor for epidermal growth factor correlates with increased dosage of chromosome 7 in malignant melanoma. Somat Cell Mol Genet 11: 297-302.

971. Korytko TP, Lowe GJ, Jimenez RE, Pohar KS, Martin DD (2012). Prostate-specific antigen response after definitive radiotherapy for Skene's gland adenocarcinoma resembling prostate adenocarcinoma. Urol Oncol 30: 602-606.

972. Kosari F, Daneshbod Y, Parwaresch R, Krams M, Wacker HH (2005). Lymphomas of the female genital tract: a study of 186 cases and review of the literature. Am J Surg Pathol 29: 1512-1520.

973. Kosary CL (1994). FIGO stage, histology, histologic grade, age and race as prognostic factors in determining survival for cancers of the female gynecological system: an analysis of 1973-87 SEER cases of cancers of the endometrium, cervix, ovary, vulva, and vagina. Semin Surg Oncol 10: 31-46.

974. Koshiyama M, Konishi I, Yoshida M, Wang DP, Mandai M, Mori T, Fujii S (1994). Transitional cell carcinoma of the fallopian tube: a light and electron microscopic study. Int J Gynecol Pathol 13: 175-180.

975. Koskas M, Uzan C, Gouy S, Pautier P, Lhomme C, Haie-Meder C, Duvillard P, Morice P (2011). Prognostic factors of a large retrospective series of mucinous borderline tumors of the ovary (excluding peritoneal pseudomyxoma). Ann Surg Oncol 18: 40-48.

976. Koss LG, Durfee GR (1956). Unusual patterns of squamous epithelium of the uterine cervix: cytologic and pathologic study of koilocytotic atypia. Ann N Y Acad Sci 63: 1245-1261.

977. Kostopoulou E, Moulla A, Giakoustidis D, Leontsini M (2004). Sclerosing stromal tumors of the ovary: a clinicopathologic, immunohistochemical and cytogenetic analysis of three cases. Eur J Gynaecol Oncol 25: 257-260.

978. Kourea HP, Adonakis G, Androutsopoulos G, Zyli P, Kourounis G, Decavalas G (2008). Fallopian tube malignant mixed mullerian tumor (carcinosarcoma): a case report with immunohistochemical profiling. Eur J Gynaecol Oncol 29: 538-542.

979. Koutsky LA, Ault KA, Wheeler CM, Brown DR, Barr E, Alvarez FB, Chiacchierini LM, Jansen KU (2002). A controlled trial of a human papillomavirus type 16 vaccine. N Engl J Med 347: 1645-1651.

980. Koutsky LA, Holmes KK, Critchlow CW, Stevens CE, Paavonen J, Beckmann AM, DeRouen TA, Galloway DA, Vernon D, Kiviat NB (1992). A cohort study of the risk of cervical intraepithelial neoplasia grade 2 or 3 in relation to papillomavirus infection. N Engl J Med 327: 1272-1278.

981. Kovacic MB, Castle PE, Herrero R, Schiffman M, Sherman ME, Wacholder S, Rodriguez AC, Hutchinson ML, Bratti MC, Hildesheim A, Morales J, Alfaro M, Burk RD (2006). Relationships of human papillomavirus type, qualitative viral load, and age with cytologic abnormality. Cancer Res 66: 10112-10119.

982. Kowalewska M, Danska-Bidzinska A, Bakula-Zalewska E, Bidzinski M (2012). Identification of suitable reference genes for gene expression measurement in uterine sarcoma and carcinosarcoma tumors. Clin Biochem 45: 368-371.

983. Kraemer BB, Silva EG, Sneige N (1984). Fibrosarcoma of ovary. A new component in the nevoid basal-cell carcinoma syndrome. Am J Surg Pathol 8: 231-236.

984. Kraggerud SM, Szymanska J, Abeler VM, Kaern J, Eknaes M, Heim S, Teixeira MR, Trope CG, Peltomaki P, Lothe RA (2000). DNA copy number changes in malignant ovarian germ cell tumors. Cancer Res 60: 3025-3030.

985. Krishnamurthy S, Jungbluth AA, Busam KJ, Rosai J (1998). Uterine tumors resembling ovarian sex-cord tumors have an immunophenotype consistent with true sex-cord differentiation. Am J Surg Pathol 22: 1078-1082.

986. Krivak TC, McBroom JW, Sundborg MJ, Crothers B, Parker MF (2001). Large cell neuroendocrine cervical carcinoma: a report of two cases and review of the literature. Gynecol Oncol 82: 187-191.

987. Krivak TC, Seidman JD, McBroom JW, MacKoul PJ, Aye LM, Rose GS (2001). Uterine adenosarcoma with sarcomatous overgrowth versus uterine carcinosarcoma: comparison of treatment and survival. Gynecol Oncol 83: 89-94.

987A. Küsters-Vandevelde HV, Van Leeuwen A, Verdijk MA, de Koning MN, Quint WG, Melchers WJ, Ligtenberg MJ, Blokx WA (2010). CDKN2A but not TP53 mutations nor HPV presence predict poor outcome in metastatic squamous cell carcinoma of the skin. Int J Cancer 126: 2123-2132.

988. Kuhn E, Kurman RJ, Vang R, Sehdev AS, Han G, Soslow R, Wang TL, Shih I (2012). TP53 mutations in serous tubal intraepithelial carcinoma and concurrent pelvic high-grade serous carcinoma--evidence supporting the clonal relationship of the two lesions. J Pathol 226: 421-426.

989. Kuhn E, Meeker A, Wang TL, Sehdev AS, Kurman RJ, Shih I (2010). Shortened telomeres in serous tubal intraepithelial carcinoma: an early event in ovarian high-grade serous carcinogenesis. Am J Surg Pathol 34: 829-836.

990. Kuhn E, Wu RC, Guan B, Wu G, Zhang J, Wang Y, Song L, Yuan X, Wei L, Roden RB, Kuo KT, Nakayama K, Clarke B, Shaw P, Olvera N, Kurman RJ, Levine DA, Wang TL, Shih I (2012). Identification of molecular pathway aberrations in uterine serous carcinoma by genome-wide analyses. J Natl Cancer Inst 104: 1503-1513.

991. Kunjoonju JP, Raitanen M, Grenman S, Tiwari N, Worsham MJ (2005). Identification of individual genes altered in squamous cell carcinoma of the vulva. Genes Chromosomes Cancer 44: 185-193.

992. Kunkel J, Peng Y, Tao Y, Krigman H, Cao D (2012). Presence of a sarcomatous component outside the ovary is an adverse prognostic factor for primary ovarian malignant mixed mesodermal/mullerian tumors: a clinicopathologic study of 47 cases. Am J Surg Pathol 36: 831-837.

993. Kuo KT, Chen MJ, Lin MC (2004). Epithelioid trophoblastic tumor of the broad ligament: a case report and review of the literature. Am J Surg Pathol 28: 405-409.

994. Kuo KT, Guan B, Feng Y, Mao TL, Chen X, Jinawath N, Wang Y, Kurman RJ, Shih I, Wang TL (2009). Analysis of DNA copy number alterations in ovarian serous tumors identifies new molecular genetic changes in low-grade and high-grade carcinomas. Cancer Res 69: 4036-4042.

995. Kuo KT, Mao TL, Jones S, Veras E, Ayhan A, Wang TL, Glas R, Slamon D, Velculescu VE, Kuman RJ, Shih I (2009). Frequent activating mutations of PIK3CA in ovarian clear cell carcinoma. Am J Pathol 174: 1597-1601.

996. Kuragaki C, Enomoto T, Ueno Y, Sun H, Fujita M, Nakashima R, Ueda Y, Wada H, Murata Y, Toki T, Konishi I, Fujii S (2003). Mutations in the STK11 gene characterize minimal deviation adenocarcinoma of the uterine cervix. Lab Invest 83: 35-45.

997. Kurihara S, Oda Y, Ohishi Y, Iwasa A, Takahira T, Kaneki E, Kobayashi H, Wake N, Tsuneyoshi M (2008). Endometrial stromal sarcomas and related high-grade sarcomas: immunohistochemical and molecular genetic study of 31 cases. Am J Surg Pathol 32: 1228-1238.

998. Kurman RJ, Kaminski PF, Norris HJ (1985). The behavior of endometrial

hyperplasia. A long-term study of "untreated" hyperplasia in 170 patients. Cancer 56: 403-412.
999. Kurman RJ, Norris HJ (1976). Embryonal carcinoma of the ovary: a clinicopathologic entity distinct from endodermal sinus tumor resembling embryonal carcinoma of the adult testis. Cancer 38: 2420-2433.
1000. Kurman RJ, Norris HJ (1976). Endodermal sinus tumor of the ovary: a clinical and pathologic analysis of 71 cases. Cancer 38: 2404-2419.
1001. Kurman RJ, Norris HJ (1976). Malignant mixed germ cell tumors of the ovary. A clinical and pathologic analysis of 30 cases. Obstet Gynecol 48: 579-589.
1002. Kurman RJ, Norris HJ (1976). Mesenchymal tumors of the uterus. VI. Epithelioid smooth muscle tumors including leiomyoblastoma and clear-cell leiomyoma: a clinical and pathologic analysis of 26 cases. Cancer 37: 1853-1865.
1003. Kurman RJ, Norris HJ (1977). Malignant germ cell tumors of the ovary. Hum Pathol 8: 551-564.
1004. Kurman RJ, Norris HJ (1982). Evaluation of criteria for distinguishing atypical endometrial hyperplasia from well-differentiated carcinoma. Cancer 49: 2547-2559.
1005. Kurman RJ, Ronnett BM, Sherman ME, Wilkinson EJ (2010). Tumors of the Cervix, Vagina, and Vulva. Third series, Fascicle four. American Registry of Pathology in collaboration with the Armed Forces Institute of Pathology: Washington, DC p. 431.
1006. Kurman RJ, Scully RE (1974). The incidence and histogenesis of vaginal adenosis. An autopsy study. Hum Pathol 5: 265-276.
1007. Kurman RJ, Scully RE (1976). Clear cell carcinoma of the endometrium: an analysis of 21 cases. Cancer 37: 872-882.
1008. Kurman RJ, Shih I (2010). The origin and pathogenesis of epithelial ovarian cancer: a proposed unifying theory. Am J Surg Pathol 34: 433-443.
1009. Kurman RJ, Shih I (2011). Molecular pathogenesis and extraovarian origin of epithelial ovarian cancer--shifting the paradigm. Hum Pathol 42: 918-931.
1010. Kurman RJ, Toki T, Schiffman MH (1993). Basaloid and warty carcinomas of the vulva. Distinctive types of squamous cell carcinoma frequently associated with human papillomaviruses. Am J Surg Pathol 17: 133-145.
1011. Kurman RJ, Vang R, Junge J, Hannibal CG, Kjaer SK, Shih I (2011). Papillary tubal hyperplasia: the putative precursor of ovarian atypical proliferative (borderline) serous tumors, noninvasive implants, and endosalpingiosis. Am J Surg Pathol 35: 1605-1614.
1012. Kuroda N, Hirano K, Inui Y, Yamasaki Y, Toi M, Nakayama H, Hiroi M, Enzan H (2001). Compound melanocytic nevus arising in a mature cystic teratoma of the ovary. Pathol Int 51: 902-904.
1013. Kusanagi Y, Kojima A, Mikami Y, Kiyokawa T, Sudo T, Yamaguchi S, Nishimura R (2010). Absence of high-risk human papillomavirus (HPV) detection in endocervical adenocarcinoma with gastric morphology and phenotype. Am J Pathol 177: 2169-2175.
1014. Kusters-Vandevelde HV, Van Leeuwen A, Verdijk MA, de Koning MN, Quint WG, Melchers WJ, Ligtenberg MJ, Blokx WA (2010). CDKN2A but not TP53 mutations nor HPV presence predict poor outcome in metastatic squamous cell carcinoma of the skin. Int J Cancer 126: 2123-2132.
1015. Kyriazi MA, Carvounis EE, Kitsou M, Arkadopoulos N, Nicolaidou E, Fotiou S, Smyrniotis V (2010). Myoepithelial carcinoma of the vulva mimicking bartholin gland abscess in a pregnant woman: case report and review of literature. Int J Gynecol Pathol 29: 501-504.
1016. La Rosa S, Sessa F, Capella C, Riva C, Leone BE, Klersy C, Rindi G, Solcia E (1996). Prognostic criteria in nonfunctioning pancreatic endocrine tumours. Virchows Arch 429: 323-333.
1017. La Vecchia C, Parazzini F, Decarli A, Franceschi S, Fasoli M, Favalli G, Negri E, Pampallona S (1984). Age of parents and risk of gestational trophoblastic disease. J Natl Cancer Inst 73: 639-642.
1018. Lacey JV Jr, Brinton LA, Barnes WA, Gravitt PE, Greenberg MD, Hadjimichael OC, McGowan L, Mortel R, Schwartz PE, Kurman RJ, Hildesheim A (2000). Use of hormone replacement therapy and adenocarcinomas and squamous cell carcinomas of the uterine cervix. Gynecol Oncol 77: 149-154.
1019. Lacey JV Jr, Chia VM, Rush BB, Carreon DJ, Richesson DA, Ioffe OB, Ronnett BM, Chatterjee N, Langholz B, Sherman ME, Glass AG (2012). Incidence rates of endometrial hyperplasia, endometrial cancer and hysterectomy from 1980 to 2003 within a large prepaid health plan. Int J Cancer 131: 1921-1929.
1020. Lacey JV Jr, Mutter GL, Nucci MR, Ronnett BM, Ioffe OB, Rush BB, Glass AG, Richesson DA, Chatterjee N, Langholz B, Sherman ME (2008). Risk of subsequent endometrial carcinoma associated with endometrial intraepithelial neoplasia classification of endometrial biopsies. Cancer 113: 2073-2081.
1021. Lack EE, Worsham GF, Callihan MD, Crawford BE, Klappenbach S, Rowden G, Chun B (1980). Granular cell tumor: a clinicopathologic study of 110 patients. J Surg Oncol 13: 301-316.
1022. Ladanyi M, Lui MY, Antonescu CR, Krause-Boehm A, Meindl A, Argani P, Healey JH, Ueda T, Yoshikawa H, Meloni-Ehrig A, Sorensen PH, Mertens F, Mandahl N, van den Berghe H, Sciot R, Dal Cin P, Bridge J (2001). The der(17)t(X;17)(p11;q25) of human alveolar soft part sarcoma fuses the TFE3 transcription factor gene to ASPL, a novel gene at 17q25. Oncogene 20: 48-57.
1023. Lagoo AS, Robboy SJ (2006). Lymphoma of the female genital tract: current status. Int J Gynecol Pathol 25: 1-21.
1024. Lai CH, Chou HH, Chang CJ, Wang CC, Hsueh S, Huang YT, Chen YR, Chang HP, Chang SC, Lin CT, Chao A, Qiu JT, Huang KG, Chen TC, Jao MS, Chen MY, Liou JD, Huang CC, Chang TC, Patsner B (2013). Clinical implications of human papillomavirus genotype in cervical adeno-adenosquamous carcinoma. Eur J Cancer 49: 633-641.
1025. Lajer CB, Garnaes E, Friis-Hansen L, Norrild B, Therkildsen MH, Glud M, Rossing M, Lajer H, Svane D, Skotte L, Specht L, Buchwald C, Nielsen FC (2012). The role of miRNAs in human papilloma virus (HPV)-associated cancers: bridging between HPV-related head and neck cancer and cervical cancer. Br J Cancer 106: 1526-1534.
1025A. Lakhani SR, Ellis IO, Schnitt SJ, Tan PH, van de Vijver MJ, Eds. (2012). WHO Classification of Tumours of the Breast. International Agency for Research on Cancer: Lyon
1026. Lallas TA, Mehaffey PC, Lager DJ, Van Voorhis BJ, Sorosky JI (1999). Malignant cervical schwannoma: An unusual pelvic tumor. Gynecol Oncol 72: 238-242.
1027. Lamarca M, Rubio P, Andres P, Rodrigo C (2011). Leiomyomatosis peritonealis disseminata with malignant degeneration. A case report. Eur J Gynaecol Oncol 32: 702-704.
1028. Lambrou NC, Mirhashemi R, Wolfson A, Thesiger P, Penalver M (2002). Malignant peripheral nerve sheath tumor of the vulva: a multimodal treatment approach. Gynecol Oncol 85: 365-371.
1029. Lamovec J, Bracko M, Cerar O (1995). Familial occurrence of small-cell carcinoma of the ovary. Arch Pathol Lab Med 119: 523-527.
1030. Lamping JD, Blythe JG (1977). Bilateral Brenner tumors: a case report and review of the literature. Hum Pathol 8: 583-585.
1031. Lan C, Huang X, Lin S, Cai M, Liu J (2012). Endometrial stromal sarcoma arising from endometriosis: a clinicopathological study and literature review. Gynecol Obstet Invest 74: 288-297.
1032. Lane BR, Ross JH, Hart WR, Kay R (2005). Mullerian papilloma of the cervix in a child with multiple renal cysts. Urology 65: 388.
1033. Lanjewar DN, Dongaonkar DD (2006). HIV-associated primary non-Hodgkin's lymphoma of ovary: a case report. Gynecol Oncol 102: 590-592.
1034. Larson AA, Liao SY, Stanbridge EJ, Cavenee WK, Hampton GM (1997). Genetic alterations accumulate during cervical tumorigenesis and indicate a common origin for multifocal lesions. Cancer Res 57: 4171-4176.
1035. Larson B, Silfversward C, Nilsson B, Pettersson F (1990). Prognostic factors in uterine leiomyosarcoma. A clinical and histopathological study of 143 cases. The Radiumhemmet series 1936-1981. Acta Oncol 29: 185-191.
1036. Larson DA, Derkay CS (2010). Epidemiology of recurrent respiratory papillomatosis. APMIS 118: 450-454.
1036A. Lash RH, Hart WR (1987). Intestinal adenocarcinomas metastatic to the ovaries. A clinicopathologic evaluation of 22 cases. Am J Surg Pathol 11: 114-121.
1037. Laskin WB, Fetsch JF, Tavassoli FA (1997). Angiomyofibroblastoma of the female genital tract: analysis of 17 cases including a lipomatous variant. Hum Pathol 28: 1046-1055.
1038. Laskin WB, Fetsch JF, Tavassoli FA (2001). Superficial cervicovaginal myofibroblastoma: fourteen cases of a distinctive mesenchymal tumor arising from the specialized subepithelial stroma of the lower female genital tract. Hum Pathol 32: 715-725.
1039. Lastra RR, Bavuso N, Randall TC, Brooks JS, Barroeta JE (2012). Neurofibroma of the cervix presenting as cervical stenosis in a patient with neurofibromatosis type 1: a case report. Int J Gynecol Pathol 31: 192-194.
1040. Lau YF, Li Y, Kido T (2009). Gonadoblastoma locus and the TSPY gene on the human Y chromosome. Birth Defects Res C Embryo Today 87: 114-122.
1041. Laury AR, Hornick JL, Perets R, Krane JF, Corson J, Drapkin R, Hirsch MS (2010). PAX8 reliably distinguishes ovarian serous tumors from malignant mesothelioma. Am J Surg Pathol 34: 627-635.
1042. Laury AR, Ning G, Quick CM, Bijron J, Parast MM, Betensky RA, Vargas SO, McKeon FD, Xian W, Nucci MR, Crum CP (2011). Fallopian tube correlates of ovarian serous borderline tumors. Am J Surg Pathol 35: 1759-1765.
1043. Lavie O, Ben-Arie A, Segev Y, Faro J, Barak F, Haya N, Auslender R, Gemer O (2010). BRCA germline mutations in women with uterine serous carcinoma--still a debate. Int J Gynecol Cancer 20: 1531-1534.
1044. Lavie O, Hornreich G, Ben-Arie A, Rennert G, Cohen Y, Keidar R, Sagi S, Lahad EL, Auslander R, Beller U (2004). BRCA germline mutations in Jewish women with uterine serous papillary carcinoma. Gynecol Oncol 92: 521-524.
1045. Lavorato-Rocha AM, de Melo MB, Rodrigues IS, Stiepcich MM, Baiocchi G, da Silva Cestari FM, Carvalho KC, Soares FA, Rocha RM (2013). Prognostication of vulvar cancer based on p14ARF status: molecular assessment of transcript and protein. Ann Surg Oncol 20: 31-39.
1046. Lawler SD, Fisher RA, Pickthall VJ, Povey S, Evans MW (1982). Genetic studies on hydatidiform moles. I. The origin of partial moles. Cancer Genet Cytogenet 5: 309-320.
1047. Lawson NW, Seifen AB, Thompson DS, Gintautas J (1982). Cyanide blood levels following nitroprusside infusion for hypotensive anesthesia. Proc West Pharmacol Soc 25: 281-283.
1048. Lax SF, Kendall B, Tashiro H, Slebos RJ, Hedrick L (2000). The frequency of p53, K-ras mutations, and microsatellite instability differs in uterine endometrioid and serous carcinoma: evidence of distinct molecular genetic pathways. Cancer 88: 814-824.
1049. Lax SF, Pizer ES, Ronnett BM, Kurman RJ (1998). Clear cell carcinoma of the endometrium is characterized by a distinctive profile of p53, Ki-67, estrogen, and progesterone receptor expression. Hum Pathol 29: 551-558.
1050. Lax SF, Pizer ES, Ronnett BM, Kurman RJ (1998). Comparison of estrogen and progesterone receptor, Ki-67, and p53 immunoreactivity in uterine endometrioid carcinoma and endometrioid carcinoma with squamous, mucinous, secretory, and ciliated cell differentiation. Hum Pathol 29: 924-931.
1051. Lea JS, Coleman RL, Garner EO, Duska LR, Miller DS, Schorge JO (2003). Adenosquamous histology predicts poor outcome in low-risk stage IB1 cervical adenocarcinoma. Gynecol Oncol 91: 558-562.
1052. Leake J, Woolas RP, Daniel J, Oram DH, Brown CL (1994). Immunocytochemical and serological expression of CA 125: a clinicopathological study of 40 malignant ovarian epithelial tumours. Histopathology 24: 57-64.
1053. Lee CH, Ali RH, Rouzbahman M, Marino-Enriquez A, Zhu M, Guo X, Brunner AL, Chiang S, Leung S, Nelnyk N, Huntsman DG, Blake Gilks C, Nielsen TO, Dal Cin P, van de Rijn M, Oliva E, Fletcher JA, Nucci MR (2012). Cyclin D1 as a diagnostic immunomarker for endometrial stromal sarcoma with YWHAE-FAM22 rearrangement. Am J Surg Pathol 36: 1562-1570.
1054. Lee CH, Marino-Enriquez A, Ou W, Zhu M, Ali RH, Chiang S, Amant F, Gilks CB, van de Rijn M, Oliva E, Debiec-Rychter M, Dal Cin P, Fletcher JA, Nucci MR (2012). The clinicopathologic features of YWHAE-FAM22 endometrial stromal sarcomas: a histologically high-grade and clinically aggressive tumor. Am J Surg Pathol 36: 641-653.
1055. Lee CH, Turbin DA, Sung YC, Espinosa I, Montgomery K, van de Rijn M, Gilks CB (2009). A panel of antibodies to determine site of origin and malignancy in smooth muscle tumors. Mod Pathol 22: 1519-1531.
1056. Lee HJ, Choi J, Kim KR (2008). Pulmonary benign metastasizing leiomyoma associated with intravenous leiomyomatosis of the uterus: clinical behavior and genomic changes supporting a transportation theory. Int J Gynecol Pathol 27: 340-345.
1057. Lee JY, Dong SM, Kim HS, Kim SY, Na EY, Shin MS, Lee SH, Park WS, Kim KM, Lee YS, Jang JJ, Yoo NJ (1998). A distinct region of chromosome 19p13.3 associated with the sporadic form of adenoma malignum of the uterine cervix. Cancer Res 58: 1140-1143.
1058. Lee KH, Lee IH, Kim BG, Nam JH, Kim WK, Kang SB, Ryu SY, Cho CH, Choi HS, Kim KT (2009). Clinicopathologic characteristics of malignant germ cell tumors in the ovaries of Korean women: a Korean Gynecologic

Oncology Group Study. Int J Gynecol Cancer 19: 84-87.
1059. Lee KR, Nucci MR (2003). Ovarian mucinous and mixed epithelial carcinomas of mullerian (endocervical-like) type: a clinicopathologic analysis of four cases of an uncommon variant associated with endometriosis. Int J Gynecol Pathol 22: 42-51.
1060. Lee KR, Scully RE (2000). Mucinous tumors of the ovary: a clinicopathologic study of 196 borderline tumors (of intestinal type) and carcinomas, including an evaluation of 11 cases with 'pseudomyxoma peritonei'. Am J Surg Pathol 24: 1447-1464.
1061. Lee KR, Young RH (2003). The distinction between primary and metastatic mucinous carcinomas of the ovary: gross and histologic findings in 50 cases. Am J Surg Pathol 27: 281-292.
1062. Lee MW, Jee KJ, Gong GY, Choi JH, Moon KC, Koh JK (2005). Comparative genomic hybridization in extramammary Paget's disease. Br J Dermatol 153: 290-294.
1063. Lee SC, Kaunitz AM, Sanchez-Ramos L, Rhatigan RM (2010). The oncogenic potential of endometrial polyps: a systematic review and meta-analysis. Obstet Gynecol 116: 1197-1205.
1063A. Lee SJ, Lee J, Lim HY, Kang WK, Choi CH, Lee JW, Kim TJ, Kim BG, Bae DS, Cho YB, Kim HC, Yun SH, Lee WY, Chun HK, Park YS (2010). Survival benefit from ovarian metastatectomy in colorectal cancer patients with ovarian metastasis: a retrospective analysis. Cancer Chemother Pharmacol 66: 229-235.
1063B. Lee S, Nelson G, Duan Q, Magliocco AM, Duggan MA (2013). Precursor lesions and prognostic factors in primary peritoneal serous carcinoma. Int J Gynecol Pathol 32: 547-555.
1064. Lee SJ, Rollason TP (1994). Argyrophilic cells in cervical intraepithelial glandular neoplasia. Int J Gynecol Pathol 13: 131-132.
1065. Lee Y, Miron A, Drapkin R, Nucci MR, Medeiros F, Saleemuddin A, Garber J, Birch C, Mou H, Gordon RW, Cramer DW, McKeon FD, Crum CP (2007). A candidate precursor to serous carcinoma that originates in the distal fallopian tube. J Pathol 211: 26-35.
1066. Leeper K, Garcia R, Swisher E, Goff B, Greer B, Paley P (2002). Pathologic findings in prophylactic oophorectomy specimens in high-risk women. Gynecol Oncol 87: 52-56.
1067. Leffers N, Gooden MJ, de Jong RA, Hoogeboom BN, ten Hoor KA, Hollema H, Boezen HM, van der Zee AG, Daemen T, Nijman HW (2009). Prognostic significance of tumor-infiltrating T-lymphocytes in primary and metastatic lesions of advanced stage ovarian cancer. Cancer Immunol Immunother 58: 449-459.
1068. Lehman MB, Hart WR (2001). Simple and complex hyperplastic papillary proliferations of the endometrium: a clinicopathologic study of nine cases of apparently localized papillary lesions with fibrovascular stromal cores and epithelial metaplasia. Am J Surg Pathol 25: 1347-1354.
1069. Leibowitch M, Neill S, Pelisse M, Moyal-Baracco M (1990). The epithelial changes associated with squamous cell carcinoma of the vulva: a review of the clinical, histological and viral findings in 78 women. Br J Obstet Gynaecol 97: 1135-1139.
1070. Leiser AL, Chi DS, Ishill NM, Tew WP (2007). Carcinosarcoma of the ovary treated with platinum and taxane: the memorial Sloan-Kettering Cancer Center experience. Gynecol Oncol 105: 657-661.
1071. Leiter U, Garbe C (2008). Epidemiology of melanoma and nonmelanoma skin cancer-the role of sunlight. Adv Exp Med Biol 624: 89-103.
1072. Lemoine NR, Hall PA (1986). Epithelial tumors metastatic to the uterine cervix. A study of 33 cases and review of the literature. Cancer 57: 2002-2005.
1073. Lenehan PM, Meffe F, Lickrish GM (1986). Vaginal intraepithelial neoplasia: biologic aspects and management. Obstet Gynecol 68: 333-337.
1074. Lennerz JK, Perry A, Mills JC, Huettner PC, Pfeifer JD (2009). Mucoepidermoid carcinoma of the cervix: another tumor with the t(11;19)-associated CRTC1-MAML2 gene fusion. Am J Surg Pathol 33: 835-843.
1075. Leon P, Daly JM, Synnestvedt M, Schultz DJ, Elder DE, Clark WH Jr (1991). The prognostic implications of microscopic satellites in patients with clinical stage I melanoma. Arch Surg 126: 1461-1468.
1076. Lerwill MF, Sung R, Oliva E, Prat J, Young RH (2004). Smooth muscle tumors of the ovary: a clinicopathologic study of 54 cases emphasizing prognostic criteria, histologic variants, and differential diagnosis. Am J Surg Pathol 28: 1436-1451.
1077. Lerwill MF, Young RH (2006). Ovarian metastases of intestinal-type gastric carcinoma: A clinicopathologic study of 4 cases with contrasting features to those of the Krukenberg tumor. Am J Surg Pathol 30: 1382-1388.
1078. Leuchter RS, Hacker NF, Voet RL, Berek JS, Townsend DE, Lagasse LD (1982). Primary carcinoma of the Bartholin gland: a report of 14 cases and review of the literature. Obstet Gynecol 60: 361-368.
1079. Levanon K, Crum C, Drapkin R (2008). New insights into the pathogenesis of serous ovarian cancer and its clinical impact. J Clin Oncol 26: 5284-5293.
1080. Levavi H, Sabah G, Kaplan B, Tytiun Y, Braslavsky D, Gutman H (2006). Granular cell tumor of the vulva: six new cases. Arch Gynecol Obstet 273: 246-249.
1081. Levine DA, Lin O, Barakat RR, Robson ME, McDermott D, Cohen L, Satagopan J, Offit K, Boyd J (2001). Risk of endometrial carcinoma associated with BRCA mutation. Gynecol Oncol 80: 395-398.
1082. Levine DA, Villella JA, Poynor EA, Soslow RA (2004). Gastrointestinal adenocarcinoma arising in a mature cystic teratoma of the ovary. Gynecol Oncol 94: 597-599.
1083. Levine PH, Abou-Nassar S, Mittal K (2001). Extrauterine low-grade endometrial stromal sarcoma with florid endometrioid glandular differentiation. Int J Gynecol Pathol 20: 395-398.
1083A. Lewis MR, Deavers MT, Silva EG, Malpica A (2006). Ovarian involvement by metastatic colorectal adenocarcinoma: still a diagnostic challenge. Am J Surg Pathol 30: 177-184.
1084. Li CC, Qian ZR, Hirokawa M, Sano T, Pan CC, Hsu CY, Yang AH, Chiang H (2004). Expression of adhesion molecules and Ki-67 in female adnexal tumor of probable Wolffian origin (FATWO): report of two cases and review of the literature. APMIS 112: 390-398.
1085. Li J, Ackerman AB (1994). "Seborrheic keratoses" that contain human papillomavirus are condylomata acuminata. Am J Dermatopathol 16: 398-405.
1086. Li JD, Zhuang Y, Li YF, Feng YL, Hou JH, Chen L, Zhu AN, Wu QL, Yun JP (2011). A clinicopathological aspect of primary small-cell carcinoma of the uterine cervix: a single-centre study of 25 cases. J Clin Pathol 64: 1102-1107.
1087. Li RF, Gupta M, McCluggage WG, Ronnett BM (2013). Embryonal rhabdomyosarcoma (botryoid type) of the uterine corpus and cervix in adult women: report of a case series and review of the literature. Am J Surg Pathol 37: 344-355.
1088. Li S, Zimmerman RL, LiVolsi VA (1999). Mixed malignant germ cell tumor of the fallopian tube. Int J Gynecol Pathol 18: 183-185.
1089. Li Y, Tabatabai ZL, Lee TL, Hatakeyama S, Ohyama C, Chan WY, Looijenga LH, Lau YF (2007). The Y-encoded TSPY protein: a significant marker potentially plays a role in the pathogenesis of testicular germ cell tumors. Hum Pathol 38: 1470-1481.
1090. Li Z, Gilbert C, Yang H, Zhao C (2012). Histologic follow-up in patients with Papanicolaou test findings of endometrial cells: results from a large academic women's hospital laboratory. Am J Clin Pathol 138: 79-84.
1091. Lialios G, Plataniotis G, Kallitsaris A, Theofanopoulou MA, Skoufi G, Messinis IE (2005). Vaginal metastasis from renal adenocarcinoma. Gynecol Oncol 98: 172-173.
1092. Liang SX, Pearl M, Liang S, Xiang L, Jia L, Yang B, Fadare O, Schwartz PE, Chambers SK, Kong B, Zheng W (2011). Personal history of breast cancer as a significant risk factor for endometrial serous carcinoma in women aged 55 years old or younger. Int J Cancer 128: 763-770.
1093. Liao X, Xin X, Lu X (2004). Primary Ewing's sarcoma-primitive neuroectodermal tumor of the vagina. Gynecol Oncol 92: 684-688.
1094. Liao XY, Xue WC, Shen DH, Ngan HY, Siu MK, Cheung AN (2007). p63 expression in ovarian tumours: a marker for Brenner tumours but not transitional cell carcinomas. Histopathology 51: 477-483.
1095. Lim D, Alvarez T, Nucci MR, Gilks B, Longacre T, Soslow RA, Oliva E (2013). Interobserver variability in the interpretation of tumor cell necrosis in uterine leiomyosarcoma. Am J Surg Pathol 37: 650-658.
1096. Lim GS, Oliva E (2011). The morphologic spectrum of uterine PEC-cell associated tumors in a patient with tuberous sclerosis. Int J Gynecol Pathol 30: 121-128.
1097. Lim KC, Thompson IW, Wiener JJ (2002). A case of primary clear cell adenocarcinoma of Bartholin's gland. BJOG 109: 1305-1307.
1098. Lim MC, Lee S, Seo SS (2010). Megestrol acetate therapy for advanced low-grade endometrial stromal sarcoma. Onkologie 33: 260-262.
1099. Lim SC, Choi SJ, Suh CH (1998). A case of small cell carcinoma arising in a mature cystic teratoma of the ovary. Pathol Int 48: 834-839.
1100. Lin MC, Lomo L, Baak JP, Eng C, Ince TA, Crum CP, Mutter GL (2009). Squamous morules are functionally inert elements of premalignant endometrial neoplasia. Mod Pathol 22: 167-174.
1101. Lin X, Lindner JL, Silverman JF, Liu Y (2008). Intestinal type and endocervical-like ovarian mucinous neoplasms are immunophenotypically distinct entities. Appl Immunohistochem Mol Morphol 16: 453-458.
1102. Lin YS, Eng HL, Jan YJ, Lee HS, Ho WL, Liou CP, Lee WY, Tzeng CC (2005). Molecular cytogenetics of ovarian granulosa cell tumors by comparative genomic hybridization. Gynecol Oncol 97: 68-73.
1103. Lindemann K, Vatten LJ, Ellstrom-Engh M, Eskild A (2008). Body mass, diabetes and smoking, and endometrial cancer risk: a follow-up study. Br J Cancer 98: 1582-1585.
1104. Linder D, McCaw BK, Hecht F (1975). Parthenogenic origin of benign ovarian teratomas. N Engl J Med 292: 63-66.
1105. Linder D, Power J (1970). Further evidence for post-meiotic origin of teratomas in the human female. Ann Hum Genet 34: 21-30.
1106. Lipata F, Parkash V, Talmor M, Bell S, Chen S, Maric V, Hui P (2010). Precise DNA genotyping diagnosis of hydatidiform mole. Obstet Gynecol 115: 784-794.
1107. Littman P, Clement PB, Henriksen B, Wang CC, Robboy SJ, Taft PD, Ulfelder H, Scully RE (1976). Glassy cell carcinoma of the cervix. Cancer 37: 2238-2246.
1108. Liu J, Albarracin CT, Chang KH, Thompson-Lanza JA, Zheng W, Gershenson DM, Broaddus R, Luthra R (2004). Microsatellite instability and expression of hMLH1 and hMSH2 proteins in ovarian endometrioid cancer. Mod Pathol 17: 75-80.
1109. Liu L, Davidson S, Singh M (2003). Mullerian adenosarcoma of vagina arising in persistent endometriosis: report of a case and review of the literature. Gynecol Oncol 90: 486-490.
1110. Lloreta J, Prat J (1992). Endometrial stromal nodule with smooth and skeletal muscle components simulating stromal sarcoma. Int J Gynecol Pathol 11: 293-298.
1111. Lobel MK, Somasundaram P, Morton CC (2006). The genetic heterogeneity of uterine leiomyomata. Obstet Gynecol Clin North Am 33: 13-39.
1112. Loddenkemper C, Mechsner S, Foss HD, Dallenbach FE, Anagnostopoulos I, Ebert AD, Stein H (2003). Use of oxytocin receptor expression in distinguishing between uterine smooth muscle tumors and endometrial stromal sarcoma. Am J Surg Pathol 27: 1458-1462.
1113. Logani S, Oliva E, Amin MB, Folpe AL, Cohen C, Young RH (2003). Immunoprofile of ovarian tumors with putative transitional cell (urothelial) differentiation using novel urothelial markers: histogenetic and diagnostic implications. Am J Surg Pathol 27: 1434-1441.
1114. Longacre TA, Chung MH, Jensen DN, Hendrickson MR (1995). Proposed criteria for the diagnosis of well-differentiated endometrial carcinoma. A diagnostic test for myoinvasion. Am J Surg Pathol 19: 371-406.
1115. Longacre TA, Chung MH, Rouse RV, Hendrickson MR (1996). Atypical polypoid adenomyofibromas (atypical polypoid adenomyomas) of the uterus. A clinicopathologic study of 55 cases. Am J Surg Pathol 20: 1-20.
1116. Longacre TA, Hendrickson MR, Kapp DS, Teng NN (1996). Lymphangioleiomyomatosis of the uterus simulating high-stage endometrial stromal sarcoma. Gynecol Oncol 63: 404-410.
1117. Longacre TA, McKenney JK, Tazelaar HD, Kempson RL, Hendrickson MR (2005). Ovarian serous tumors of low malignant potential (borderline tumors): outcome-based study of 276 patients with long-term (> or =5-year) follow-up. Am J Surg Pathol 29: 707-723.
1118. Longy M, Toulouse C, Mage P, Chauvergne J, Trojani M (1996). Familial cluster of ovarian small cell carcinoma: a new mendelian entity? J Med Genet 33: 333-335.
1119. Look KY, Brunetto VL, Clarke-Pearson DL, Averette HE, Major FJ, Alvarez RD, Homesley HD, Zaino RJ (1996). An analysis of cell type in patients with surgically staged stage IB carcinoma of the cervix: a Gynecologic Oncology Group study. Gynecol Oncol 63: 304-311.
1120. Lopez-Garcia MA, Palacios J (2010). Pathologic and molecular features of uterine carcinosarcomas. Semin Diagn Pathol 27: 274-286.
1121. Lopez-Rios F, Miguel PS, Bellas C, Ballestin C, Hernandez L (2000). Lymphoepithelioma-like carcinoma of the uterine cervix: a case report studied by in situ hybridization and polymerase chain reaction for Epstein-Barr virus. Arch Pathol Lab Med 124: 746-747.
1122. Lorincz AT, Reid R, Jenson AB, Greenberg MD, Lancaster W, Kurman RJ

(1992). Human papillomavirus infection of the cervix: relative risk associations of 15 common anogenital types. Obstet Gynecol 79: 328-337.
1123. Lotocki RJ, Krepart GV, Paraskevas M, Vadas G, Heywood M, Fung FK (1992). Glassy cell carcinoma of the cervix: a bimodal treatment strategy. Gynecol Oncol 44: 254-259.
1124. Lovell MA, Ross GW, Cooper PH (1989). Gliomatosis peritonei associated with a ventriculoperitoneal shunt. Am J Clin Pathol 91: 485-487.
1125. Loverro G, Cormio G, Renzulli G, Lepera A, Ricco R, Selvaggi L (1997). Serous papillary cystadenoma of borderline malignancy of the broad ligament. Eur J Obstet Gynecol Reprod Biol 74: 211-213.
1126. Lu FI, Gilks CB, Mulligan AM, Ryan P, Allo G, Sy K, Shaw PA, Pollett A, Clarke BA (2012). Prevalence of loss of expression of DNA mismatch repair proteins in primary epithelial ovarian tumors. Int J Gynecol Pathol 31: 524-531.
1127. Lu L, Risch H, Irwin ML, Mayne ST, Cartmel B, Schwartz P, Rutherford T, Yu H (2011). Long-term overweight and weight gain in early adulthood in association with risk of endometrial cancer. Int J Cancer 129: 1237-1243.
1128. Lucia SP, Mills H, Lowenhaupt E, Hunt ML (1952). Visceral involvement in primary neoplastic diseases of the reticulo-endothelial system. Cancer 5: 1193-1200.
1129. Ludwick C, Gilks CB, Miller D, Yaziji H, Clement PB (2005). Aggressive behavior of stage I ovarian mucinous tumors lacking extensive infiltrative invasion: a report of four cases and review of the literature. Int J Gynecol Pathol 24: 205-217.
1130. Luft F, Gebert J, Schneider A, Melsheimer P, von Knebel Doeberitz M (1999). Frequent allelic imbalance of tumor suppressor gene loci in cervical dysplasia. Int J Gynecol Pathol 18: 374-380.
1131. Lurain JR (2011). Gestational trophoblastic disease II: classification and management of gestational trophoblastic neoplasia. Am J Obstet Gynecol 204: 11-18.
1132. Lurain JR, Brewer JI, Torok EE, Halpern B (1983). Natural history of hydatidiform mole after primary evacuation. Am J Obstet Gynecol 145: 591-595.
1133. Lv L, Yang K, Wu H, Lou J, Peng Z (2011). Pure choriocarcinoma of the ovary: a case report. J Gynecol Oncol 22: 135-139.
1134. Ly A, Mills AM, McKenney JK, Balzer BL, Kempson RL, Hendrickson MR, Longacre TA (2013). Atypical leiomyomas of the uterus: a clinicopathologic study of 51 cases. Am J Surg Pathol 37: 643-649.
1135. Lyth J, Hansson J, Ingvar C, Mansson-Brahme E, Naredi P, Stierner U, Wagenius G, Lindholm C (2013). Prognostic subclassifications of T1 cutaneous melanomas based on ulceration, tumour thickness and Clark's level of invasion: results of a population-based study from the Swedish Melanoma Register. Br J Dermatol 168: 779-786.
1136. Ma J, Shi QL, Zhou XJ, Meng K, Chen JY, Huang WB (2007). Lymphoma-like lesion of the uterine cervix: report of 12 cases of a rare entity. Int J Gynecol Pathol 26: 194-198.
1137. Mabuchi S, Okazawa M, Kinose Y, Matsuo K, Fujiwara M, Suzuki O, Morii E, Kamiura S, Ogawa K, Kimura T (2012). Comparison of the prognoses of FIGO stage I to stage II adenosquamous carcinoma and adenocarcinoma of the uterine cervix treated with radical hysterectomy. Int J Gynecol Cancer 22: 1389-1397.
1138. Amador-Ortiz C, Roma AA, Huettner PC, Becker N, Pfeifer JD (2011). JAZF1 and JJAZ1 gene fusion in primary extrauterine endometrial stromal sarcoma. Hum Pathol 42: 939-946.
1139. Maeda D, Shibahara J, Sakuma T, Isobe M, Teshima S, Mori M, Oda K, Nakagawa S, Taketani Y, Ishikawa S, Fukayama M (2011). beta-catenin (CTNNB1) S33C mutation in ovarian microcystic stromal tumors. Am J Surg Pathol 35: 1429-1440.
1140. Maggiani F, Debiec-Rychter M, Vanbockrijck M, Sciot R (2007). Cellular angiofibroma: another mesenchymal tumour with 13q14 involvement, suggesting a link with spindle cell lipoma and (extra)-mammary myofibroblastoma. Histopathology 51: 410-412.
1141. Maglione MA, Tricarico OD, Calandria L (2002). Malignant peripheral nerve sheath tumor of the vulva. A case report. J Reprod Med 47: 721-724.
1142. Magrina JF, Gonzalez-Bosquet J, Weaver AL, Gaffey TA, Leslie KO, Webb MJ, Podratz KC (2000). Squamous cell carcinoma of the vulva stage IA: long-term results. Gynecol Oncol 76: 24-27.
1143. Magro G, Caltabiano R, Kacerovska D, Vecchio GM, Kazakov D, Michal M (2012). Vulvovaginal myofibroblastoma: expanding the morphological and immunohistochemical spectrum. A clinicopathologic study of 10 cases. Hum Pathol 43: 243-253.
1144. Magro G, Righi A, Casorzo L, Antonietta T, Salvatorelli L, Kacerovska D, Kazakov D, Michal M (2012). Mammary and vaginal myofibroblastomas are genetically related lesions: fluorescence in situ hybridization analysis shows deletion of 13q14 region. Hum Pathol 43: 1887-1893.
1145. Mahdavi A, Silberberg B, Malviya VK, Braunstein AH, Shapiro J (2003). Gangliocytic paraganglioma arising from mature cystic teratoma of the ovary. Gynecol Oncol 90: 482-485.
1146. Majmudar B, Castellano PZ, Wilson RW, Siegel RJ (1990). Granular cell tumors of the vulva. J Reprod Med 35: 1008-1014.
1147. Major FJ, Blessing JA, Silverberg SG, Morrow CP, Creasman WT, Currie JL, Yordan E, Brady MF (1993). Prognostic factors in early-stage uterine sarcoma. A Gynecologic Oncology Group study. Cancer 71: 1702-1709.
1148. Makinen N, Vahteristo P, Kampjarvi K, Arola J, Butzow R, Aaltonen LA (2013). MED12 exon 2 mutations in histopathological uterine leiomyoma variants. Eur J Hum Genet 21: 1300-1303.
1149. Maleki Z, Kim HS, Thonse VR, Judson K, Vinh TN, Vang R (2010). Uterine artery embolization with trisacryl gelatin microspheres in women treated for leiomyomas: a clinicopathologic analysis of alterations in gynecologic surgical specimens. Int J Gynecol Pathol 29: 260-268.
1150. Malinowska I, Kwiatkowski DJ, Weiss S, Martignoni G, Netto G, Argani P (2012). Perivascular epithelioid cell tumors (PEComas) harboring TFE3 gene rearrangements lack the TSC2 alterations characteristic of conventional PEComas: further evidence for a biological distinction. Am J Surg Pathol 36: 783-784.
1151. Malpica A, Deavers MT (2011). Ovarian low-grade serous carcinoma involving the cervix mimicking a cervical primary. Int J Gynecol Pathol 30: 613-619.
1152. Malpica A, Deavers MT, Lu K, Bodurka DC, Atkinson EN, Gershenson DM, Silva EG (2004). Grading ovarian serous carcinoma using a two-tier system. Am J Surg Pathol 28: 496-504.
1153. Malpica A, Deavers MT, Tornos C, Kurman RJ, Soslow R, Seidman JD, Munsell MF, Gaertner E, Frishberg D, Silva EG (2007). Interobserver and intraobserver variability of a two-tier system for grading ovarian serous carcinoma. Am J Surg Pathol 31: 1168-1174.
1154. Malpica A, Sant'Ambrogio S, Deavers MT, Silva EG (2012). Well-differentiated papillary mesothelioma of the female peritoneum: a clinicopathologic study of 26 cases. Am J Surg Pathol 36: 117-127.
1155. Manawapat A, Stubenrauch F, Russ R, Munk C, Kjaer SK, Iftner T (2012). Physical state and viral load as predictive biomarkersfor persistence and progression of HPV16-positive cervical lesions: results from a population based long-term prospective cohort study. Am J Cancer Res 2: 192-203.
1156. Mandai M, Konishi I, Kuroda H, Komatsu T, Yamamoto S, Nanbu K, Matsushita K, Fukumoto M, Yamabe H, Mori T (1998). Heterogeneous distribution of K-ras-mutated epithelia in mucinous ovarian tumors with special reference to histopathology. Hum Pathol 29: 34-40.
1157. Mangili G, Taccagni G, Garavaglia E, Carnelli M, Montoli S (2004). An unusual admixture of neoplastic and metaplastic lesions of the female genital tract in the Peutz-Jeghers Syndrome. Gynecol Oncol 92: 337-342.
1158. Mani H, Merino MJ (2010). Mesothelial neoplasms presenting as, and mimicking, ovarian cancer. Int J Gynecol Pathol 29: 523-528.
1159. Maniar KP, Ronnett BM, Vang R, Yemelyanova A (2013). Coexisting high-grade vulvar intraepithelial neoplasia (VIN) and condyloma acuminatum: independent lesions due to different HPV types occurring in immunocompromised patients. Am J Surg Pathol 37: 53-60.
1160. Maniar KP, Wang Y, Visvanathan K, Shih IM, Kurman RJ (2014). Evaluation of microinvasion and lymph node involvement in ovarian serous borderline/atypical proliferative serous tumors: a morphologic and immunohistochemical analysis of 37 cases. Am J Surg Pathol; Epub ahead of print.
1161. Mannion C, Park WS, Man YG, Zhuang Z, Albores-Saavedra J, Tavassoli FA (1998). Endocrine tumors of the cervix: morphologic assessment, expression of human papillomavirus, and evaluation for loss of heterozygosity on 1p,3p, 11q, and 17p. Cancer 83: 1391-1400.
1162. Manoharan M, Azmi MA, Soosay G, Mould T, Weekes AR (2007). Mullerian adenosarcoma of uterine cervix: report of three cases and review of literature. Gynecol Oncol 105: 256-260.
1163. Mansouri H, Sifat H, Gaye M, Hassouni K, Mansouri A, El GB (2000). Primary malignant lymphoma of the ovary: an unusual presentation of a rare disease. Eur J Gynaecol Oncol 21: 616-618.
1164. Mao TL, Kurman RJ, Huang CC, Lin MC, Shih I (2007). Immunohistochemistry of choriocarcinoma: an aid in differential diagnosis and in elucidating pathogenesis. Am J Surg Pathol 31: 1726-1732.
1165. Mao TL, Seidman JD, Kurman RJ, Shih I (2006). Cyclin E and p16 immunoreactivity in epithelioid trophoblastic tumor--an aid in differential diagnosis. Am J Surg Pathol 30: 1105-1110.
1165A. Mardi K, Gupta N, Bindra R (2011). Primary yolk sac tumor of cervix and vagina in an adult female: a rare case report. Indian J Cancer 48: 515-516.
1166. Mariani A, Nascimento AG, Webb MJ, Sim FH, Podratz KC (2000). Surgical management of desmoid tumors of the female pelvis. J Am Coll Surg 191: 175-183.
1167. Markowski DN, Huhle S, Nimzyk R, Stenman G, Loning T, Bullerdiek J (2013). MED12 mutations occurring in benign and malignant mammalian smooth muscle tumors. Genes Chromosomes Cancer 52: 297-304.
1168. Marsden JR, Newton-Bishop JA, Burrows L, Cook M, Corrie PG, Cox NH, Gore ME, Lorigan P, MacKie R, Nathan P, Peach H, Powell B, Walker C (2010). Revised U.K. guidelines for the management of cutaneous melanoma 2010. Br J Dermatol 163: 238-256.
1169. Marshall RJ, Braye SG, Jones DB (1986). Leiomyosarcoma of the uterus with giant cells resembling osteoclasts. Int J Gynecol Pathol 5: 260-268.
1169A. Masand RP, Malpica A, Ramalingam P (2013). PAX-8 and ER in mucinous tumours in the ovary: Are they useful in distinguishing primary from metastasis? Lab Investigation 93: 288A.
1169B. Masand RP, Euscher ED, Deavers MT, Malpica A (2013). Endometrioid stromal sarcoma: a clinicopathologic study of 63 cases. Am J Surg Pathol 37:1635-1647.
1170. Martignoni G, Pea M, Reghellin D, Gobbo S, Zamboni G, Chilosi M, Bonetti F (2010). Molecular pathology of lymphangioleiomyomatosis and other perivascular epithelioid cell tumors. Arch Pathol Lab Med 134: 33-40.
1171. Martin PM (1978). High frequency of hydatidiform mole in native Alaskans. Int J Gynaecol Obstet 15: 395-396.
1172. Martinez-Roman S, Frumovitz M, Deavers MT, Ramirez PT (2005). Metastatic carcinoma of the gallbladder mimicking an advanced cervical carcinoma. Gynecol Oncol 97: 942-945.
1173. Martorell MA, Julian JM, Calabuig C, Garcia-Garcia JA, Perez-Valles A (2002). Lymphoepithelioma-like carcinoma of the uterine cervix. Arch Pathol Lab Med 126: 1501-1505.
1174. Marzano DA, Haefner HK (2004). The bartholin gland cyst: past, present, and future. J Low Genit Tract Dis 8: 195-204.
1175. Mashal RD, Fejzo ML, Friedman AJ, Mitchner N, Nowak RA, Rein MS, Morton CC, Sklar J (1994). Analysis of androgen receptor DNA reveals the independent clonal origins of uterine leiomyomata and the secondary nature of cytogenetic aberrations in the development of leiomyomata. Genes Chromosomes Cancer 11: 1-6.
1176. Masih AS, Stoler MH, Farrow GM, Wooldridge TN, Johansson SL (1992). Penile verrucous carcinoma: a clinicopathologic, human papillomavirus typing and flow cytometric analysis. Mod Pathol 5: 48-55.
1177. Massad LS, Jeronimo J, Katki HA, Schiffman M (2009). The accuracy of colposcopic grading for detection of high-grade cervical intraepithelial neoplasia. J Low Genit Tract Dis 13: 137-144.
1178. Massad LS, Xie X, Darragh T, Minkoff H, Levine AM, Watts DH, Wright RL, D'Souza G, Colie C, Strickler HD (2011). Genital warts and vulvar intraepithelial neoplasia: natural history and effects of treatment and human immunodeficiency virus infection. Obstet Gynecol 118: 831-839.
1179. Matias-Guiu X, Catasus L, Bussaglia E, Lagarda H, Garcia A, Pons C, Munoz J, Arguelles R, Machin P, Prat J (2001). Molecular pathology of endometrial hyperplasia and carcinoma. Hum Pathol 32: 569-577.
1180. Matias-Guiu X, Prat J (2013). Molecular pathology of endometrial carcinoma. Histopathology 62: 111-123.
1181. Matsui H, Iizuka Y, Sekiya S (1996). Incidence of invasive mole and choriocarcinoma following partial hydatidiform mole. Int J Gynaecol Obstet 53: 63-64.
1182. Matsumoto T, Hiura M, Baba T, Ishiko O, Shiozawa T, Yaegashi N, Kobayashi H, Yoshikawa H, Kawamura N, Kaku T (2013). Clinical management of atypical polypoid adenomyoma of the uterus. A clinicopathological review of 29 cases. Gynecol Oncol 129: 54-57.
1183. Matsuno RK, Sherman ME, Visvanathan

K, Goodman MT, Hernandez BY, Lynch CF, Ioffe OB, Horio D, Platz C, Altekruse SF, Pfeiffer RM, Anderson WF (2013). Agreement for tumor grade of ovarian carcinoma: analysis of archival tissues from the surveillance, epidemiology, and end results residual tissue repository. Cancer Causes Control 24: 749-757.
1184. Matsuura J, Chiu D, Jacobs PA, Szulman AE (1984). Complete hydatidiform mole in Hawaii: an epidemiological study. Genet Epidemiol 1: 271-284.
1185. Matsuura Y, Murakami N, Nagashio E, Toki N, Kashimura M (2001). Glassy cell carcinoma of the uterine cervix: combination chemotherapy with paclitaxel and carboplatin in recurrent tumor. J Obstet Gynaecol Res 27: 129-132.
1186. Matsuura Y, Robertson G, Marsden DE, Kim SN, Gebski V, Hacker NF (2007). Thromboembolic complications in patients with clear cell carcinoma of the ovary. Gynecol Oncol 104: 406-410.
1187. Matsuzaki S, Murakami T, Sato S, Moriya T, Sasano H, Yajima A (2000). Endomyometriosis arising in the uterosacral ligament: a case report including a literature review and immunohistochemical analysis. Pathol Int 50: 493-496.
1188. Matthews T, Amanuel B, Tsokos N (2003). Atypical leiomyoma of the broad ligament. Aust N Z J Obstet Gynaecol 43: 326-328.
1189. Mauland KK, Trovik J, Wik E, Raeder MB, Njolstad TS, Stefansson IM, Oyan AM, Kalland KH, Bjorge T, Akslen LA, Salvesen HB (2011). High BMI is significantly associated with positive progesterone receptor status and clinico-pathological markers for non-aggressive disease in endometrial cancer. Br J Cancer 104: 921-926.
1189A. Mauz-Körholz C, Harms D, Calaminus G, Göbel U (2000). Primary chemotherapy and conservative surgery for vaginal yolk-sac tumour. Maligne Keimzelltumoren Study Group. Lancet 355: 625.
1190. Mavaddat N, Barrowdale D, Andrulis IL, Domchek SM, Eccles D, Nevanlinna H, Ramus SJ, Spurdle A, Robson M, Sherman M, Mulligan AM, Couch FJ, Engel C, McGuffog L, Healey S, Sinilnikova OM, Southey MC, Terry MB, Goldgar D, O'Malley F, John EM, Janavicius R, Tihomirova L, Hansen TV, Nielsen FC, Osorio A, Stavropoulou A, Benitez J, Manoukian S, Peissel B, Barile M, Volorio S, Pasini B, Dolcetti R, Putignano AL, Ottini L, Radice P, Hamann U, Rashid MU, Hogervorst FB, Kriege M, van der Luijt RB, Peock S, Frost D, Evans DG, Brewer C, Walker L, Rogers MT, Side LE, Houghton C, Weaver J, Godwin AK, Schmutzler RK, Wappenschmidt B, Meindl A, Kast K, Arnold N, Niederacher D, Sutter C, Deissler H, Gadzicki D, Preisler-Adams S, Varon-Mateeva R, Schonbuchner I, Gevensleben H, Stoppa-Lyonnet D, Belotti M, Barjhoux L, Isaacs C, Peshkin BN, Caldes T, de la Hoya M, Canadas C, Heikkinen T, Heikkila P, Aittomaki K, Blanco I, Lazaro C, Brunet J, Agnarsson BA, Arason A, Barkardottir RB, Dumont M, Simard J, Montagna M, Agata S, D'Andrea E, Yan M, Fox S, Rebbeck TR, Rubinstein W, Tung N, Garber JE, Wang X, Fredericksen Z, Pankratz VS, Lindor NM, Szabo C, Offit K, Sakr R, Gaudet MM, Singer CF, Tea MK, Rappaport C, Mai PL, Greene MH, Sokolenko A, Imyanitov E, Toland AE, Senter L, Sweet K, Thomassen M, Gerdes AM, Kruse T, Caligo M, Aretini P, Rantala J, von Wachenfeld A, Henriksson K, Steele L, Neuhausen SL, Nussbaum R, Beattie M, Odunsi K, Sucheston L, Gayther SA, Nathanson K, Gross J, Walsh C, Karlan B, Chenevix-Trench G, Easton DF, Antoniou AC (2012). Pathology of breast and ovarian cancers among BRCA1 and BRCA2 mutation carriers: results from the Consortium of Investigators of Modifiers of BRCA1/2 (CIMBA). Cancer Epidemiol Biomarkers Prev 21: 134-147.
1190A. May T, Virtanen C, Sharma M, Milea A, Begley H, Rosen B, Murphy KJ, Brown TJ, Shaw PA (2010). Low malignant potential tumors with micropapillary features are molecularly similar to low-grade serous carcinoma of the ovary. Gynecol Oncol 117: 9-17.
1191. Mayerhofer K, Obermair A, Windbichler G, Petru E, Kaider A, Hefler L, Czerwenka K, Leodolter S, Kainz C (1999). Leiomyosarcoma of the uterus: a clinicopathologic multicenter study of 71 cases. Gynecol Oncol 74: 196-201.
1192. Mayr D, Hirschmann A, Lohrs U, Diebold J (2006). KRAS and BRAF mutations in ovarian tumors: a comprehensive study of invasive carcinomas, borderline tumors and extraovarian implants. Gynecol Oncol 103: 883-887.
1193. Mazur MT (1981). Atypical polypoid adenomyomas of the endometrium. Am J Surg Pathol 5: 473-482.
1194. Mazur MT, Hsueh S, Gersell DJ (1984). Metastases to the female genital tract. Analysis of 325 cases. Cancer 53: 1978-1984.
1195. Mazur MT, Kurman RJ (2005). Diagnosis of Endometrial Biopsies and Curettings: A Practical Approach. 2nd Ed. Springer: New York.
1196. Mazur MT, Shultz JJ, Myers JL (1990). Granular cell tumor. Immunohistochemical analysis of 21 benign tumors and one malignant tumor. Arch Pathol Lab Med 114: 692-696.
1197. McAdam JA, Stewart F, Reid R (1998). Vaginal epithelioid angiosarcoma. J Clin Pathol 51: 928-930.
1198. McCarter MD, Quan SH, Busam K, Paty PP, Wong D, Guillem JG (2003). Long-term outcome of perianal Paget's disease. Dis Colon Rectum 46: 612-616.
1199. McCarthy DM, Hruban RH, Argani P, Howe JR, Conlon KC, Brennan MF, Zahurak M, Wilentz RE, Cameron JL, Yeo CJ, Kern SE, Klimstra DS (2003). Role of the DPC4 tumor suppressor gene in adenocarcinoma of the ampulla of Vater: analysis of 140 cases. Mod Pathol 16: 272-278.
1200. McCaughey WT, Kirk ME, Lester W, Dardick I (1984). Peritoneal epithelial lesions associated with proliferative serous tumours of ovary. Histopathology 8: 195-208.
1201. McClean GE, Kurian S, Walter N, Kekre A, McCluggage WG (2007). Cervical embryonal rhabdomyosarcoma and ovarian Sertoli-Leydig cell tumour: a more than coincidental association of two rare neoplasms? J Clin Pathol 60: 326-328.
1202. McCluggage WG (2002). Malignant biphasic uterine tumours: carcinosarcomas or metaplastic carcinomas? J Clin Pathol 55: 321-325.
1203. McCluggage WG (2003). Endocervical glandular lesions: controversial aspects and ancillary techniques. J Clin Pathol 56: 164-173.
1204. McCluggage WG (2005). Immunoreactivity of ovarian juvenile granulosa cell tumours with epithelial membrane antigen. Histopathology 46: 235-236.
1205. McCluggage WG (2008). My approach to and thoughts on the typing of ovarian carcinomas. J Clin Pathol 61: 152-163.
1206. McCluggage WG (2010). Miscellaneous disorders involving the endometrium. Semin Diagn Pathol 27: 287-310.
1207. McCluggage WG (2010). Mullerian adenosarcoma of the female genital tract. Adv Anat Pathol 17: 122-129.
1208. McCluggage WG (2013). New developments in endocervical glandular lesions. Histopathology 62: 138-160.
1209. McCluggage WG, Abdulkader M, Price JH, Kelehan P, Hamilton S, Beattie J, Al-Nafussi A (2000). Uterine carcinosarcomas in patients receiving tamoxifen. A report of 19 cases. Int J Gynecol Cancer 10: 280-284.
1210. McCluggage WG, Aydin NE, Wong NA, Cooper K (2009). Low-grade epithelial-myoepithelial carcinoma of bartholin gland: report of 2 cases of a distinctive neoplasm arising in the vulvovaginal region. Int J Gynecol Pathol 28: 286-291.
1211. McCluggage WG, Bissonnette JP, Young RH (2006). Primary malignant melanoma of the ovary: a report of 9 definite or probable cases with emphasis on their morphologic diversity and mimicry of other primary and secondary ovarian neoplasms. Int J Gynecol Pathol 25: 321-329.
1212. McCluggage WG, Connolly L, McBride HA (2010). HMGA2 is a sensitive but not specific immunohistochemical marker of vulvovaginal aggressive angiomyxoma. Am J Surg Pathol 34: 1037-1042.
1213. McCluggage WG, Cromie AJ, Bryson C, Traub AI (2001). Uterine endometrial stromal sarcoma with smooth muscle and glandular differentiation. J Clin Pathol 54: 481-483.
1214. McCluggage WG, Date A, Bharucha H, Toner PG (1996). Endometrial stromal sarcoma with sex cord-like areas and focal rhabdoid differentiation. Histopathology 29: 369-374.
1215. McCluggage WG, Ganesan R, Herrington CS (2009). Endometrial stromal sarcomas with extensive endometrioid glandular differentiation: report of a series with emphasis on the potential for misdiagnosis and discussion of the differential diagnosis. Histopathology 54: 365-373.
1216. McCluggage WG, Ganesan R, Hirschowitz L, Rollason TP (2004). Cellular angiofibroma and related fibromatous lesions of the vulva: report of a series of cases with a morphological spectrum wider than previously described. Histopathology 45: 360-368.
1217. McCluggage WG, Harley I, Houghton JP, Geyer FC, MacKay A, Reis-Filho JS (2010). Composite cervical adenocarcinoma composed of adenoma malignum and gastric type adenocarcinoma (dedifferentiated adenoma malignum) in a patient with Peutz Jeghers syndrome. J Clin Pathol 63: 935-941.
1218. McCluggage WG, Jamieson T, Dobbs SP, Grey A (2006). Aggressive angiomyxoma of the vulva: Dramatic response to gonadotropin-releasing hormone agonist therapy. Gynecol Oncol 100: 623-625.
1219. McCluggage WG, Kennedy K, Busam KJ (2010). An immunohistochemical study of cervical neuroendocrine carcinomas: Neoplasms that are commonly TTF1 positive and which may express CK20 and P63. Am J Surg Pathol 34: 525-532.
1220. McCluggage WG, Lioe TF, McClelland HR, Lamki H (2002). Rhabdomyosarcoma of the uterus: report of two cases, including one of the spindle cell variant. Int J Gynecol Cancer 12: 128-132.
1221. McCluggage WG, Nielsen GP, Young RH (2008). Massive vulval edema secondary to obesity and immobilization: a potential mimic of aggressive angiomyxoma. Int J Gynecol Pathol 27: 447-452.
1222. McCluggage WG, Nirmala V, Radhakumari K (1999). Intramural mullerian papilloma of the vagina. Int J Gynecol Pathol 18: 94-95.
1223. McCluggage WG, Oliva E, Connolly LE, McBride HA, Young RH (2004). An immunohistochemical analysis of ovarian small cell carcinoma of hypercalcemic type. Int J Gynecol Pathol 23: 330-336.
1224. McCluggage WG, Oliva E, Herrington CS, McBride H, Young RH (2003). CD10 and calretinin staining of endocervical glandular lesions, endocervical stroma and endometrioid adenocarcinomas of the uterine corpus: CD10 positivity is characteristic of, but not specific for, mesonephric lesions and is not specific for endometrial stroma. Histopathology 43: 144-150.
1225. McCluggage WG, Patterson A, Maxwell P (2000). Aggressive angiomyxoma of pelvic parts exhibits oestrogen and progesterone receptor positivity. J Clin Pathol 53: 603-605.
1226. McCluggage WG, Price JH, Dobbs SP (2001). Primary adenocarcinoma of the vagina arising in endocervicosis. Int J Gynecol Pathol 20: 399-402.
1227. McCluggage WG, Smith JH (2011). Reactive fibroblastic and myofibroblastic proliferation of the vulva (Cyclist's Nodule): A hitherto poorly described vulval lesion occurring in cyclists. Am J Surg Pathol 35: 110-114.
1228. McCluggage WG, Sumathi VP, Nucci MR, Hirsch M, Dal Cin P, Wells M, Flanagan AM, Fisher C (2007). Ewing family of tumours involving the vulva and vagina: report of a series of four cases. J Clin Pathol 60: 674-680.
1229. McCluggage WG, Young RH (2006). Paraganglioma of the ovary: report of three cases of a rare ovarian neoplasm, including two exhibiting inhibin positivity. Am J Surg Pathol 30: 600-605.
1230. McCluggage WG, Young RH (2007). Ovarian sertoli-leydig cell tumors with pseudoendometrioid tubules (pseudoendometrioid sertoli-leydig cell tumors). Am J Surg Pathol 31: 592-597.
1231. McCluggage WG, Young RH (2008). Endometrial stromal sarcomas with true papillae and pseudopapillae. Int J Gynecol Pathol 27: 555-561.
1232. McCluggage WG, Young RH (2008). Primary ovarian mucinous tumors with signet ring cells: report of 3 cases with discussion of so-called primary Krukenberg tumor. Am J Surg Pathol 32: 1373-1379.
1233. McConechy MK, Ding J, Cheang MC, Wiegand KC, Senz J, Tone AA, Yang W, Prentice LM, Tse K, Zeng T, McDonald H, Schmidt AP, Mutch DG, McAlpine JN, Hirst M, Shah SP, Lee CH, Goodfellow PJ, Gilks CB, Huntsman DG (2012). Use of mutation profiles to refine the classification of endometrial carcinomas. J Pathol 228: 20-30.
1234. McConnell TG, Murphy KM, Hafez M, Vang R, Ronnett BM (2009). Diagnosis and subclassification of hydatidiform moles using p57 immunohistochemistry and molecular genotyping: validation and prospective analysis in routine and consultation practice settings with development of an algorithmic approach. Am J Surg Pathol 33: 805-817.
1235. McCoubrey A, Houghton O, McCallion K, McCluggage WG (2005). Serous adenocarcinoma of the sigmoid mesentery arising in cystic endosalpingiosis. J Clin Pathol 58: 1221-1223.
1236. McCredie MR, Sharples KJ, Paul C, Baranyai J, Medley G, Jones RW, Skegg DC (2008). Natural history of cervical neoplasia and risk of invasive cancer in women with cervical intraepithelial neoplasia 3: a retrospective cohort study. Lancet Oncol 9: 425-434.
1237. McCullough ML, Patel AV, Patel R, Rodriguez C, Feigelson HS, Bandera EV, Gansler T, Thun MJ, Calle EE (2008). Body mass and endometrial cancer risk by hormone replacement therapy and cancer subtype. Cancer Epidemiol Biomarkers Prev 17: 73-79.
1238. McDonald AG, Dal Cin P, Ganguly A, Campbell S, Imai Y, Rosenberg AE, Oliva E (2011). Liposarcoma arising in uterine lipoleiomyoma: a report of 3 cases and review of the literature. Am J Surg Pathol 35: 221-227.

1239. McFadden DE, Clement PB (1986). Peritoneal inclusion cysts with mural mesothelial proliferation. A clinicopathological analysis of six cases. Am J Surg Pathol 10: 844-854.
1240. McKenney JK, Balzer BL, Longacre TA (2006). Patterns of stromal invasion in ovarian serous tumors of low malignant potential (borderline tumors): a reevaluation of the concept of stromal microinvasion. Am J Surg Pathol 30: 1209-1221.
1241. McKenney JK, Soslow RA, Longacre TA (2008). Ovarian mature teratomas with mucinous epithelial neoplasms: morphologic heterogeneity and association with pseudomyxoma peritonei. Am J Surg Pathol 32: 645-655.
1242. McLachlin CM, Kozakewich H, Craighill M, O'Connell B, Crum CP (1994). Histologic correlates of vulvar human papillomavirus infection in children and young adults. Am J Surg Pathol 18: 728-735.
1243. McMeekin DS, Alektiar KM, Sabbatini PJ, Zaino R (2009). Corpus: epithelial tumours. In: Principles and practice of gynecologic oncology. Principles and practice of gynecologic oncology. 683-732.
1244. Medeiros F, Erickson-Johnson MR, Keeney GL, Clayton AC, Nascimento AG, Wang X, Oliveira AM (2007). Frequency and characterization of HMGA2 and HMGA1 rearrangements in mesenchymal tumors of the lower genital tract. Genes Chromosomes Cancer 46: 981-990.
1245. Medeiros F, Muto MG, Lee Y, Elvin JA, Callahan MJ, Feltmate C, Garber JE, Cramer DW, Crum CP (2006). The tubal fimbria is a preferred site for early adenocarcinoma in women with familial ovarian cancer syndrome. Am J Surg Pathol 30: 230-236.
1246. Medeiros F, Nascimento AF, Crum CP (2005). Early vulvar squamous neoplasia: advances in classification, diagnosis, and differential diagnosis. Adv Anat Pathol 12: 20-26.
1247. Meenakshi M, McCluggage WG (2009). Myoepithelial neoplasms involving the vulva and vagina: report of 4 cases. Hum Pathol 40: 1747-1753.
1248. Mehes G, Hegyi K, Csonka T, Fazakas F, Kocsis Z, Radvanyi G, Vadnay I, Bagdi E, Krenacs L (2012). Primary uterine NK-cell lymphoma, nasal-type: a unique malignancy of a prominent cell type of the endometrium. Pathol Oncol Res 18: 519-522.
1249. Mehrad M, Ning G, Chen EY, Mehra KK, Crum CP (2010). A pathologist's road map to benign, precancerous, and malignant intraepithelial proliferations in the fallopian tube. Adv Anat Pathol 17: 293-302.
1250. Meisels A, Fortin R (1976). Condylomatous lesions of the cervix and vagina. I. Cytologic patterns. Acta Cytol 20: 505-509.
1251. Melhem MF, Tobon H (1987). Mucinous adenocarcinoma of the endometrium: a clinico-pathological review of 18 cases. Int J Gynecol Pathol 6: 347-355.
1252. Mendez LE, Joy S, Angioli R, Estape R, Penalver M (1999). Primary uterine angiosarcoma. Gynecol Oncol 75: 272-276.
1253. Meriden Z, Yemelyanova AV, Vang R, Ronnett BM (2011). Ovarian metastases of pancreaticobiliary tract adenocarcinomas: analysis of 35 cases, with emphasis on the ability of metastases to simulate primary ovarian mucinous tumors. Am J Surg Pathol 35: 276-288.
1254. Meydanli MM, Kucukali T, Usubutun A, Ataoglu O, Kafkasli A (2002). Epithelioid trophoblastic tumor of the endocervix: a case report. Gynecol Oncol 87: 219-224.
1255. Meyer LA, Broaddus RR, Lu KH (2009). Endometrial cancer and Lynch syndrome: clinical and pathologic considerations. Cancer Control 16: 14-22.
1256. Micci F, Panagopoulos I, Bjerkehagen B, Heim S (2006). Consistent rearrangement of chromosomal band 6p21 with generation of fusion genes JAZF1/PHF1 and EPC1/PHF1 in endometrial stromal sarcoma. Cancer Res 66: 107-112.
1257. Micci F, Panagopoulos I, Bjerkehagen B, Heim S (2006). Deregulation of HMGA2 in an aggressive angiomyxoma with t(11;12)(q23;q15). Virchows Arch 448: 838-842.
1258. Micci F, Teixeira MR, Scheistroen M, Abeler VM, Heim S (2003). Cytogenetic characterization of tumors of the vulva and vagina. Genes Chromosomes Cancer 38: 137-148.
1259. Micci F, Walter CU, Teixeira MR, Panagopoulos I, Bjerkehagen B, Saeter G, Heim S (2003). Cytogenetic and molecular genetic analyses of endometrial stromal sarcoma: nonrandom involvement of chromosome arms 6p and 7p and confirmation of JAZF1/JJAZ1 gene fusion in t(7;17). Cancer Genet Cytogenet 144: 119-124.
1260. Michal M, Kacerovska D, Mukensnabl P, Petersson F, Danis D, Adamkov M, Kazakov DV (2009). Ovarian fibromas with heavy deposition of hyaline globules: a diagnostic pitfall. Int J Gynecol Pathol 28: 356-361.
1261. Michal M, Vanecek T, Sima R, Mukensnabl P, Hes O, Kazakov DV, Matoska J, Zuntova A, Dvorak V, Talerman A (2006). Mixed germ cell sex cord-stromal tumors of the testis and ovary. Morphological, immunohistochemical, and molecular genetic study of seven cases. Virchows Arch 448: 612-622.
1262. Micheletti L, Preti M, Bogliatto F, Chieppa P (2000). [Vestibular papillomatosis]. Minerva Ginecol 52: 87-91.
1263. Miettinen M, Sobin LH, Lasota J (2009). Gastrointestinal stromal tumors presenting as omental masses--a clinicopathologic analysis of 95 cases. Am J Surg Pathol 33: 1267-1275.
1264. Mihajlovic M, Vlajkovic S, Jovanovic P, Stefanovic V (2012). Primary mucosal melanomas: a comprehensive review. Int J Clin Exp Pathol 5: 739-753.
1265. Mikami M, Ezawa S, Sakaiya N, Komuro Y, Tei C, Fukuchi T, Mukai M (2000). Response of glassy-cell carcinoma of the cervix to cisplatin, epirubicin, and mitomycin C. Lancet 355: 1159-1160.
1266. Mikami Y, Kiyokawa T, Hata S, Fujiwara K, Moriya T, Sasano H, Manabe T, Akahira J, Ito K, Tase T, Yaegashi N, Sato I, Tateno H, Naganuma H (2004). Gastrointestinal immunophenotype in adenocarcinomas of the uterine cervix and related glandular lesions: a possible link between lobular endocervical glandular hyperplasia/pyloric gland metaplasia and 'adenoma malignum'. Mod Pathol 17: 962-972.
1267. Mikami Y, Maehata K, Fujiwara K, Manabe T (2001). Endocervical adenomyoma. A case report with histochemical and immunohistochemical studies. APMIS 109: 546-550.
1268. Mikami Y, McCluggage WG (2013). Endocervical glandular lesions exhibiting gastric differentiation: an emerging spectrum of benign, premalignant, and malignant lesions. Adv Anat Pathol 20: 227-237.
1269. Miksanek T, Reyes CV, Semkiw Z, Molnar ZV (1983). Granulocytic sarcoma of the peritoneum. CA Cancer J Clin 33: 40-43.
1270. Milam MR, Atkinson JB, Currie JL (2006). Adenosarcoma arising in inguinal endometriosis. Obstet Gynecol 108: 753-755.
1271. Miles PA, Norris HJ (1972). Proliferative and malignant brenner tumors of the ovary. Cancer 30: 174-186.
1272. Mills AM, Karamchandani JR, Vogel H, Longacre TA (2011). Endocervical fibroblastic malignant peripheral nerve sheath tumor (neurofibrosarcoma): report of a novel entity possibly related to endocervical CD34 fibrocytes. Am J Surg Pathol 35: 404-412.
1273. Mills AM, Ly A, Balzer BL, Hendrickson MR, Kempson RL, McKenney JK, Longacre TA (2013). Cell cycle regulatory markers in uterine atypical leiomyoma and leiomyosarcoma: immunohistochemical study of 68 cases with clinical follow-up. Am J Surg Pathol 37: 634-642.
1274. Miner TJ, Delgado R, Zeisler J, Busam K, Alektiar K, Barakat R, Poynor E (2004). Primary vaginal melanoma: a critical analysis of therapy. Ann Surg Oncol 11: 34-39.
1275. Mingels MJ, Roelofsen T, van der Laak JA, de Hullu JA, van Ham MA, Massuger LF, Bulten J, Bol M (2012). Tubal epithelial lesions in salpingo-oophorectomy specimens of BRCA-mutation carriers and controls. Gynecol Oncol 127: 88-93.
1276. Minicozzi A, Borzellino G, Momo R, Steccanella F, Pitoni F, de Manzoni G (2010). Perianal Paget's disease: presentation of six cases and literature review. Int J Colorectal Dis 25: 1-7.
1277. Mink PJ, Sherman ME, Devesa SS (2002). Incidence patterns of invasive and borderline ovarian tumors among white women and black women in the United States. Results from the SEER Program, 1978-1998. Cancer 95: 2380-2389.
1278. Mitchell HS (2004). Outcome after a cytological prediction of glandular abnormality. Aust N Z J Obstet Gynaecol 44: 436-440.
1279. Mitra D, Luo X, Morgan A, Wang J, Hoang MP, Lo J, Guerrero CR, Lennerz JK, Mihm MC, Wargo JA, Robinson KC, Devi SP, Vanover JC, D'Orazio JA, McMahon M, Bosenberg MW, Haigis KM, Haber DA, Wang Y, Fisher DE (2012). An ultraviolet-radiation-independent pathway to melanoma carcinogenesis in the red hair/fair skin background. Nature 491: 449-453.
1280. Mitsuhashi A, Nagai Y, Suzuka K, Yamazawa K, Nojima T, Nikaido T, Ishikura H, Matsui H, Shozu M (2007). Primary synovial sarcoma in fallopian tube: case report and literature review. Int J Gynecol Pathol 26: 34-37.
1281. Mochizuki K, Obatake M, Taura Y, Inamura Y, Takatsuki M, Nagayasu T, Eguchi S (2012). Yolk sac tumor of the vulva: a case report with recurrence after long-term follow-up. Pediatr Surg Int 28: 931-934.
1282. Modugno F, Ness RB, Wheeler JE (2001). Reproductive risk factors for epithelial ovarian cancer according to histologic type and invasiveness. Ann Epidemiol 11: 568-574.
1283. Mohit M, Mosallai A, Monabbati A, Mortazavi H (2009). Merkel cell carcinoma of the vulva. Saudi Med J 30: 717-718.
1284. Moinfar F, Regitnig P, Tabrizi AD, Denk H, Tavassoli FA (2004). Expression of androgen receptors in benign and malignant endometrial stromal neoplasms. Virchows Arch 444: 410-414.
1285. Mok SC, Bell DA, Knapp RC, Fishbaugh PM, Welch WR, Muto MG, Berkowitz RS, Tsao SW (1993). Mutation of K-ras protooncogene in human ovarian epithelial tumors of borderline malignancy. Cancer Res 53: 1489-1492.
1286. Molinie V, Paniel BJ, Lessana-Leibowitch M, Moyal-Barracco M, Pelisse M, Escande JP (1993). [Paget disease of the vulva. 36 cases]. Ann Dermatol Venereol 120: 522-527.
1287. Moloshok T, Pearce G, Ryan CA (1992). Oligouronide signaling of proteinase inhibitor genes in plants: structure-activity relationships of Di- and trigalacturonic acids and their derivatives. Arch Biochem Biophys 294: 731-734.
1288. Moniaga NC, Randall LM (2011). Malignant mixed ovarian germ cell tumor with embryonal component. J Pediatr Adolesc Gynecol 24: e1-e3.
1289. Montag TW, D'ablaing G, Schlaerth JB, Gaddis O Jr, Morrow CP (1986). Embryonal rhabdomyosarcoma of the uterine corpus and cervix. Gynecol Oncol 25: 171-194.
1290. Monte NM, Webster KA, Neuberg D, Dressler GR, Mutter GL (2010). Joint loss of PAX2 and PTEN expression in endometrial precancers and cancer. Cancer Res 70: 6225-6232.
1291. Montz FJ, Schlaerth JB, Morrow CP (1988). The natural history of theca lutein cysts. Obstet Gynecol 72: 247-251.
1292. Mooney EE, Man YG, Bratthauer GL, Tavassoli FA (1999). Evidence that Leydig cells in Sertoli-Leydig cell tumors have a reactive rather than a neoplastic profile. Cancer 86: 2312-2319.
1293. Mooney EE, Nogales FF, Bergeron C, Tavassoli FA (2002). Retiform Sertoli-Leydig cell tumours: clinical, morphological and immunohistochemical findings. Histopathology 41: 110-117.
1294. Mooney EE, Nogales FF, Tavassoli FA (1999). Hepatocytic differentiation in retiform Sertoli-Leydig cell tumors: distinguishing a heterologous element from Leydig cells. Hum Pathol 30: 611-617.
1295. Mooney EE, Vaidya KP, Tavassoli FA (2000). Ossifying well-differentiated Sertoli-Leydig cell tumor of the ovary. Ann Diagn Pathol 4: 34-38.
1296. Mooney J, Silva E, Tornos C, Gershenson D (1997). Unusual features of serous neoplasms of low malignant potential during pregnancy. Gynecol Oncol 65: 30-35.
1297. Moore G, Fetterman B, Cox JT, Poitras N, Lorey T, Kinney W, Castle PE (2010). Lessons from practice: risk of CIN 3 or cancer associated with an LSIL or HPV-positive ASC-US screening result in women aged 21 to 24. J Low Genit Tract Dis 14: 97-102.
1298. Moore RG, Chung M, Granai CO, Gajewski W, Steinhoff MM (2004). Incidence of metastasis to the ovaries from nongenital tract primary tumors. Gynecol Oncol 93: 87-91.
1299. Morch LS, Lokkegaard E, Andreasen AH, Kjaer SK, Lidegaard O (2012). Hormone therapy and ovarian borderline tumors: a national cohort study. Cancer Causes Control 23: 113-120.
1300. Moreno-Bueno G, Gamallo C, Perez-Gallego L, de Mora JC, Suarez A, Palacios J (2001). beta-Catenin expression pattern, beta-catenin gene mutations, and microsatellite instability in endometrioid ovarian carcinomas and synchronous endometrial carcinomas. Diagn Mol Pathol 10: 116-122.
1301. Moreno-Bueno G, Hardisson D, Sarrio D, Sanchez C, Cassia R, Prat J, Herman JG, Esteller M, Matias-Guiu X, Palacios J (2003). Abnormalities of E- and P-cadherin and catenin (beta-, gamma-catenin, and p120ctn) expression in endometrial cancer and endometrial atypical hyperplasia. J Pathol 199: 471-478.
1302. Morgan JM, Lurain JR (2008). Gestational trophoblastic neoplasia: an update. Curr Oncol Rep 10: 497-504.
1303. Moritani S, Kushima R, Ichihara S, Okabe H, Hattori T, Kobayashi TK, Silverberg SG (2005). Eosinophilic cell change of the endometrium: a possible relationship to mucinous differentiation. Mod Pathol 18: 1243-1248.
1304. Morovic A, Damjanov I (2008). Neuroectodermal ovarian tumors: a brief overview. Histol Histopathol 23: 765-771.
1305. Moscicki AB, Schiffman M, Burchell A, Albero G, Giuliano AR, Goodman MT, Kjaer SK, Palefsky J (2012). Updating the natural history of human papillomavirus and anogenital cancers. Vaccine 30 Suppl 5: F24-F33.

1306. Moss EL, Pearmain P, Askew S, Dawson P, Singh K, Hirschowitz L, Ganesan R (2011). Neuroendocrine carcinoma of the cervix: a review of clinical management and survival. International Journal of Gynecological Cancer 21, supplement 3.
1307. Mostoufizadeh M, Scully RE (1980). Malignant tumors arising in endometriosis. Clin Obstet Gynecol 23: 951-963.
1308. Mousavi A, Akhavan S (2010). Sarcoma botryoides (embryonal rhabdomyosarcoma) of the uterine cervix in sisters. J Gynecol Oncol 21: 273-275.
1309. Moxley KM, Fader AN, Rose PG, Case AS, Mutch DG, Berry E, Schink JC, Kim CH, Chi DS, Moore KN (2011). Malignant melanoma of the vulva: an extension of cutaneous melanoma? Gynecol Oncol 122: 612-617.
1310. Mrad K, Driss M, Abdelmoula S, Sassi S, Hechiche M, Ben RK (2005). Primary broad ligament cystadenocarcinoma with mucinous component: a case report with immunohistochemical study. Arch Pathol Lab Med 129: 244-246.
1311. Mueck AO, Seeger H, Rabe T (2010). Hormonal contraception and risk of endometrial cancer: a systematic review. Endocr Relat Cancer 17: R263-R271.
1312. Mulvany NJ, Ostor AG, Ross I (1995). Diffuse leiomyomatosis of the uterus. Histopathology 27: 175-179.
1313. Mulvany NJ, Rayoo M, Allen DG (2012). Basal cell carcinoma of the vulva: a case series. Pathology 44: 528-533.
1314. Mulvany NJ, Slavin JL, Ostor AG, Fortune DW (1994). Intravenous leiomyomatosis of the uterus: a clinicopathologic study of 22 cases. Int J Gynecol Pathol 13: 1-9.
1315. Mumba E, Ali H, Turton D, Cooper K, Grayson W (2008). Human papillomaviruses do not play an aetiological role in Mullerian adenosarcomas of the uterine cervix. J Clin Pathol 61: 1041-1044.
1316. Munksgaard PS, Blaakaer J (2012). The association between endometriosis and ovarian cancer: a review of histological, genetic and molecular alterations. Gynecol Oncol 124: 164-169.
1317. Munoz N, Franceschi S, Bosetti C, Moreno V, Herrero R, Smith JS, Shah KV, Meijer CJ, Bosch FX (2002). Role of parity and human papillomavirus in cervical cancer: the IARC multicentric case-control study. Lancet 359: 1093-1101.
1318. Murdoch F, Sharma R, Al-Nafussi A (2003). Benign mixed tumor of the vagina: case report with expanded immunohistochemical profile. Int J Gynecol Cancer 13: 543-547.
1319. Murdoch S, Djuric U, Mazhar B, Seoud M, Khan R, Kuick R, Bagga R, Kircheisen R, Ao A, Ratti B, Hanash S, Rouleau GA, Slim R (2006). Mutations in NALP7 cause recurrent hydatidiform moles and reproductive wastage in humans. Nat Genet 38: 300-302.
1320. Murphy KM, Descipio C, Wagenfuehr J, Tandy S, Mabray J, Beierl K, Micetich K, Libby AL, Ronnett BM (2012). Tetraploid partial hydatidiform mole: a case report and review of the literature. Int J Gynecol Pathol 31: 73-79.
1321. Mutter GL, Baak JP, Crum CP, Richart RM, Ferenczy A, Faquin WC (2000). Endometrial precancer diagnosis by histopathology, clonal analysis, and computerized morphometry. J Pathol 190: 462-469.
1322. Mutter GL, Ince TA, Baak JP, Kust GA, Zhou XP, Eng C (2001). Molecular identification of latent precancers in histologically normal endometrium. Cancer Res 61: 4311-4314.
1323. Mutter GL, Kauderer J, Baak JP, Alberts D (2008). Biopsy histomorphometry predicts uterine myoinvasion by endometrial carcinoma: a Gynecologic Oncology Group study. Hum Pathol 39: 866-874.
1324. Myhre-Jensen O (1981). A consecutive 7-year series of 1331 benign soft tissue tumours. Clinicopathologic data. Comparison with sarcomas. Acta Orthop Scand 52: 287-293.
1325. Nagai Y, Kishimoto T, Kato K, Ozaki D, Kondo F, Kobayashi A, Shimizu H, Ishikura H (2002). Uterine adenosarcoma with sarcomatous overgrowth: a case report with cytology of overgrown poorly differentiated sarcoma and immunohistochemical identification of epithelial microinvasion. Int J Gynecol Cancer 12: 501-505.
1326. Nagai Y, Kishimoto T, Nikaido T, Nishihara K, Matsumoto T, Suzuki C, Ogishima T, Kuwahara Y, Hurukata Y, Mizunuma M, Nakata Y, Ishikura H (2003). Squamous predominance in mixed-epithelial papillary cystadenomas of borderline malignancy of mullerian type arising in endometriotic cysts: a study of four cases. Am J Surg Pathol 27: 242-247.
1327. Nakano T, Oka K, Ishikawa A, Morita S (1997). Correlation of cervical carcinoma c-erb B-2 oncogene with cell proliferation parameters in patients treated with radiation therapy for cervical carcinoma. Cancer 79: 513-520.
1328. Nakashima N, Fukatsu T, Nagasaka T, Sobue M, Takeuchi J (1987). The frequency and histology of hepatic tissue in germ cell tumors. Am J Surg Pathol 11: 682-692.
1329. Nakashima N, Murakami S, Fukatsu T, Nagasaka T, Fukata S, Ohiwa N, Nara Y, Sobue M, Takeuchi J (1988). Characteristics of "embryoid body" in human gonadal germ cell tumors. Hum Pathol 19: 1144-1154.
1330. Nara M, Hashi A, Murata S, Kondo T, Yuminamochi T, Nakazawa K, Katoh R, Hoshi K (2007). Lobular endocervical glandular hyperplasia as a presumed precursor of cervical adenocarcinoma independent of human papillomavirus infection. Gynecol Oncol 106: 289-298.
1331. Nardi V, Song Y, Santamaria-Barria JA, Cosper AK, Lam Q, Faber AC, Boland GM, Yeap BY, Bergethon K, Scialabba VL, Tsao H, Settleman J, Ryan DP, Borger DR, Bhan AK, Hoang MP, Iafrate AJ, Cusack JC, Engelman JA, Dias-Santagata D (2012). Activation of PI3K signaling in Merkel cell carcinoma. Clin Cancer Res 18: 1227-1236.
1332. Narita F, Takeuchi K, Hamana S, Ohbayashi C, Ayata M, Maruo T (2003). Epithelioid trophoblastic tumor (ETT) initially interpreted as cervical cancer. Int J Gynecol Cancer 13: 551-554.
1333. Nascimento AF, Granter SR, Cviko A, Yuan L, Hecht JL, Crum CP (2004). Vulvar acanthosis with altered differentiation: a precursor to verrucous carcinoma? Am J Surg Pathol 28: 638-643.
1334. Nascimento AF, Ruiz R, Hornick JL, Fletcher CD (2002). Calcifying fibrous 'pseudotumor': clinicopathologic study of 15 cases and analysis of its relationship to inflammatory myofibroblastic tumor. Int J Surg Pathol 10: 189-196.
1335. Nasiell K, Nasiell M, Vaclavinkova V (1983). Behavior of moderate cervical dysplasia during long-term follow-up. Obstet Gynecol 61: 609-614.
1335A. Navani SS, Alvarado-Cabrero I, Young RH, Scully RE (1996). Endometrioid carcinoma of the fallopian tube: a clinicopathologic analysis of 26 cases. Gynecol Oncol 63: 371-408.
1336. Naves AE, Monti JA, Chichoni E (1980). Basal cell-like carcinoma in the upper third of the vagina. Am J Obstet Gynecol 137: 136-137.
1337. Nayar R, Siriaunkgul S, Robbins KM, McGowan L, Ginzan S, Silverberg SG (1996). Microinvasion in low malignant potential tumors of the ovary. Hum Pathol 27: 521-527.
1337A. Nazer A, Al-Badawi I, Chebbo W, Chaudhri N, El-Gohary G (2012). Myeloid sarcoma of the vulva post-bone marrow transplant presenting as isolated extramedullary relapse in a patient with acute myeloid leukemia. Hematol Oncol Stem Cell Ther 5: 118-121.
1338. Neesham D, Kerdemelidis P, Scurry J (1998). Primary malignant mixed Mullerian tumor of the vagina. Gynecol Oncol 70: 303-307.
1339. Negri G, Bellisano G, Zannoni GF, Rivasi F, Kasal A, Vittadello F, Antoniazzi S, Faa G, Ambu R, Egarter-Vigl E (2008). p16 ink4a and HPV L1 immunohistochemistry is helpful for estimating the behavior of low-grade dysplastic lesions of the cervix uteri. Am J Surg Pathol 32: 1715-1720.
1340. Neto AG, Deavers MT, Silva EG, Malpica A (2003). Metastatic tumors of the vulva: a clinicopathologic study of 66 cases. Am J Surg Pathol 27: 799-804.
1341. Neuhauser TS, Tavassoli FA, Abbondanzo SL (2000). Follicle center lymphoma involving the female genital tract: a morphologic and molecular genetic study of three cases. Ann Diagn Pathol 4: 293-299.
1342. Newlands ES (2003). The management of recurrent and drug-resistant gestational trophoblastic neoplasia (GTN). Best Pract Res Clin Obstet Gynaecol 17: 905-923.
1343. Ngan HY, Fisher C, Blake P, Shepherd JH (1994). Vaginal sarcoma: the Royal Marsden experience. Int J Gynecol Cancer 4: 337-341.
1344. Ngan HY, Kohorn EI, Cole LA, Kurman RJ, Kim SJ, Lurain JR, Seckl MJ, Sasaki S, Soper JT (2012). Trophoblastic disease. Int J Gynaecol Obstet 119 Suppl 2: S130-S136.
1345. Ngan HY, Liu SS, Yu H, Liu KL, Cheung AN (1999). Proto-oncogenes and p53 protein expression in normal cervical stratified squamous epithelium and cervical intra-epithelial neoplasia. Eur J Cancer 35: 1546-1550.
1346. Ngan S, Seckl MJ (2007). Gestational trophoblastic neoplasia management: an update. Curr Opin Oncol 19: 486-491.
1347. Angeles-Angeles A, Gutierrez-Villalobos LI, Lome-Maldonado C, Jimenez-Moreno A (2002). Polypoid Brenner tumor of the uterus. Int J Gynecol Pathol 21: 86-87.
1348. Ngwalle KE, Hirakawa T, Tsuneyoshi M, Enjoji M (1990). Osteosarcoma arising in a benign dermoid cyst of the ovary. Gynecol Oncol 37: 143-147.
1349. Nicolas MM, Tamboli P, Gomez JA, Czerniak BA (2010). Pleomorphic and dedifferentiated leiomyosarcoma: clinicopathologic and immunohistochemical study of 41 cases. Hum Pathol 41: 663-671.
1350. Nielsen GP, Oliva E, Young RH, Rosenberg AE, Dickersin GR, Scully RE (1995). Alveolar soft-part sarcoma of the female genital tract: a report of nine cases and review of the literature. Int J Gynecol Pathol 14: 283-292.
1351. Nielsen GP, Oliva E, Young RH, Rosenberg AE, Prat J, Scully RE (1998). Primary ovarian rhabdomyosarcoma: a report of 13 cases. Int J Gynecol Pathol 17: 113-119.
1352. Nielsen GP, Rosenberg AE, Koerner FC, Young RH, Scully RE (1996). Smooth-muscle tumors of the vulva. A clinicopathological study of 25 cases and review of the literature. Am J Surg Pathol 20: 779-793.
1353. Nielsen GP, Rosenberg AE, Young RH, Dickersin GR, Clement PB, Scully RE (1996). Angiomyofibroblastoma of the vulva and vagina. Mod Pathol 9: 284-291.
1354. Nielsen GP, Young RH (1997). Fibromatosis of soft tissue type involving the female genital tract: a report of two cases. Int J Gynecol Pathol 16: 383-386.
1355. Nielsen GP, Young RH (2001). Mesenchymal tumors and tumor-like lesions of the female genital tract: a selective review with emphasis on recently described entities. Int J Gynecol Pathol 20: 105-127.
1356. Nielsen GP, Young RH, Dickersin GR, Rosenberg AE (1997). Angiomyofibroblastoma of the vulva with sarcomatous transformation ("angiomyofibrosarcoma"). Am J Surg Pathol 21: 1104-1108.
1357. Nielsen GP, Young RH, Prat J, Scully RE (1997). Primary angiosarcoma of the ovary: a report of seven cases and review of the literature. Int J Gynecol Pathol 16: 378-382.
1358. Niwa K, Onogi K, Wu Y, Mori H, Tamaya T (2007). Primary endodermal sinus tumor of the vulva in a 52-year-old woman with long-term survival: a case report. Eur J Gynaecol Oncol 28: 506-508.
1359. Diniz da Costa AT, Coelho AM, Lourenco AV, Bernardino M, Ribeirinho AL, Jorge CC (2012). Primary breast cancer of the vulva: a case report. J Low Genit Tract Dis 16: 155-157.
1360. Noack F, Lange K, Lehmann V, Caselitz J, Merz H (2002). Primary extranodal marginal zone B-cell lymphoma of the fallopian tube. Gynecol Oncol 86: 384-386.
1361. Noel J, Lespagnard L, Fayt I, Verhest A, Dargent J (2001). Evidence of human papilloma virus infection but lack of Epstein-Barr virus in lymphoepithelioma-like carcinoma of uterine cervix: report of two cases and review of the literature. Hum Pathol 32: 135-138.
1362. Nofech-Mozes S, Rasty G, Ismiil N, Covens A, Khalifa MA (2006). Immunohistochemical characterization of endocervical papillary serous carcinoma. Int J Gynecol Cancer 16 Suppl 1: 286-292.
1363. Nogales FF, Aguilar D (2002). Florid vascular proliferation in grade 0 glial implants from ovarian immature teratoma. Int J Gynecol Pathol 21: 305-307.
1364. Nogales FF, Ayala A, Ruiz-Avila I, Sirvent JJ (1991). Myxoid leiomyosarcoma of the ovary: analysis of three cases. Hum Pathol 22: 1268-1273.
1365. Nogales FF, Bergeron C, Carvia RE, Alvaro T, Fulwood HR (1996). Ovarian endometrioid tumors with yolk sac tumor component, an unusual form of ovarian neoplasm. Analysis of six cases. Am J Surg Pathol 20: 1056-1066.
1366. Nogales FF, Carvia RE, Donne C, Campello TR, Vidal M, Martin A (1997). Adenomas of the rete ovarii. Hum Pathol 28: 1428-1433.
1367. Nogales FF, Dulcey I (2012). The secondary human yolk sac has an immunophenotype indicative of both hepatic and intestinal differentiation. Int J Dev Biol 56: 755-760.
1368. Nogales FF Jr, Favara BE, Major FJ, Silverberg SG (1976). Immature teratoma of the ovary with a neural component ("solid" teratoma). A clinicopathologic study of 20 cases. Hum Pathol 7: 625-642.
1369. Nogales FF, Goyenaga P, Preda O, Nicolae A, Vieites B, Ruiz-Marcellan MC, Pedrosa A, Merino MJ (2012). An analysis of five clear cell papillary cystadenomas of mesosalpinx and broad ligament: four associated with von Hippel-Lindau disease and one aggressive sporadic type. Histopathology 60: 748-757.
1370. Nogales FF, Isaac MA, Hardisson D, Bosincu L, Palacios J, Ordi J, Mendoza E, Manzarbeitia F, Olivera H, O'Valle F, Krasevic M, Marquez M (2002). Adenomatoid tumors of the uterus: an analysis of 60 cases. Int J Gynecol Pathol 21: 34-40.
1371. Nogales FF, Martin-Sances L, Mendoza-Garcia E, Salamanca A, Gonzalez-Nunez MA, Pardo Mindan FJ (1996). Massive ovarian oedema. Histopathology 28: 229-234.
1372. Nogales FF Jr, Matilla A, Nogales O,

galera-Davidson HL (1978). Yolk sac tumors with pure and mixed polyvesicular vitelline patterns. Hum Pathol 9: 553-566.

1373. Nogales FF, Preda O, Nicolae A (2012). Yolk sac tumours revisited. A review of their many faces and names. Histopathology 60: 1023-1033.

1374. Nogales FF, Stolnicu S, Harilal KR, Mooney E, Garcia-Galvis OF (2009). Retiform uterine tumours resembling ovarian sex cord tumours. A comparative immunohistochemical study with retiform structures of the female genital tract. Histopathology 54: 471-477.

1375. Nola M, Babic D, Ilic J, Marusic M, Uzarevic B, Petrovecki M, Sabioncello A, Kovac D, Jukic S (1996). Prognostic parameters for survival of patients with malignant mesenchymal tumors of the uterus. Cancer 78: 2543-2550.

1376. Nordal RR, Kristensen GB, Kaern J, Stenwig AE, Pettersen EO, Trope CG (1995). The prognostic significance of stage, tumor size, cellular atypia and DNA ploidy in uterine leiomyosarcoma. Acta Oncol 34: 797-802.

1377. Nordal RR, Kristensen GB, Stenwig AE, Nesland JM, Pettersen EO, Trope CG (1997). An evaluation of prognostic factors in uterine carcinosarcoma. Gynecol Oncol 67: 316-321.

1378. Nordin AJ (1994). Primary carcinoma of the fallopian tube: a 20-year literature review. Obstet Gynecol Surv 49: 349-361.

1379. Norris HJ, Parmley T (1975). Mesenchymal tumors of the uterus. V. Intravenous leiomyomatosis. A clinical and pathologic study of 14 cases. Cancer 36: 2164-2178.

1380. Norris HJ, Taylor HB (1966). Mesenchymal tumors of the uterus. I. A clinical and pathological study of 53 endometrial stromal tumors. Cancer 19: 755-766.

1381. Norris HJ, Taylor HB (1967). Nodular theca-lutein hyperplasia of pregnancy (so-called "pregnancy luteoma"). A clinical and pathologic study of 15 cases. Am J Clin Pathol 47: 557-566.

1382. Norris HJ, Zirkin HJ, Benson WL (1976). Immature (malignant) teratoma of the ovary: a clinical and pathologic study of 58 cases. Cancer 37: 2359-2372.

1383. Nozawa S, Iwata T, Yamashita H, Banno K, Kubushiro K, Aoki R, Tsukazaki K (2000). Gonadotropin-releasing hormone analogue therapy for peritoneal inclusion cysts after gynecological surgery. J Obstet Gynaecol Res 26: 389-393.

1384. Ansari-Lari MA, Staebler A, Zaino RJ, Shah KV, Ronnett BM (2004). Distinction of endocervical and endometrial adenocarcinomas: immunohistochemical p16 expression correlated with human papillomavirus (HPV) DNA detection. Am J Surg Pathol 28: 160-167.

1385. Nucci MR, Drapkin R, Dal Cin P, Fletcher CD, Fletcher JA (2007). Distinctive cytogenetic profile in benign metastasizing leiomyoma: pathogenetic implications. Am J Surg Pathol 31: 737-743.

1386. Nucci MR, Fletcher CD (1998). Liposarcoma (atypical lipomatous tumors) of the vulva: a clinicopathologic study of six cases. Int J Gynecol Pathol 17: 17-23.

1387. Nucci MR, Fletcher CD (2000). Vulvovaginal soft tissue tumours: update and review. Histopathology 36: 97-108.

1388. Nucci MR, Genest DR, Tate JE, Sparks CK, Crum CP (1996). Pseudobowenoid change of the vulva: a histologic variant of untreated condylata acuminatum. Mod Pathol 9: 375-379.

1389. Nucci MR, Granter SR, Fletcher CD (1997). Cellular angiofibroma: a benign neoplasm distinct from angiomyofibroblastoma and spindle cell lipoma. Am J Surg Pathol 21: 636-644.

1390. Nucci MR, Harburger D, Koontz J, Dal Cin P, Sklar J (2007). Molecular analysis of the JAZF1-JJAZ1 gene fusion by RT-PCR and fluorescence in situ hybridization in endometrial stromal neoplasms. Am J Surg Pathol 31: 65-70.

1391. Nucci MR, Krausz T, Lifschitz-Mercer B, Chan JK, Fletcher CD (1998). Angiosarcoma of the ovary: clinicopathologic and immunohistochemical analysis of four cases with a broad morphologic spectrum. Am J Surg Pathol 22: 620-630.

1392. Nucci MR, O'Connell JT, Huettner PC, Cviko A, Sun D, Quade BJ (2001). h-Caldesmon expression effectively distinguishes endometrial stromal tumors from uterine smooth muscle tumors. Am J Surg Pathol 25: 455-463.

1393. Nucci MR, Prasad CJ, Crum CP, Mutter GL (1999). Mucinous endometrial epithelial proliferations: a morphologic spectrum of changes with diverse clinical significance. Mod Pathol 12: 1137-1142.

1394. Nucci MR, Weremowicz S, Neskey DM, Sornberger K, Tallini G, Morton CC, Quade BJ (2001). Chromosomal translocation t(8;12) induces aberrant HMGIC expression in aggressive angiomyxoma of the vulva. Genes Chromosomes Cancer 32: 172-176.

1395. Nucci MR, Young RH (2004). Arias-Stella reaction of the endocervix: a report of 18 cases with emphasis on its varied histology and differential diagnosis. Am J Surg Pathol 28: 608-612.

1396. Nucci MR, Young RH, Fletcher CD (2000). Cellular pseudosarcomatous fibroepithelial stromal polyps of the lower female genital tract: an underrecognized lesion often misdiagnosed as sarcoma. Am J Surg Pathol 24: 231-240.

1397. Nuciforo PG, Fraggetta F, Fasani R, Braidotti P, Nuciforo G (2004). Neuroendocrine carcinoma of the vulva with paraganglioma-like features. Histopathology 44: 304-306.

1398. Nugent EK, Brooks RA, Barr CD, Case AS, Mutch DG, Massad LS (2011). Clinical and pathologic features of vulvar intraepithelial neoplasia in premenopausal and postmenopausal women. J Low Genit Tract Dis 15: 15-19.

1399. O'Brien PC, Noller KL, Robboy SJ, Barnes AB, Kaufman RH, Tilley BC, Townsend DE (1979). Vaginal epithelial changes in young women enrolled in the National Cooperative Diethylstilbestrol Adenosis (DESAD) project. Obstet Gynecol 53: 300-308.

1400. O'Connor DM, Norris HJ (1990). Mitotically active leiomyomas of the uterus. Hum Pathol 21: 223-227.

1401. O'Connor DM, Norris HJ (1994). The influence of grade on the outcome of stage I ovarian immature (malignant) teratomas and the reproducibility of grading. Int J Gynecol Pathol 13: 283-289.

1402. O'Neill CJ, McBride HA, Connolly LE, McCluggage WG (2007). Uterine leiomyosarcomas are characterized by high p16, p53 and MIB1 expression in comparison with usual leiomyomas, leiomyoma variants and smooth muscle tumours of uncertain malignant potential. Histopathology 50: 851-858.

1403. Obata K, Morland SJ, Watson RH, Hitchcock A, Chenevix-Trench G, Thomas EJ, Campbell IG (1998). Frequent PTEN/MMAC mutations in endometrioid but not serous or mucinous epithelial ovarian tumors. Cancer Res 58: 2095-2097.

1404. Ober WB, Edgcomb JH, Price EB Jr (1971). The pathology of choriocarcinoma. Ann N Y Acad Sci 172: 299-426.

1405. Ober WB, Maier RC (1981). Gestational choriocarcinoma of the fallopian tube. Diagn Gynecol Obstet 3: 213-231.

1406. Oda K, Stokoe D, Taketani Y, McCormick F (2005). High frequency of coexistent mutations of PIK3CA and PTEN genes in endometrial carcinoma. Cancer Res 65: 10669-10673.

1407. Offman SL, Longacre TA (2012). Clear cell carcinoma of the female genital tract (not everything is as clear as it seems). Adv Anat Pathol 19: 296-312.

1408. Ogawa S, Kaku T, Amada S, Kobayashi H, Hirakawa T, Ariyoshi K, Kamura T, Nakano H (2000). Ovarian endometriosis associated with ovarian carcinoma: a clinicopathological and immunohistochemical study. Gynecol Oncol 77: 298-304.

1409. Oh JT, Choi SH, Ahn SG, Kim MJ, Yang WI, Han SJ (2009). Vulvar lipomas in children: an analysis of 7 cases. J Pediatr Surg 44: 1920-1923.

1410. Ohishi Y, Oda Y, Kurihara S, Kaku T, Yasunaga M, Nishimura I, Okuma E, Kobayashi H, Wake N, Tsuneyoshi M (2009). Hobnail-like cells in serous borderline tumor do not represent concomitant incipient clear cell neoplasms. Hum Pathol 40: 1168-1175.

1411. Olah KS, Dunn JA, Gee H (1992). Leiomyosarcomas have a poorer prognosis than mixed mesodermal tumours when adjusting for known prognostic factors: the result of a retrospective study of 423 cases of uterine sarcoma. Br J Obstet Gynaecol 99: 590-594.

1412. Oliva E, Alvarez T, Young RH (2005). Sertoli cell tumors of the ovary: a clinicopathologic and immunohistochemical study of 54 cases. Am J Surg Pathol 29: 143-156.

1413. Oliva E, Andrada E, Pezzica E, Prat J (1993). Ovarian carcinomas with choriocarcinomatous differentiation. Cancer 72: 2441-2446.

1414. Oliva E, Clement PB, Young RH (1995). Tubal and tubo-endometrioid metaplasia of the uterine cervix. Unemphasized features that may cause problems in differential diagnosis: a report of 25 cases. Am J Clin Pathol 103: 618-623.

1415. Oliva E, Clement PB, Young RH (2000). Endometrial stromal tumors: an update on a group of tumors with a protean phenotype. Adv Anat Pathol 7: 257-281.

1416. Oliva E, Clement PB, Young RH (2002). Epithelioid endometrial and endometrioid stromal tumors: a report of four cases emphasizing their distinction from epithelioid smooth muscle tumors and other oxyphilic uterine and extrauterine tumors. Int J Gynecol Pathol 21: 48-55.

1417. Oliva E, Clement PB, Young RH, Scully RE (1998). Mixed endometrial stromal and smooth muscle tumors of the uterus: a clinicopathologic study of 15 cases. Am J Surg Pathol 22: 997-1005.

1418. Oliva E, de Leval L, Soslow RA, Herens C (2007). High frequency of JAZF1-JJAZ1 gene fusion in endometrial stromal tumors with smooth muscle differentiation by interphase FISH detection. Am J Surg Pathol 31: 1277-1284.

1418A. Oliva E, Egger J-F, Young RH (2014). Primary endometrioid stromal sarcoma of the ovary. A clinicopathologic study of 27 cases with morphologic and behavioral features similar to those of uterine low-grade endometrial stromal sarcoma. Am J. Surg Pathol (in press).

1419. Oliva E, Ferry JA, Young RH, Prat J, Srigley JR, Scully RE (1997). Granulocytic sarcoma of the female genital tract: a clinicopathologic study of 11 cases. Am J Surg Pathol 21: 1156-1165.

1420. Oliva E, Garcia-Miralles N, Vu Q, Young RH (2007). CD10 expression in pure stromal and sex cord-stromal tumors of the ovary: an immunohistochemical analysis of 101 cases. Int J Gynecol Pathol 26: 359-367.

1421. Oliva E, Gonzalez L, Dionigi A, Young RH (2004). Mixed tumors of the vagina: an immunohistochemical study of 13 cases with emphasis on the cell of origin and potential aid in differential diagnosis. Mod Pathol 17: 1243-1250.

1422. Oliva E, Young RH, Amin MB, Clement PB (2002). An immunohistochemical analysis of endometrial stromal and smooth muscle tumors of the uterus: a study of 54 cases emphasizing the importance of using a panel because of overlap in immunoreactivity for individual antibodies. Am J Surg Pathol 26: 403-412.

1423. Oliva E, Young RH, Clement PB, Scully RE (1999). Myxoid and fibrous endometrial stromal tumors of the uterus: a report of 10 cases. Int J Gynecol Pathol 18: 310-319.

1424. Olson DJ, Fujimura M, Swanson P, Okagaki T (1991). Immunohistochemical features of Paget's disease of the vulva with and without adenocarcinoma. Int J Gynecol Pathol 10: 285-295.

1425. Omholt K, Grafstrom E, Kanter-Lewensohn L, Hansson J, Ragnarsson-Olding BK (2011). KIT pathway alterations in mucosal melanomas of the vulva and other sites. Clin Cancer Res 17: 3933-3942.

1426. Onderoglu LS, Gultekin M, Dursun P, Karcaaltincaba M, Usubutun A, Akata D, Ayhan A (2004). Bilateral ovarian fibromatosis presenting with ascites and hirsutism. Gynecol Oncol 94: 223-225.

1427. Oner UU, Tokar B, Acikalin MF, Ilhan H, Tel N (2002). Wilms' tumor of the ovary: A case report. J Pediatr Surg 37: 127-129.

1428. Ong AC, Lim TY, Tan TC, Wang S, Raju GC (2012). Proximal epithelioid sarcoma of the vulva: a case report and review of current medical literature. J Obstet Gynaecol Res 38: 1032-1035.

1428A. Oparka R, Herrington CS (2012). Precursors of vulvovaginal squamous cell carcinoma. In: Brown L (Ed) Pathology of the Vulva and Vagina. Essentials of Diagnostic Gynecological Pathology. Springer-Verlag: London.

1429. Oparka R, McCluggage WG, Herrington CS (2011). Peritoneal mesothelial hyperplasia associated with gynaecological disease: a potential diagnostic pitfall that is commonly associated with endometriosis. J Clin Pathol 64: 313-318.

1430. Ordi J, Alejo M, Fuste V, Lloveras B, Del Pino M, Alonso I, Torne A (2009). HPV-negative vulvar intraepithelial neoplasia (VIN) with basaloid histologic pattern: an unrecognized variant of simplex (differentiated) VIN. Am J Surg Pathol 33: 1659-1665.

1431. Ordi J, Schammel DP, Rasekh L, Tavassoli FA (1999). Sertoliform endometrioid carcinomas of the ovary: a clinicopathologic and immunohistochemical study of 13 cases. Mod Pathol 12: 933-940.

1432. Ordi J, Stamatakos MD, Tavassoli FA (1997). Pure pleomorphic rhabdomyosarcomas of the uterus. Int J Gynecol Pathol 16: 369-377.

1433. Ordonez JL, Osuna D, Garcia-Dominguez DJ, Amaral AT, Otero-Motta AP, Mackintosh C, Sevillano MV, Barbado MV, Hernandez T, de Alava E (2010). The clinical relevance of molecular genetics in soft tissue sarcomas. Adv Anat Pathol 17: 162-181.

1434. Ordonez NG (1998). Role of immunohistochemistry in distinguishing epithelial peritoneal mesotheliomas from peritoneal and ovarian serous carcinomas. Am J Surg Pathol 22: 1203-1214.

1435. Ordonez NG (2006). Value of immunohistochemistry in distinguishing peritoneal mesothelioma from serous carcinoma of the ovary and peritoneum: a review and update. Adv Anat Pathol 13: 16-25.

1436. Ordonez NG, Ro JY, Ayala AG (1998). Lesions described as nodular mesothelial hyperplasia are primarily composed of histiocytes. Am J Surg Pathol 22: 285-292.
1437. Oshima H, Miyagawa H, Sato Y, Satake M, Shiraki N, Nishikawa H, Arakawa A, Ogino H, Hara M (2002). Adenofibroma of the endometrium after tamoxifen therapy for breast cancer: MR findings. Abdom Imaging 27: 592-594.
1438. Ostor AG (1993). Natural history of cervical intraepithelial neoplasia: a critical review. Int J Gynecol Pathol 12: 186-192.
1439. Ostor AG, Fortune DW, Riley CB (1988). Fibroepithelial polyps with atypical stromal cells (pseudosarcoma botryoides) of vulva and vagina. A report of 13 cases. Int J Gynecol Pathol 7: 351-360.
1440. Ostor AG, Rollason TP (2003). Mixed tumours of the uterus. In: Haines & Taylor Obstetrical and Gynaecological Pathology. Fox H, Wells M, eds. Churchill Livingstone: 549-584.
1441. Ota S, Catasus L, Matias-Guiu X, Bussaglia E, Lagarda H, Pons C, Munoz J, Kamura T, Prat J (2003). Molecular pathology of atypical polypoid adenomyoma of the uterus. Hum Pathol 34: 784-788.
1442. Ota S, Ushijima K, Fujiyoshi N, Fujimoto T, Hayashi R, Murakami F, Komai K, Fujiyoshi K, Hori D, Kamura T (2010). Desmoplastic small round cell tumor in the ovary: Report of two cases and literature review. J Obstet Gynaecol Res 36: 430-434.
1443. Ouansafi I, Arabadjief M, Mathew S, Srivastara S, Orazi A (2011). Myeloid sarcoma with t(11;19)(q23;p13.3) (MLL-ELL) in the uterine cervix. Br J Haematol 153: 679.
1444. Ozaki S, Zen Y, Inoue M (2011). Biomarker expression in cervical intraepithelial neoplasia: potential progression predictive factors for low-grade lesions. Hum Pathol 42: 1007-1012.
1445. Pai RK, Longacre TA (2007). Pseudomyxoma peritonei syndrome: classification of appendiceal mucinous tumours. Cancer Treat Res 134: 71-107.
1446. Palacios J, Suarez MA, Ruiz VA, Burgos LE, Gamallo AC (1991). Cystic adenomatoid tumor of the uterus. Int J Gynecol Pathol 10: 296-301.
1447. Palmer JE, Macdonald M, Wells M, Hancock BW, Tidy JA (2008). Epithelioid trophoblastic tumor: a review of the literature. J Reprod Med 53: 465-475.
1448. Palmer JR (1994). Advances in the epidemiology of gestational trophoblastic disease. J Reprod Med 39: 155-162.
1449. Palmer PE, Bogojavlensky S, Bhan AK, Scully RE (1990). Prolactinoma in wall of ovarian dermoid cyst with hyperprolactinemia. Obstet Gynecol 75: 540-543.
1450. Pang B, Leong CC, Salto-Tellez M, Petersson F (2011). Desmoplastic small round cell tumor of major salivary glands: report of 1 case and a review of the literature. Appl Immunohistochem Mol Morphol 19: 70-75.
1451. Papachatzopoulos S, Theodoridis TD, Zafrakas M, Nikolakopoulos P, Molibas E (2009). Broad ligament leiomyosarcoma in a premenopausal nulliparous woman: case report and review of the literature. Eur J Gynaecol Oncol 30: 452-454.
1452. Papadopoulos AJ, Foskett M, Seckl MJ, McNeish I, Paradinas FJ, Rees H, Newlands ES (2002). Twenty-five years' clinical experience with placental site trophoblastic tumors. J Reprod Med 47: 460-464.
1453. Parada D, Pena KB, Riu F (2012). Coexisting malignant melanoma and blue nevus of the uterine cervix: an unusual combination. Case Rep Pathol 2012: 986542.
1454. Paraskevas M, Scully RE (1989). Hilus cell tumor of the ovary. A clinicopathological analysis of 12 Reinke crystal-positive and nine crystal-negative cases. Int J Gynecol Pathol 8: 299-310.
1455. Parazzini F, La VC, Bocciolone L, Franceschi S (1991). The epidemiology of endometrial cancer. Gynecol Oncol 41: 1-16.
1456. Parikh H, Lesseps A (2000). Intravenous leiomyomatosis. J Obstet Gynaecol 20: 439-440.
1457. Park HJ, Choi YM, Chung CK, Lee SH, Yim GW, Kim SW, Nam EJ, Kim YT (2011). Pap smear screening for small cell carcinoma of the uterine cervix: a case series and review of the literature. J Gynecol Oncol 22: 39-43.
1458. Park JJ, Genest DR, Sun D, Crum CP (1999). Atypical immature metaplastic-like proliferations of the cervix: diagnostic reproducibility and viral (HPV) correlates. Hum Pathol 30: 1161-1165.
1459. Park JJ, Sun D, Quade BJ, Flynn C, Sheets EE, Yang A, McKeon F, Crum CP (2000). Stratified mucin-producing intraepithelial lesions of the cervix: adenosquamous or columnar cell neoplasia? Am J Surg Pathol 24: 1414-1419.
1460. Park KJ, Kiyokawa T, Soslow RA, Lamb CA, Oliva E, Zivanovic O, Juretzka MM, Pirog EC (2011). Unusual endocervical adenocarcinomas: an immunohistochemical analysis with molecular detection of human papillomavirus. Am J Surg Pathol 35: 633-646.
1461. Park SH, Park A, Kim JY, Kwon JH, Koh SB (2009). A case of non-gestational choriocarcinoma arising in the ovary of a postmenopausal woman. J Gynecol Oncol 20: 192-194.
1462. Parker LP, Duong JL, Wharton JT, Malpica A, Silva EG, Deavers MT (2002). Desmoplastic small round cell tumor: report of a case presenting as a primary ovarian neoplasm. Eur J Gynaecol Oncol 23: 199-202.
1463. Parker RL, Dadmanesh F, Young RH, Clement PB (2004). Polypoid endometriosis: a clinicopathologic analysis of 24 cases and a review of the literature. Am J Surg Pathol 28: 285-297.
1464. Parker RL, Young RH, Clement PB (2005). Skeletal muscle-like and rhabdoid cells in uterine leiomyomas. Int J Gynecol Pathol 24: 319-325.
1465. Parker WH, Fu YS, Berek JS (1994). Uterine sarcoma in patients operated on for presumed leiomyoma and rapidly growing leiomyoma. Obstet Gynecol 83: 414-418.
1466. Parkes SE, Raafat F, Morland BJ (1998). Paraganglioma of the vagina: the first report of a rare tumor in a child. Pediatr Hematol Oncol 15: 545-551.
1467. Parrington JM, West LF, Povey S (1984). The origin of ovarian teratomas. J Med Genet 21: 4-12.
1468. Parwani AV, Smith Sehdev AE, Kurman RJ, Ronnett BM (2005). Cervical adenoid basal tumors comprised of adenoid basal epithelioma associated with various types of invasive carcinoma: clinicopathologic features, human papillomavirus DNA detection, and P16 expression. Hum Pathol 36: 82-90.
1469. Patel DS, Bhagavan BS (1985). Blue nevus of the uterine cervix. Hum Pathol 16: 79-86.
1470. Patel RM, Weiss SW, Folpe AL (2006). Heterotopic mesenteric ossification: a distinctive pseudosarcoma commonly associated with intestinal obstruction. Am J Surg Pathol 30: 119-122.
1471. Patil DT, Laskin WB, Fetsch JF, Miettinen M (2011). Inguinal smooth muscle tumors in women-a dichotomous group consisting of Mullerian-type leiomyomas and soft tissue leiomyosarcomas: an analysis of 55 cases. Am J Surg Pathol 35: 315-324.
1472. Patrelli TS, Silini EM, Berretta R, Thai E, Gizzo S, Bacchi MA, Nardelli GB (2011). Squamotransitional cell carcinoma of the vagina: diagnosis and clinical management: a literature review starting from a rare case report. Pathol Oncol Res 17: 149-153.
1473. Pattee SF, Silvis NG (2003). Keratoacanthoma developing in sites of previous trauma: a report of two cases and review of the literature. J Am Acad Dermatol 48: S35-S38.
1474. Patton KT, Cheng L, Papavero V, Blum MG, Yeldandi AV, Adley BP, Luan C, Diaz LK, Hui P, Yang XJ (2006). Benign metastasizing leiomyoma: clonality, telomere length and clinicopathologic analysis. Mod Pathol 19: 130-140.
1475. Pautier P, Genestie C, Rey A, Morice P, Roche B, Lhomme C, Haie-Meder C, Duvillard P (2000). Analysis of clinicopathologic prognostic factors for 157 uterine sarcomas and evaluation of a grading score validated for soft tissue sarcoma. Cancer 88: 1425-1431.
1476. Pauwels P, Ambros P, Hattinger C, Lammens M, Dal Cin P, Ribot J, Struyk A, van Den Berghe H (2000). Peripheral primitive neuroectodermal tumour of the cervix. Virchows Arch 436: 68-73.
1477. Pawar R, Vijayalakshmy AR, Khan S, al Lawati FA (2005). Primary neuroendocrine carcinoma (Merkel's cell carcinoma) of the vulva mimicking as a Bartholin's gland abscess. Ann Saudi Med 25: 161-164.
1478. Pawelec M, Karmowski A, Karmowski M (2010). A rare case of vulvar melanoma in a young woman who frequently tanned in tanning parlors. Arch Dermatol 146: 347-348.
1479. Peacock G, Archer S (1989). Myxoid leiomyosarcoma of the uterus: case report and review of the literature. Am J Obstet Gynecol 160: 1515-1518.
1480. Pearce CL, Chung K, Pike MC, Wu AH (2009). Increased ovarian cancer risk associated with menopausal estrogen therapy is reduced by adding a progestin. Cancer 115: 531-539.
1481. Pearl ML, Johnston CM, Frank TS, Roberts JA (1993). Synchronous dual primary ovarian and endometrial carcinomas. Int J Gynaecol Obstet 43: 305-312.
1482. Peitsidis P, Akrivos T, Vecchini G, Rodolakis A, Akrivos N, Markaki S (2007). Splenosis of the peritoneal cavity resembling an adnexal tumor: case report. Clin Exp Obstet Gynecol 34: 120-122.
1483. Pejovic T, Burki N, Odunsi K, Fiedler P, Achong N, Schwartz PE, Ward DC (1999). Well-differentiated mucinous carcinoma of the ovary and a coexisting Brenner tumor both exhibit amplification of 12q14-21 by comparative genomic hybridization. Gynecol Oncol 74: 134-137.
1484. Pelmus M, Penault-Llorca F, Guillou L, Collin F, Bertrand G, Trassard M, Leroux A, Floquet A, Stoeckle E, Thomas L, MacGrogan G (2009). Prognostic factors in early-stage leiomyosarcoma of the uterus. Int J Gynecol Cancer 19: 385-390.
1485. Pelucchi C, Galeone C, Talamini R, Bosetti C, Montella M, Negri E, Franceschi S, La Vecchia C (2007). Lifetime ovulatory cycles and ovarian cancer risk in 2 Italian case-control studies. Am J Obstet Gynecol 196: 83-87.
1486. Pena-Fernandez M, Abdulkader-Nallib I, Novo-Dominguez A, Turrado-Sanchez EM, Brea-Fernandez A, Sebio-Lago L, Ruiz-Ponte C, Cameselle-Teijeiro J (2013). Vaginal tubulovillous adenoma: a clinicopathologic and molecular study with review of the literature. Int J Gynecol Pathol 32: 131-136.
1487. Pepas L, Kaushik S, Bryant A, Nordin A, Dickinson HO (2011). Medical interventions for high grade vulval intraepithelial neoplasia. Cochrane Database Syst Rev CD007924.
1488. Pereira F, Carrascal E, Canas C, Florez L (2000). Extrarenal Wilms tumor of the left ovary: a case report. J Pediatr Hematol Oncol 22: 88-89.
1489. Permuth-Wey J, Sellers TA (2009). Epidemiology of ovarian cancer. Methods Mol Biol 472: 413-437.
1490. Perri T, Korach J, Sadetzki S, Oberman B, Fridman E, Ben-Baruch G (2009). Uterine leiomyosarcoma: does the primary surgical procedure matter? Int J Gynecol Cancer 19: 257-260.
1491. Perrin L, Ward B (1995). Small cell carcinoma of the cervix. Int J Gynecol Cancer 5: 200-203.
1492. Perrone T, Dehner LP (1988). Prognostically favorable "mitotically active" smooth-muscle tumors of the uterus. A clinicopathologic study of ten cases. Am J Surg Pathol 12: 1-8.
1493. Peters WA 3rd, Kumar NB, Andersen WA, Morley GW (1985). Primary sarcoma of the adult vagina: a clinicopathologic study. Obstet Gynecol 65: 699-704.
1494. Peters WA 3rd, Kumar NB, Morley GW (1985). Microinvasive carcinoma of the vagina: a distinct clinical entity? Am J Obstet Gynecol 153: 505-507.
1495. Peterson WF (1956). Solid, histologically benign teratomas of the ovary; a report of four cases and review of the literature. Am J Obstet Gynecol 72: 1094-1102.
1496. Peterson WF (1957). Malignant degeneration of benign cystic teratomas of the overy; a collective review of the literature. Obstet Gynecol Surv 12: 793-830.
1497. Peterson WF, Prevost EC, Edmunds FT, Hundley JM Jr, Morris FK (1955). Benign cystic teratomas of the ovary; a clinico-statistical study of 1,007 cases with a review of the literature. Am J Obstet Gynecol 70: 368-382.
1498. Peto J, Collins N, Barfoot R, Seal S, Warren W, Rahman N, Easton DF, Evans C, Deacon J, Stratton MR (1999). Prevalence of BRCA1 and BRCA2 gene mutations in patients with early-onset breast cancer. J Natl Cancer Inst 91: 943-949.
1499. Petry KU, Luyten A, Justus A, Iftner A, Strehlke S, Schulze-Rath R, Iftner T (2012). Prevalence of low-risk HPV types and genital warts in women born 1988/89 or 1983/84 -results of WOLVES, a population-based epidemiological study in Wolfsburg, Germany. BMC Infect Dis 12: 367.
1500. Philippe-Chomette P, Kabbara N, Andre N, Pierron G, Coulomb A, Laurence V, Blay JY, Delattre O, Schleiermacher G, Orbach D (2012). Desmoplastic small round cell tumors with EWS-WT1 fusion transcript in children and young adults. Pediatr Blood Cancer 58: 891-897.
1501. Phillips V, McCluggage WG, Young RH (2007). Oxyphilic adenomatoid tumor of the ovary: a case report with discussion of the differential diagnosis of ovarian tumors with vacuoles and related spaces. Int J Gynecol Pathol 26: 16-20.
1502. Photopulos GJ, Carney CN, Edelman DA, Hughes RR, Fowler WC Jr, Walton LA (1979). Clear cell carcinoma of the endometrium. Cancer 43: 1448-1456.
1503. Pickel H, Thalhammer M (1971). [Chondrosarcoma of the Fallopian tube]. Geburtshilfe Frauenheilkd 31: 1243-1248.
1504. Piek JM, van Diest PJ, Zweemer RP, Jansen JW, Poort-Keesom RJ, Menko FH, Gille JJ, Jongsma AP, Pals G, Kenemans P, Verheijen RH (2001). Dysplastic changes in prophylactically removed Fallopian tubes of women predisposed to developing ovarian cancer. J Pathol 195: 451-456.
1505. Pierce Campbell CM, Menezes LJ,

Paskett ED, Giuliano AR (2012). Prevention of invasive cervical cancer in the United States: past, present, and future. Cancer Epidemiol Biomarkers Prev 21: 1402-1408.
1506. Pins MR, Young RH, Daly WJ, Scully RE (1996). Primary squamous cell carcinoma of the ovary. Report of 37 cases. Am J Surg Pathol 20: 823-833.
1507. Pinto AP, Miron A, Yassin Y, Monte N, Woo TY, Mehra KK, Medeiros F, Crum CP (2010). Differentiated vulvar intraepithelial neoplasia contains Tp53 mutations and is genetically linked to vulvar squamous cell carcinoma. Mod Pathol 23: 404-412.
1508. Pitman MB, Triratanachat S, Young RH, Oliva E (2004). Hepatocyte paraffin 1 antibody does not distinguish primary ovarian tumors with hepatoid differentiation from metastatic hepatocellular carcinoma. Int J Gynecol Pathol 23: 58-64.
1509. Pitman MB, Young RH, Clement PB, Dickersin GR, Scully RE (1994). Endometrioid carcinoma of the ovary and endometrium, oxyphilic cell type: a report of nine cases. Int J Gynecol Pathol 13: 290-301.
1510. Piura B, Rabinovich A, Yanai-Inbar I (2002). Primary malignant melanoma of the vagina: case report and review of literature. Eur J Gynaecol Oncol 23: 195-198.
1510A. Plaza JA, Kacerovska D, Stockman DL, Buonaccorsi JN, Baillargeon P, Suster S, Kazakov DV (2011). The histomorphologic spectrum of primary cutaneous diffuse large B-cell lymphoma: a study of 79 cases. Am J Dermatopathol 33: 649-655; quiz 656-658.
1511. Pocobelli G, Doherty JA, Voigt LF, Beresford SA, Hill DA, Chen C, Rossing MA, Holmes RS, Noor ZS, Weiss NS (2011). Pregnancy history and risk of endometrial cancer. Epidemiology 22: 638-645.
1512. Poen HT, Djojopranoto M (1965). The possible etiologic factors of hydatidiform mole and choriocarcinoma: preliminary report. Am J Obstet Gynecol 92: 510-513.
1513. Policarpio-Nicolas ML, Valente PT, Aune GJ, Higgins RA (2012). Isolated vaginal myeloid sarcoma in a 16-year-old girl. Ann Diagn Pathol 16: 374-379.
1514. Pollard RR, Goldberg JM (2001). Prolapsed cervical myoma after uterine artery embolization. A case report. J Reprod Med 46: 499-500.
1515. Pongtippan A, Malpica A, Levenback C, Deavers MT, Silva EG (2004). Skene's gland adenocarcinoma resembling prostatic adenocarcinoma. Int J Gynecol Pathol 23: 71-74.
1516. Pothuri B, Leitao MM, Levine DA, Viale A, Olshen AB, Arroyo C, Bogomolniy F, Olvera N, Lin O, Soslow RA, Robson ME, Offit K, Barakat RR, Boyd J (2010). Genetic analysis of the early natural history of epithelial ovarian carcinoma. PLoS One 5: e10358.
1517. Powell CB, Chen LM, McLennan J, Crawford B, Zaloudek C, Rabban JT, Moore DH, Ziegler J (2011). Risk-reducing salpingo-oophorectomy (RRSO) in BRCA mutation carriers: experience with a consecutive series of 111 patients using a standardized surgical-pathological protocol. Int J Gynecol Cancer 21: 846-851.
1518. Powell CB, Kenley E, Chen LM, Crawford B, McLennan J, Zaloudek C, Komaromy M, Beattie M, Ziegler J (2005). Risk-reducing salpingo-oophorectomy in BRCA mutation carriers: role of serial sectioning in the detection of occult malignancy. J Clin Oncol 23: 127-132.
1519. Powell CB, Swisher EM, Cass I, McLennan J, Norquist B, Garcia RL, Lester J, Karlan BY, Chen L (2013). Long term follow up of BRCA1 and BRCA2 mutation carriers with unsuspected neoplasia identified at risk reducing salpingo-oophorectomy. Gynecol Oncol 129: 364-371.
1520. Prat J, Bhan AK, Dickersin GR, Robboy SJ, Scully RE (1982). Hepatoid yolk sac tumor of the ovary (endodermal sinus tumor with hepatoid differentiation): a light microscopic, ultrastructural and immunohistochemical study of seven cases. Cancer 50: 2355-2368.
1521. Prat J, De Nictolis M (2002). Serous borderline tumors of the ovary: a long-term follow-up study of 137 cases, including 18 with a micropapillary pattern and 20 with microinvasion. Am J Surg Pathol 26: 1111-1128.
1521A. Prat J, FIGO Committee on Gynecologic Oncology (2014). Staging classification for cancer of the ovary, fallopian tube, and peritoneum. Int J Gynaecol Obstet 124:1-5.
1522. Prat J, Matias-Guiu X, Barreto J (1991). Simultaneous carcinoma involving the endometrium and the ovary. A clinicopathologic, immunohistochemical, and DNA flow cytometric study of 18 cases. Cancer 68: 2455-2459.
1523. Prat J, Scully RE (1979). Sarcomas in ovarian mucinous tumors: a report of two cases. Cancer 44: 1327-1331.
1524. Prat J, Scully RE (1981). Cellular fibromas and fibrosarcomas of the ovary: a comparative clinicopathologic analysis of seventeen cases. Cancer 47: 2663-2670.
1525. Prayson RA, Goldblum JR, Hart WR (1997). Epithelioid smooth-muscle tumors of the uterus: a clinicopathologic study of 18 patients. Am J Surg Pathol 21: 383-391.
1526. Prayson RA, Hart WR (1992). Mitotically active leiomyomas of the uterus. Am J Clin Pathol 97: 14-20.
1527. Preda O, Nicolae A, Aneiros-Fernandez J, Borda A, Nogales FF (2011). Glypican 3 is a sensitive, but not a specific, marker for the diagnosis of yolk sac tumours. Histopathology 58: 312-314.
1528. Prempree T, Tang CK, Hatef A, Forster S (1983). Angiosarcoma of the vagina: a clinicopathologic report. A reappraisal of the radiation treatment of angiosarcomas of the female genital tract. Cancer 51: 618-622.
1529. Prentice L, Stewart A, Mohiuddin S, Johnson NP (2012). What is endosalpingiosis? Fertil Steril 98: 942-947.
1530. Proppe KH, Scully RE, Rosai J (1984). Postoperative spindle cell nodules of genitourinary tract resembling sarcomas. A report of eight cases. Am J Surg Pathol 8: 101-108.
1531. Provenza C, Young RH, Prat J (2008). Anaplastic carcinoma in mucinous ovarian tumors: a clinicopathologic study of 34 cases emphasizing the crucial impact of stage on prognosis, their histologic spectrum, and overlap with sarcomalike mural nodules. Am J Surg Pathol 32: 383-389.
1532. Przybycin CG, Kurman RJ, Ronnett BM, Shih I, Vang R (2010). Are all pelvic (nonuterine) serous carcinomas of tubal origin? Am J Surg Pathol 34: 1407-1416.
1533. Pschera H, Wikstrom B (1991). Extraovarian Brenner tumor coexisting with serous cystadenoma. Case report. Gynecol Obstet Invest 31: 185-187.
1534. Pueblitz-Peredo S, Luevano-Flores E, Rincon-Taracena R, Ochoa-Carrillo FJ (1985). Uteruslike mass of the ovary: endomyometriosis or congenital malformation? A case with a discussion of histogenesis. Arch Pathol Lab Med 109: 361-364.
1535. Puig-Butille JA, Badenas C, Ogbah Z, Carrera C, Aguilera P, Malvehy J, Puig S (2013). Genetic alterations in RAS-regulated pathway in acral lentiginous melanoma. Exp Dermatol 22: 148-150.
1536. Pullarkat V, Veliz L, Chang K, Mohrbacher A, Teotico AL, Forman SJ, Slovak ML (2007). Therapy-related, mixed-lineage leukaemia translocation-positive, monoblastic myeloid sarcoma of the uterus. J Clin Pathol 60: 562-564.
1537. Purola E, Savia E (1977). Cytology of gynecologic condyloma acuminatum. Acta Cytol 21: 26-31.
1538. Pusceddu S, Bajetta E, Buzzoni R, Carcangiu ML, Platania M, Del VM, Ditto A (2008). Primary uterine cervix melanoma resembling malignant peripheral nerve sheath tumor: a case report. Int J Gynecol Pathol 27: 596-600.
1539. Pusceddu S, Bajetta E, Carcangiu ML, Formisano B, Ducceschi M, Buzzoni R (2012). A literature overview of primary cervical malignant melanoma: an exceedingly rare cancer. Crit Rev Oncol Hematol 81: 185-195.
1540. Pusiol T, Morichetti D, Zorzi MG (2011). Sebaceous carcinoma of the vulva: critical approach to grading and review of the literature. Pathologica 103: 64-67.
1541. Quade BJ (1995). Pathology, cytogenetics and molecular biology of uterine leiomyomas and other smooth muscle lesions. Curr Opin Obstet Gynecol 7: 35-42.
1542. Quade BJ, Pinto AP, Howard DR, Peters WA 3rd, Crum CP (1999). Frequent loss of heterozygosity for chromosome 10 in uterine leiomyosarcoma in contrast to leiomyoma. Am J Pathol 154: 945-950.
1543. Quddus MR, Sung CJ, Zhang C, Lawrence WD (2010). Minor serous and clear cell components adversely affect prognosis in "mixed-type" endometrial carcinomas: a clinicopathologic study of 36 stage-I cases. Reprod Sci 17: 673-678.
1544. Quick CM, Ning G, Bijron J, Laury A, Wei TS, Chen EY, Vargas SO, Betensky RA, McKeon FD, Xian W, Crum CP (2012). PAX2-null secretory cell outgrowths in the oviduct and their relationship to pelvic serous cancer. Mod Pathol 25: 449-455.
1545. Quint KD, de Koning MN, van Doorn LJ, Quint WG, Pirog EC (2010). HPV genotyping and HPV16 variant analysis in glandular and squamous neoplastic lesions of the uterine cervix. Gynecol Oncol 117: 297-301.
1546. Quint W, Jenkins D, Molijn A, Struijk L, van de Sandt M, Doorbar J, Mols J, Van Hoof C, Hardt K, Struyf F, Colau B (2012). One virus, one lesion--individual components of CIN lesions contain a specific HPV type. J Pathol 227: 62-71.
1547. Qureshi A, Raza A, Kayani N (2010). The morphologic and immunohistochemical spectrum of 16 cases of sclerosing stromal tumor of the ovary. Indian J Pathol Microbiol 53: 658-660.
1548. Qureshi SS, Shrikhande S, Ramadwar M, Desai S, Visvanathan S, Medhi SS, Laskar S, Muckaden MA, Pai SK, Desai S, Kurkure PA (2011). Desmoplastic small round cell tumor of the pancreas: An unusual primary site for an uncommon tumor. J Indian Assoc Pediatr Surg 16: 66-68.
1549. Rabban JT, Dal Cin P, Oliva E (2006). HMGA2 rearrangement in a case of vulvar aggressive angiomyxoma. Int J Gynecol Pathol 25: 403-407.
1550. Rabban JT, Lerwill MF, McCluggage WG, Grenert JP, Zaloudek CJ (2009). Primary ovarian carcinoid tumors may express CDX-2: a potential pitfall in distinction from metastatic intestinal carcinoid tumors involving the ovary. Int J Gynecol Pathol 28: 41-48.
1551. Rabban JT, Zaloudek CJ (2013). A practical approach to immunohistochemical diagnosis of ovarian germ cell tumours and sex cord-stromal tumours. Histopathology 62: 71-88.
1552. Rabban JT, Zaloudek CJ, Shekitka KM, Tavassoli FA (2005). Inflammatory myofibroblastic tumor of the uterus: a clinicopathologic study of 6 cases emphasizing distinction from aggressive mesenchymal tumors. Am J Surg Pathol 29: 1348-1355.
1553. Ragnarsson-Olding B, Johansson H, Rutqvist LE, Ringborg U (1993). Malignant melanoma of the vulva and vagina. Trends in incidence, age distribution, and long-term survival among 245 consecutive cases in Sweden 1960-1984. Cancer 71: 1893-1897.
1554. Ragnarsson-Olding BK, Kanter-Lewensohn LR, Lagerlof B, Nilsson BR, Ringborg UK (1999). Malignant melanoma of the vulva in a nationwide, 25-year study of 219 Swedish females: clinical observations and histopathologic features. Cancer 86: 1273-1284.
1555. Rahilly MA, Al-Nafussi A (1991). Uterus-like mass of the ovary associated with endometrioid carcinoma. Histopathology 18: 549-551.
1556. Rahimi S, Marani C, Renzi C, Natale ME, Giovannini P, Zeloni R (2009). Endometrial polyps and the risk of atypical hyperplasia on biopsies of unremarkable endometrium: a study on 694 patients with benign endometrial polyps. Int J Gynecol Pathol 28: 522-528.
1557. Ramirez PT, Wolf JK, Malpica A, Deavers MT, Liu J, Broaddus R (2002). Wolffian duct tumors: case reports and review of the literature. Gynecol Oncol 86: 225-230.
1558. Ramos P, Ruiz A, Carabias E, Pinero I, Garzon A, Alvarez I (2002). Mullerian adenosarcoma of the cervix with heterologous elements: report of a case and review of the literature. Gynecol Oncol 84: 161-166.
1559. Randall BJ, Ritchie C, Hutchison RS (1991). Paget's disease and invasive undifferentiated carcinoma occurring in a mature cystic teratoma of the ovary. Histopathology 18: 469-470.
1560. Randall ME, Kim JA, Mills SE, Hahn SS, Constable WC (1986). Uncommon variants of cervical carcinoma treated with radical irradiation. A clinicopathologic study of 66 cases. Cancer 57: 816-822.
1561. Rashad MN, Fathalla MF, Kerr MG (1966). Sex chromatin and chromosome analysis in ovarian teratomas. Am J Obstet Gynecol 96: 461-465.
1562. Raspollini MR, Pinzani P, Simi L, Amunni G, Villanucci A, Paglierani M, Taddei GL (2005). Uterine leiomyosarcomas express KIT protein but lack mutation(s) in exon 9 of c-KIT. Gynecol Oncol 98: 334-335.
1563. Rauh-Hain JA, Growdon WB, Rodriguez N, Goodman AK, Boruta DM, Schorge JO, Horowitz NS, del Carmen MG (2011). Carcinosarcoma of the ovary: a case-control study. Gynecol Oncol 121: 477-481.
1564. Rawlinson NJ, West WW, Nelson M, Bridge JA (2008). Aggressive angiomyxoma with t(12;21) and HMGA2 rearrangement: report of a case and review of the literature. Cancer Genet Cytogenet 181: 119-124.
1565. Redman R, Wilkinson EJ, Massoll NA (2005). Uterine-like mass with features of an extrauterine adenomyoma presenting 22 years after total abdominal hysterectomy-bilateral salpingo-oophorectomy: a case report and review of the literature. Arch Pathol Lab Med 129: 1041-1043.
1566. Reed SD, Newton KM, Clinton WL, Epplein M, Garcia R, Allison K, Voigt LF, Weiss NS (2009). Incidence of endometrial hyperplasia. Am J Obstet Gynecol 200: 678.e1-6.
1567. Reeves KW, Carter GC, Rodabaugh RJ, Lane D, McNeeley SG, Stefanick ML, Paskett ED (2011). Obesity in relation to endometrial cancer risk and disease characteristics in the

Women's Health Initiative. Gynecol Oncol 121: 376-382.

1568. Regauer S (2005). Immune dysregulation in lichen sclerosus. Eur J Cell Biol 84: 273-277.

1569. Regauer S (2011). Residual anogenital lichen sclerosus after cancer surgery has a high risk for recurrence: a clinicopathological study of 75 women. Gynecol Oncol 123: 289-294.

1570. Regauer S, Reich O, Beham-Schmid C (2002). Monoclonal gamma-T-cell receptor rearrangement in vulvar lichen sclerosus and squamous cell carcinomas. Am J Pathol 160: 1035-1045.

1571. Reich O, Regauer S (2004). Aromatase expression in low-grade endometrial stromal sarcomas: an immunohistochemical study. Mod Pathol 17: 104-108.

1572. Reich O, Tamussino K, Lahousen M, Pickel H, Haas J, Winter R (2000). Clear cell carcinoma of the uterine cervix: pathology and prognosis in surgically treated stage IB-IIB disease in women not exposed in utero to diethylstilbestrol. Gynecol Oncol 76: 331-335.

1573. Reichert RA (2007). Primary ovarian adenofibromatous neoplasms with mucin-containing signet-ring cells: a report of 2 cases. Int J Gynecol Pathol 26: 165-172.

1574. Rein MS, Barbieri RL, Welch W, Gleason RE, Caulfield JP, Friedman AJ (1993). The concentrations of collagen-associated amino acids are higher in GnRH agonist-treated uterine myomas. Obstet Gynecol 82: 901-905.

1575. Reis-Filho JS, Milanezi F, Soares MF, Fillus-Neto J, Schmitt FC (2002). Intradermal spindle cell/pleomorphic lipoma of the vulva: case report and review of the literature. J Cutan Pathol 29: 59-62.

1576. Reith JD, Goldblum JR, Lyles RH, Weiss SW (2000). Extragastrointestinal (soft tissue) stromal tumors: an analysis of 48 cases with emphasis on histologic predictors of outcome. Mod Pathol 13: 577-585.

1577. Reitsma W, de Bock GH, Oosterwijk JC, Bart J, Hollema H, Mourits MJ (2013). Support of the 'fallopian tube hypothesis' in a prospective series of risk-reducing salpingo-oophorectomy specimens. Eur J Cancer 49: 132-141.

1578. Rescorla F, Billmire D, Vinocur C, Colombani P, London W, Giller R, Cushing B, Lauer S, Cullen J, Davis M, Hawkins E (2003). The effect of neoadjuvant chemotherapy and surgery in children with malignant germ cell tumors of the genital region: a pediatric intergroup trial. J Pediatr Surg 38: 910-912.

1579. Rhemtula H, Grayson W, van Iddekinge B, Tiltman A (2001). Large-cell neuroendocrine carcinoma of the uterine cervix--a clinicopathological study of five cases. S Afr Med J 91: 525-528.

1580. Arias-Stella J (2002). The Arias-Stella reaction: facts and fancies four decades after. Adv Anat Pathol 9: 12-23.

1581. Ribe A (2008). Melanocytic lesions of the genital area with attention given to atypical genital nevi. J Cutan Pathol 35 Suppl 2: 24-27.

1582. Ribeiro F, Figueiredo A, Paula T, Borrego J (2012). Vulvar intraepithelial neoplasia: evaluation of treatment modalities. J Low Genit Tract Dis 16: 313-317.

1583. Ribeiro-Silva A, Chang D, Bisson FW, Re LO (2003). Clinicopathological and immunohistochemical features of a sebaceous carcinoma arising within a benign dermoid cyst of the ovary. Virchows Arch 443: 574-578.

1584. Rice BF, Barclay DL, Sternberg WH (1969). Luteoma of pregnancy: steroidogenic and morphologic considerations. Am J Obstet Gynecol 104: 871-878.

1585. Rice LW, Berkowitz RS, Lage JM, Goldstein DP, Bernstein MR (1990). Persistent

gestational trophoblastic tumor after partial hydatidiform mole. Gynecol Oncol 36: 358-362.

1586. Richart RM (1973). Cervical intraepithelial neoplasia. Pathol Annu 8: 301-328.

1587. Riedel I, Czernobilsky B, Lifschitz-Mercer B, Roth LM, Wu XR, Sun TT, Moll R (2001). Brenner tumors but not transitional cell carcinomas of the ovary show urothelial differentiation: immunohistochemical staining of urothelial markers, including cytokeratins and uroplakins. Virchows Arch 438: 181-191.

1588. Ries LAG, Melbert D, Krapcho M, et al (2013). SEER Cancer Statistics Review, 1975-2005. National Cancer Institute

1589. Riethdorf S, Neffen EF, Cviko A, Loning T, Crum CP, Riethdorf L (2004). p16INK4A expression as biomarker for HPV 16-related vulvar neoplasias. Hum Pathol 35: 1477-1483.

1590. Rietveld L, Nieboer TE, Kluivers KB, Schreuder HW, Bulten J, Massuger LF (2009). First case of juvenile granulosa cell tumor in an adult with Ollier disease. Int J Gynecol Pathol 28: 464-467.

1591. Riman T, Dickman PW, Nilsson S, Correia N, Nordlinder H, Magnusson CM, Persson IR (2001). Risk factors for epithelial borderline ovarian tumors: results of a Swedish case-control study. Gynecol Oncol 83: 575-585.

1592. Ringertz N (1970). Hydatidiform mole, invasive mole and choriocarcinoma in Sweden 1958-1965. Acta Obstet Gynecol Scand 49: 195-203.

1593. Rio FT, Bahubeshi A, Kanellopoulou C, Hamel N, Niedziela M, Sabbaghian N, Pouchet C, Gilbert L, O'Brien PK, Serfas K, Broderick P, Houlston RS, Lesueur F, Bonora E, Muljo S, Schimke RN, Bouron-Dal SD, Arseneau J, Schultz KA, Priest JR, Nguyen VH, Harach HR, Livingston DM, Foulkes WD, Tischkowitz M (2011). DICER1 mutations in familial multinodular goiter with and without ovarian Sertoli-Leydig cell tumors. JAMA 305: 68-77.

1594. Riopel MA, Perlman EJ, Seidman JD, Kurman RJ, Sherman ME (1998). Inhibin and epithelial membrane antigen immunohistochemistry assist in the diagnosis of sex cord-stromal tumors and provide clues to the histogenesis of hypercalcemic small cell carcinomas. Int J Gynecol Pathol 17: 46-53.

1595. Riopel MA, Ronnett BM, Kurman RJ (1999). Evaluation of diagnostic criteria and behavior of ovarian intestinal-type mucinous tumors: atypical proliferative (borderline) tumors and intraepithelial, microinvasive, invasive, and metastatic carcinomas. Am J Surg Pathol 23: 617-635.

1596. Riopel MA, Spellerberg A, Griffin CA, Perlman EJ (1998). Genetic analysis of ovarian germ cell tumors by comparative genomic hybridization. Cancer Res 58: 3105-3110.

1597. Robboy SJ, Hill EC, Sandberg EC, Czernobilsky B (1986). Vaginal adenosis in women born prior to the diethylstilbestrol era. Hum Pathol 17: 488-492.

1598. Robboy SJ, Noller KL, O'Brien P, Kaufman RH, Townsend D, Barnes AB, Gundersen J, Lawrence WD, Bergstrahl E, McGorray S, . (1984). Increased incidence of cervical and vaginal dysplasia in 3,980 diethylstilbestrol-exposed young women. Experience of the National Collaborative Diethylstilbestrol Adenosis Project. JAMA 252: 2979-2983.

1599. Robboy SJ, Norris HJ, Scully RE (1975). Insular carcinoid primary in the ovary. A clinicopathologic analysis of 48 cases. Cancer 36: 404-418.

1600. Robboy SJ, Ross JS, Prat J, Keh PC, Welch WR (1978). Urogenital sinus origin of mucinous and ciliated cysts of the vulva. Obstet Gynecol 51: 347-351.

1601. Robboy SJ, Scully RE (1970). Ovarian

teratoma with glial implants on the peritoneum. An analysis of 12 cases. Hum Pathol 1: 643-653.

1602. Robboy SJ, Scully RE (1980). Strumal carcinoid of the ovary: an analysis of 50 cases of a distinctive tumor composed of thyroid tissue and carcinoid. Cancer 46: 2019-2034.

1603. Robboy SJ, Scully RE, Norris HJ (1977). Primary trabecular carcinoid of the ovary. Obstet Gynecol 49: 202-207.

1604. Robboy SJ, Shaco-Levy R, Peng RY, Snyder MJ, Donahue J, Bentley RC, Bean S, Krigman HR, Roth LM, Young RH (2009). Malignant struma ovarii: an analysis of 88 cases, including 27 with extraovarian spread. Int J Gynecol Pathol 28: 405-422.

1605. Robboy SJ, Young RH, Welch WR, Truslow GY, Prat J, Herbst AL, Scully RE (1984). Atypical vaginal adenosis and cervical ectropion. Association with clear cell adenocarcinoma in diethylstilbestrol-exposed offspring. Cancer 54: 869-875.

1606. Robles-Frias A, Severin CE, Robles-Frias MJ, Garrido JL (2001). Diffuse uterine leiomyomatosis with ovarian and parametrial involvement. Obstet Gynecol 97: 834-835.

1607. Rockville Merkel Cell Carcinoma Group (2009). Merkel cell carcinoma: recent progress and current priorities on etiology, pathogenesis, and clinical management. J Clin Oncol 27: 4021-4026.

1608. Rodien P, Beau I, Vasseur C (2010). Ovarian hyperstimulation syndrome (OHSS) due to mutations in the follicle-stimulating hormone receptor. Ann Endocrinol (Paris) 71: 206-209.

1609. Rodke G, Friedrich EG Jr, Wilkinson EJ (1988). Malignant potential of mixed vulvar dystrophy (lichen sclerosus associated with squamous cell hyperplasia). J Reprod Med 33: 545-550.

1610. Rodriguez E, Melamed J, Reuter V, Chaganti RS (1995). Chromosomal abnormalities in choriocarcinomas of the female. Cancer Genet Cytogenet 80: 9-12.

1611. Rodriguez HA, Ackerman LV (1968). Cellular blue nevus. Clinicopathologic study of forty-five cases. Cancer 21: 393-405.

1612. Rodriguez IM, Irving JA, Prat J (2004). Endocervical-like mucinous borderline tumors of the ovary: a clinicopathologic analysis of 31 cases. Am J Surg Pathol 28: 1311-1318.

1613. Rodriguez IM, Prat J (2002). Mucinous tumors of the ovary: a clinicopathologic analysis of 75 borderline tumors (of intestinal type) and carcinomas. Am J Surg Pathol 26: 139-152.

1614. Roma A, Malpica AA, Deavers MT, Silva EG (2008). Ovarian serous borderline tumors with a predominant micropapillary pattern are aggressive neoplasms with an increased risk of low grade serous carcinoma. Modern Pathology 21: 221A.

1615. Roma AA, Yang B, Senior ME, Goldblum JR (2005). TFE3 immunoreactivity in alveolar soft part sarcoma of the uterine cervix: case report. Int J Gynecol Pathol 24: 131-135.

1616. Romero-Perez L, Castilla MA, Lopez-Garcia MA, Diaz-Martin J, Biscuola M, Ramiro-Fuentes S, Oliva E, Matias-Guiu X, Prat J, Cano A, Moreno-Bueno G, Palacios J (2013). Molecular events in endometrial carcinosarcomas and the role of high mobility group AT-hook 2 in endometrial carcinogenesis. Hum Pathol 44: 244-254.

1617. Ronnett BM, Descipio C, Murphy KM (2011). Hydatidiform moles: ancillary techniques to refine diagnosis. Int J Gynecol Pathol 30: 101-116.

1618. Ronnett BM, Kajdacsy-Balla A, Gilks CB, Merino MJ, Silva E, Werness BA, Young RH (2004). Mucinous borderline ovarian

tumors: points of general agreement and persistent controversies regarding nomenclature, diagnostic criteria, and behavior. Hum Pathol 35: 949-960.

1619. Ronnett BM, Kurman RJ, Shmookler BM, Sugarbaker PH, Young RH (1997). The morphologic spectrum of ovarian metastases of appendiceal adenocarcinomas: a clinicopathologic and immunohistochemical analysis of tumors often misinterpreted as primary ovarian tumors or metastatic tumors from other gastrointestinal sites. Am J Surg Pathol 21: 1144-1155.

1620. Ronnett BM, Kurman RJ, Zahn CM, Shmookler BM, Jablonski KA, Kass ME, Sugarbaker PH (1995). Pseudomyxoma peritonei in women: a clinicopathologic analysis of 30 cases with emphasis on site of origin, prognosis, and relationship to ovarian mucinous tumors of low malignant potential. Hum Pathol 26: 509-524.

1621. Ronnett BM, Shmookler BM, Diener-West M, Sugarbaker PH, Kurman RJ (1997). Immunohistochemical evidence supporting the appendiceal origin of pseudomyxoma peritonei in women. Int J Gynecol Pathol 16: 1-9.

1622. Ronnett BM, Yan H, Kurman RJ, Shmookler BM, Wu L, Sugarbaker PH (2001). Patients with pseudomyxoma peritonei associated with disseminated peritoneal adenomucinosis have a significantly more favorable prognosis than patients with peritoneal mucinous carcinomatosis. Cancer 92: 85-91.

1623. Ronnett BM, Yemelyanova AV, Vang R, Gilks CB, Miller D, Gravitt PE, Kurman RJ (2008). Endocervical adenocarcinomas with ovarian metastases: analysis of 29 cases with emphasis on minimally invasive cervical tumors and the ability of the metastases to simulate primary ovarian neoplasms. Am J Surg Pathol 32: 1835-1853.

1624. Ronnett BM, Zahn CM, Kurman RJ, Kass ME, Sugarbaker PH, Shmookler BM (1995). Disseminated peritoneal adenomucinosis and peritoneal mucinous carcinomatosis. A clinicopathologic analysis of 109 cases with emphasis on distinguishing pathologic features, site of origin, prognosis, and relationship to "pseudomyxoma peritonei". Am J Surg Pathol 19: 1390-1408.

1625. Rose PG, Ali S, Watkins E, Thigpen JT, Deppe G, Clarke-Pearson DL, Insalaco S (2007). Long-term follow-up of a randomized trial comparing concurrent single agent cisplatin, cisplatin-based combination chemotherapy, or hydroxyurea during pelvic irradiation for locally advanced cervical cancer: a Gynecologic Oncology Group Study. J Clin Oncol 25: 2804-2810.

1626. Rose PG, Stoler MH, Abdul-Karim FW (1998). Papillary squamotransitional cell carcinoma of the vagina. Int J Gynecol Pathol 17: 372-375.

1627. Rosenfeld WD, Rose E, Vermund SH, Schreiber K, Burk RD (1992). Follow-up evaluation of cervicovaginal human papillomavirus infection in adolescents. J Pediatr 121: 307-311.

1628. Ross JC, Eifel PJ, Cox RS, Kempson RL, Hendrickson MR (1983). Primary mucinous adenocarcinoma of the endometrium. A clinicopathologic and histochemical study. Am J Surg Pathol 7: 715-729.

1629. Ross MJ, Welch WR, Scully RE (1989). Multilocular peritoneal inclusion cysts (so-called cystic mesotheliomas). Cancer 64: 1336-1346.

1630. Roth LM (1974). The Brenner tumor and the Walthard cell nest. An electron microscopic study. Lab Invest 31: 15-23.

1631. Roth LM, Czernobilsky B (1985). Ovarian Brenner tumors. II. Malignant. Cancer 56: 592-601.

1632. Roth LM, Davis MM, Sutton GP (1996). Steroid cell tumor of the broad ligament arising in an accessory ovary. Arch Pathol Lab Med 120: 405-409.
1633. Roth LM, Deaton RL, Sternberg WH (1979). Massive ovarian edema. A clinicopathologic study of five cases including ultrastructural observations and review of the literature. Am J Surg Pathol 3: 11-21.
1634. Roth LM, Emerson RE, Ulbright TM (2003). Ovarian endometrioid tumors of low malignant potential: a clinicopathologic study of 30 cases with comparison to well-differentiated endometrioid adenocarcinoma. Am J Surg Pathol 27: 1253-1259.
1635. Roth LM, Karseladze AI (2008). Highly differentiated follicular carcinoma arising from struma ovarii: a report of 3 cases, a review of the literature, and a reassessment of so-called peritoneal strumosis. Int J Gynecol Pathol 27: 213-222.
1636. Roth LM, Langley FA, Fox H, Wheeler JE, Czernobilsky B (1984). Ovarian clear cell adenofibromatous tumors. Benign, of low malignant potential, and associated with invasive clear cell carcinoma. Cancer 53: 1156-1163.
1637. Roth LM, Dallenbach-Hellweg G, Czernobilsky B (1985). Ovarian Brenner tumors. I. Metaplastic, proliferating, and of low malignant potential. Cancer 56: 582-591.
1638. Roth LM, Liban E, Czernobilsky B (1982). Ovarian endometrioid tumors mimicking Sertoli and Sertoli-Leydig cell tumors: Sertoliform variant of endometrioid carcinoma. Cancer 50: 1322-1331.
1639. Roth LM, Look KY (2000). Inverted follicular keratosis of the vulvar skin: a lesion that can be confused with squamous cell carcinoma. Int J Gynecol Pathol 19: 369-373.
1640. Roth LM, Miller AW 3rd, Talerman A (2008). Typical thyroid-type carcinoma arising in struma ovarii: a report of 4 cases and review of the literature. Int J Gynecol Pathol 27: 496-506.
1641. Roth LM, Reed RJ (1999). Dissecting leiomyomas of the uterus other than cotyledonoid dissecting leiomyomas: a report of eight cases. Am J Surg Pathol 23: 1032-1039.
1642. Roth LM, Reed RJ, Sternberg WH (1996). Cotyledonoid dissecting leiomyoma of the uterus. The Sternberg tumor. Am J Surg Pathol 20: 1455-1461.
1643. Roth LM, Sternberg WH (1973). Ovarian stromal tumors containing Leydig cells. II. Pure Leydig cell tumor, non-hilar type. Cancer 32: 952-960.
1644. Roth LM, Talerman A (2006). Recent advances in the pathology and classification of ovarian germ cell tumors. Int J Gynecol Pathol 25: 305-320.
1645. Roth LM, Talerman A (2007). The enigma of struma ovarii. Pathology 39: 139-146.
1646. Roth LM, Talerman A, Levy T, Sukmanov O, Czernobilsky B (2011). Ovarian yolk sac tumors in older women arising from epithelial ovarian tumors or with no detectable epithelial component. Int J Gynecol Pathol 30: 442-451.
1647. Roth LM, Talerman A, Wadsley J, Karseladze AI (2010). Risk factors in thyroid-type carcinoma arising in ovarian struma: a report of 15 cases with comparison to ordinary struma ovarii. Histopathology 57: 148-152.
1648. Rudd ML, Price JC, Fogoros S, Godwin AK, Sgroi DC, Merino MJ, Bell DW (2011). A unique spectrum of somatic PIK3CA (p110alpha) mutations within primary endometrial carcinomas. Clin Cancer Res 17: 1331-1340.
1649. Ruggiero S, Ripetti V, Bianchi A, La Vaccara V, Alloni R, Coppola R (2011). A singular observation of a giant benign Brenner tumor of the ovary. Arch Gynecol Obstet 284: 513-516.
1650. Ruiz-Casado A, Miliani C, Lopez C, Lopez M, Martin T, Pereira F (2012). Round ligament metastatic gastric cancer as a finding in an inguinal surgery. Gastrointest Cancer Res 5: 137-138.
1651. Rushing RS, Shajahan S, Chendil D, Wilder JL, Pulliam J, Lee EY, Ueland FR, van Nagell Jr, Ahmed MM, Lele SM (2003). Uterine sarcomas express KIT protein but lack mutation(s) in exon 11 or 17 of c-KIT. Gynecol Oncol 91: 9-14.
1652. Russell MJ, Fadare O (2006). Adenoid basal lesions of the uterine cervix: evolving terminology and clinicopathological concepts. Diagn Pathol 1: 18.
1653. Russell P (1984). Borderline epithelial tumours of the ovary: a conceptual dilemma. Clin Obstet Gynaecol 11: 259-277.
1654. Rutgers JL, Scully RE (1988). Cysts (cystadenomas) and tumors of the rete ovarii. Int J Gynecol Pathol 7: 330-342.
1655. Rutgers JL, Scully RE (1988). Ovarian mixed-epithelial papillary cystadenomas of borderline malignancy of mullerian type. A clinicopathologic analysis. Cancer 61: 546-554.
1656. Rutgers JL, Scully RE (1988). Ovarian mullerian mucinous papillary cystadenomas of borderline malignancy. A clinicopathologic analysis. Cancer 61: 340-348.
1657. Rydholm A, Berg NO (1983). Size, site and clinical incidence of lipoma. Factors in the differential diagnosis of lipoma and sarcoma. Acta Orthop Scand 54: 929-934.
1658. Ryu SY, Park SI, Nam BH, Kim I, Yoo CW, Nam JH, Lee KH, Cho CH, Kim JH, Park SY, Kim BG, Kang SB (2009). Prognostic significance of histological grade in clear-cell carcinoma of the ovary: a retrospective study of Korean Gynecologic Oncology Group. Ann Oncol 20: 1032-1036.
1659. Rywlin AM, Simmons RJ, Robinson MJ (1969). Leiomyoma of vagina recurrent in pregnancy: a case with apparent hormone dependency. South Med J 62: 1449-1451.
1660. Saad RS, Mashhour M, Noftech-Mozes S, Ismiil N, Dube V, Ghorab Z, Faragalla H, Khalifa MA (2012). P16INK4a expression in undifferentiated carcinoma of the uterus does not exclude its endometrial origin. Int J Gynecol Pathol 31: 57-65.
1661. Sadeghi B, Arvieux C, Glehen O, Beaujard AC, Rivoire M, Baulieux J, Fontaumard E, Brachet A, Caillot JL, Faure JL, Porcheron J, Peix JL, Francois Y, Vignal J, Gilly FN (2000). Peritoneal carcinomatosis from non-gynecologic malignancies: results of the EVOCAPE 1 multicentric prospective study. Cancer 88: 358-363.
1662. Saegusa M, Hashimura M, Kuwata T, Okayasu I (2009). Requirement of the Akt/beta-catenin pathway for uterine carcinosarcoma genesis, modulating E-cadherin expression through the transactivation of slug. Am J Pathol 174: 2107-2115.
1663. Saegusa M, Okayasu I (2001). Frequent nuclear beta-catenin accumulation and associated mutations in endometrioid-type endometrial and ovarian carcinomas with squamous differentiation. J Pathol 194: 59-67.
1664. Saffos RO, Rhatigan RM, Scully RE (1980). Metaplastic papillary tumor of the fallopian tube--a distinctive lesion of pregnancy. Am J Clin Pathol 74: 232-236.
1665. Sagae S, Kobayashi K, Nishioka Y, Sugimura M, Ishioka S, Nagata M, Terasawa K, Tokino T, Kudo R (1999). Mutational analysis of beta-catenin gene in Japanese ovarian carcinomas: frequent mutations in endometrioid carcinomas. Jpn J Cancer Res 90: 510-515.
1666. Sah SP, McCluggage WG (2013). DOG1 immunoreactivity in uterine leiomyosarcomas. J Clin Pathol 66: 40-43.
1667. Sahin A, Benda JA (1988). Primary ovarian Wilms' tumor. Cancer 61: 1460-1463.
1668. Salawu A, Ul-Hassan A, Hammond D, Fernando M, Reed M, Sisley K (2012). High quality genomic copy number data from archival formalin-fixed paraffin-embedded leiomyosarcoma: optimisation of universal linkage system labelling. PLoS One 7: e50415.
1669. Salvador S, Rempel A, Soslow RA, Gilks B, Huntsman D, Miller D (2008). Chromosomal instability in fallopian tube precursor lesions of serous carcinoma and frequent monoclonality of synchronous ovarian and fallopian tube mucosal serous carcinoma. Gynecol Oncol 110: 408-417.
1670. Samanth KK, Black WC 3rd (1970). Benign ovarian stromal tumors associated with free peritoneal fluid. Am J Obstet Gynecol 107: 538-545.
1671. Samlal RA, Ten Kate FJ, Hart AA, Lammes FB (1998). Do mucin-secreting squamous cell carcinomas of the uterine cervix metastasize more frequently to pelvic lymph nodes? A case-control study? Int J Gynecol Pathol 17: 201-204.
1672. Sandberg AA (2005). Updates on the cytogenetics and molecular genetics of bone and soft tissue tumors: leiomyosarcoma. Cancer Genet Cytogenet 161: 1-19.
1673. Sangoi AR, McKenney JK, Schwartz EJ, Rouse RV, Longacre TA (2009). Adenomatoid tumors of the female and male genital tracts: a clinicopathological and immunohistochemical study of 44 cases. Mod Pathol 22: 1228-1235.
1674. Sanjeevi CB, Hjelmstrom P, Hallmans G, Wiklund F, Lenner P, Angstrom T, Dillner J, Lernmark A (1996). Different HLA-DR-DQ haplotypes are associated with cervical intraepithelial neoplasia among human papillomavirus type-16 seropositive and seronegative Swedish women. Int J Cancer 68: 409-414.
1675. Sankaranarayanan R, Black RJ, Swaminathan R, Parkin DM (1998). An overview of cancer survival in developing countries. IARC Sci Publ 135-173.
1676. Sano T, Oyama T, Kashiwabara K, Fukuda T, Nakajima T (1998). Expression status of p16 protein is associated with human papillomavirus oncogenic potential in cervical and genital lesions. Am J Pathol 153: 1741-1748.
1677. Santala M, Suonio S, Syrjanen K, Uronen MT, Saarikoski S (1987). Malignant fibrous histiocytoma of the vulva. Gynecol Oncol 27: 121-126.
1678. Santegoets LA, Helmerhorst TJ, van der Meijden WI (2010). A retrospective study of 95 women with a clinical diagnosis of genital lichen planus. J Low Genit Tract Dis 14: 323-328.
1679. Santini D, Gelli MC, Mazzoleni G, Ricci M, Severi B, Pasquinelli G, Pelusi G, Martinelli G (1989). Brenner tumor of the ovary: a correlative histologic, histochemical, immunohistochemical, and ultrastructural investigation. Hum Pathol 20: 787-795.
1680. Santos LD, Kennerson AR, Killingsworth MC (2006). Nodular hyperplasia of Bartholin's gland. Pathology 38: 223-228.
1681. Santoso JT, Long M, Crigger M, Wan JY, Haefner HK (2010). Anal intraepithelial neoplasia in women with genital intraepithelial neoplasia. Obstet Gynecol 116: 578-582.
1682. Sanz-Ortega J, Vocke C, Stratton P, Linehan WM, Merino MJ (2013). Morphologic and molecular characteristics of uterine leiomyomas in hereditary leiomyomatosis and renal cancer (HLRCC) syndrome. Am J Surg Pathol 37: 74-80.
1683. Sargenti-Neto S, Brazao-Silva MT, do Nascimento Souza KC, de Faria PR, Durighetto-Junior AF, Loyola AM, Cardoso SV (2009). Multicentric granular cell tumor: report of a patient with oral and cutaneous lesions. Br J Oral Maxillofac Surg 47: 62-64.
1684. Sasano H, Fukunaga M, Rojas M, Silverberg SG (1989). Hyperthecosis of the ovary. Clinicopathologic study of 19 cases with immunohistochemical analysis of steroidogenic enzymes. Int J Gynecol Pathol 8: 311-320.
1685. Sasano H, Sato S, Yajima A, Akama J, Nagura H (1997). Adrenal rest tumor of the broad ligament: case report with immunohistochemical study of steroidogenic enzymes. Pathol Int 47: 493-496.
1686. Sasieni P, Castanon A, Cuzick J (2009). Screening and adenocarcinoma of the cervix. Int J Cancer 125: 525-529.
1687. Sato K, Ueda Y, Sugaya J, Ozaki M, Hisaoka M, Katsuda S (2007). Extrauterine endometrial stromal sarcoma with JAZF1/JJAZ1 fusion confirmed by RT-PCR and interphase FISH presenting as an inguinal tumor. Virchows Arch 450: 349-353.
1688. Sato N, Tsunoda H, Nishida M, Morishita Y, Takimoto Y, Kubo T, Noguchi M (2000). Loss of heterozygosity on 10q23.3 and mutation of the tumor suppressor gene PTEN in benign endometrial cyst of the ovary: possible sequence progression from benign endometrial cyst to endometrioid carcinoma and clear cell carcinoma of the ovary. Cancer Res 60: 7052-7056.
1689. Savvari P, Peitsidis P, Alevizaki M, Dimopoulos MA, Antsaklis A, Papadimitriou CA (2009). Paraneoplastic humorally mediated hypercalcemia induced by parathyroid hormone-related protein in gynecologic malignancies: a systematic review. Onkologie 32: 517-523.
1690. Scanlon R, Kelehan P, Flannelly G, McDonald D, McCluggage WG (2004). Ischemic fasciitis: an unusual vulvovaginal spindle cell lesion. Int J Gynecol Pathol 23: 65-67.
1691. Schammel DP, Tavassoli FA (1998). Uterine angiosarcomas: a morphologic and immunohistochemical study of four cases. Am J Surg Pathol 22: 246-250.
1692. Schiavone MB, Herzog TJ, Lewin SN, Deutsch I, Sun X, Burke WM, Wright JD (2011). Natural history and outcome of mucinous carcinoma of the ovary. Am J Obstet Gynecol 205: 480-488.
1693. Schiffman M, Wentzensen N, Wacholder S, Kinney W, Gage JC, Castle PE (2011). Human papillomavirus testing in the prevention of cervical cancer. J Natl Cancer Inst 103: 368-383.
1694. Schiller JT, Lowy DR (2012). Understanding and learning from the success of prophylactic human papillomavirus vaccines. Nat Rev Microbiol 10: 681-692.
1695. Schmandt RE, Iglesias DA, Co NN, Lu KH (2011). Understanding obesity and endometrial cancer risk: opportunities for prevention. Am J Obstet Gynecol 205: 518-525.
1696. Schmeler KM, Sun CC, Bodurka DC, Deavers MT, Malpica A, Coleman RL, Ramirez PT, Gershenson DM (2008). Neoadjuvant chemotherapy for low-grade serous carcinoma of the ovary or peritoneum. Gynecol Oncol 108: 510-514.
1697. Schmid P, Nagai Y, Agarwal R, Hancock B, Savage PM, Sebire NJ, Lindsay I, Wells M, Fisher RA, Short D, Newlands ES, Wischnewsky MB, Seckl MJ (2009). Prognostic markers and long-term outcome of placental-site trophoblastic tumours: a retrospective observational study. Lancet 374: 48-55.
1698. Schmidt J, Derr V, Heinrich MC, Crum CP, Fletcher JA, Corless CL, Nose V (2007). BRAF in papillary thyroid carcinoma

of ovary (struma ovarii). Am J Surg Pathol 31: 1337-1343.
1699. Schneider DT, Calaminus G, Harms D, Gobel U (2005). Ovarian sex cord-stromal tumors in children and adolescents. J Reprod Med 50: 439-446.
1700. Schofield DE, Fletcher JA (1992). Trisomy 12 in pediatric granulosa-stromal cell tumors. Demonstration by a modified method of fluorescence in situ hybridization on paraffin-embedded material. Am J Pathol 141: 1265-1269.
1701. Schorge JO, Muto MG, Lee SJ, Huang LW, Welch WR, Bell DA, Keung EZ, Berkowitz RS, Mok SC (2000). BRCA1-related papillary serous carcinoma of the peritoneum has a unique molecular pathogenesis. Cancer Res 60: 1361-1364.
1702. Schorge JO, Muto MG, Welch WR, Bandera CA, Rubin SC, Bell DA, Berkowitz RS, Mok SC (1998). Molecular evidence for multifocal papillary serous carcinoma of the peritoneum in patients with germline BRCA1 mutations. J Natl Cancer Inst 90: 841-845.
1703. Schultz KA, Pacheco MC, Yang J, Williams GM, Messinger Y, Hill DA, Dehner LP, Priest JR (2011). Ovarian sex cord-stromal tumors, pleuropulmonary blastoma and DICER1 mutations: a report from the International Pleuropulmonary Blastoma Registry. Gynecol Oncol 122: 246-250.
1704. Schwartz DR, Kardia SL, Shedden KA, Kuick R, Michailidis G, Taylor JM, Misek DE, Wu R, Zhai Y, Darrah DM, Reed H, Ellenson LH, Giordano TJ, Fearon ER, Hanash SM, Cho KR (2002). Gene expression in ovarian cancer reflects both morphology and biological behavior, distinguishing clear cell from other poor-prognosis ovarian carcinomas. Cancer Res 62: 4722-4729.
1705. Schwartz EJ, Longacre TA (2004). Adenomatoid tumors of the female and male genital tracts express WT1. Int J Gynecol Pathol 23: 123-128.
1706. Scinicariello F, Rady P, Hannigan E, Dinh TV, Tyring SK (1992). Human papillomavirus type 16 found in primary transitional cell carcinoma of the Bartholin's gland and in a lymph node metastasis. Gynecol Oncol 47: 263-266.
1707. Scully RE (1970). Gonadoblastoma. A review of 74 cases. Cancer 25: 1340-1356.
1708. Scully RE, Bonfiglio TA, Kurman RJ, Silverberg SG, Wilkinson EJ (Eds.) (1994). Histological Typing of Female Genital Tract Tumours. International Histological Classification of Tumours. 2nd Ed. Springer: Berlin, Heidelberg.
1709. Scully RE, Young RH (1981). Trophoblastic pseudotumor: a reappraisal. Am J Surg Pathol 5: 75-76.
1710. Scully RE, Young RH, Clement PB (Eds.) (1998). Tumors of the Ovary, Maldeveloped Gonads, Fallopian Tube and Broad Ligament. Atlas of Tumor Pathology. 3rd Series, Fascicle 23. Armed Forces Institute of Pathology: Washington, DC.
1711. Scurry J, Brand A, Planner R, Dowling J, Rode J (1996). Vulvar Merkel cell tumor with glandular and squamous differentiation. Gynecol Oncol 62: 292-297.
1712. Scurry J, van der Putte SC, Pyman J, Chetty N, Szabo R (2009). Mammary-like gland adenoma of the vulva: review of 46 cases. Pathology 41: 372-378.
1713. Sebenik M, Yan Z, Khalbuss WE, Mittal K (2007). Malignant mixed mullerian tumor of the vagina: case report with review of the literature, immunohistochemical study, and evaluation for human papilloma virus. Hum Pathol 38: 1282-1288.
1714. Sebire NJ, Fisher RA, Foskett M, Rees H, Seckl MJ, Newlands ES (2003). Risk of recurrent hydatidiform mole and subsequent pregnancy outcome following complete or partial hydatidiform molar pregnancy. BJOG 110: 22-26.
1715. Sebire NJ, Fisher RA, Rees HC (2003). Histopathological diagnosis of partial and complete hydatidiform mole in the first trimester of pregnancy. Pediatr Dev Pathol 6: 69-77.
1716. Sebire NJ, Foskett M, Fisher RA, Rees H, Seckl M, Newlands E (2002). Risk of partial and complete hydatidiform molar pregnancy in relation to maternal age. BJOG 109: 99-102.
1717. Sebire NJ, Lindsay I, Fisher RA, Seckl MJ (2005). Intraplacental choriocarcinoma: experience from a tertiary referral center and relationship with infantile choriocarcinoma. Fetal Pediatr Pathol 24: 21-29.
1718. Seckl MJ, Fisher RA, Salerno G, Rees H, Paradinas FJ, Foskett M, Newlands ES (2000). Choriocarcinoma and partial hydatidiform moles. Lancet 356: 36-39.
1719. Seckl MJ, Mulholland PJ, Bishop AE, Teale JD, Hales CN, Glaser M, Watkins S, Seckl JR (1999). Hypoglycemia due to an insulin-secreting small-cell carcinoma of the cervix. N Engl J Med 341: 733-736.
1720. Seckl MJ, Sebire NJ, Berkowitz RS (2010). Gestational trophoblastic disease. Lancet 376: 717-729.
1721. Sedlacek TV, Riva JM, Magen AB, Mangan CE, Cunnane MF (1990). Vaginal and vulvar adenosis. An unsuspected side effect of CO2 laser vaporization. J Reprod Med 35: 995-1001.
1722. Segev Y, Iqbal J, Lubinski J, Gronwald J, Lynch HT, Moller P, Ghadirian P, Rosen B, Tung N, Kim-Sing C, Foulkes WD, Neuhausen SL, Senter L, Singer CF, Karlan B, Ping S, Narod SA (2013). The incidence of endometrial cancer in women with BRCA1 and BRCA2 mutations: an international prospective cohort study. Gynecol Oncol 130: 127-131.
1723. Seidman JD (1996). Unclassified ovarian gonadal stromal tumors. A clinicopathologic study of 32 cases. Am J Surg Pathol 20: 699-706.
1724. Seidman JD, Chauhan S (2003). Evaluation of the relationship between adenosarcoma and carcinosarcoma and a hypothesis of the histogenesis of uterine sarcomas. Int J Gynecol Pathol 22: 75-82.
1724A. Seidman JD, Cho KR, Ronnett BM, Kurman RJ (2011). Surface epithelial tumors of the ovary. In: Blaustein's Pathology of female genital tract. Kurman RJ, Ellenson HK, Ronnett BM (Eds) Springer: New York, 679-784.
1725. Seidman JD, Khedmati F (2008). Exploring the histogenesis of ovarian mucinous and transitional cell (Brenner) neoplasms and their relationship with Walthard cell nests: a study of 120 tumors. Arch Pathol Lab Med 132: 1753-1760.
1726. Seidman JD, Kurman RJ (1996). Subclassification of serous borderline tumors of the ovary into benign and malignant types. A clinicopathologic study of 65 advanced stage cases. Am J Surg Pathol 20: 1331-1345.
1727. Seidman JD, Kurman RJ (2000). Ovarian serous borderline tumors: a critical review of the literature with emphasis on prognostic indicators. Hum Pathol 31: 539-557.
1728. Seidman JD, Kurman RJ, Ronnett BM (2003). Primary and metastatic mucinous adenocarcinomas in the ovaries: incidence in routine practice with a new approach to improve intraoperative diagnosis. Am J Surg Pathol 27: 985-993.
1729. Seidman JD, Soslow RA, Vang R, Berman JJ, Stoler MH, Sherman ME, Oliva E, Kajdacsy-Balla A, Berman DM, Copeland LJ (2004). Borderline ovarian tumors: diverse contemporary viewpoints on terminology and diagnostic criteria with illustrative images. Hum Pathol 35: 918-933.
1730. Seidman JD, Yemelyanova A, Zaino RJ, Kurman RJ (2011). The fallopian tube-peritoneal junction: a potential site of carcinogenesis. Int J Gynecol Pathol 30: 4-11.
1731. Seltzer VL, Levine A, Spiegel G, Rosenfeld D, Coffey EL (1990). Adenofibroma of the uterus: multiple recurrences following wide local excision. Gynecol Oncol 37: 427-431.
1732. Semere LG, Ko E, Johnson NR, Vitonis AF, Phang LJ, Cramer DW, Mutter GL (2011). Endometrial intraepithelial neoplasia: clinical correlates and outcomes. Obstet Gynecol 118: 21-28.
1733. Senzaki H, Osaki T, Uemura Y, Kiyozuka Y, Ogura E, Okamura A, Tsubura A (1997). Adenoid basal carcinoma of the uterine cervix: immunohistochemical study and literature review. Jpn J Clin Oncol 27: 437-441.
1734. Seoud M, Tjalma WA, Ronsse V (2011). Cervical adenocarcinoma: moving towards better prevention. Vaccine 29: 9148-9158.
1735. Scully R.E., Bonfiglio T.A., Kurman R.J., Silverberg S.G., Wilkinson E.J. (Eds.) (1975). Histological Typing of Female Genital Tract Tumours. International Histological Classification of Tumours. World Health Organization: Geneva.
1736. Setiawan VW, Pike MC, Karageorgi S, Deming SL, Anderson K, Bernstein L, Brinton LA, Cai H, Cerhan JR, Cozen W, Chen C, Doherty J, Freudenheim JL, Goodman MT, Hankinson SE, Lacey JV Jr, Liang X, Lissowska J, Lu L, Lurie G, Mack T, Matsuno RK, McCann S, Moysich KB, Olson SH, Rastogi R, Rebbeck TR, Risch H, Robien K, Schairer C, Shu XO, Spurdle AB, Strom BL, Thompson PJ, Ursin G, Webb PM, Weiss NS, Wentzensen N, Xiang YB, Yang HP, Yu H, Horn-Ross PL, De Vivo I (2012). Age at last birth in relation to risk of endometrial cancer: pooled analysis in the epidemiology of endometrial cancer consortium. Am J Epidemiol 176: 269-278.
1737. Sever M, Jones TD, Roth LM, Karim FW, Zheng W, Michael H, Hattab EM, Emerson RE, Baldridge LA, Cheng L (2005). Expression of CD117 (c-kit) receptor in dysgerminoma of the ovary: diagnostic and therapeutic implications. Mod Pathol 18: 1411-1416.
1738. Seward S, Ali-Fehmi R, Munkarah AR, Semaan A, Al-Wahab ZR, Elshaikh MA, Cote ML, Morris RT, Bandyopadhyay S (2012). Outcomes of patients with uterine serous carcinoma using the revised FIGO staging system. Int J Gynecol Cancer 22: 452-456.
1739. Shaco-Levy R, Bean SM, Bentley RC, Robboy SJ (2010). Natural history of biologically malignant struma ovarii: analysis of 27 cases with extraovarian spread. Int J Gynecol Pathol 29: 212-227.
1740. Shaco-Levy R, Peng RY, Snyder MJ, Osmond GW, Veras E, Bean SM, Bentley RC, Robboy SJ (2012). Malignant struma ovarii: a blinded study of 86 cases assessing which histologic features correlate with aggressive clinical behavior. Arch Pathol Lab Med 136: 172-178.
1741. Shah SP, Köbel M, Senz J, Morin RD, Clarke BA, Wiegand KC, Leung G, Zayed A, Mehl E, Kalloger SE, Sun M, Giuliany R, Yorida E, Jones S, Varhol R, Swenerton KD, Miller D, Clement PB, Crane C, Madore J, Provencher D, Leung P, deFazio A, Khattra J, Turashvili G, Zhao Y, Zeng T, Glover JN, Vanderhyden B, Zhao C, Parkinson CA, Jimenez-Linan M, Bowtell DD, Mes-Masson AM, Brenton JD, Aparicio SA, Boyd N, Hirst M, Gilks CB, Marra M, Huntsman DG (2009). Mutation of FOXL2 in granulosa-cell tumors of the ovary. N Engl J Med 360: 2719-2729.
1742. Shankar AG, Ashley S, Craft AW, Pinkerton CR (2003). Outcome after relapse in an unselected cohort of children and adolescents with Ewing sarcoma. Med Pediatr Oncol 40: 141-147.
1743. Shappell HW, Riopel MA, Smith Sehdev AE, Ronnett BM, Kurman RJ (2002). Diagnostic criteria and behavior of ovarian seromucinous (endocervical-type mucinous and mixed cell-type) tumors: atypical proliferative (borderline) tumors, intraepithelial, microinvasive, and invasive carcinomas. Am J Surg Pathol 26: 1529-1541.
1744. Sharma P, Chaturvedi KU, Gupta R, Nigam S (2004). Leiomyomatosis peritonealis disseminata with malignant change in a post-menopausal woman. Gynecol Oncol 95: 742-745.
1745. Shatz P, Bergeron C, Wilkinson EJ, Arseneau J, Ferenczy A (1989). Vulvar intraepithelial neoplasia and skin appendage involvement. Obstet Gynecol 74: 769-774.
1746. Sheikh ZA, Nair I, Vijaykumar DK, Jojo A, Nandeesh M (2010). Neuroendocrine tumor of vulva: a case report and review of literature. J Cancer Res Ther 6: 365-366.
1747. Shen DH, Khoo US, Ngan HY, Ng TY, Chau MT, Xue WC, Cheung AN (2003). Coexisting epithelioid trophoblastic tumor and choriocarcinoma of the uterus following a chemoresistant hydatidiform mole. Arch Pathol Lab Med 127: e291-e293.
1748. Shen JG, Chen YX, Xu DY, Feng YF, Tong ZH (2008). Vaginal paraganglioma presenting as a gynecologic mass: case report. Eur J Gynaecol Oncol 29: 184-185.
1749. Shen JT, D'ablaing G, Morrow CP (1982). Alveolar soft part sarcoma of the vulva: report of first case and review of literature. Gynecol Oncol 13: 120-128.
1750. Shenjere P, Salman WD, Singh M, Mangham DC, Williams A, Eyden BP, Howard N, Knight B, Banerjee SS (2012). Intra-abdominal clear-cell sarcoma: a report of 3 cases, including 1 case with unusual morphological features, and review of the literature. Int J Surg Pathol 20: 378-385.
1751. Sheppard DM, Fisher RA, Lawler SD (1985). Karyotypic analysis and chromosome polymorphisms in four choriocarcinoma cell lines. Cancer Genet Cytogenet 16: 251-258.
1752. Sherman ME (2000). Theories of endometrial carcinogenesis: a multidisciplinary approach. Mod Pathol 13: 295-308.
1753. Sherman ME, Guido R, Wentzensen N, Yang HP, Mai PL, Greene MH (2012). New views on the pathogenesis of high-grade pelvic serous carcinoma with suggestions for advancing future research. Gynecol Oncol 127: 645-650.
1754. Sherman ME, Solomon D, Schiffman M (2001). Qualification of ASCUS. A comparison of equivocal LSIL and equivocal HSIL cervical cytology in the ASCUS LSIL Triage Study. Am J Clin Pathol 116: 386-394.
1755. Sheu BC, Lin HH, Chen CK, Chao KH, Shun CT, Huang SC (1995). Synchronous primary carcinomas of the endometrium and ovary. Int J Gynaecol Obstet 51: 141-146.
1756. Shevchuk MM, Fenoglio CM, Richart RM (1980). Histogenesis of Brenner tumors, I: histology and ultrastructure. Cancer 46: 2607-2616.
1757. Shibata R, Umezawa A, Takehara K, Aoki D, Nozawa S, Hata J (2003). Primary carcinosarcoma of the vagina. Pathol Int 53: 106-110.
1758. Shih IM, Kurman RJ (1997). New concepts in trophoblastic growth and differentiation

with practical application for the diagnosis of gestational trophoblastic disease. Verh Dtsch Ges Pathol 81: 266-272.

1759. Shih IM, Kurman RJ (1998). Epithelioid trophoblastic tumor: a neoplasm distinct from choriocarcinoma and placental site trophoblastic tumor simulating carcinoma. Am J Surg Pathol 22: 1393-1403.

1760. Shih IM, Kurman RJ (1998). Ki-67 labeling index in the differential diagnosis of exaggerated placental site, placental site trophoblastic tumor, and choriocarcinoma: a double immunohistochemical staining technique using Ki-67 and Mel-CAM antibodies. Hum Pathol 29: 27-33.

1761. Shih IM, Kurman RJ (2001). The pathology of intermediate trophoblastic tumors and tumor-like lesions. Int J Gynecol Pathol 20: 31-47.

1762. Shih IM, Seidman JD, Kurman RJ (1999). Placental site nodule and characterization of distinctive types of intermediate trophoblast. Hum Pathol 30: 687-694.

1763. Shih I (2007). Gestational trophoblastic neoplasia--pathogenesis and potential therapeutic targets. Lancet Oncol 8: 642-650.

1764. Shih I (2007). Trophogram, an immunohistochemistry-based algorithmic approach, in the differential diagnosis of trophoblastic tumors and tumorlike lesions. Ann Diagn Pathol 11: 228-234.

1765. Shih I, Chen L, Wang CC, Gu J, Davidson B, Cope L, Kurman RJ, Xuan J, Wang TL (2010). Distinct DNA methylation profiles in ovarian serous neoplasms and their implications in ovarian carcinogenesis. Am J Obstet Gynecol 203: 584-22.

1766. Shih I, Kurman RJ (2004). Ovarian tumorigenesis: a proposed model based on morphological and molecular genetic analysis. Am J Pathol 164: 1511-1518.

1767. Shingleton HM, Bell MC, Fremgen A, Chmiel JS, Russell AH, Jones WB, Winchester DP, Clive RE (1995). Is there really a difference in survival of women with squamous cell carcinoma, adenocarcinoma, and adenosquamous cell carcinoma of the cervix? Cancer 76: 1948-1955.

1768. Short NJ, Hayes TG, Bhargava P (2011). Intra-abdominal splenosis mimicking metastatic cancer. Am J Med Sci 341: 246-249.

1769. Shutter J (2005). Uterus-like ovarian mass presenting near menarche. Int J Gynecol Pathol 24: 382-384.

1770. Shvartsman HS, Sun CC, Bodurka DC, Mahajan V, Crispens M, Lu KH, Deavers MT, Malpica A, Silva EG, Gershenson DM (2007). Comparison of the clinical behavior of newly diagnosed stages II-IV low-grade serous carcinoma of the ovary with that of serous ovarian tumors of low malignant potential that recur as low-grade serous carcinoma. Gynecol Oncol 105: 625-629.

1771. Sideri M, Jones RW, Heller DS, Haefner H, Neill S, Preti M, Scurry J, Wilkinson EJ, Edwards L (2007). Comment on the Article: Srodon M, Stoler MH, Baber GB, et al. The distribution of low and high-risk HPV types in vulvar and vaginal intraepithelial neoplasia (VIN and VaIN) Am J Surg Pathol. 2006;30:1513-1518. Am J Surg Pathol 31: 1452-1454.

1772. Sieben NL, Macropoulos P, Roemen GM, Kolkman-Uljee SM, Jan Fleuren G, Houmadi R, Diss T, Warren B, Al Adnani M, De Goeij AP, Krausz T, Flanagan AM (2004). In ovarian neoplasms, BRAF, but not KRAS, mutations are restricted to low-grade serous tumours. J Pathol 202: 336-340.

1772A. Sieh W, Köbel M, Longacre TA, Bowtell DD, deFazio A, Goodman MT, Høgdall E, Deen S, Wentzensen N, Moysich KB, Brenton JD, Clarke BA, Menon U, Gilks CB, Kim A,

Madore J, Fereday S, George J, Galletta L, Lurie G, Wilkens LR, Carney ME, Thompson PJ, Matsuno RK, Kjær SK, Jensen A, Høgdall C, Kalli KR, Fridley BL, Keeney GL, Vierkant RA, Cunningham JM, Brinton LA, Yang HP, Sherman ME, García-Closas M, Lissowska J, Odunsi K, Morrison C, Lele S, Bshara W, Sucheston L, Jimenez-Linan M, Driver K, Alsop J, Mack M, McGuire V, Rothstein JH, Rosen BP, Bernardini MQ, Mackay H, Oza A, Wozniak EL, Benjamin E, Gentry-Maharaj A, Gayther SA, Tinker AV, Prentice LM, Chow C, Anglesio MS, Johnatty SE, Chenevix-Trench G, Whittemore AS, Pharoah PD, Goode EL, Huntsman DG, Ramus SJ (2013). Hormone-receptor expression and ovarian cancer survival: an Ovarian Tumor Tissue Analysis consortium study. Lancet Oncol 14: 853-862.

1773. Sigismondi C, Gadducci A, Lorusso D, Candiani M, Breda E, Raspagliesi F, Cormio G, Marinaccio M, Mangili G (2012). Ovarian Sertoli-Leydig cell tumors. a retrospective MITO study. Gynecol Oncol 125: 673-676.

1774. Sikov WM, Schiffman FJ, Weaver M, Dyckman J, Shulman R, Torgan P (2000). Splenosis presenting as occult gastrointestinal bleeding. Am J Hematol 65: 56-61.

1775. Sillman FH, Fruchter RG, Chen YS, Camilien L, Sedlis A, McTigue E (1997). Vaginal intraepithelial neoplasia: risk factors for persistence, recurrence, and invasion and its management. Am J Obstet Gynecol 176: 93-99.

1776. Silva EG, Deavers MT, Bodurka DC, Malpica A (2006). Association of low-grade endometrioid carcinoma of the uterus and ovary with undifferentiated carcinoma: a new type of dedifferentiated carcinoma? Int J Gynecol Pathol 25: 52-58.

1777. Silva EG, Deavers MT, Malpica A (2010). Patterns of low-grade serous carcinoma with emphasis on the nonepithelial-lined spaces pattern of invasion and the disorganized orphan papillae. Int J Gynecol Pathol 29: 507-512.

1778. Silva EG, Gershenson DM, Malpica A, Deavers M (2006). The recurrence and the overall survival rates of ovarian serous borderline neoplasms with noninvasive implants is time dependent. Am J Surg Pathol 30: 1367-1371.

1779. Silva EG, Robey-Cafferty SS, Smith TL, Gershenson DM (1990). Ovarian carcinomas with transitional cell carcinoma pattern. Am J Clin Pathol 93: 457-465.

1780. Silva EG, Tornos C, Malpica A, Deavers MT, Tortolero-Luna G, Gershenson DM (2002). The association of benign and malignant ovarian adenofibromas with breast cancer and thyroid disorders. Int J Surg Pathol 10: 33-39.

1781. Silver SA, Tavassoli FA (2000). Glomus tumor arising in a mature teratoma of the ovary: report of a case simulating a metastasis from cervical squamous carcinoma. Arch Pathol Lab Med 124: 1373-1375.

1782. Silver SA, Devouassoux-Shisheboran M, Mezzetti TP, Tavassoli FA (2001). Mesonephric adenocarcinomas of the uterine cervix: a study of 11 cases with immunohistochemical findings. Am J Surg Pathol 25: 379-387.

1783. Silverberg SG, Kurman RJ, Kubik-Huch RA, Nogales F, Tavassoli FA (2013). Tumors of the uterine corpus: epithelial tumors and related lesions. In: Tumours of the Breast and Female Genital Organs. Tavassoli FA, Devilee P, eds. IARC Press: Lyon, pp. 221-232.

1784. Silverberg SG, Major FJ, Blessing JA, Fetter B, Askin FB, Liao SY, Miller A (1990). Carcinosarcoma (malignant mixed mesodermal tumor) of the uterus. A Gynecologic Oncology Group pathologic study of 203 cases. Int J Gynecol Pathol 9: 1-19.

1785. Simeone S, Laterza MM, Scaravilli G,

Capuano S, Serao M, Orabona P, Rossi R, Balbi C (2009). Malignant melanoma metastasizing to the uterus in a patient with atypical postmenopause metrorrhagia. A case report. Minerva Ginecol 61: 77-80.

1786. Simpson RC, Littlewood SM, Cooper SM, Cruickshank ME, Green CM, Derrick E, Yell J, Chiang N, Bell H, Owen C, Javed A, Wilson CL, McLelland J, Murphy R (2012). Real-life experience of managing vulval erosive lichen planus: a case-based review and U.K. multicentre case note audit. Br J Dermatol 167: 85-91.

1787. Sims SM, Stinson K, McLean FW, Davis JD, Wilkinson EJ (2012). Angiomyofibroblastoma of the vulva: a case report of a pedunculated variant and review of the literature. J Low Genit Tract Dis 16: 149-154.

1788. Singer G, Oldt R, III, Cohen Y, Wang BG, Sidransky D, Kurman RJ, Shih I (2003). Mutations in BRAF and KRAS characterize the development of low-grade ovarian serous carcinoma. J Natl Cancer Inst 95: 484-486.

1789. Singer G, Stohr R, Cope L, Dehari R, Hartmann A, Cao DF, Wang TL, Kurman RJ, Shih I (2005). Patterns of p53 mutations separate ovarian serous borderline tumors and low- and high-grade carcinomas and provide support for a new model of ovarian carcinogenesis: a mutational analysis with immunohistochemical correlation. Am J Surg Pathol 29: 218-224.

1790. Sinniah R, O'Brien FV (1973). Pigmented progonoma in a dermoid cyst of the ovary. J Pathol 109: 357-359.

1791. Siriaunkgul S, Robbins KM, McGowan L, Silverberg SG (1995). Ovarian mucinous tumors of low malignant potential: a clinicopathologic study of 54 tumors of intestinal and mullerian type. Int J Gynecol Pathol 14: 198-208.

1792. Sisodia SM, Khan WA, Goel A (2012). Ovarian ligament adenomyoma: report of a rare entity with review of the literature. J Obstet Gynaecol Res 38: 724-728.

1793. Siu SS, Tam WH, To KF, Yuen PM (2003). Is vaginal dermoid cyst a rare occurrence or a misnomer? A case report and review of the literature. Ultrasound Obstet Gynecol 21: 404-406.

1794. Skeete DH, Cesar-Rittenberg P, Jong R, Murray SK, Colgan TJ (2010). Myeloid sarcoma of the vagina: a report of 2 cases. J Low Genit Tract Dis 14: 136-141.

1795. Skirnisdottir I, Garmo H, Holmberg L (2007). Non-genital tract metastases to the ovaries presented as ovarian tumors in Sweden 1990-2003: occurrence, origin and survival compared to ovarian cancer. Gynecol Oncol 105: 166-171.

1796. Skov BG, Broholm H, Engel U, Franzmann MB, Nielsen AL, Lauritzen AF, Skov T (1997). Comparison of the reproducibility of the WHO classifications of 1975 and 1994 of endometrial hyperplasia. Int J Gynecol Pathol 16: 33-37.

1797. Slim R, Mehio A (2007). The genetics of hydatidiform moles: new lights on an ancient disease. Clin Genet 71: 25-34.

1798. Smith Sehdev AE, Sehdev PS, Kurman RJ (2003). Noninvasive and invasive micropapillary (low-grade) serous carcinoma of the ovary: a clinicopathologic analysis of 135 cases. Am J Surg Pathol 27: 725-736.

1799. Smith CJ, Ferrier AJ, Russell P, Danieletto S (2005). Primary synovial sarcoma of the ovary: first reported case. Pathology 37: 385-387.

1800. Smith EM, Ritchie JM, Yankowitz J, Swarnavel S, Wang D, Haugen TH, Turek LP (2004). Human papillomavirus prevalence and types in newborns and parents: concordance and modes of transmission. Sex Transm Dis 31: 57-62.

1801. Smith HO (2003). Gestational trophoblastic disease epidemiology and trends. Clin Obstet Gynecol 46: 541-556.

1802. Smith HO, Berwick M, Verschraegen CF, Wiggins C, Lansing L, Muller CY, Qualls CR (2006). Incidence and survival rates for female malignant germ cell tumors. Obstet Gynecol 107: 1075-1085.

1803. Smith HO, Kohorn E, Cole LA (2005). Choriocarcinoma and gestational trophoblastic disease. Obstet Gynecol Clin North Am 32: 661-684.

1804. Smith JS, Green J, Berrington de GA, Appleby P, Peto J, Plummer M, Franceschi S, Beral V (2003). Cervical cancer and use of hormonal contraceptives: a systematic review. Lancet 361: 1159-1167.

1805. Soga J, Osaka M, Yakuwa Y (2000). Carcinoids of the ovary: an analysis of 329 reported cases. J Exp Clin Cancer Res 19: 271-280.

1806. Soga J, Osaka M, Yakuwa Y (2001). Gut-endocrinomas (carcinoids and related endocrine variants) of the uterine cervix: an analysis of 205 reported cases. J Exp Clin Cancer Res 20: 327-334.

1807. Soliman PT, Slomovitz BM, Broaddus RR, Sun CC, Oh JC, Eifel PJ, Gershenson DM, Lu KH (2004). Synchronous primary cancers of the endometrium and ovary: a single institution review of 84 cases. Gynecol Oncol 94: 456-462.

1808. Song JY, Lee JK, Lee NW, Jung HH, Kim SH, Lee KW (2008). Microarray analysis of normal cervix, carcinoma in situ, and invasive cervical cancer: identification of candidate genes in pathogenesis of invasion in cervical cancer. Int J Gynecol Cancer 18: 1051-1059.

1809. Song W, Conner M (2012). Squamous cell carcinoma arising within a mature cystic teratoma with invasion into the adjacent small intestine: a case report. Int J Gynecol Pathol 31: 272-275.

1810. Song YJ, Ryu SY, Choi SC, Lee ED, Lee KH, Cho SY (2009). Adenocarcinoma arising from the respiratory ciliated epithelium in a benign cystic teratoma of the ovary. Arch Gynecol Obstet 280: 659-662.

1811. Sonoda Y, Saigo PE, Federici MG, Boyd J (2000). Carcinosarcoma of the ovary in a patient with a germline BRCA2 mutation: evidence for monoclonal origin. Gynecol Oncol 76: 226-229.

1812. Soper JT (2006). Gestational trophoblastic disease. Obstet Gynecol 108: 176-187.

1813. Sornberger KS, Weremowicz S, Williams AJ, Quade BJ, Ligon AH, Pedeutour F, Vanni R, Morton CC (1999). Expression of HMGIY in three uterine leiomyomata with complex rearrangements of chromosome 6. Cancer Genet Cytogenet 114: 9-16.

1814. Soslow RA, Ali A, Oliva E (2008). Mullerian adenosarcomas: an immunophenotypic analysis of 35 cases. Am J Surg Pathol 32: 1013-1021.

1815. Soslow RA, Chung MH, Rouse RV, Hendrickson MR, Longacre TA (1996). Atypical polypoid adenomyofibroma (APA) versus well-differentiated endometrial carcinoma with prominent stromal matrix: an immunohistochemical study. Int J Gynecol Pathol 15: 209-216.

1816. Sotiropoulou M, Haidopoulos D, Vlachos G, Pilalis A, Rodolakis A, Diakomanolis E (2005). Primary malignant mixed mullerian tumor of the vagina immunohistochemically confirmed. Arch Gynecol Obstet 271: 264-266.

1817. Sreenan JJ, Hart WR (1995). Carcinosarcomas of the female genital tract. A pathologic study of 29 metastatic tumors: further evidence for the dominant role of the epithelial component and the conversion theory of histogenesis. Am J Surg Pathol 19: 666-674.

1818. Srodon M, Stoler MH, Baber GB, Kurman RJ (2006). The distribution of low and high-risk HPV types in vulvar and vaginal intraepithelial neoplasia (VIN and VaIN). Am J Surg Pathol 30: 1513-1518.

1819. St Pierre-Robson K, Dunn PJ, Cooper E, Tofazzal N, Hirschowitz L, McCluggage WG, Ganesan R (2013). Three cases of an unusual pattern of invasion in malignant Brenner tumors. Int J Gynecol Pathol 32: 31-34.

1820. Staats PN, Garcia JJ, Dias-Santagata DC, Kuhlmann G, Stubbs H, McCluggage WG, De Nictolis M, Kommoss F, Soslow RA, Iafrate AJ, Oliva E (2009). Uterine tumors resembling ovarian sex cord tumors (UTROSCT) lack the JAZF1-JJAZ1 translocation frequently seen in endometrial stromal tumors. Am J Surg Pathol 33: 1206-1212.

1821. Staats PN, McCluggage WG, Clement PB, Young RH (2008). Luteinized thecomas (thecomatosis) of the type typically associated with sclerosing peritonitis: a clinical, histopathologic, and immunohistochemical analysis of 27 cases. Am J Surg Pathol 32: 1273-1290.

1822. Stang A, Streller B, Eisinger B, Jockel KH (2005). Population-based incidence rates of malignant melanoma of the vulva in Germany. Gynecol Oncol 96: 216-221.

1823. Steeper TA, Piscioli F, Rosai J (1983). Squamous cell carcinoma with sarcoma-like stroma of the female genital tract. Clinicopathologic study of four cases. Cancer 52: 890-898.

1824. Steeper TA, Rosai J (1983). Aggressive angiomyxoma of the female pelvis and perineum. Report of nine cases of a distinctive type of gynecologic soft-tissue neoplasm. Am J Surg Pathol 7: 463-475.

1825. Stehman FB, Bundy BN, DiSaia PJ, Keys HM, Larson JE, Fowler WC (1991). Carcinoma of the cervix treated with radiation therapy. I. A multi-variate analysis of prognostic variables in the Gynecologic Oncology Group. Cancer 67: 2776-2785.

1826. Stelow EB, Jo VY, Stoler MH, Mills SE (2010). Human papillomavirus-associated squamous cell carcinoma of the upper aerodigestive tract. Am J Surg Pathol 34: e15-e24.

1827. Stephen JK, Chen KM, Raitanen M, Grenman S, Worsham MJ (2009). DNA hypermethylation profiles in squamous cell carcinoma of the vulva. Int J Gynecol Pathol 28: 63-75.

1828. Stephenson RD, Denehy TR (2012). Rapid spontaneous regression of acute-onset vulvar intraepithelial neoplasia 3 in young women: a case series. J Low Genit Tract Dis 16: 56-58.

1829. Stephenson TJ, Mills PM (1986). Adenomatoid tumours: an immunohistochemical and ultrastructural appraisal of their histogenesis. J Pathol 148: 327-335.

1830. Stern RC, Dash R, Bentley RC, Snyder MJ, Haney AF, Robboy SJ (2001). Malignancy in endometriosis: frequency and comparison of ovarian and extraovarian types. Int J Gynecol Pathol 20: 133-139.

1831. Sternberg WH, Barclay DL (1966). Luteoma of pregnancy. Am J Obstet Gynecol 95: 165-184.

1832. Sternberg WH, Roth LM (1973). Ovarian stromal tumors containing Leydig cells. I. Stromal-Leydig cell tumor and non-neoplastic transformation of ovarian stroma to Leydig cells. Cancer 32: 940-951.

1833. Stevens VL, Jacobs EJ, Sun J, McCullough ML, Patel AV, Gaudet MM, Teras LR, Gapstur SM (2012). Weight cycling and risk of endometrial cancer. Cancer Epidemiol Biomarkers Prev 21: 747-752.

1834. Stewart CJ (2009). Tubulo-squamous vaginal polyp with basaloid epithelial differentiation. Int J Gynecol Pathol 28: 563-566.

1835. Stewart CJ, Amanuel B, Brennan BA, Jain S, Rajakaruna R, Wallace S (2005). Superficial cervico-vaginal myofibroblastoma: a report of five cases. Pathology 37: 144-148.

1835A. Stewart CJ, Ardakani NM, Doherty DA, Young RH (2014). An evaluation of the morphologic features of low-grade mucinous neoplasms of the appendix metastatic in the ovary, and comparison with primary ovarian mucinous tumors. Int J Gynecol Pathol. 33:1-10

1836. Stewart CJ, Farquharson MA, Foulis AK (1992). Characterization of the inflammatory infiltrate in ovarian dysgerminoma: an immunocytochemical study. Histopathology 20: 491-497.

1837. Stewart SL, Wike JM, Foster SL, Michaud F (2007). The incidence of primary fallopian tube cancer in the United States. Gynecol Oncol 107: 392-397.

1838. Stoler MH (1997). The Biology of Human Papillomavirus. In: Pathology Case Reviews. Pathology Case Reviews. 1-13.

1839. Stoler MH (2000). Human papillomaviruses and cervical neoplasia: a model for carcinogenesis. Int J Gynecol Pathol 19: 16-28.

1840. Stoler MH (2002). New Bethesda terminology and evidence-based management guidelines for cervical cytology findings. JAMA 287: 2140-2141.

1841. Stoler MH (2004). The Pathology of Cervical Neoplasia. In: Cervical Cancer: From Etiology to Prevention. Rohan TE, Shah KV, eds. Kluwer Academic Publishers.

1842. Stoler MH, Mills SE (2010). The Vulva and Vagina. In: Diagnostic Surgical Pathology. Mills SE, ed. Lippincott, Williams & Wilkins: Philadelphia, PA, pp. 2096-2131.

1843. Stoler MH, Mills SE, Gersell DJ, Walker AN (1991). Small-cell neuroendocrine carcinoma of the cervix. A human papillomavirus type 18-associated cancer. Am J Surg Pathol 15: 28-32.

1844. Stoler MH, Schiffman M (2001). Interobserver reproducibility of cervical cytologic and histologic interpretations: realistic estimates from the ASCUS-LSIL Triage Study. JAMA 285: 1500-1505.

1845. Stoler MH, Vichnin MD, Ferenczy A, Ferris DG, Perez G, Paavonen J, Joura EA, Djursing H, Sigurdsson K, Jefferson L, Alvarez F, Sings HL, Lu S, James MK, Saah A, Haupt RM (2011). The accuracy of colposcopic biopsy: analyses from the placebo arm of the Gardasil clinical trials. Int J Cancer 128: 1354-1362.

1846. Stoler MH, Wolinsky SM, Whitbeck A, Broker TR, Chow LT (1989). Differentiation-linked human papillomavirus types 6 and 11 transcription in genital condylomata revealed by in situ hybridization with message-specific RNA probes. Virology 172: 331-340.

1847. Stoler MH, Wright TC Jr, Cuzick J, Dockter J, Reid JL, Getman D, Giachetti C (2013). APTIMA HPV assay performance in women with atypical squamous cells of undetermined significance cytology results. Am J Obstet Gynecol 208: 144-148.

1848. Stolnicu S, Furtado A, Sanches A, Nicolae A, Preda O, Hincu M, Nogales FF (2011). Ovarian ependymomas of extra-axial type or central immunophenotypes. Hum Pathol 42: 403-408.

1849. Storey DJ, Rush R, Stewart M, Rye T, Al-Nafussi A, Williams AR, Smyth JF, Gabra H (2008). Endometrioid epithelial ovarian cancer : 20 years of prospectively collected data from a single center. Cancer 112: 2211-2220.

1850. Straughn JM Jr, Richter HE, Conner MG, Meleth S, Barnes MN (2001). Predictors of outcome in small cell carcinoma of the cervix--a case series. Gynecol Oncol 83: 216-220.

1851. Stuart GC, Flagler EA, Nation JG, Duggan M, Robertson DI (1988). Laser vaporization of vaginal intraepithelial neoplasia. Am J Obstet Gynecol 158: 240-243.

1852. Sturegard E, Johansson H, Ekstrom J, Hansson BG, Johnsson A, Gustafsson E, Dillner J, Forslund O (2013). Human papillomavirus typing in reporting of condyloma. Sex Transm Dis 40: 123-129.

1853. Sturgeon SR, Brinton LA, Devesa SS, Kurman RJ (1992). In situ and invasive vulvar cancer incidence trends (1973 to 1987). Am J Obstet Gynecol 166: 1482-1485.

1854. Suarez-Vilela D, Izquierdo-Garcia FM (2002). Nodular histiocytic/mesothelial hyperplasia: a process mediated by adhesion molecules? Histopathology 40: 299-300.

1855. Sueblinvong T, Carney ME (2009). Current understanding of risk factors for ovarian cancer. Curr Treat Options Oncol 10: 67-81.

1856. Sugiyama T, Kamura T, Kigawa J, Terakawa N, Kikuchi Y, Kita T, Suzuki M, Sato I, Taguchi K (2000). Clinical characteristics of clear cell carcinoma of the ovary: a distinct histologic type with poor prognosis and resistance to platinum-based chemotherapy. Cancer 88: 2584-2589.

1857. Sugiyama VE, Chan JK, Shin JY, Berek JS, Osann K, Kapp DS (2007). Vulvar melanoma: a multivariable analysis of 644 patients. Obstet Gynecol 110: 296-301.

1858. Suh MJ, Park DC (2008). Leiomyosarcoma of the vagina: a case report and review from the literature. J Gynecol Oncol 19: 261-264.

1859. Sulak P, Barnhill D, Heller P, Weiser E, Hoskins W, Park R, Woodward J (1988). Nonsquamous cancer of the vagina. Gynecol Oncol 29: 309-320.

1860. Sumathi VP, Al-Hussaini M, Connolly LE, Fullerton L, McCluggage WG (2004). Endometrial stromal neoplasms are immunoreactive with WT-1 antibody. Int J Gynecol Pathol 23: 241-247.

1861. Sumathi VP, Fisher C, Williams A, Meis JM, Ganesan R, Kindblom LG, McCluggage WG (2011). Synovial sarcoma of the vulva and vagina: a clinicopathologic and molecular genetic study of 4 cases. Int J Gynecol Pathol 30: 84-91.

1862. Sumathi VP, Murnaghan M, Dobbs SP, McCluggage WG (2002). Extragenital mullerian carcinosarcoma arising from the peritoneum: report of two cases. Int J Gynecol Cancer 12: 764-767.

1863. Sumi T, Ishiko O, Maeda K, Haba T, Wakasa K, Ogita S (2002). Adenocarcinoma arising from respiratory ciliated epithelium in mature ovarian cystic teratoma. Arch Gynecol Obstet 267: 107-109.

1864. Sun HD, Lin H, Jao MS, Wang KL, Liou WS, Hung YC, Chiang YC, Lu CH, Lai HC, Yu MH (2012). A long-term follow-up study of 176 cases with adult-type ovarian granulosa cell tumors. Gynecol Oncol 124: 244-249.

1865. Sung CO, Ahn G, Song SY, Choi YL, Bae DS (2009). Atypical leiomyomas of the uterus with long-term follow-up after myomectomy with immunohistochemical analysis for p16INK4A, p53, Ki-67, estrogen receptors, and progesterone receptors. Int J Gynecol Pathol 28: 529-534.

1866. Suva ML, Riggi N, Stehle JC, Baumer K, Tercier S, Joseph JM, Suva D, Clement V, Provero P, Cironi L, Osterheld MC, Guillou L, Stamenkovic I (2009). Identification of cancer stem cells in Ewing's sarcoma. Cancer Res 69: 1776-1781.

1867. Suzuki A, Shiozawa T, Mori A, Kimura K, Konishi I (2006). Cystic clear cell tumor of borderline malignancy of the ovary lacking fibromatous components: report of two cases and a possible new histological subtype. Gynecol Oncol 101: 540-544.

1868. Symonds RP, Habeshaw T, Paul J, Kerr DJ, Darling A, Burnett RA, Sotsiou F, Linardopoulos S, Spandidos DA (1992). No correlation between ras, c-myc and c-jun proto-oncogene expression and prognosis in advanced carcinoma of cervix. Eur J Cancer 28A: 1615-1617.

1869. Syriac S, Durie N, Kesterson J, Lele S, Mhawech-Fauceglia P (2011). Female adnexal tumor of probable Wolffian origin (FATWO) with recurrence 3 years postsurgery. Int J Gynecol Pathol 30: 231-235.

1870. Syriac S, Kesterson J, Izevbaye I, de Mesy Bentley KL, Lele S, Mhawech-Fauceglia P (2012). Clinically aggressive primary solid pseudopapillary tumor of the ovary in a 45-year-old woman. Ann Diagn Pathol 16: 498-503.

1871. Szukala SA, Marks JR, Burchette JL, Elbendary AA, Krigman HR (1999). Co-expression of p53 by epithelial and stromal elements in carcinosarcoma of the female genital tract: an immunohistochemical study of 19 cases. Int J Gynecol Cancer 9: 131-136.

1872. Szulman AE (1984). Syndromes of hydatidiform moles. Partial vs. complete. J Reprod Med 29: 788-791.

1873. Szyfelbein WM, Young RH, Scully RE (1994). Cystic struma ovarii: a frequently unrecognized tumor. A report of 20 cases. Am J Surg Pathol 18: 785-788.

1874. Szyfelbein WM, Young RH, Scully RE (1995). Struma ovarii simulating ovarian tumors of other types. A report of 30 cases. Am J Surg Pathol 19: 21-29.

1875. Tafe LJ, Garg K, Chew I, Tornos C, Soslow RA (2010). Endometrial and ovarian carcinomas with undifferentiated components: clinically aggressive and frequently underrecognized neoplasms. Mod Pathol 23: 781-789.

1876. Tahlan A, Nanda A, Mohan H (2006). Uterine adenomyoma: a clinicopathologic review of 26 cases and a review of the literature. Int J Gynecol Pathol 25: 361-365.

1877. Tahmasbi M, Nguyen J, Ghayouri M, Shan Y, Hakam A (2012). Primary uterine cervix schwannoma: a case report and review of the literature. Case Rep Pathol 2012: 353049.

1878. Takai N, Nakamura S, Goto K, Hayashita C, Kira N, Urabe S, Narahara H, Matsumoto H (2009). Lymphoepithelioma-like carcinoma of the uterine cervix. Arch Gynecol Obstet 280: 725-727.

1879. Takano M, Yoshikawa T, Kato M, Aida S, Goto T, Furuya K, Kikuchi Y (2009). Primary clear cell carcinoma of the peritoneum: report of two cases and a review of the literature. Eur J Gynaecol Oncol 30: 575-578.

1880. Takashina T, Ito E, Kudo R (1985). Cytologic diagnosis of primary tubal cancer. Acta Cytol 29: 367-372.

1881. Takeda A, Imoto S, Mori M, Yamada J, Nakamura H (2011). Uterus-like mass of ovarian ligament: Image diagnosis and management by laparoendoscopic single-site surgery. J Obstet Gynaecol Res 37: 1895-1899.

1882. Takeda T, Masuhara K, Kamiura S (2008). Successful management of a leiomyomatosis peritonealis disseminata with an aromatase inhibitor. Obstet Gynecol 112: 491-493.

1883. Takeshima Y, Amatya VJ, Nakayori F, Nakano T, Iwaoki Y, Daitoku K, Inai K (2002). Co-existent carcinosarcoma and adenoid basal carcinoma of the uterine cervix and correlation with human papillomavirus infection. Int J Gynecol Pathol 21: 186-190.

1884. Takeuchi S, Hirano H, Ichio T, Taniguchi H, Toyoda N (1999). A case report: rare case of primary transitional cell carcinoma of the

fallopian tube. J Obstet Gynaecol Res 25: 29-32.
1885. Takeuchi T, Ohishi Y, Imamura H, Aman M, Shida K, Kobayashi H, Kato K, Oda Y (2013). Ovarian transitional cell carcinoma represents a poorly differentiated form of high-grade serous or endometrioid adenocarcinoma. Am J Surg Pathol 37: 1091-1099.
1886. Taki M, Baba T, Mandai M, Suzuki A, Mikami Y, Matsumura N, Konishi I (2012). Solitary fibrous tumor arising slowly in the vulva over 10 years: case report and review. J Obstet Gynaecol Res 38: 884-888.
1887. Talerman A (1984). Carcinoid tumors of the ovary. J Cancer Res Clin Oncol 107: 125-135.
1888. Talerman A, Evans MI (1982). Primary trabecular carcinoid tumor of the ovary. Cancer 50: 1403-1407.
1889. Talerman A, Roth LM (2007). Recent advances in the pathology and classification of gonadal neoplasms composed of germ cells and sex cord derivatives. Int J Gynecol Pathol 26: 313-321.
1890. Talerman A, van der Harten JJ (1977). Mixed germ cell-sex cord stroma tumor of the ovary associated with isosexual precocious puberty in a normal girl. Cancer 40: 889-894.
1891. Tallini G, Price FV, Carcangiu ML (1993). Epithelioid angiosarcoma arising in uterine leiomyomas. Am J Clin Pathol 100: 514-518.
1892. Tambouret R, Clement PB, Young RH (2003). Endometrial endometrioid adenocarcinoma with a deceptive pattern of spread to the uterine cervix: a manifestation of stage IIb endometrial carcinoma liable to be misinterpreted as an independent carcinoma or a benign lesion. Am J Surg Pathol 27: 1080-1088.
1893. Tan MH, Mester JL, Ngeow J, Rybicki LA, Orloff MS, Eng C (2012). Lifetime cancer risks in individuals with germline PTEN mutations. Clin Cancer Res 18: 400-407.
1894. Tan SS, Peng XC, Cao Y (2011). Primary precursor B cell lymphoblastic lymphoma of uterine corpus: case report and review of the literature. Arch Gynecol Obstet 284: 1289-1292.
1895. Tanahashi J, Kashima K, Daa T, Kondo Y, Kitano S, Yokoyama S (2006). Florid cystic endosalpingiosis of the spleen. APMIS 114: 393-398.
1896. Tanaka H, Kobayashi T, Yoshida K, Asakura T, Taniguchi H, Mikami Y (2011). Low-grade appendiceal mucinous neoplasm with disseminated peritoneal adenomucinosis involving the uterus, mimicking primary mucinous endometrial adenocarcinoma: a case report. J Obstet Gynaecol Res 37: 1726-1730.
1897. Tanaka M, Sawai H, Okada Y, Yamamoto M, Funahashi H, Hayakawa T, Takeyama H, Manabe T (2006). Malignant solitary fibrous tumor originating from the peritoneum and review of the literature. Med Sci Monit 12: CS95-CS98.
1898. Tanaka Y, Sasaki Y, Nishihira H, Izawa T, Nishi T (1992). Ovarian juvenile granulosa cell tumor associated with Maffucci's syndrome. Am J Clin Pathol 97: 523-527.
1899. Tanas MR, Goldblum JR (2009). Fluorescence in situ hybridization in the diagnosis of soft tissue neoplasms: a review. Adv Anat Pathol 16: 383-391.
1900. Tang S, Onuma K, Deb P, Wang E, Lytwyn A, Sur M, Daya D (2012). Frequency of serous tubal intraepithelial carcinoma in various gynecologic malignancies: a study of 300 consecutive cases. Int J Gynecol Pathol 31: 103-110.
1901. Tang Z, Zou S, Hao Y, Wang B, Yang X, Qiu F (2002). Frequency of loss expression of the DPC4 protein in various locations of biliary tract carcinoma. Zhonghua Yu Fang Yi Xue Za Zhi 36: 481-484.
1902. Tanner EJ, Garg K, Leitao MM Jr, Soslow RA, Hensley ML (2012). High grade undifferentiated uterine sarcoma: surgery, treatment, and survival outcomes. Gynecol Oncol 127: 27-31.
1903. Tao T, Yang J, Cao D, Guo L, Chen J, Lang J, Shen K (2012). Conservative treatment and long-term follow up of endodermal sinus tumor of the vagina. Gynecol Oncol 125: 358-361.
1904. Taraif SH, Deavers MT, Malpica A, Silva EG (2009). The significance of neuroendocrine expression in undifferentiated carcinoma of the endometrium. Int J Gynecol Pathol 28: 142-147.
1905. Tasci Y, Kayikcioglu F, Cavusoglu D, Gokcin H (2005). Splenosis mimicking pelvic mass. Obstet Gynecol 106: 1167-1169.
1906. Tashiro H, Blazes MS, Wu R, Cho KR, Bose S, Wang SI, Li J, Parsons R, Ellenson LH (1997). Mutations in PTEN are frequent in endometrial carcinoma but rare in other common gynecological malignancies. Cancer Res 57: 3935-3940.
1906A. Tavassoli FA , Devilee P (2003). Pathology and Genetics of Tumours of the Breast and Female Genital Organs (IARC WHO Classification of Tumours). IARC: Lyon.
1907. Tavassoli FA, Norris HJ (1979). Smooth muscle tumors of the vagina. Obstet Gynecol 53: 689-693.
1908. Tavassoli FA, Norris HJ (1979). Smooth muscle tumors of the vulva. Obstet Gynecol 53: 213-217.
1909. Tavassoli FA, Norris HJ (1980). Sertoli tumors of the ovary. A clinicopathologic study of 28 cases with ultrastructural observations. Cancer 46: 2281-2297.
1910. Tavassoli FA, Norris HJ (1981). Mesenchymal tumours of the uterus. VII. A clinicopathological study of 60 endometrial stromal nodules. Histopathology 5: 1-10.
1911. Taylor ES, Droegemeuller W (1962). Choriocarcinoma, chorioadenoma destruens, and syncytial endometritis. Am J Obstet Gynecol 83: 958-968.
1912. Taylor NP, Zighelboim I, Huettner PC, Powell MA, Gibb RK, Rader JS, Mutch DG, Edmonston TB, Goodfellow PJ (2006). DNA mismatch repair and TP53 defects are early events in uterine carcinosarcoma tumorigenesis. Mod Pathol 19: 1333-1338.
1913. Tchang F, Okagaki T, Richart RM (1973). Adenocarcinoma of Bartholin's gland associated with Paget's disease of vulvar area. Cancer 31: 221-225.
1914. Terlou A, Blok LJ, Helmerhorst TJ, van Beurden M. (2010). Premalignant epithelial disorders of the vulva: squamous vulvar intraepithelial neoplasia, vulvar Paget's disease and melanoma in situ. Acta Obstet Gynecol Scand 89: 741-748.
1915. Tewari K, Cappuccini F, DiSaia PJ, Berman ML, Manetta A, Kohler MF (2000). Malignant germ cell tumors of the ovary. Obstet Gynecol 95: 128-133.
1916. The Atypical Squamous Cells of Undetermined Significance/Low-Grade Squamous Intraepithelial Lesions Triage Study (ALTS) Grou (2003). A randomized trial on the management of low-grade squamous intraepithelial lesion cytology interpretations. Am J Obstet Gynecol 188: 1393-1400.
1917. The Writing Group for the PEPI Trial (1996). Effects of hormone replacement therapy on endometrial histology in postmenopausal women. The Postmenopausal Estrogen/Progestin Interventions (PEPI) Trial. JAMA 275: 370-375.
1918. Thomas CC, Wingo PA, Dolan MS, Lee NC, Richardson LC (2009). Endometrial cancer risk among younger, overweight women. Obstet Gynecol 114: 22-27.
1919. Thomason RW, Rush W, Dave H (1995). Transitional cell carcinoma arising within a paratubal cyst: report of a case. Int J Gynecol Pathol 14: 270-273.
1920. Thrall MM, Paley P, Pizer E, Garcia R, Goff BA (2011). Patterns of spread and recurrence of sex cord-stromal tumors of the ovary. Gynecol Oncol 122: 242-245.
1921. Tidbury P, Singer A, Jenkins D (1992). CIN 3: the role of lesion size in invasion. Br J Obstet Gynaecol 99: 583-586.
1922. Tietze L, Gunther K, Horbe A, Pawlik C, Klosterhalfen B, Handt S, Merkelbach-Bruse S (2000). Benign metastasizing leiomyoma: a cytogenetically balanced but clonal disease. Hum Pathol 31: 126-128.
1923. Tilling T, Moll I (2012). Which are the cells of origin in merkel cell carcinoma? J Skin Cancer 2012: 680410.
1924. Tiltman AJ (1998). Leiomyomas of the uterine cervix: a study of frequency. Int J Gynecol Pathol 17: 231-234.
1925. Tiltman AJ, Allard U (2001). Female adnexal tumours of probable Wolffian origin: an immunohistochemical study comparing tumours, mesonephric remnants and paramesonephric derivatives. Histopathology 38: 237-242.
1926. Tirode F, Laud-Duval K, Prieur A, Delorme B, Charbord P, Delattre O (2007). Mesenchymal stem cell features of Ewing tumors. Cancer Cell 11: 421-429.
1927. Tjalma WA, Colpaert CG (2005). Myxoid leiomyosarcoma of the vulva. Gynecol Oncol 96: 548-551.
1927A. Tjalma WA, Van de Velde AL, Schroyens WA (2002). Primary non-Hodgkin's lymphoma in Bartholin's gland. Gynecol Oncol 87: 308-309.
1928. Toki T, Kurman RJ, Park JS, Kessis T, Daniel RW, Shah KV (1991). Probable nonpapillomavirus etiology of squamous cell carcinoma of the vulva in older women: a clinicopathologic study using in situ hybridization and polymerase chain reaction. Int J Gynecol Pathol 10: 107-125.
1929. Tori M, Akamatsu H, Mizutani S, Yoshidome K, Oyama T, Ueshima S, Tsujimoto M, Nakahara M (2008). Multiple benign metastasizing leiomyomas in the pelvic lymph nodes and biceps muscle: report of a case. Surg Today 38: 432-435.
1930. Tornos C, Silva EG, Ordonez NG, Gershenson DM, Young RH, Scully RE (1995). Endometrioid carcinoma of the ovary with a prominent spindle-cell component, a source of diagnostic confusion. A report of 14 cases. Am J Surg Pathol 19: 1343-1353.
1931. Trimble CL, Kauderer J, Zaino R, Silverberg S, Lim PC, Burke JJ, Alberts D, Curtin J (2006). Concurrent endometrial carcinoma in women with a biopsy diagnosis of atypical endometrial hyperplasia: a Gynecologic Oncology Group study. Cancer 106: 812-819.
1932. Trimble CL, Method M, Leitao M, Lu K, Ioffe O, Hampton M, Higgins R, Zaino R, Mutter GL (2012). Management of endometrial precancers. Obstet Gynecol 120: 1160-1175.
1933. Trzyna W, McHugh M, McCue P, McHugh KM (1997). Molecular determination of the malignant potential of smooth muscle neoplasms. Cancer 80: 211-217.
1934. Tsai HW, Lin CP, Chou CY, Li CF, Chow NH, Shih IM, Ho CL (2008). Placental site nodule transformed into a malignant epithelioid trophoblastic tumour with pelvic lymph node and lung metastasis. Histopathology 53: 601-604.
1935. Tseng CJ, Pao CC, Tseng LH, Chang CT, Lai CH, Soong YK, Hsueh S, Jyu-Jen H (1997). Lymphoepithelioma-like carcinoma of the uterine cervix: association with Epstein-Barr virus and human papillomavirus. Cancer 80: 91-97.
1936. Tsoi D, Buck M, Hammond I, White J (2005). Gastric adenocarcinoma presenting as uterine metastasis--a case report. Gynecol Oncol 97: 932-934.
1937. Tsoumpou I, Arbyn M, Kyrgiou M, Wentzensen N, Koliopoulos G, Martin-Hirsch P, Malamou-Mitsi V, Paraskevaidis E (2009). p16(INK4a) immunostaining in cytological and histological specimens from the uterine cervix: a systematic review and meta-analysis. Cancer Treat Rev 35: 210-220.
1938. Tsuji T, Catasus L, Prat J (2005). Is loss of heterozygosity at 9q22.3 (PTCH gene) and 19p13.3 (STK11 gene) involved in the pathogenesis of ovarian stromal tumors? Hum Pathol 36: 792-796.
1939. Tsuji T, Kawauchi S, Utsunomiya T, Nagata Y, Tsuneyoshi M (1997). Fibrosarcoma versus cellular fibroma of the ovary: a comparative study of their proliferative activity and chromosome aberrations using MIB-1 immunostaining, DNA flow cytometry, and fluorescence in situ hybridization. Am J Surg Pathol 21: 52-59.
1940. Tsujimura T, Kawano K (1992). Rhabdomyosarcoma coexistent with ovarian mucinous cystadenocarcinoma: a case report. Int J Gynecol Pathol 11: 58-62.
1941. Turan T, Aykan B, Koc S, Boran N, Tulunay G, Karacay O, Erdogan Z, Kose F (2006). Analysis of metastatic ovarian tumors from extragenital primary sites. Tumori 92: 491-495.
1942. Ud Din N, Memon A, Aftab K, Ahmad Z, Ahmed R, Hassan S (2012). Oligodendroglioma arising in the glial component of ovarian teratomas: a series of six cases and review of literature. J Clin Pathol 65: 631-634.
1943. Ueda A, Matsumoto T, Komuro Y (2011). Lymphangiogenesis is a predictor of nodal metastasis in extramammary Paget's disease. Histopathology 58: 870-874.
1944. Ueda G, Fujita M, Ogawa H, Sawada M, Inoue M, Tanizawa O (1993). Adenocarcinoma in a benign cystic teratoma of the ovary: report of a case with a long survival period. Gynecol Oncol 48: 259-263.
1945. Ueda T, Emoto M, Fukuoka M, Miyahara D, Horiuchi S, Tsujioka H, Kawarabayashi T (2010). Primary leiomyosarcoma of the fallopian tube. Int J Clin Oncol 15: 206-209.
1946. Ulbright TM, Roth LM, Brodhecker CA (1986). Yolk sac differentiation in germ cell tumors. A morphologic study of 50 cases with emphasis on hepatic, enteric, and parietal yolk sac features. Am J Surg Pathol 10: 151-164.
1947. Ulker V, Yavuz E, Gedikbasi A, Numanoglu C, Sudolmus S, Gulkilik A (2011). Uterine adenosarcoma with ovarian sex cord-like differentiation: a case report and review of the literature. Taiwan J Obstet Gynecol 50: 518-521.
1948. Underwood M, Arbyn M, Parry-Smith W, De Bellis-Ayres S, Todd R, Redman CW, Moss EL (2012). Accuracy of colposcopy-directed punch biopsies: a systematic review and meta-analysis. BJOG 119: 1293-1301.
1949. Ungerleider RS, Donaldson SS, Warnke RA, Wilbur JR (1978). Endodermal sinus tumor: the Stanford experience and the first reported case arising in the vulva. Cancer 41: 1627-1634.
1950. Urick ME, Rudd ML, Godwin AK, Sgroi D, Merino M, Bell DW (2011). PIK3R1 (p85alpha) is somatically mutated at high frequency in primary endometrial cancer. Cancer Res 71: 4061-4067.
1951. Utsugi K, Shimizu Y, Akiyama F, Hasumi K (2002). Villoglandular papillary

adenocarcinoma of the uterine cervix with bulky lymph node metastases. Eur J Obstet Gynecol Reprod Biol 105: 186-188.

1952. Uzan C, Dufeu-Lefebvre M, Fauvet R, Gouy S, Duvillard P, Darai E, Morice P (2012). Management and prognosis of clear cell borderline ovarian tumor. Int J Gynecol Cancer 22: 993-999.

1953. Vakiani E, Young RH, Carcangiu ML, Klimstra DS (2008). Acinar cell carcinoma of the pancreas metastatic to the ovary: a report of 4 cases. Am J Surg Pathol 32: 1540-1545.

1954. Vallerie AM, Lerner JP, Wright JD, Baxi LV (2009). Peritoneal inclusion cysts: a review. Obstet Gynecol Surv 64: 321-334.

1955. van de Rijn M, Kamel OW, Chang PP, Lee A, Warnke RA, Salhany KE (1997). Primary low-grade endometrial B-cell lymphoma. Am J Surg Pathol 21: 187-194.

1956. van den Einden LC, de Hullu JA, Massuger LF, Grefte JM, Bult P, Wiersma A, van Engen-van Grunsven AC, Sturm B, Bosch SL, Hollema H, Bulten J (2013). Interobserver variability and the effect of education in the histopathological diagnosis of differentiated vulvar intraepithelial neoplasia. Mod Pathol 26: 874-880.

1957. van der Aa MA, Helmerhorst TJ, Siesling S, Riemersma S, Coebergh JW (2010). Vaginal and (uncommon) cervical cancers in the Netherlands, 1989-2003. Int J Gynecol Cancer 20: 638-645.

1957A. van der Avoort I, van de Nieuwenhof HP, Otte-Holler I, Nirmala E, Bulten J, Massuger LF, van der Laak JA, Slootweg PJ, de Hullu JA, van Kempen LC (2010). High levels of p53 expression correlate with DNA aneuploidy in (pre)malignancies of the vulva. Hum Pathol 41: 1475-1485.

1957B. van der Avoort I, van der Laak JA, Paffen A, Grefte JM, Massuger LF, de Wilde PC, de Hullu JA, Bulten J (2007). MIB1 expression in basal cell layer: a diagnostic tool to identify premalignancies of the vulva. Mod Pathol 20: 770-778.

1958. van der Putte SC (1994). Mammary-like glands of the vulva and their disorders. Int J Gynecol Pathol 13: 150-160.

1959. van Hoeven KH, Hudock JA, Woodruff JM, Suhrland MJ (1995). Small cell neuroendocrine carcinoma of the endometrium. Int J Gynecol Pathol 14: 21-29.

1960. van der Avoort I, van de Nieuwenhof HP, Otte-Holler I, Nirmala E, Bulten J, Massuger LF, van der Laak JA, Slootweg PJ, de Hullu JA, van Kempen LC (2010). High levels of p53 expression correlate with DNA aneuploidy in (pre)malignancies of the vulva. Hum Pathol 41: 1475-1485.

1961. van der Avoort I, van der Laak JA, Paffen A, Grefte JM, Massuger LF, de Wilde PC, de Hullu JA, Bulten J (2007). MIB1 expression in basal cell layer: a diagnostic tool to identify premalignancies of the vulva. Mod Pathol 20: 770-778.

1962. Vang R, Bague S, Tavassoli FA, Prat J (2004). Signet-ring stromal tumor of the ovary: clinicopathologic analysis and comparison with Krukenberg tumor. Int J Gynecol Pathol 23: 45-51.

1963. Vang R, Gown AM, Barry TS, Wheeler DT, Ronnett BM (2006). Immunohistochemistry for estrogen and progesterone receptors in the distinction of primary and metastatic mucinous tumors in the ovary: an analysis of 124 cases. Mod Pathol 19: 97-105.

1964. Vang R, Gown AM, Barry TS, Wheeler DT, Ronnett BM (2006). Ovarian atypical proliferative (borderline) mucinous tumors: gastrointestinal and seromucinous (endocervical-like)

types are immunophenotypically distinctive. Int J Gynecol Pathol 25: 83-89.

1965. Vang R, Gown AM, Barry TS, Wheeler DT, Yemelyanova A, Seidman JD, Ronnett BM (2006). Cytokeratins 7 and 20 in primary and secondary mucinous tumors of the ovary: analysis of coordinate immunohistochemical expression profiles and staining distribution in 179 cases. Am J Surg Pathol 30: 1130-1139.

1966. Vang R, Gown AM, Farinola M, Barry TS, Wheeler DT, Yemelyanova A, Seidman JD, Judson K, Ronnett BM (2007). p16 expression in primary ovarian mucinous and endometrioid tumors and metastatic adenocarcinomas in the ovary: utility for identification of metastatic HPV-related endocervical adenocarcinomas. Am J Surg Pathol 31: 653-663.

1967. Vang R, Gown AM, Wu LS, Barry TS, Wheeler DT, Yemelyanova A, Seidman JD, Ronnett BM (2006). Immunohistochemical expression of CDX2 in primary ovarian mucinous tumors and metastatic mucinous carcinomas involving the ovary: comparison with CK20 and correlation with coordinate expression of CK7. Mod Pathol 19: 1421-1428.

1968. Vang R, Gown AM, Zhao C, Barry TS, Isacson C, Richardson MS, Ronnett BM (2007). Ovarian mucinous tumors associated with mature cystic teratomas: morphologic and immunohistochemical analysis identifies a subset of potential teratomatous origin that shares features of lower gastrointestinal tract mucinous tumors more commonly encountered as secondary tumors in the ovary. Am J Surg Pathol 31: 854-869.

1969. Vang R, Kempson RL (2002). Perivascular epithelioid cell tumor ('PEComa') of the uterus: a subset of HMB-45-positive epithelioid mesenchymal neoplasms with an uncertain relationship to pure smooth muscle tumors. Am J Surg Pathol 26: 1-13.

1970. Vang R, Medeiros LJ, Fuller GN, Sarris AH, Deavers M (2001). Non-Hodgkin's lymphoma involving the gynecologic tract: a review of 88 cases. Adv Anat Pathol 8: 200-217.

1971. Vang R, Medeiros LJ, Ha CS, Deavers M (2000). Non-Hodgkin's lymphomas involving the uterus: a clinicopathologic analysis of 26 cases. Mod Pathol 13: 19-28.

1971A. Vang R, Medeiros LJ, Malpica A, Levenback C, Deavers M (2000). Non-Hodgkin's lymphoma involving the vulva. Int J Gynecol Pathol 19: 236-242.

1972. Vang R, Medeiros LJ, Silva EG, Gershenson DM, Deavers M (2000). Non-Hodgkin's lymphoma involving the vagina: a clinicopathologic analysis of 14 patients. Am J Surg Pathol 24: 719-725.

1973. Vang R, Medeiros LJ, Warnke RA, Higgins JP, Deavers MT (2001). Ovarian non-Hodgkin's lymphoma: a clinicopathologic study of eight primary cases. Mod Pathol 14: 1093-1099.

1974. Vang R, Shih I, Kurman RJ (2009). Ovarian low-grade and high-grade serous carcinoma: pathogenesis, clinicopathologic and molecular biologic features, and diagnostic problems. Adv Anat Pathol 16: 267-282.

1975. Alvarado-Cabrero I, Navani SS, Young RH, Scully RE (1997). Tumors of the fimbriated end of the fallopian tube: a clinicopathologic analysis of 20 cases, including nine carcinomas. Int J Gynecol Pathol 16: 189-196.

1976. Vargas SO, Kozakewich HP, Boyd TK, Ecklund K, Fishman SJ, Laufer MR, Perez-Atayde AR (2005). Childhood asymmetric labium majus enlargement: mimicking a neoplasm. Am J Surg Pathol 29: 1007-1016.

1977. Vasseur C, Rodien P, Beau I, Desroches A, Gerard C, de Poncheville L, Chaplot S, Savagner F, Croue A, Mathieu E, Lahlou N,

Descamps P, Misrahi M (2003). A chorionic gonadotropin-sensitive mutation in the follicle-stimulating hormone receptor as a cause of familial gestational spontaneous ovarian hyperstimulation syndrome. N Engl J Med 349: 753-759.

1978. Veger HT, Ravensbergen NJ, Ottenhof A, da Costa SA (2010). Familial multiple lipomatosis: a case report. Acta Chir Belg 110: 98-100.

1979. Velasco-Oses A, Alonso-Alvaro A, Blanco-Pozo A, Nogales FF Jr (1988). Ollier's disease associated with ovarian juvenile granulosa cell tumor. Cancer 62: 222-225.

1980. Veras E, Mao TL, Ayhan A, Ueda S, Lai H, Hayran M, Shih I, Kurman RJ (2009). Cystic and adenofibromatous clear cell carcinomas of the ovary: distinctive tumors that differ in their pathogenesis and behavior: a clinicopathologic analysis of 122 cases. Am J Surg Pathol 33: 844-853.

1981. Veras E, Zivanovic O, Jacks L, Chiappetta D, Hensley M, Soslow R (2011). "Low-grade leiomyosarcoma" and late-recurring smooth muscle tumors of the uterus: a heterogenous collection of frequently misdiagnosed tumors associated with an overall favorable prognosis relative to conventional uterine leiomyosarcomas. Am J Surg Pathol 35: 1626-1637.

1982. Verhest A, Simonart T, Noel JC (1996). A unique clonal chromosome 2 deletion in endomyometriosis. Cancer Genet Cytogenet 86: 174-176.

1983. Verschraegen CF, Vasuratna A, Edwards C, Freedman R, Kudelka AP, Tornos C, Kavanagh JJ (1998). Clinicopathologic analysis of mullerian adenosarcoma: the M.D. Anderson Cancer Center experience. Oncol Rep 5: 939-944.

1984. Vicus D, Beiner ME, Klachook S, Le LW, Laframboise S, Mackay H (2010). Pure dysgerminoma of the ovary 35 years on: a single institutional experience. Gynecol Oncol 117: 23-26.

1985. Vinokurova S, Wentzensen N, Kraus I, Klaes R, Driesch C, Melsheimer P, Kisseljov F, Durst M, Schneider A, von Knebel Doeberitz M (2008). Type-dependent integration frequency of human papillomavirus genomes in cervical lesions. Cancer Res 68: 307-313.

1986. Visvanathan K, Vang R, Shaw P, Gross A, Soslow R, Parkash V, Shih I, Kurman RJ (2011). Diagnosis of serous tubal intraepithelial carcinoma based on morphologic and immunohistochemical features: a reproducibility study. Am J Surg Pathol 35: 1766-1775.

1987. Vlahos NF, Economopoulos KP, Creatsas G (2010). Fertility drugs and ovarian cancer risk: a critical review of the literature. Ann N Y Acad Sci 1205: 214-219.

1988. Vos A, Oosterhuis JW, de Jong B, Castedo SM, Hollema H, Buist J, Aalders JG (1990). Karyotyping and DNA flow cytometry of metastatic ovarian yolk sac tumor. Cancer Genet Cytogenet 44: 223-228.

1989. Devouassoux-Shisheboran M, Silver SA, Tavassoli FA (1999). Wolffian adnexal tumor, so-called female adnexal tumor of probable Wolffian origin (FATWO): immunohistochemical evidence in support of a Wolffian origin. Hum Pathol 30: 856-863.

1990. Vydianath B, Ganesan R, McCluggage WG (2008). Displaced granulosa cells in the fallopian tube mimicking small cell carcinoma. J Clin Pathol 61: 1323-1325.

1991. Waggoner SE, Mittendorf R, Biney N, Anderson D, Herbst AL (1994). Influence of in utero diethylstilbestrol exposure on the prognosis and biologic behavior of vaginal clear-cell adenocarcinoma. Gynecol Oncol 55: 238-244.

1992. Wagner AJ, Malinowska-Kolodziej I, Morgan JA, Qin W, Fletcher CD, Vena N, Ligon AH, Antonescu CR, Ramaiya NH, Demetri GD,

Kwiatkowski DJ, Maki RG (2010). Clinical activity of mTOR inhibition with sirolimus in malignant perivascular epithelioid cell tumors: targeting the pathogenic activation of mTORC1 in tumors. J Clin Oncol 28: 835-840.

1993. Wajda KJ, Lucas JG, Marsh WL Jr (1989). Hyperreactio luteinalis. Benign disorder masquerading as an ovarian neoplasm. Arch Pathol Lab Med 113: 921-925.

1994. Walboomers JM, Jacobs MV, Manos MM, Bosch FX, Kummer JA, Shah KV, Snijders PJ, Peto J, Meijer CJ, Munoz N (1999). Human papillomavirus is a necessary cause of invasive cervical cancer worldwide. J Pathol 189: 12-19.

1995. Waldhorn RE (1990). Surgical treatment of obstructive sleep apnea. Is mandibular surgery an advance? Chest 98: 1315-1316.

1996. Wallace DC, Surti U, Adams CW, Szulman AE (1982). Complete moles have paternal chromosomes but maternal mitochondrial DNA. Hum Genet 61: 145-147.

1997. Wallbillich JJ, Rhodes HE, Milbourne AM, Munsell MF, Frumovitz M, Brown J, Trimble CL, Schmeler KM (2012). Vulvar intraepithelial neoplasia (VIN 2/3): comparing clinical outcomes and evaluating risk factors for recurrence. Gynecol Oncol 127: 312-315.

1998. Walsh T, Casadei S, Lee MK, Pennil CC, Nord AS, Thornton AM, Roeb W, Agnew KJ, Stray SM, Wickramanayake A, Norquist B, Pennington KP, Garcia RL, King MC, Swisher EM (2011). Mutations in 12 genes for inherited ovarian, fallopian tube, and peritoneal carcinoma identified by massively parallel sequencing. Proc Natl Acad Sci U S A 108: 18032-18037.

1999. Wang F, Liu A, Peng Y, Rakheja D, Wei L, Xue D, Allan RW, Molberg KH, Li J, Cao D (2009). Diagnostic utility of SALL4 in extragonadal yolk sac tumors: an immunohistochemical study of 59 cases with comparison to placental-like alkaline phosphatase, alpha-fetoprotein, and glypican-3. Am J Surg Pathol 33: 1529-1539.

2000. Wang LY, Zhong YQ, Li HG, Zeng YJ, Zhang SN, Chen WX, Chen QK, Zhan J, Zhu ZH (2005). [Adenomatoid tumor of peritoneum--a case report]. Zhonghua Yi Xue Za Zhi 85: 495-497.

2001. Wang PH, Liu YC, Lai CR, Chao HT, Yuan CC, Yu KJ (1998). Small cell carcinoma of the cervix: analysis of clinical and pathological findings. Eur J Gynaecol Oncol 19: 189-192.

2002. Wang R, Titley JC, Lu YJ, Summersgill BM, Bridge JA, Fisher C, Shipley J (2003). Loss of 13q14-q21 and gain of 5p14-pter in the progression of leiomyosarcoma. Mod Pathol 16: 778-785.

2003. Wang WL, Soslow R, Hensley M, Asad H, Zannoni GF, de Nictolis M, Branton P, Muzikansky A, Oliva E (2011). Histopathologic prognostic factors in stage I leiomyosarcoma of the uterus: a detailed analysis of 27 cases. Am J Surg Pathol 35: 522-529.

2004. Wang X, Kumar D, Seidman JD (2006). Uterine lipoleiomyomas: a clinicopathologic study of 50 cases. Int J Gynecol Pathol 25: 239-242.

2005. Ward BE, Saleh AM, Williams JV, Zitz JC, Crum CP (1992). Papillary immature metaplasia of the cervix: a distinct subset of exophytic cervical condyloma associated with HPV-6/11 nucleic acids. Mod Pathol 5: 391-395.

2006. Watanabe K, Ogura G, Suzuki T (2003). Leiomyoblastoma of the uterus: an immunohistochemical and electron microscopic study of distinctive tumours with immature smooth muscle cell differentiation mimicking fetal uterine myocytes. Histopathology 42: 379-386.

2007. Waxman M (1979). Pure and mixed Brenner tumors of the ovary: clinicopathologic and histogenetic observations. Cancer 43: 1830-1839.

2008. Waxman M, Vuletin JC, Urcuyo R, Belling CG (1979). Ovarian low-grade stromal sarcoma with thecomatous features: a critical reappraisal of the so-called "malignant thecoma". Cancer 44: 2206-2217.

2009. Webb GA, Lagios MD (1987). Clear cell carcinoma of the endometrium. Am J Obstet Gynecol 156: 1486-1491.

2010. Wei EX, Albores-Saavedra J, Fowler MR (2005). Plexiform neurofibroma of the uterine cervix: a case report and review of the literature. Arch Pathol Lab Med 129: 783-786.

2011. Wei J, Wu H, Sun M, Liu W, Meng L (2012). Primary endometrial natural killer (NK)/T cell lymphoma: case report and review of literature. Eur J Gynaecol Oncol 33: 425-427.

2012. Weichert W, Denkert C, Gauruder-Burmester A, Kurzeja R, Hamm B, Dietel M, Kroencke TJ (2005). Uterine arterial embolization with tris-acryl gelatin microspheres: a histopathologic evaluation. Am J Surg Pathol 29: 955-961.

2013. Weinberg E, Hoisington S, Eastman AY, Rice DK, Malfetano J, Ross JS (1993). Uterine cervical lymphoepithelial-like carcinoma. Absence of Epstein-Barr virus genomes. Am J Clin Pathol 99: 195-199.

2014. Weinstein D, Rabinowitz R, Malach D, Mor-Yosef S, Eldor A, Schenker JG (1983). Ovarian hemorrhage in women with Von Willebrand's disease. A report of two cases. J Reprod Med 28: 500-502.

2015. Weinstock MA (1994). Malignant melanoma of the vulva and vagina in the United States: patterns of incidence and population-based estimates of survival. Am J Obstet Gynecol 171: 1225-1230.

2016. Weir MM, Bell DA, Young RH (1997). Transitional cell metaplasia of the uterine cervix and vagina: an underrecognized lesion that may be confused with high-grade dysplasia. A report of 59 cases. Am J Surg Pathol 21: 510-517.

2017. Weir MM, Bell DA, Young RH (1998). Grade 1 peritoneal serous carcinomas: a report of 14 cases and comparison with 7 peritoneal serous psammocarcinomas and 19 peritoneal serous borderline tumors. Am J Surg Pathol 22: 849-862.

2018. Weiss SW, Tavassoli FA (1988). Multicystic mesothelioma. An analysis of pathologic findings and biologic behavior in 37 cases. Am J Surg Pathol 12: 737-746.

2019. Wentzensen N, du Bois A, Kommoss S, Pfisterer J, von Knebel Doeberitz M, Schmidt D, Kommoss F (2008). No metastatic cervical adenocarcinomas in a series of p16INK4a-positive mucinous or endometrioid advanced ovarian carcinomas: an analysis of the AGO Ovarian Cancer Study Group. Int J Gynecol Pathol 27: 18-23.

2020. Wentzensen N, Schwartz L, Zuna RE, Smith K, Mathews C, Gold MA, Allen RA, Zhang R, Dunn ST, Walker JL, Schiffman M (2012). Performance of p16/Ki-67 immunostaining to detect cervical cancer precursors in a colposcopy referral population. Clin Cancer Res 18: 4154-4162.

2021. Wentzensen N, Zuna RE, Sherman ME, Gold MA, Schiffman M, Dunn ST, Jeronimo J, Zhang R, Walker J, Wang SS (2009). Accuracy of cervical specimens obtained for biomarker studies in women with CIN3. Gynecol Oncol 115: 493-496.

2022. Weyers W (2013). Hypertrophic Lichen Sclerosus With Dyskeratosis and Parakeratosis-A Common Presentation of Vulvar Lichen Sclerosus Not Associated With a Significant Risk of Malignancy. Am J Dermatopathol 35:713-21.

2023. Wheeler CM (2010). HPV genotypes: implications for worldwide cervical cancer screening and vaccination. Lancet Oncol 11: 1013-1014.

2024. Wheeler DT, Bell KA, Kurman RJ, Sherman ME (2000). Minimal uterine serous carcinoma: diagnosis and clinicopathologic correlation. Am J Surg Pathol 24: 797-806.

2025. Wheelock JB, Goplerud DR, Dunn LJ, Oates JF, III (1984). Primary carcinoma of the Bartholin gland: a report of ten cases. Obstet Gynecol 63: 820-824.

2026. Wick MR, Goellner JR, Wolfe JT 3rd, Su WP (1985). Vulvar sweat gland carcinomas. Arch Pathol Lab Med 109: 43-47.

2027. Wiegand KC, Lee AF, Al-Agha OM, Chow C, Kalloger SE, Scott DW, Steidl C, Wiseman SM, Gascoyne RD, Gilks B, Huntsman DG (2011). Loss of BAF250a (ARID1A) is frequent in high-grade endometrial carcinomas. J Pathol 224: 328-333.

2028. Wiegand KC, Shah SP, Al-Agha OM, Zhao Y, Tse K, Zeng T, Senz J, McConechy MK, Anglesio MS, Kalloger SE, Yang W, Heravi-Moussavi A, Giuliany R, Chow C, Fee J, Zayed A, Prentice L, Melnyk N, Turashvili G, Delaney AD, Madore J, Yip S, McPherson AW, Ha G, Bell L, Fereday S, Tam A, Galletta L, Tonin PN, Provencher D, Miller D, Jones SJ, Moore RA, Morin GB, Oloumi A, Boyd N, Aparicio SA, Shih I, Mes-Masson AM, Bowtell DD, Hirst M, Gilks B, Marra MA, Huntsman DG (2010). ARID1A mutations in endometriosis-associated ovarian carcinomas. N Engl J Med 363: 1532-1543.

2029. Wilbur DC, Reichman RC, Stoler MH (1988). Detection of infection by human papillomavirus in genital condylomata. A comparison study using immunocytochemistry and in situ nucleic acid hybridization. Am J Clin Pathol 89: 505-510.

2030. Wilkinson EJ, Brown HM (2002). Vulvar Paget disease of urothelial origin: a report of three cases and a proposed classification of vulvar Paget disease. Hum Pathol 33: 549-554.

2031. Wilkinson EJ, Croker BP, Friedrich EG Jr, Franzini DA (1988). Two distinct pathologic types of giant cell tumor of the vulva. A report of two cases. J Reprod Med 33: 519-522.

2032. Willett GD, Kurman RJ, Reid R, Greenberg M, Jenson AB, Lorincz AT (1989). Correlation of the histologic appearance of intraepithelial neoplasia of the cervix with human papillomavirus types. Emphasis on low grade lesions including so-called flat condyloma. Int J Gynecol Pathol 8: 18-25.

2033. Willner J, Wurz K, Allison KH, Galic V, Garcia RL, Goff BA, Swisher EM (2007). Alternate molecular genetic pathways in ovarian carcinomas of common histological types. Hum Pathol 38: 607-613.

2034. Willson JR, Peale AR (1952). Multiple peritoneal leiomyomas associated with a granulosa-cell tumor of the ovary. Am J Obstet Gynecol 64: 204-208.

2035. Wilting SM, de Wilde J, Meijer CJ, Berkhof J, Yi Y, van Wieringen WN, Braakhuis BJ, Meijer GA, Ylstra B, Snijders PJ, Steenbergen RD (2008). Integrated genomic and transcriptional profiling identifies chromosomal loci with altered gene expression in cervical cancer. Genes Chromosomes Cancer 47: 890-905.

2036. Winfield HL, De Las Casas LE, Greenfield WW, Santin AD, McKenney JK (2007). Low-grade fibromyxoid sarcoma presenting clinically as a primary ovarian neoplasm: a case report. Int J Gynecol Pathol 26: 173-176.

2036A. Winnicki M, Gariepy G, Sauthier PG, Funaro D (2009). Hodgkin lymphoma presenting as a vulvar mass in a patient with Crohn disease: a case report and literature review. J Low Genit Tract Dis 13: 110-114.

2037. Wisniewski M, Deppisch LM (1973). Solid teratomas of the ovary. Cancer 32: 440-446.

2038. Wistuba II, Thomas B, Behrens C, Onuki N, Lindberg G, Albores-Saavedra J, Gazdar AF (1999). Molecular abnormalities associated with endocrine tumors of the uterine cervix. Gynecol Oncol 72: 3-9.

2039. Witkiewicz AK, Hecht JL, Cviko A, McKeon FD, Ince TA, Crum CP (2005). Microglandular hyperplasia: a model for the de novo emergence and evolution of endocervical reserve cells. Hum Pathol 36: 154-161.

2040. Woelber L, Mahner S, Voelker K, Eulenburg CZ, Gieseking F, Choschzick M, Jaenicke F, Schwarz J (2009). Clinicopathological prognostic factors and patterns of recurrence in vulvar cancer. Anticancer Res 29: 545-552.

2041. Wojnar A, Drozdz K, Dziegiel P (2010). Cavernous haemangioma of the oviduct. Pol J Pathol 61: 103-104.

2042. Wolber RA, Talerman A, Wilkinson EJ, Clement PB (1991). Vulvar granular cell tumors with pseudocarcinomatous hyperplasia: a comparative analysis with well-differentiated squamous carcinoma. Int J Gynecol Pathol 10: 59-66.

2043. Wolfson AH, Wolfson DJ, Sittler SY, Breton L, Markoe AM, Schwade JG, Houdek PV, Averette HE, Sevin BU, Penalver M, . (1994). A multivariate analysis of clinicopathologic factors for predicting outcome in uterine sarcomas. Gynecol Oncol 52: 56-62.

2044. Wong AK, Seidman JD, Barbuto DA, McPhaul LW, Silva EG (2011). Mucinous metaplasia of the fallopian tube: a diagnostic pitfall mimicking metastasis. Int J Gynecol Pathol 30: 36-40.

2045. Wong CW, Fan YS, Chan TL, Chan AS, Ho LC, Ma TK, Yuen ST, Leung SY (2005). BRAF and NRAS mutations are uncommon in melanomas arising in diverse internal organs. J Clin Pathol 58: 640-644.

2046. Wong KK, Tsang YT, Deavers MT, Mok SC, Zu Z, Sun C, Malpica A, Wolf JK, Lu KH, Gershenson DM (2010). BRAF mutation is rare in advanced-stage low-grade ovarian serous carcinomas. Am J Pathol 177: 1611-1617.

2047. Woodruff JD, Parmley TH, Julian CG (1975). Topical 5-fluorouracil in the treatment of vaginal carcinoma-in-situ. Gynecol Oncol 3: 124-132.

2048. Woodruff JD, Rauh JT, Markley RL (1966). Ovarian struma. Obstet Gynecol 27: 194-201.

2049. Worsham MJ, Van Dyke DL, Grenman SE, Grenman R, Hopkins MP, Roberts JA, Gasser KM, Schwartz DR, Carey TE (1991). Consistent chromosome abnormalities in squamous cell carcinoma of the vulva. Genes Chromosomes Cancer 3: 420-432.

2050. Wright K, Wilson P, Morland S, Campbell I, Walsh M, Hurst T, Ward B, Cummings M, Chenevix-Trench G (1999). beta-catenin mutation and expression analysis in ovarian cancer: exon 3 mutations and nuclear translocation in 16% of endometrioid tumours. Int J Cancer 82: 625-629.

2051. Wright TC Jr, Massad LS, Dunton CJ, Spitzer M, Wilkinson EJ, Solomon D (2007). 2006 consensus guidelines for the management of women with cervical intraepithelial neoplasia or adenocarcinoma in situ. Am J Obstet Gynecol 197: 340-345.

2052. Wright TC, Jr., Stoler MH, Behrens CM, Apple R, Derion T, Wright TL (2012). The ATHENA human papillomavirus study: design, methods, and baseline results. Am J Obstet Gynecol 206: 46-46.

2053. Wu CH, Mao TL, Vang R, Ayhan A, Wang TL, Kurman RJ, Shih I (2012). Endocervical-type mucinous borderline tumors are related to endometrioid tumors based on mutation and loss of expression of ARID1A. Int J Gynecol Pathol 31: 297-303.

2054. Wu R, Hendrix-Lucas N, Kuick R, Zhai Y, Schwartz DR, Akyol A, Hanash S, Misek DE, Katabuchi H, Williams BO, Fearon ER, Cho KR (2007). Mouse model of human ovarian endometrioid adenocarcinoma based on somatic defects in the Wnt/beta-catenin and PI3K/Pten signaling pathways. Cancer Cell 11: 321-333.

2055. Wu R, Zhai Y, Fearon ER, Cho KR (2001). Diverse mechanisms of beta-catenin deregulation in ovarian endometrioid adenocarcinomas. Cancer Res 61: 8247-8255.

2056. Wu X, Matanoski G, Chen VW, Saraiya M, Coughlin SS, King JB, Tao XG (2008). Descriptive epidemiology of vaginal cancer incidence and survival by race, ethnicity, and age in the United States. Cancer 113: 2873-2882.

2057. Wuntakal R, Lawrence A (2013). Are oestrogens and genetic predisposition etiologic factors in the development of clear cell carcinoma of the peritoneum? Med Hypotheses 80: 167-171.

2058. Xie YP, Yao HX, Shen YM (2012). Mullerian adenosarcoma of the uterus with heterologous elements: two case reports and literature review. Arch Gynecol Obstet 286: 537-540.

2059. Xu JY, Hashi A, Kondo T, Yuminamochi T, Nara M, Hashi K, Murata S, Katoh R, Hoshi K (2005). Absence of human papillomavirus infection in minimal deviation adenocarcinoma and lobular endocervical glandular hyperplasia. Int J Gynecol Pathol 24: 296-302.

2060. Xu ML, Yang B, Carcangiu ML, Hui P (2009). Epithelioid trophoblastic tumor: comparative genomic hybridization and diagnostic DNA genotyping. Mod Pathol 22: 232-238.

2061. Xue D, Peng Y, Wang F, Allan RW, Cao D (2011). RNA-binding protein LIN28 is a sensitive marker of ovarian primitive germ cell tumours. Histopathology 59: 452-459.

2062. Xue WC, Guan XY, Ngan HY, Shen DH, Khoo US, Cheung AN (2002). Malignant placental site trophoblastic tumor: a cytogenetic study using comparative genomic hybridization and chromosome in situ hybridization. Cancer 94: 2288-2294.

2063. Yada-Hashimoto N, Yamamoto T, Kamiura S, Seino H, Ohira H, Sawai K, Kimura T, Saji F (2003). Metastatic ovarian tumors: a review of 64 cases. Gynecol Oncol 89: 314-317.

2064. Yahata T, Kawasaki T, Serikawa T, Suzuki M, Tanaka K (2008). Adenocarcinoma arising from respiratory ciliated epithelium in benign cystic teratoma of the ovary: a case report with analyzes of the CT, MRI, and pathological findings. J Obstet Gynaecol Res 34: 408-412.

2065. Yamada SD, Burger RA, Brewster WR, Anton D, Kohler MF, Monk BJ (2000). Pathologic variables and adjuvant therapy as predictors of recurrence and survival for patients with surgically evaluated carcinosarcoma of the uterus. Cancer 88: 2782-2786.

2066. Yamaguchi T, Imamura Y, Yamamoto T, Fukuda M (2003). Leiomyomatosis peritonealis disseminata with malignant change in a man. Pathol Int 53: 179-185.

2067. Yamamoto H, Kojima A, Nagata S, Tomita Y, Takahashi S, Oda Y (2011). KIT-negative gastrointestinal stromal tumor of the abdominal soft tissue: a clinicopathologic and genetic study of 10 cases. Am J Surg Pathol 35: 1287-1295.

2068. Yamamoto H, Oda Y, Kawaguchi K, Nakamura N, Takahira T, Tamiya S, Saito T, Oshiro Y, Ohta M, Yao T, Tsuneyoshi M (2004).

c-kit and PDGFRA mutations in extragastrointestinal stromal tumor (gastrointestinal stromal tumor of the soft tissue). Am J Surg Pathol 28: 479-488.

2069. Yamamoto S, Tsuda H, Takano M, Hase K, Tamai S, Matsubara O (2008). Clear-cell adenofibroma can be a clonal precursor for clear-cell adenocarcinoma of the ovary: a possible alternative ovarian clear-cell carcinogenic pathway. J Pathol 216: 103-110.

2070. Yamamoto S, Tsuda H, Takano M, Iwaya K, Tamai S, Matsubara O (2011). PIK3CA mutation is an early event in the development of endometriosis-associated ovarian clear cell adenocarcinoma. J Pathol 225: 189-194.

2071. Yamamoto S, Tsuda H, Takano M, Tamai S, Matsubara O (2012). Loss of ARID1A protein expression occurs as an early event in ovarian clear-cell carcinoma development and frequently coexists with PIK3CA mutations. Mod Pathol 25: 615-624.

2072. Yamamoto S, Tsuda H, Takano M, Tamai S, Matsubara O (2012). PIK3CA mutations and loss of ARID1A protein expression are early events in the development of cystic ovarian clear cell adenocarcinoma. Virchows Arch 460: 77-87.

2073. Yamamoto S, Tsuda H, Yoshikawa T, Kudoh K, Kita T, Furuya K, Tamai S, Matsubara O (2007). Clear cell adenocarcinoma associated with clear cell adenofibromatous components: a subgroup of ovarian clear cell adenocarcinoma with distinct clinicopathologic characteristics. Am J Surg Pathol 31: 999-1006.

2074. Yanai-Inbar I, Scully RE (1987). Relation of ovarian dermoid cysts and immature teratomas: an analysis of 350 cases of immature teratoma and 10 cases of dermoid cyst with microscopic foci of immature tissue. Int J Gynecol Pathol 6: 203-212.

2075. Yanai-Inbar I, Silverberg SG (2000). Mucosal epithelial proliferation of the fallopian tube: prevalence, clinical associations, and optimal strategy for histopathologic assessment. Int J Gynecol Pathol 19: 139-144.

2076. Yang B, Hart WR (2000). Vulvar intraepithelial neoplasia of the simplex (differentiated) type: a clinicopathologic study including analysis of HPV and p53 expression. Am J Surg Pathol 24: 429-441.

2077. Yang HP, Zuna RE, Schiffman M, Walker JL, Sherman ME, Landrum LM, Moxley K, Gold MA, Dunn ST, Allen RA, Zhang R, Long R, Wang SS, Wentzensen N (2012). Clinical and pathological heterogeneity of cervical intraepithelial neoplasia grade 3. PLoS One 7: e29051.

2078. Yang SY, Lee JW, Kim WS, Jung KL, Lee SJ, Lee JH, Bae DS, Kim BG (2006). Adenoid cystic carcinoma of the Bartholin's gland: report of two cases and review of the literature. Gynecol Oncol 100: 422-425.

2079. Yang TY, Cairns BJ, Allen N, Sweetland S, Reeves GK, Beral V (2012). Postmenopausal endometrial cancer risk and body size in early life and middle age: prospective cohort study. Br J Cancer 107: 169-175.

2080. Yap KL, Hafez MJ, Mao TL, Kurman RJ, Murphy KM, Shih I (2010). Lack of a y-chromosomal complement in the majority of gestational trophoblastic neoplasms. J Oncol 2010: 364508.

2081. Yasunaga M, Ohishi Y, Oda Y, Misumi M, Iwasa A, Kurihara S, Nishimura I, Okuma E, Kobayashi H, Wake N, Tsuneyoshi M (2009). Immunohistochemical characterization of mullerian mucinous borderline tumors: possible histogenetic link with serous borderline tumors and low-grade endometrioid tumors. Hum Pathol 40: 965-974.

2082. Ye HY, Chen JG, Luo DL, Jiang ZM, Chen ZH (2012). Perivascular epithelioid cell tumor (PEComa) of gynecologic origin: a clinicopathological study of three cases. Eur J Gynaecol Oncol 33: 105-108.

2083. Yeh CJ, Chuang WY, Chou HH, Jung SM, Hsueh S (2008). Multiple extragenital adenomatoid tumors in the mesocolon and omentum. APMIS 116: 1016-1019.

2084. Yemelyanova A, Mao TL, Nakayama N, Shih I, Kurman RJ (2008). Low-grade serous carcinoma of the ovary displaying a macropapillary pattern of invasion. Am J Surg Pathol 32: 1800-1806.

2085. Yemelyanova A, Vang R, Kshirsagar M, Lu D, Marks MA, Shih I, Kurman RJ (2011). Immunohistochemical staining patterns of p53 can serve as a surrogate marker for TP53 mutations in ovarian carcinoma: an immunohistochemical and nucleotide sequencing analysis. Mod Pathol 24: 1248-1253.

2086. Yemelyanova AV, Vang R, Judson K, Wu LS, Ronnett BM (2008). Distinction of primary and metastatic mucinous tumors involving the ovary: analysis of size and laterality data by primary site with reevaluation of an algorithm for tumor classification. Am J Surg Pathol 32: 128-138.

2087. Yilmaz A, Rush DS, Soslow RA (2002). Endometrial stromal sarcomas with unusual histologic features: a report of 24 primary and metastatic tumors emphasizing fibroblastic and smooth muscle differentiation. Am J Surg Pathol 26: 1142-1150.

2088. Yilmaz F, Ozdemir N, Akalin T, Veral A, Dikmen Y, Erhan Y (2000). Uterine adenosarcoma with rhabdomyosarcomatous overgrowth. Brief communication. Eur J Gynaecol Oncol 21: 430-432.

2089. Yingna S, Yang X, Xiuyu Y, Hongzhao S (2002). Clinical characteristics and treatment of gestational trophoblastic tumor with vaginal metastasis. Gynecol Oncol 84: 416-419.

2090. Yoder BJ, Rufforny I, Massoll NA, Wilkinson EJ (2008). Stage IA vulvar squamous cell carcinoma: an analysis of tumor invasive characteristics and risk. Am J Surg Pathol 32: 765-772.

2091. Yoo SH, Park BH, Choi J, Yoo J, Lee SW, Kim YM, Kim KR (2012). Papillary mucinous metaplasia of the endometrium as a possible precursor of endometrial mucinous adenocarcinoma. Mod Pathol 25: 1496-1507.

2092. Yoon NR, Lee JW, Kim BG, Bae DS, Sohn I, Sung CO, Song SY (2012). Gliomatosis peritonei is associated with frequent recurrence, but does not affect overall survival in patients with ovarian immature teratoma. Virchows Arch 461: 299-304.

2093. Yoonessi M, Abell MR (1979). Brenner tumors of the ovary. Obstet Gynecol 54: 90-96.

2094. Yoong WC, Shakya R, Sanders BT, Lind J (2004). Clitoral inclusion cyst: a complication of type I female genital mutilation. J Obstet Gynaecol 24: 98-99.

2095. Yoshida M, Obayashi C, Tachibana M, Minami R (2004). Coexisting Brenner tumor and struma ovarii in the right ovary: case report and review of the literature. Pathol Int 54: 793-797.

2096. Yoshida T, Sano T, Oyama T, Kanuma T, Fukuda T (2009). Prevalence, viral load, and physical status of HPV 16 and 18 in cervical adenosquamous carcinoma. Virchows Arch 455: 253-259.

2097. Yoshida Y, Kurokawa T, Fukuno N, Nishikawa Y, Kamitani N, Kotsuji F (2000). Markers of apoptosis and angiogenesis indicate that carcinomatous components play an important role in the malignant behavior of uterine carcinosarcoma. Hum Pathol 31: 1448-1454.

2098. Yoshida Y, Sato K, Katayama K, Yamaguchi A, Imamura Y, Kotsuji F (2011). Atypical metastatic carcinoid of the uterine cervix and review of the literature. J Obstet Gynaecol Res 37: 636-640.

2099. Yoshinaga K, Akahira J, Niikura H, Ito K, Moriya T, Murakami T, Kameoka J, Ichinohasama R, Okamura K, Yaegashi N (2004). A case of primary mucosa-associated lymphoid tissue lymphoma of the vagina. Hum Pathol 35: 1164-1166.

2100. Young RH (2004). Pseudomyxoma peritonei and selected other aspects of the spread of appendiceal neoplasms. Semin Diagn Pathol 21: 134-150.

2101. Young RH (2007). From Krukenberg to today: the ever present problems posed by metastatic tumors in the ovary. Part II. Adv Anat Pathol 14: 149-177.

2102. Young RH (2007). Neoplasms of the fallopian tube and broad ligament: a selective survey including historical perspective and emphasising recent developments. Pathology 39: 112-124.

2103. Young RH (2010). Ovarian tumors of the young. Int J Surg Pathol 18: 156S-161S.

2104. Young RH, Carey RW, Robboy SJ (1981). Breast carcinoma masquerading as primary ovarian neoplasm. Cancer 48: 210-212.

2105. Young RH, Clement PB (2000). Endocervicosis involving the uterine cervix: a report of four cases of a benign process that may be confused with deeply invasive endocervical adenocarcinoma. Int J Gynecol Pathol 19: 322-328.

2106. Young RH, Clement PB (2002). Endocervical adenocarcinoma and its variants: their morphology and differential diagnosis. Histopathology 41: 185-207.

2107. Young RH, Clement PB, McCaughey WT (1990). Solitary fibrous tumors ('fibrous mesotheliomas') of the peritoneum. A report of three cases and a review of the literature. Arch Pathol Lab Med 114: 493-495.

2108. Young RH, Clement PB, Scully RE (1988). Calcified thecomas in young women. A report of four cases. Int J Gynecol Pathol 7: 343-350.

2109. Young RH, Dickersin GR, Scully RE (1983). A distinctive ovarian sex cord-stromal tumor causing sexual precocity in the Peutz-Jeghers syndrome. Am J Surg Pathol 7: 233-243.

2110. Young RH, Dickersin GR, Scully RE (1984). Juvenile granulosa cell tumor of the ovary. A clinicopathological analysis of 125 cases. Am J Surg Pathol 8: 575-596.

2111. Young RH, Dudley AG, Scully RE (1984). Granulosa cell, Sertoli-Leydig cell, and unclassified sex cord-stromal tumors associated with pregnancy: a clinicopathological analysis of thirty-six cases. Gynecol Oncol 18: 181-205.

2112. Young RH, Harris NL, Scully RE (1985). Lymphoma-like lesions of the lower female genital tract: a report of 16 cases. Int J Gynecol Pathol 4: 289-299.

2113. Young RH, Hart WR (1989). Metastases from carcinomas of the pancreas simulating primary mucinous tumors of the ovary. A report of seven cases. Am J Surg Pathol 13: 748-756.

2114. Young RH, Kurman RJ, Scully RE (1988). Proliferations and tumors of intermediate trophoblast of the placental site. Semin Diagn Pathol 5: 223-237.

2115. Young RH, Kurman RJ, Scully RE (1990). Placental site nodules and plaques. A clinicopathologic analysis of 20 cases. Am J Surg Pathol 14: 1001-1009.

2116. Young RH, Oliva E, Scully RE (1994). Small cell carcinoma of the ovary, hypercalcemic type. A clinicopathological analysis of 150 cases. Am J Surg Pathol 18: 1102-1116.

2117. Young RH, Prat J, Scully RE (1982). Ovarian endometrioid carcinomas resembling sex cord-stromal tumors. A clinicopathological analysis of 13 cases. Am J Surg Pathol 6: 513-522.

2118. Young RH, Prat J, Scully RE (1984). Endometrioid stromal sarcomas of the ovary. A clinicopathologic analysis of 23 cases. Cancer 53: 1143-1155.

2119. Young RH, Scully RE (1983). Ovarian stromal tumors with minor sex cord elements: a report of seven cases. Int J Gynecol Pathol 2: 227-234.

2120. Young RH, Scully RE (1983). Ovarian tumors of probable wolffian origin. A report of 11 cases. Am J Surg Pathol 7: 125-135.

2121. Young RH, Scully RE (1984). Endodermal sinus tumor of the vagina: a report of nine cases and review of the literature. Gynecol Oncol 18: 380-392.

2122. Young RH, Scully RE (1984). Fibromatosis and massive edema of the ovary, possibly related entities: a report of 14 cases of fibromatosis and 11 cases of massive edema. Int J Gynecol Pathol 3: 153-178.

2123. Young RH, Scully RE (1984). Placental-site trophoblastic tumor: current status. Clin Obstet Gynecol 27: 248-258.

2124. Young RH, Scully RE (1985). Ovarian Sertoli-Leydig cell tumors. A clinicopathological analysis of 207 cases. Am J Surg Pathol 9: 543-569.

2125. Young RH, Scully RE (1989). Villoglandular papillary adenocarcinoma of the uterine cervix. A clinicopathologic analysis of 13 cases. Cancer 63: 1773-1779.

2126. Young RH, Scully RE (1990). Ovarian metastases from carcinoma of the gallbladder and extrahepatic bile ducts simulating primary tumors of the ovary. A report of six cases. Int J Gynecol Pathol 9: 60-72.

2127. Young RH, Scully RE (1993). Minimal-deviation endometrioid adenocarcinoma of the uterine cervix. A report of five cases of a distinctive neoplasm that may be misinterpreted as benign. Am J Surg Pathol 17: 660-665.

2128. Young RH, Silva EG, Scully RE (1991). Ovarian and juxtaovarian adenomatoid tumors: a report of six cases. Int J Gynecol Pathol 10: 364-371.

2129. Young RH, Treger T, Scully RE (1986). Atypical polypoid adenomyoma of the uterus. A report of 27 cases. Am J Clin Pathol 86: 139-145.

2130. Young RH, Ulbright TM, Policarpio-Nicolas ML (2013). Yolk sac tumor with a prominent polyvesicular vitelline pattern: a report of three cases. Am J Surg Pathol 37: 393-398.

2131. Young RH, Welch WR, Dickersin GR, Scully RE (1982). Ovarian sex cord tumor with annular tubules: review of 74 cases including 27 with Peutz-Jeghers syndrome and four with adenoma malignum of the cervix. Cancer 50: 1384-1402.

2132. Youngs LA, Taylor HB (1967). Adenomatoid tumors of the uterus and fallopian tube. Am J Clin Pathol 48: 537-545.

2133. Yuan CC, Wang PH, Lai CR, Yen MS, Chen CY, Juang CM (1998). Prognosis-predicting system based on factors related to survival of cervical carcinoma. Int J Gynaecol Obstet 63: 163-167.

2134. Zahn CM, Kendall BS, Liang CY (2001). Spindle cell lipoma of the female genital tract. A report of two cases. J Reprod Med 46: 769-772.

2135. Zaino R (2000). Conventional and Novel Prognostic Factors in Endometrial Adenocarcinoma: A Critical Appraisal. Pathology Case Reviews 138-152.

2136. Zaino RJ (2002). Symposium part I: adenocarcinoma in situ, glandular dysplasia, and early invasive adenocarcinoma of the uterine cervix. Int J Gynecol Pathol 21: 314-326.

2137. Zaino RJ, Brady MF, Lele SM, Michael H, Greer B, Bookman MA (2011). Advanced stage mucinous adenocarcinoma of the ovary is both rare and highly lethal: a Gynecologic Oncology Group study. Cancer 117: 554-562.

2138. Zaino RJ, Kauderer J, Trimble CL, Silverberg SG, Curtin JP, Lim PC, Gallup DG (2006). Reproducibility of the diagnosis of atypical endometrial hyperplasia: a Gynecologic Oncology Group study. Cancer 106: 804-811.

2139. Zaino RJ, Kurman RJ, Diana KL, Morrow CP (1995). The utility of the revised International Federation of Gynecology and Obstetrics histologic grading of endometrial adenocarcinoma using a defined nuclear grading system. A Gynecologic Oncology Group study. Cancer 75: 81-86.

2140. Zaino RJ, Kurman RJ, Diana KL, Morrow CP (1996). Pathologic models to predict outcome for women with endometrial adenocarcinoma: the importance of the distinction between surgical stage and clinical stage--a Gynecologic Oncology Group study. Cancer 77: 1115-1121.

2141. Zaino RJ, Nucci M, Kurman RJ (2011). Diseases of the vagina. In: Blaustein's Pathology of female genital tract. Kurman RJ, Ellenson HK, Ronnett BM, eds. Springer: New York, pp. 144-145.

2142. Zaino RJ, Unger ER, Whitney C (1984). Synchronous carcinomas of the uterine corpus and ovary. Gynecol Oncol 19: 329-335.

2143. Zaloudek C, Norris HJ (1982). Granulosa tumors of the ovary in children: a clinical and pathologic study of 32 cases. Am J Surg Pathol 6: 503-512.

2144. Zaloudek C, Norris HJ (1984). Sertoli-Leydig tumors of the ovary. A clinicopathologic study of 64 intermediate and poorly differentiated neoplasms. Am J Surg Pathol 8: 405-418.

2145. Zaloudek CJ, Norris HJ (1981). Adenofibroma and adenosarcoma of the uterus: a clinicopathologic study of 35 cases. Cancer 48: 354-366.

2146. Zaman SS, Mazur MT (1993). Endometrial papillary syncytial change. A nonspecific alteration associated with active breakdown. Am J Clin Pathol 99: 741-745.

2147. Zanagnolo V, Pasinetti B, Sartori E (2004). Clinical review of 63 cases of sex cord stromal tumors. Eur J Gynaecol Oncol 25: 431-438.

2148. Zanetta G, Maggi R, Colombo M, Bratina G, Mangioni C (1997). Choriocarcinoma coexistent with intrauterine pregnancy: two additional cases and a review of the literature. Int J Gynecol Cancer 7: 66-77.

2149. Zannoni GF, Prisco MG, Vellone VG, De Stefano I, Vizzielli G, Tortorella L, Fagotti A, Scambia G, Gallo D (2011). Cytoplasmic expression of oestrogen receptor beta (ERbeta) as a prognostic factor in vulvar squamous cell carcinoma in elderly women. Histopathology 59: 909-917.

2150. Zaviacic M, Sidlo J, Borovsky M (1993). Prostate specific antigen and prostate specific acid phosphatase in adenocarcinoma of Skene's paraurethral glands and ducts. Virchows Arch A Pathol Anat Histopathol 423: 503-505.

2151. Zekioglu O, Ozdemir N, Terek C, Ozsaran A, Dikmen Y (2010). Clinicopathological and immunohistochemical analysis of sclerosing stromal tumours of the ovary. Arch Gynecol Obstet 282: 671-676.

2151A. Zeller C, Dai W, Curry E, Siddiq A, Walley A, Masrour N, Kitsou-Mylona I, Anderson G, Ghaem-Maghami S, Brown R, El-Bahrawy M (2013). The DNA methylomes of

serous borderline tumors reveal subgroups with malignant- or benign-like profiles. Am J Pathol 182: 668-677.

2152. Zeng HA, Cartun R, Ricci A Jr (2005). Potential diagnostic utility of CDX-2 immunophenotyping in extramammary Paget's disease. Appl Immunohistochem Mol Morphol 13: 342-346.

2153. Zhang C, Zhang P, Sung CJ, Lawrence WD (2003). Overexpression of p53 is correlated with stromal invasion in extramammary Paget's disease of the vulva. Hum Pathol 34: 880-885.

2154. Zhang H, Li L, Hao J, Liu M, Shi M, Mu Y (2011). Granular cell tumor from a 7-year swelling of the vulva: a case report. Arch Gynecol Obstet 284: 1293-1294.

2155. Zhang HK, Chen WD (2012). Atypical polypoid adenomyomas progressed to endometrial endometrioid adenocarcinomas. Arch Gynecol Obstet 286: 707-710.

2156. Zhang J, Chen Y, Wang K, Xi M, Yang K, Liu H (2011). Prepubertal vulval fibroma with a coincidental ectopic breast fibroadenoma: report of an unusual case with literature review. J Obstet Gynaecol Res 37: 1720-1725.

2157. Zhang J, Sun Y, Peng ZL (2009). Malignant peripheral nerve sheath tumor of the vagina. Saudi Med J 30: 705-707.

2158. Zhang J, Young RH, Arseneau J, Scully RE (1982). Ovarian stromal tumors containing lutein or Leydig cells (luteinized thecomas and stromal Leydig cell tumors)--a clinicopathological analysis of fifty cases. Int J Gynecol Pathol 1: 270-285.

2159. Zhang L, Conejo-Garcia JR, Katsaros D, Gimotty PA, Massobrio M, Regnani G, Makrigiannakis A, Gray H, Schlienger K, Liebman MN, Rubin SC, Coukos G (2003). Intratumoral T cells, recurrence, and survival in epithelial ovarian cancer. N Engl J Med 348: 203-213.

2160. Zhao C, Barner R, Vinh TN, McManus K, Dabbs D, Vang R (2008). SF-1 is a diagnostically useful immunohistochemical marker and comparable to other sex cord-stromal tumor markers for the differential diagnosis of ovarian sertoli cell tumor. Int J Gynecol Pathol 27: 507-514.

2161. Zhao C, Bratthauer GL, Barner R, Vang R (2007). Comparative analysis of alternative and traditional immunohistochemical markers for the distinction of ovarian sertoli cell tumor from endometrioid tumors and carcinoid tumor: A study of 160 cases. Am J Surg Pathol 31: 255-266.

2162. Zhao C, Bratthauer GL, Barner R, Vang R (2007). Diagnostic utility of WT1 immunostaining in ovarian sertoli cell tumor. Am J Surg Pathol 31: 1378-1386.

2163. Zhao C, Vinh TN, McManus K, Dabbs D, Barner R, Vang R (2009). Identification of the most sensitive and robust immunohistochemical markers in different categories of ovarian sex cord-stromal tumors. Am J Surg Pathol 33: 354-366.

2164. Zhao C, Wu LS, Barner R (2011). Pathogenesis of ovarian clear cell adenofibroma, atypical proliferative (borderline) tumor, and carcinoma: clinicopathologic features of tumors with endometriosis or adenofibromatous components support two related pathways of tumor development. J Cancer 2: 94-106.

2165. Zhao XY, Hong XN, Cao JN, Leaw SJ, Guo Y, Li ZT, Chang JH (2011). Clinical features and treatment outcomes of 14 cases of primary ovarian non-Hodgkin's lymphoma: a single-center experience. Med Oncol 28: 1559-1564.

2166. Zheng W, Schwartz PE (2005). Serous EIC as an early form of uterine papillary serous carcinoma: recent progress in understanding its

pathogenesis and current opinions regarding pathologic and clinical management. Gynecol Oncol 96: 579-582.

2167. Zheng W, Wolf S, Kramer EE, Cox KA, Hoda SA (1996). Borderline papillary serous tumour of the fallopian tube. Am J Surg Pathol 20: 30-35.

2168. Zhong YP, Zhang JJ, Huang XN (2012). Multiple myeloma with rupture of ovarian plasmacytoma. Chin Med J (Engl) 125: 2948-2950.

2169. Zhou B, Yang L, Sun Q, Cong R, Gu H, Tang N, Zhu H, Wang B (2008). Cigarette smoking and the risk of endometrial cancer: a meta-analysis. Am J Med 121: 501-508.

2170. Zhou C, Gilks CB, Hayes M, Clement PB (1998). Papillary serous carcinoma of the uterine cervix: a clinicopathologic study of 17 cases. Am J Surg Pathol 22: 113-120.

2171. Zhou J, Tomashefski J Jr, Khiyami A (2007). Diagnostic value of the thin-layer, liquid-based Pap test in endometrial cancer: a retrospective study with emphasis on cytomorphologic features. Acta Cytol 51: 735-741.

2172. Zhuang Z, Devouassoux-Shisheboran M, Lubensky IA, Tavassoli F, Vortmeyer AO (2005). Premeiotic origin of teratomas: is meiosis required for differentiation into mature tissues? Cell Cycle 4: 1683-1687.

2173. Zielinski GD, Snijders PJ, Rozendaal L, Daalmeijer NF, Risse EK, Voorhorst FJ, Jiwa NM, van der Linden HC, de Schipper FA, Runsink AP, Meijer CJ (2003). The presence of high-risk HPV combined with specific p53 and p16INK4a expression patterns points to high-risk HPV as the main causative agent for adenocarcinoma in situ and adenocarcinoma of the cervix. J Pathol 201: 535-543.

2174. Zinsser KR, Wheeler JE (1982). Endosalpingiosis in the omentum: a study of autopsy and surgical material. Am J Surg Pathol 6: 109-117.

2175. Zivanovic O, Sima CS, Iasonos A, Bell-McGuinn KM, Sabbatini PJ, Leitao MM, Levine DA, Gardner GJ, Barakat RR, Chi DS (2009). Exploratory analysis of serum CA-125 response to surgery and the risk of relapse in patients with FIGO stage IIIC ovarian cancer. Gynecol Oncol 115: 209-214.

2176. Zuna RE, Wang SS, Rosenthal DL, Jeronimo J, Schiffman M, Solomon D (2005). Determinants of human papillomavirus-negative, low-grade squamous intraepithelial lesions in the atypical squamous cells of undetermined significance/low-grade squamous intraepithelial lesions triage study (ALTS). Cancer 105: 253-262.

2177. Zynger DL, Everton MJ, Dimov ND, Chou PM, Yang XJ (2008). Expression of glypican 3 in ovarian and extragonadal germ cell tumors. Am J Clin Pathol 130: 224-230.

Subject index

Endocervical-type mucinous and mixed epithelial carcinomas of Müllerian type 39
Endocervical-type mucinous borderline tumour 38
Endocervicosis 170, **193**, 208, **216**
Endodermal sinus tumour 59, 225, 252
Endolymphatic stromal myosis 142
Endometrioid intraepithelial neoplasia 9, **125**
Endometrial stromal and related tumours 122
Endometrial stromal nodule 122, **141**
Endometrioid adenocarcinoma 170, 187, 208, 214
Endometrioid adenofibroma 12, **29**
Endometrioid borderline tumour / Atypical proliferative endometrioid tumour 30
Endometrioid carcinoma 12, **31**, 32, 93, 104, **108**, 114, **116**, 122, **126**–128, 170, **187**, 208, **214**
Endometrioid carcinoma resembling sex cord-stromal tumour 32
Endometrioid carcinoma, secretory 122, 126, 134
Endometrioid carcinoma, squamous 126
Endometrioid carcinoma, villoglandular 122, **126**, 170, 186, 187
Endometrioid cystadenoma 12, **29**
Endometrioid intraepithelial neoplasia 122, **125**
Endometrioid metaplasia 193
Endometrioid stromal tumour 88, **97**
Endometrioid tumours of low malignant potential 30
Endometriomas 29
Endometriosis 88, **98**, 99, 104, **110**, 114, 116, 120, 170, **193**, 208, **216**
Endometriotic cyst 12, **29**
Endomyometriosis 116, 117
Endosalpingiosis 19, 88, 92, 94, **99**, 104, 110, 114, 120
Eosinophilic and ciliated cell metaplasias 134
Eosinophilic metaplasia 134
EPC1-PHF1 fusion gene 41, 141, 143
Ependymoblastoma 65, 152
Ependymoma 65, 114, **119**
Epidermal growth factor receptor 37, 181, 251
Epidermoid carcinoma 211
Epithelial borderline tumour 104
Epithelioid leiomyosarcoma 122, 139, **140**
Epithelioid sarcoma 230, **249**
Epithelioid sarcoma, proximal variant 249
Epithelioid trophoblastic tumour 159, 160, **161**, 162
Epstein-Barr virus 81, 180
ERG 201
ETT *See* Epithelioid trophoblastic tumour

Ewing sarcoma 64, 152, 170, 201, 208, **226**, 230, **242**
EWS/FLI fusion gene 152, 226, 242
Exaggerated implantation site 162
Exaggerated placental site 156, **162**
Extra-gastrointestinal stromal tumour 88, **96**
Extramammary Paget disease 236
Extramedullary myeloid tumour 82, 112, 153, 205, 223, 253
Extranodal marginal zone lymphoma of mucosa-associated lymphoid tissue (MALT lymphoma) 80
Extranodal NK/T-cell lymphoma, nasal-type 81
Extraskeletal Ewing sarcoma 152

F
Familial atypical mole-melanoma 251
Familial multinodular goitre 56
FAMM *See* Familial atypical mole-melanoma
Fanconi anaemia pathway 24
FATWO *See* Female adnexal tumour of Wolffian origin
FBXW7 130
Female adnexal tumour of probable Wolffian origin 69, 108, 117
Fibroadenoma 230, **240**
Fibroepithelial polyp 182, 208, **213**, 243
Fibroepithelial stromal polyp 230, **243**
Fibrolipoma 243
Fibroma 12, **44**
Fibromatosis 13, **77**, 95
Fibrosarcoma 12, **46**, 230, 249
Flat condyloma 9, 172, 210, 232
Flexner-Wintersteiner rosettes 144
Fli-1 152, 201
Follicle cyst 13, **75**
Follicular lymphoma **80**, 112, 205
FOXL2 49–53, 55, 67
FOXO1A 200
Frasier syndrome 68
Fumarate hydratase 137, 138

G
Galectin-3 247
Gartner duct cysts 216
GATA3 35, 86
GBY locus 68
GCDFP-15 86, 236
GDF3 62
Genital rhabdomyoma 218
Genital wart 181, 235
Genital wart of the cervix 181
Germ cell tumour 7, 11, 13, 57, 103, 104, 111, 122, **152**, 208, 225
Glassy cell carcinoma 170, **194**, 195
Glioblastoma multiforme 65
Gliomatosis 62, 88, **101**
Glomus tumour 66
Glypican 3 59, 62, 225, 252

Gonadal dysgenesis 58–60, 67, 68
Gonadoblastoma including gonadoblastoma with malignant germ cell tumour 13, **67**
Gorlin syndrome 44
Granular cell myoblastoma 247
Granular cell tumour 230, **247**
Granulocytic sarcoma 82, 97, **112**, **153**, 205, 223, 253

H
H3D3B1 161
HAIR-AN syndrome 77
HBME1 73, 74, 90, 247
h-caldesmon 74, 95, 138, 140, 143, 147, 199
HDAC8 140, 143
HER2 28, 181, 236, 237
Hereditary nonpolyposis colorectal cancer 128
HG-CGIN *See* Adenocarcinoma in situ / High-grade cervical glandular intraepithelial neoplasia
HGPSC *See* High-grade peritoneal serous carcinomas
HGSC *See* High-grade serous carcinoma
Hidradenoma papilliferum 239
High-grade cervical glandular intraepithelial neoplasia 183
High-grade endometrial stromal sarcoma 88, 97, 122, **144**
High-grade endometrioid stromal sarcoma 12, **41**, **97**
High-grade neuroendocrine carcinoma 122, **131**, 170, **197**, 198, 208, **217**, 230, **241**
High-grade peritoneal serous carcinomas 92
High-grade serous carcinoma 8, 12, 18, **22**–24, 88, **92**, 104, 106–108, 114, 115
High-grade squamous intraepithelial lesion 9, 170, 172, 173, **174**–177, 179, 180, 182, 183, 208, **210**–213, 230, **232**–235
High-grade tubal intraepithelial neoplasia 106
HIK1083 186
Hilar cell hyperplasia 78
Hilus cell tumour 48
Hirsuties papillaris genitalis 236
Histiocytic nodule 88, **99**
Histone deacetylase 8 138, 140
HLA-G 159, 160, 161
HMB-45 147, 204, 225, 236, 241, 251
HMBE-1 151
HMGA2 141, 151, 220, 245, 246
HMGI-C 246
hMLH1 32
hMSH2 32

List of abbreviations

5-FU	5-fluorouracil
ACTH	adrenocorticotropic hormone
ADH	antidiuretic hormone
AFP	alpha-fetoprotein
AJCC	American Joint Committee on Cancer
ALK	anaplastic lymphoma kinase
CEA	carcinoembryonic antigen
CGH	comparative genomic hybridization
CIN	cervical intraepithelial neoplasia
CNS	central nervous system
DES	diethylstilbestrol
EBV	Epstein-Barr virus
EGFR	epidermal growth factor receptor
EMA	epithelial membrane antigen
ER	oestrogen receptor
FIGO	International Federation of Gynecology and Obstetrics
FISH	fluorescence in situ hybridization
FSH	follicle stimulating hormone
GFAP	glial-fibrillary acidic protein
GnRH	gonadotropin-releasing hormone
H&E	haematoxylin and eosin
hCG	human chorionic gonadotrophan
HIV	human immunodeficiency virus
HPF	high-power field
HPV	human papilloma virus
IGF2	insulin-like growth factor 2
LDH	lactate dehydrogenase
LEEP	loop electrosurgical excision procedure
LH	luteinizing hormone
MSA	muscle-specific actin
NCI	National Cancer Institute
NOS	not otherwise specified
NSE	neuronal-specific enolase
PAS	periodic acid-Schiff
PAS-D	periodic acid-Schiff-diastase
PCR	polymerase chain reaction
PLAP	placental alkaline phosphatase
PR	progesterone receptor
RT-PCR	reverse-transcriptase polymerase chain reaction
SMA	smooth-muscle actin
ST-1	steroidogenic factor-1
UICC	International Union against Cancer
VEGF3	vascular endothelial growth factor receptor-3
WT-1	Wilms tumour-1 protein